Oxford Textbook of

Shared Decision Making in Healthcare

Oxford Textbook of

Shared Decision Making in Healthcare

FOURTH EDITION

EDITED BY

Glyn Elwyn

Professor and Physician Researcher, The Dartmouth Institute for Health Policy and Clinical Practice, Dartmouth College, Hanover, New Hampshire, USA

Natalie Joseph-Williams

Reader in Improving Patient Care and Associate Director for the Health and Care Research, Wales Evidence Centre, School of Medicine, Cardiff University, Cardiff, UK

Adrian Edwards

Professor of General Practice, Director of Health and Care Research Wales Evidence Centre, Division of Population Medicine, Cardiff University, Cardiff, UK

OXFORD
UNIVERSITY PRESS

OXFORD
UNIVERSITY PRESS

Great Clarendon Street, Oxford, OX2 6DP,
United Kingdom

Oxford University Press is a department of the University of Oxford.
It furthers the University's objective of excellence in research, scholarship,
and education by publishing worldwide. Oxford is a registered trade mark of
Oxford University Press in the UK and in certain other countries.

First Edition published in 2001
Second Edition published in 2009
Third Edition published in 2016
Fourth Edition published in 2025

Published in the United States of America by Oxford University Press
198 Madison Avenue, New York, NY 10016, United States of America.

British Library Cataloguing in Publication Data
Data available

Library of Congress Control Number: 2025934113

ISBN 978–0–19–889780–4

DOI: 10.1093/med/9780198897804.001.0001

Printed and bound by
CPI Group (UK) Ltd., Croydon, CR0 4YY

Foreword 1

I am delighted and honoured to provide this foreword from the perspective of both a patient and a solicitor on the crucially important topic of shared decision making for the *Oxford Textbook of Shared Decision Making in Healthcare*.

It has now been a lengthy 25 years since my own personal tragedy that led to the unanimous Supreme Court judgment, which was handed down 10 years ago, in *Montgomery v Lanarkshire Health Board*. My case finally brought the UK into line with other common law jurisdictions by establishing a new test for questions in relation to information disclosure and consent in medical negligence claims. It is one of the most significant clinical negligence judgments of our time, finally upholding the patient's common law right to autonomy. At the very heart of the judgment is choice and the Supreme Court made clear that if there is a choice to be made then that it is ultimately for the patient to make that choice and not the doctor.

As human beings, we desire to determine our own lives by making our own decisions. Each individual comes with their own unique set of circumstances that influences them towards certain decisions. The same must be said for patients when it comes to decisions regarding medical treatment that could affect their bodily integrity. The doctrine of informed consent is considered central to the doctor–patient relationship and is highly valued out of respect for the fundamental ethical principle of autonomy. The concept that each patient has the right to make their own decisions based on factors that are important to them must be respected. Only by respecting this can we achieve a valid consent to treatment.

It has been an incredibly slow process to get here, but what astounds me is that the right of a patient to make their own decision is by no means a revolutionary principle in medicine. Most people are familiar with the phrase 'first do no harm' from the Hippocratic oath, but I suspect less familiar with the fact that the physician and 'father of medicine', Hippocrates, was already practising using consent techniques over two thousand years ago.

While I am delighted with the progress we are making in this area, we still have a long way to go. I hope this textbook will become prescribed reading for all healthcare and legal professionals, and will become core to their curriculum, so that they may learn, reflect, and understand the importance of the communication process between doctors and patients, making their decisions together.

Out of our own tragedy do we find our life's work.

Nadine Montgomery Allam,
Solicitor, Levy & McRae Solicitors LLP, Glasgow, UK

Foreword 2

It is an honour and privilege to be asked to write a foreword to this immensely important new textbook on shared decision making and to do so together with Nadine Montgomery Allam is such a joy to me. In my opinion, shared decision making is the core value of good clinical practice. The fruitful meeting between the clinical expert and the personal expert.

I was trained in clinical genetics myself. As a young doctor, I was eager to learn and understand the discipline and the many new possibilities for patients and families. I wanted to be as clever and competent as possible to explain the many advantages of knowing the risk of a genetic disease to people referred for genetic counselling. I remember being so persistent when a patient or a family seemed reluctant to opt for testing. I thought I had not explained the benefits well enough and would tell it all again trying to persuade the person in front of me to accept. I thought I knew what was best for them. I could not have been more wrong. Luckily, I had a wonderful teacher and mentor. A senior leader who took me under his wings and taught me about ethics, about human autonomy, about listening to the patients, and more than anything about respecting everyone for who they are and for their preferences and values. It changed me and my way of practising and it became the foundation of my work ever since.

Many of us who decided to train and work within healthcare did it on the grounds of a strong wish to help and support other people. We wanted to do good. And like me, many of us thought that the patients came to us to be diagnosed and treated with the best clinical guidelines. But we must always remember that guidelines are just guidelines. At best they are the optimal treatment for an average patient. But very few if any of us are in fact average. Our life situations, abilities, and preferences are very different and unique. So, we must be humble about the reality that in many clinical situations we actually don't know what the best decision would be for the person in front of us. However, if we get to know the person by listening and trying to understand their situation, their reasons, and their preferences and values we might be able to help and support them in making decisions that are right for them. And by doing so we may succeed with our own wish to help and support patients and their relatives in the best way possible.

Therefore, my hope is that this substantial textbook will be a mandatory read for everyone within healthcare. Of course, my hope includes leaders at all levels too. Leaders have the responsibility to create and support an organizational culture where we respect people whether they are patients, relatives, or employees. Shared decision making is much more than just a decision tool or a new procedure. It's a human value and as such it must be embedded in the culture of all healthcare institutions. May this wonderful textbook teach us how to succeed.

Dorthe Crüger, MD, PhD
Expert Advisor to the Danish Health Authority.
Former CEO of Lillebaelt University Hospital of Southern Denmark and founder of the National Centre for Shared Decision Making

Contents

PART 7
The view from allied disciplines

PART 8
The way forward

Contributors

Johanna (Annemijn) W.M. Aarts, Department of Obstetrics and Gynaecology, Amsterdam University Medical Centers, Amsterdam, The Netherlands

Samira Abbasgholizadeh Rahimi, Department of Family Medicine, McGill University, Montreal, Canada; Mila Quebec-AI Institute, Montreal, Canada; Lady Davis Institute for Medical Research, Jewish General Hospital, Montreal, Canada; Faculty of Dental Medicine and Oral Sciences, McGill University, Montreal, Canada

Eman Abukmail, PhD student, Faculty of Health Sciences & Medicine, Bond University, Queensland, Australia

Thomas Agoritsas, The MAGIC Evidence Ecosystem Foundation; Department of Medicine, University Hospitals of Geneva, Geneva, Switzerland; Department of Health Research Methods, Evidence, and Impact, McMaster University, Hamilton, Canada

Olawale A. Akinrogunde, Patient Partner, UK

Nadine Montgomery Allam, Solicitor, Levy & McRae Solicitors LLP, Glasgow, UK

Yumi Aoki, Associate Professor, Psychiatric and Mental Health Nursing, Graduate School of Nursing Science, St. Luke's International University, Tokyo, Japan

Kenny Ardouin, Lecturer, School of Psychology, Speech and Hearing, University of Canterbury, Christchurch, New Zealand

Julie Ayre, Sydney Health Literacy Lab, School of Public Health, Faculty of Medicine and Health, The University of Sydney, Sydney, Australia

Katherine Baker, Associate Professor, Department of Sport, Exercise and Rehabilitation, Northumbria University, Newcastle upon Tyne, UK

Mina Bakhit, Assistant Professor of Public Health, Faculty of Health Sciences and Medicine, Bond University, Gold Coast, Australia

Jennifer L. Barton, Professor of Medicine, Division of Arthritis and Rheumatology, Oregon Health & Science University, Portland, Oregon, USA

Paul B. Batalden, Emeritus Professor, The Dartmouth Institute for Health Policy & Clinical Practice, Geisel School of Medicine at Dartmouth, Lebanon, New Hampshire, USA

Hilary L. Bekker, Professor of Medical Decision Making, Unit of Complex Intervention Development (LUCID), Leeds Institute of Health Sciences, School of Medicine, University of Leeds, Leeds, UK

Fernanda Bellolio, Professor of Emergency Medicine, Research Chair, Department of Emergency Medicine, Mayo Clinic, Rochester, Minnesota, USA

Jan Faldt Bentsen, Patient and Relative Board, Lillebaelt Hospital, University Hospital of Southern Denmark, Kolding, Denmark

Zackary Berger, Associate Professor of Medicine, Johns Hopkins School of Medicine; Core Faculty, Johns Hopkins Berman Institute of Bioethics; and Associate Professor, Johns Hopkins School of Public Health, Baltimore, Maryland, USA

Roger Bertozzi, Patient Partnership, 3P Program, Geneva University Hospital (HUG), Geneva, Switzerland

Kasey Boehmer, Knowledge and Evaluation Research (KER) Unit, Division of Nephrology & Hypertension, and Health Care Delivery Research, Mayo Clinic, Rochester, Minnesota, USA; Patient representative, patient with lived experience

Liesbeth Boersma, Department of Radiation Oncology (Maastro), GROW-Research Institute for Oncology and Reproduction, Maastricht University Medical Center+, Maastricht, The Netherlands

Carissa Bonner, Associate Professor, Sydney Health Literacy Lab, School of Public Health, The University of Sydney, Sydney, Australia; Wiser Healthcare, Australia

Willem Jan W. Bos, Department of Internal Medicine, Leiden University Medical Center, The Netherlands; Department of Internal Medicine, St. Antonius Hospital Nieuwegein, The Netherlands

David C. Bosanquet, Consultant Vascular Surgeon, South East Wales Vascular Network, Aneurin Bevan University Health Board, Newport, UK

Emily F. Boss, Professor, Department of Otolaryngology–Head and Neck Surgery, Johns Hopkins University, Baltimore, Maryland, USA

Gemma Bradley, Assistant Professor, Department of Social Work, Education and Community Wellbeing, Northumbria University, Newcastle upon Tyne, UK

Paulina Bravo, Director of Patient Education and Involvement, Fundación Arturo López Pérez, Santiago, Chile

Alessandro Brunelli, Consultant Thoracic Surgeon and Honorary Clinical Associate Professor, Department of Thoracic Surgery, St James's University Hospital, Leeds, UK

Sam Brunsden, Patient Advocate; Trustee, Flat Friends UK

E. Chandlee Bryan, Career Services Manager, Geisel School of Medicine at Dartmouth, Hanover, New Hampshire, USA

Helen Bulbeck, Patient Leader, Director of Services and Policy, Brains Trust, UK

Angie Burke, Retired, Formerly of The Ross Memorial Hospital, Lindsay, Ontario, Canada

Bianca Buurman, Professor of Acute Geriatric Care, University of Amsterdam, The Netherlands

Hugo Campos, Patient Advocate, Oakland, California, USA

Valerie C. Cates, McCaig Institute for Bone and Joint Health, University of Calgary, Calgary, Alberta, Canada; Department of Medical Sciences, University of Calgary, Calgary, Alberta, Canada

Marty Chakoian, Patient Advocate, Seattle, Washington, USA

Ivor G. Chestnutt, Professor and Honorary Consultant, Dental Public Health, School of Dentistry, Cardiff University, Cardiff, UK

Wiebe Cnossen, Patient, Dutch Haematology patient association 'Hematon', Utrecht, The Netherlands

Alf Collins, Independent Health Consultant, UK

Joan Collison, Patient Partner, UK

Anwen Cope, Senior Clinical Lecturer and Honorary Consultant, Dental Public Health, School of Dentistry, Cardiff University, Cardiff, UK

Carrie C. Coughlin, Division of Dermatology, Departments of Medicine and Pediatrics, Washington University in St. Louis School of Medicine, St. Louis, Missouri, USA

Craig Craggs, Expert by Lived Experience, Newcastle upon Tyne, UK

Craig Creelman, Owner/Operator, AllServe Self-Storage, Wilder, Vermont, USA

Cheryl Crow, Founder, CEO, and Patient Educator, Arthritis Life, Bellevue, Washington, USA

Deirdre Daly, Professor in Midwifery, School of Nursing and Midwifery, Trinity College Dublin, Dublin, Ireland

Martin Dando, Principal Physiotherapist, Physiotherapy Department, Cardiff and Vale University Health Board, Cardiff, UK

Eileen Davidson, Rheumatoid arthritis, Vancouver, British Columbia, Canada

Saam Dilmaghani, Instructor in Medicine, Division of Gastroenterology & Hepatology, Mayo Clinic, Rochester, Minnesota, USA

Marie-Anne Durand, Associate Professor, Unisanté, University Center for Primary Care and Public Health, Department of Ambulatory Care, Lausanne, Switzerland; Adjunct Associate Professor, The Dartmouth Institute for Health Policy & Clinical Practice, Dartmouth College, Lebanon, New Hampshire, USA

Adrian Edwards, Professor of General Practice, Director of Health and Care Research Wales Evidence Centre, Division of Population Medicine, Cardiff University, Cardiff, UK

Anna Edwards, Associate Director of Transformation and Change, South East Coast Ambulance Service, NHS Foundation Trust, Brabourne, UK

Glyn Elwyn, Professor and Physician Researcher, The Dartmouth Institute for Health Policy and Clinical Practice, Dartmouth College, Hanover, New Hampshire, USA

Jeanette Finderup, Clinical Nurse Specialist, Department of Renal Medicine, Aarhus University Hospital, Aarhus, Denmark; Associate Professor, Department of Clinical Medicine, Aarhus University, Aarhus, Denmark

Darren Flynn, Professor of Applied Health and Social Care, Department of Nursing, Midwifery and Health, Northumbria University, Newcastle upon Tyne, UK

Rachel C. Forcino, Assistant Professor, Department of Population Health, University of Kansas School of Medicine, Kansas City, Kansas, USA

Erin Foster, Assistant Professor, Department of Dermatology, Oregon Health and Science University, Oregon, USA

Tina C. Foster, Department of Obstetrics and Gynaecology, Dartmouth Hitchcock Medical Center, Lebanon, New Hampshire, USA

Jean Fox, Assistant Professor of Medicine, Division of Gastroenterology & Hepatology, Mayo Clinic, Rochester, Minnesota, USA

Juan V. A. Franco, Family Physician, Institute of General Practice, Medical Faculty of the Heinrich-Heine-University Düsseldorf, Düsseldorf, Germany

Susannah Fraser, Person with Lived Experience and Communication & Media Manager, Bladder Health UK, Birmingham, UK

Wiebke Frerichs, Senior Researcher, Department of Medical Psychology, Medical Center Hamburg-Eppendorf, Hamburg, Germany

Melanie Fritz, Resident, Department of Surgery, University of Wisconsin, Madison, Wisconsin, USA

Paulus A.F. Geerts, Internist-Haematologist, Department of Internal Medicine, Isala, Zwolle, The Netherlands

Anik Giguere, Professor, Department of Family Medicine and Emergency Medicine, Université Laval, Quebec City, Canada

Yuko Goto, Contract Researcher, Department of Home Care and Regional Liaison Promotion, National Center for Geriatrics and Gerontology, Nagoya, Japan

Matthijs Graner-Baars, Expert by Experience, Founder ééndiabetes Foundation, Amsterdam, The Netherlands

Paul Grundy, Consultant Neurosurgeon and Chief Medical Officer, University Hospital Southampton NHS Foundation Trust, Southampton, UK

Pål Gulbrandsen, Professor, Institute of Clinical Medicine, University of Oslo, Oslo, Norway

Pola Hahlweg, Research Group Leader, 'Patient-Centered Care: Evaluation and Implementation', Department of Medical Psychology, University Medical Center Hamburg-Eppendorf, Hamburg, Germany

Paul K.J. Han, Senior Scientist, Division of Cancer Control and Population Sciences, National Cancer Institute, Rockville, Maryland, USA

Désirée Hairwassers, MS Health Sciences, Patient Advocate, Hereditary Cancer Foundation, The Netherlands

Ian Hargraves, Assistant Professor of Medicine, Knowledge and Evaluation Research Unit, Mayo Clinic, Rochester, Minnesota, USA

Adina Harri, Senior Medical Student, Geisel School of Medicine at Dartmouth, Hanover, New Hampshire, USA

Martin Härter, Professor of Medical Psychology, Department of Medical Psychology and Institute for Psychotherapy, University Medical Center Hamburg-Eppendorf, Hamburg, Germany

Alexander T. Hawkins, Vanderbilt University Medical Center, Division of General Surgery, Section of Colon & Rectal Surgery, Nashville, Tennessee, USA

Glen Hazlewood, McCaig Institute for Bone and Joint Health, University of Calgary, Calgary, Alberta, Canada; Departments of Medicine and Community Health Sciences, Cumming School of Medicine, University of Calgary, Calgary, Canada

Anja Fog Heen, The MAGIC Evidence Ecosystem Foundation; Department of Medicine, Lovisenberg Diaconal Hospital, Oslo, Norway

Christoph Heesen, Head Multiple Sclerosis Day Hospital, Institute of Neuroimmunology and Multiple Sclerosis, UMC Hamburg, Germany

Jolyn Hersch, Senior Research Fellow, Sydney Health Literacy Lab, School of Public Health, The University of Sydney, Sydney, Australia; Wiser Healthcare, Australia

Gérard Hendriks, Informal Caregiver, The Netherlands

Erik Hess, Professor of Emergency Medicine, Chair, Department of Emergency Medicine, Vanderbilt University, Nashville, Tennessee, USA

Tammy C. Hoffmann, Professor of Clinical Epidemiology, Institute for Evidence-Based Healthcare, Bond University, Gold Coast, Australia

Paul Hong, Professor, Department of Surgery, Dalhousie University, Halifax, Canada

May Hua, Department of Anesthesiology, College of Physicians and Surgeons, Department of Epidemiology, Mailman School of Public Health, Columbia University, New York City, New York, USA

Libby Humphris, Patient Partner, and Honorary Research Associate, Cardiff University, Cardiff, UK

Giulia M. Ippolito, Assistant Professor, Urology, University of Michigan, Ann Arbor, Michigan, USA

Mayuko Ito Fukunaga, Assistant Professor, Department of Medicine, University of Massachusetts Chan Medical School, Worcester, Massachusetts, USA

Srinivas Joga Ivatury, University of Texas at Austin Dell Medical School, Division of Colon and Rectal Surgery, Austin, Texas, USA

Christopher R. Jacobs, Patient Representative, The Dartmouth Institute for Health Policy and Clinical Practice, Dartmouth College, Hanover, New Hampshire, USA

Rakhshan Kamran, NIHR Doctoral Research Fellow, University of Oxford, Oxford, UK

Robert M. Kaplan, Clinical Excellence Research Center, Stanford University School of Medicine, Stanford, California, USA

Kathy Kastner, Best Endings, Toronto, Ontario, Canada

Julie Kenealy, Patient Partner, UK

Adele Ketley, Medical Student, Department of Clinical Medicine, University of Sheffield, Sheffield, UK

Chris Knoepke, Associate Professor, Department of Medicine, University of Colorado, Aurora, Colorado, USA

Valerie Gutmann Koch, Professor of Law, University of Houston Law Center, Houston, Texas USA

Otmar Kodalle, Patient Representative, Lead of Regional Self-help Group for Patients with Esophageal Cancer, Member of Patient Advisory Board of the University Cancer Center Hamburg, Hamburg, Germany

Elizabeth A. Kroll, Senior Medical Student, Geisel School of Medicine at Dartmouth, Hanover, New Hampshire, USA

Nancy Kuemin, Office of Patient Experience, University of Michigan Health, Ann Arbor, Michigan, USA

Marleen Kunneman, Assistant Professor of Medicine, Biomedical Data Sciences, Leiden University Medical Center, Leiden, The Netherlands; Knowledge and Evaluation Research Unit, Mayo Clinic, Rochester, Minnesota, USA

Lindsay M. Kuroki, Division of Gynecologic Oncology, Department of Obstetrics and Gynecology, Washington University in St. Louis School of Medicine, St. Louis, Missouri, USA

Naomi Laventhal, University of Michigan Medical School, Ann Arbor, Michigan, USA; Committee on Bioethics, American Academy of Pediatrics, Itasca, Illinois, USA

Tim Lahey, The Robert Larner, M.D. College of Medicine at The University of Vermont, and the University of Vermont Medical Center, Burlington, Vermont, USA

Hannah Leavitt, Patient Representative, The Dartmouth Institute for Health Policy and Clinical Practice, Geisel School of Medicine at Dartmouth College, Lebanon, New Hampshire, USA

Thomas W. LeBlanc, Haematologic Oncologist, Division of Haematologic Malignancies and Cellular Therapy, Department of Medicine, Duke University School of Medicine, Durham, North Carolina, USA

France Légaré, Tier 1 Canada Research Chair in Shared Decision Making and Knowledge Mobilization, Department of Family Medicine and Emergency Medicine, Faculty of Medicine, Laval University, Québec, Canada

Arne Lein, Patient Advocate, Norway

Helen Leonard, Parent Carer, UK

Rob Letchford, Consultant Physiotherapist, Physiotherapy Department, Cardiff and Vale University Health Board, Cardiff; Honorary Senior Lecturer, Healthcare Sciences, Cardiff University, Cardiff; Clinical Lead National Strategic Clinical Network Musculoskeletal, NHS Wales, UK

Krystina B. Lewis, Associate Professor, Faculty of Health Sciences, University of Ottawa and Affiliate Investigator, Ottawa Hospital Research Institute, Ottawa, Canada

Sally Lewis, Welsh Value in Health Centre, Cardiff; Welsh Government, Cardiff; Swansea School of Medicine, Swansea, UK

Anja Lindig, Research Assistant, Department of Medical Psychology, University Medical Center Hamburg-Eppendorf, Hamburg, Germany

Kirsten Lomborg, Professor Emeritus, Department of Clinical Medicine, University of Copenhagen, Copenhagen, Denmark

Carrie J. MacEwen, Consultant Ophthalmologist, Ninewells Hospital, Dundee, UK

Meredith MacMartin, Assistant Professor of Medicine and Health Policy & Clinical Practice, Geisel School of Medicine at Dartmouth, Lebanon, New Hampshire, USA

Walter Maetzler, Department of Neurology, University Hospital Schleswig-Holstein and Kiel University, Kiel, Germany

Danil V. Makarov, Associate Professor, Urology & Population Health, NYU Grossman School of Medicine, New York City, New York, USA

Christine M. Marx, Washington University School of Medicine, Department of Surgery, Division of Public Health Sciences, St. Louis, Missouri, USA

Neal Maskrey, Visiting Professor, Keele University, Keele, UK

Rashmi G. Mathew, Consultant Ophthalmologist, Moorfields Eye Hospital/University College London, London, UK

Dan D. Matlock, Professor, Department of Medicine, University of Colorado, Aurora, USA

Hidetoshi Matsuura, Lived Experience Contributor, Bipolar-Work Lab, Liva Incorporated, Tokyo, Japan

Kirsten J. McCaffery, Sydney Health Literacy Lab, School of Public Health, Faculty of Medicine and Health, The University of Sydney, Sydney, Australia

Ruth McCullars, Patient Partner, USA

Ellen McEvoy, Lived Experience Contributor, Ireland

Michael Mcloughlin, Lived Experience Contributor, UK

Jessica Miller, Patient Partner, Oak Ridge, Missouri, USA

Myrtle Mitchell, Patient Partner, USA

Victor M. Montori, Knowledge and Evaluation Research Unit, Division of Endocrinology, Mayo Clinic, USA

Andrew Mooney, Consultant Renal Physician, Renal Unit, St James's University Hospital, Leeds Teaching Hospital Trust, Leeds, UK; Honorary Associate Professor, Leeds Unit of Complex Intervention Development (LUCID), Leeds Institute of Health Sciences, School of Medicine, University of Leeds, Leeds, UK

Jenna Morgan, NIHR Advanced Fellow in Surgery, Department of Clinical Medicine, University of Sheffield, UK; Honorary Consultant Oncoplastic Breast Surgeon, Doncaster and Bassetlaw Teaching Hospitals NHS Foundation Trust, Doncaster, UK

Tessalyn Morrison, Resident Physician, Department of Medicine, University of Vermont Medical Center, Burlington, Vermont, USA

Cordula Mühr, Honorary Patient Representative, on the Federal Joint Committee of Physicians and Health Insurance Funds (G-BA) and the Institute for Quality Assurance and Transparency in Healthcare (IQTiG)

Eugene C. Nelson, Professor, The Dartmouth Institute for Health Policy & Clinical Practice, Geisel School of Medicine at Dartmouth, Lebanon, New Hampshire, USA

Mark D. Neuman, Professor, Department of Anesthesiology and Critical Care, University of Pennsylvania, Pennsylvania, USA

Marianne Nieuwenhuijze, Professor of Midwifery, Care and Public Health Research Institute (CAPHRI), Maastricht University, Maastricht, The Netherlands

Simon Noble, Marie Curie Professor of Supportive and Palliative Medicine, Cardiff University, Cardiff, UK

Daniel C. Norvell, Senior Epidemiologist, Center for Limb Loss and MoBility, VA Puget Sound Health Care System, Seattle, Washington, USA; Research Associate Professor, University of Washington, Department of Rehabilitation Medicine, Seattle, Washington, USA

Karina Olling, Center for Shared Decision Making, Lillebaelt Hospital, University Hospital of Southern Denmark, Vejle, Denmark; Institute of Regional Health Sciences, Faculty of Health Sciences, University of Southern Denmark, Odense, Denmark

Douglas J. Opel, Treuman Katz Center for Pediatric Bioethics and Palliative Care, Seattle Children's Research Institute; Department of Pediatrics, University of Washington School of Medicine, Seattle, Washington, USA

Naykky Singh Ospina, Division of Endocrinology, Department of Medicine, University of Florida; Knowledge and Evaluation Research Unit, Division of Endocrinology, Mayo Clinic, USA

Tod Papageorge, Lived Experience Contributor, USA

Kai-Uwe Parsons-Galka, 1st Chairman of the Board, of the Förderverein für Knochenmarktransplantation in Hamburg e.V. (Bone Marrow Transplant Patient Support Association), Hamburg, Germany

Roshan Paudel, Research Fellow, Medical Oncology, Dana-Farber Cancer Institute, Boston, Massachusetts, USA

Liam J. Peck, Doctor, Ashford and St Peter's Hospitals NHS Foundation Trust, Surrey, UK

Ruth E. Pel-Littel, Professor of Shared Decision Making with older adults, The University of Applied Sciences Arnhem/Nijmegen, The Netherlands

Vincent D. Pellegrini Jr, Professor and Vice Chair of Education and Research Affairs, Department of Orthopaedics, Dartmouth-Hitchcock Medical Center, Lebanon, New Hampshire, USA; Professor of The Dartmouth Institute and Immediate Past Chair, Faculty Council, Geisel School of Medicine at Dartmouth, Hanover, New Hampshire, USA

Lilisbeth Perestelo-Pérez, Director of Unit, Evaluation Unit (SESCS), Canary Islands Health Service (SCS), Tenerife, Spain; Network for Research on Chronicity, Primary Care, and Health Promotion (RICAPPS), Tenerife, Spain

Mona Muusmann Petersen, Patient Representative, Denmark

Arwen H. Pieterse, Associate Professor, Leiden University Medical Center, The Netherlands, and Visiting Professor, University of Oslo, Oslo, Norway

Rita Pipes, Patient Advocate, USA

Carole Pitkeathley, Standing Lay Member and Patient Advocate for NICE guideline Development and Technology Appraisal Committees and NHS England Strategic Boards, UK

Dan Poenaru, Institute of Health Sciences Education, McGill University, Montreal, Quebec, Canada; Department of Pediatric Surgery, McGill University, Montreal, Canada

Mary C. Politi, Professor, School of Public Health, Washington University in St Louis, St. Louis, Missouri, USA

Thaddeus Mason Pope, Professor of Law, Mitchell Hamline School of Law, Saint Paul, Minnesota, USA

Karina Prévost, Patient Partner, Unité de Soutien, SSA, Québec, Canada

Amy Price, Senior Research Scientist, The Dartmouth Institute for Health Policy and Clinical Practice, Dartmouth College, Hanover, New Hampshire, USA

Michaela Prigge, Intensive Care Nurse, Paedagogical Specialist, Patient Representative, Germany

Joshua B. Rager, Assistant Professor of Medicine, Indiana University School of Medicine, Indianapolis, Indiana, USA

Janette Rawlinson, Patient Advocate/ Representative, European Lung Foundation Lung Cancer Advisory Group, European Respiratory Society Lung Cancer Task forces, European Organisation for Research and Treatment of Cancer Lung Cancer Group, British Thoracic Oncology Group Steering Committee, NHS England Lung Screening Advisory Group, Sandwell, West Midlands, UK

Dawn P. Richards, Five02 Labs Inc., Toronto, Canada; Canada Arthritis Patient Alliance, Toronto, Canada

Sara Riggare, Participatory eHealth and Health Data Research Group, Uppsala University, Uppsala, Sweden; Uppsala University Centre for Disability Studies, Uppsala, Sweden

Jeremy N. Rodrigues, Associate Professor, Clinical Trials Unit, The University of Warwick, Coventry, UK, Aylesbury, UK

Rene Rodriguez-Gutierrez, Knowledge and Evaluation Research Unit, Division of Endocrinology, Mayo Clinic, USA; Plataforma INVEST Medicina UANL—KER Unit (KER Unit México), Subdireccion de Investigacion, Universidad Autónoma de Nuevo León, Mexico

Wim Roelofs, Informal Caregiver, The Netherlands

Johannah Ruddy, The Rome Foundation, Raleigh, USA

Leigh Sanyaolu, General Practitioner and Health and Care Research Wales, NIHR Doctoral Fellow, Division of Population Medicine and PRIME Centre Wales, Cardiff University, Cardiff, UK

Catherine H. Saunders, Scientist, Assistant Professor of Medicine and Health Policy and Clinical Practice, Dartmouth Health, The Geisel School of Medicine at Dartmouth, Hanover, New Hampshire, USA

Robert Schlegel, Patient Partner and Lived Experience Contributor, Retired US Navy, Beaufort, South Carolina, USA

Fülöp Scheibler, Head of Evidence Team, National Competency Center for Shared Decision Making, University Hospital Schleswig Holstein; Partner, SHARE TO CARE, Patient Centered Care, GmbH, Cologne, Germany

Isabelle Scholl, Professor of Psycho-Oncology and Patient-Centered Medicine, Department of Medical Psychology, University Medical Center Hamburg-Eppendorf, Hamburg, Germany

Danielle Schubbe, The Dartmouth Institute for Health Policy and Clinical Practice, Geisel School of Medicine, Dartmouth College, New Hampshire, USA

Jason Scott, Associate Professor of Health and Social Care Quality, Department of Social Work, Education and Community Wellbeing, Northumbria University, Newcastle upon Tyne, UK

Margaret Schwarze, Professor, Department of Surgery and Department of Medical History and Bioethics, University of Wisconsin, Madison, Wisconsin, USA

Karen R. Sepucha, Associate Professor of Medicine, Massachusetts General Hospital, Harvard Medical School, Boston, Massachusetts, USA

Seema K. Shah, Department of Pediatrics, Northwestern University Feinberg School of Medicine; Bioethics Program, Lurie Children's Hospital, Chicago, Illinois, USA

Zoe Silsbury, Clinical Lead Physiotherapist, Physiotherapy Department, Cwm Taff Morgannwg University Health Board, Merthyr Tydfil, UK

Scout Silverstein, Lived Experience Contributor and Doctoral Candidate, The Shared Decision Making Laboratory, College of Public Health, Temple University, Philadelphia, Pennsylvania, USA

Namrata Singh, Assistant Professor, Division of Rheumatology, University of Washington, Seattle, Washington, USA

Elisabeth Smith, Clinical Research Fellow in Vascular Surgery, Gwent Vascular Institute, Aneurin Bevan University Health Board, Newport, UK

Lowri Smith, Patient Representative, UK

Maureen Smith, Health Consumer, and Patient Partner, Ottawa, Canada

Valerie Smith, Professor of Midwifery, School of Nursing, Midwifery and Health Systems, University College Dublin, Dublin, Ireland

Henning Søndergaard, Patient Partner with Kidney Services, Department of Clinical Medicine, Aarhus University, Aarhus, Denmark, and Aarhus University Hospital, Denmark

Erica S. Spatz, Associate Professor, Section of Cardiovascular Medicine, Department of Medicine, Yale School of Medicine, New Haven, Connecticut, USA

Laura Spinnewijn, Department of Obstetrics and Gynaecology, Radboudumc, Nijmegen, The Netherlands

Dominique Sprengers, Senior Advisor Patient Interests, Netherlands Patients Federation, Utrecht, The Netherlands

Dawn Stacey, Distinguished Professor, School of Nursing, University of Ottawa, Ottawa, Canada; Senior Scientist, Centre for Implementation Research, Ottawa Hospital Research Institute, Ottawa, Canada

Karina Dahl Steffensen, Professor in Shared Decision Making, Center for Shared Decision Making, Lillebaelt Hospital, University Hospital of Southern Denmark, Vejle, Denmark; Institute of Regional Health Sciences, Faculty of Health Sciences, University of Southern Denmark, Odense, Denmark

Anne M. Stiggelbout, Department of Biomedical Data Sciences, Leiden University Medical Center, Leiden, The Netherlands

Rikke Nicoline Stokholm, PhD Student, Department of Public Health Programmes and University Research Clinic for Cancer Screening, Randers Regional Hospital, Randers, Denmark; Department of Clinical Medicine, Aarhus University, Aarhus, Denmark

Constanze Stolz-Klingenberg, National Competency Center for Shared Decision Making, University Hospital Schleswig-Holstein, Kiel, Germany

Susan Strong, Director of Patient Engagement, Heart Valve Voice, Washington, D.C., USA

Henning Søndergaard, Patient representative, The Danish Kidney Association, Denmark

Elaine Taylor, Lived Experience Contributor, UK

Jerry Thomas, Research Coordinator, Urology & Population Health, NYU Grossman School of Medicine, New York City, New York, USA

Elaine C. Thompson, Resident, Department of Otolaryngology–Head and Neck Surgery, Johns Hopkins University, Baltimore, Maryland, USA

Sally Thorne, Professor Emeritus, School of Nursing, University of British Columbia, Vancouver, Canada

Hannah M. Timlin, Consultant Ophthalmologist, Moorfields Eye Hospital/University College London, London, UK

Lyndal Trevena, Professor Emerita, University of Sydney, Sydney, Australia

Janice Tufte, Patient Partner and PCORI Ambassador, Patient-Centered Outcomes Research Institute (PCORI), USA; Cochrane Consumer Network

Dirk T. Ubbink, Professor in Evidence-Based Medicine and Shared Decision-Making, Department of Surgery, Amsterdam University Medical Center, Amsterdam, The Netherlands

Jonathan Underhill, Director, JLU Associates; Honorary Lecturer, Keele University School of Pharmacy; formerly Medicines Consultant Clinical Adviser, NICE, UK

K.D. Valentine, Faculty, Department of General Internal Medicine, Massachusetts General Hospital; Instructor, Harvard Medical School, Boston, Massachusetts, USA

Trudy van der Weijden, Professor, Department of Family Medicine, CAPHRI, Maastricht University, Maastricht, The Netherlands

Haske van Veenendaal, Erasmus School of Health Policy & Management, Erasmus University Rotterdam, Rotterdam, The Netherlands

Irma Vargas, Health Professional, Division of Primary Care, Ministry of Health, Santiago, Chile

Robert J. Volk, Professor, Department of Health Services Research, The University of

Texas MD Anderson Cancer Center, Houston, Texas, USA

Christian von Plessen, Consultant and Senior Lecturer, Center for Primary Care and Public Health, Unisanté & Faculty of Biology & Medicine, University of Lausanne, Lausanne, Switzerland

Anna Waters, Simulated Participant, Faculty of Health Sciences and Medicine, Bond University, Gold Coast, Australia

Jolanda Wellen, Lived Experience Contributor

Angela Williams, Patient Advocate, USA

Denitza Williams, Lecturer, Division of Population Medicine, College of Biomedical and Life Sciences, School of Medicine, Cardiff University, Cardiff, UK

Natalie Joseph-Williams, Reader in Improving Patient Care and Associate Director for the Health and Care Research, Wales Evidence Centre, School of Medicine, Cardiff University, Cardiff, UK

Steven D. Williams, Lead Clinical Pharmacist, Poole Bay and Bournemouth Primary Care Network; Honorary Clinical Lecturer, University of Manchester Pharmacy School, Manchester, UK

Jennifer Wilson, Lived Experience Contributor, UK

Anna E. Winterbottom, Senior Health Services Researcher, Renal Unit, St James's University Hospital, Leeds Teaching Hospital Trust, Leeds, UK; Visiting Senior Research Fellow, Leeds Unit of Complex Intervention Development (LUCID), Leeds Institute of Health Sciences, School of Medicine, University of Leeds, Leeds, UK

Marlene Würgler, Center for Patient Involvement, Capital Region, Copenhagen, Denmark

Helene Juul Würtz, Lillebaelt University Hospital of Southern Denmark, Vejle, Denmark

Lynda Wyld, Professor of Surgical Oncology, Department of Clinical Medicine, University of Sheffield, UK; Honorary Consultant Oncoplastic Breast Surgeon, Doncaster and Bassetlaw Teaching Hospitals NHS Foundation Trust, UK

Amy Zelenski, Associate Professor, Department of Medicine, University of Wisconsin, Madison, Wisconsin, USA

Yaara Zisman-Ilani, Associate Professor, Department of Social and Behavioral Sciences, College of Public HealthTemple University, Philadelphia, PA, USA; Associate Professor (Honorary), Department of Clinical, Educational and Health Psychology, Division of Psychology and Language Sciences, University College London (UCL), London, UK

Laura Zwaan, Associate Professor, Institute of Medical Education Research Rotterdam (iMERR), Erasmus Medical Center, Rotterdam, The Netherlands

Abbreviations

A3Q	Ask 3 Questions
AAA	abdominal aortic aneurysm
AF	atrial fibrillation
AI	artificial intelligence
AML	acute myeloid leukaemia
APN	Advanced Practice Nursing
BCS	breast-conserving surgery
BRAN	Benefits of the medicine; Risks of the medicine; Alternatives to the medicine; No change from current management
CLL	chronic lymphocytic leukaemia
CMS	Centers for Medicare and Medicaid Services
DA	decision aid
ED	emergency department
EM	emergency medicine
ENT	ear, nose, and throat
FIGO	International Federation of Gynecology and Obstetrics
FMS	fibromyalgia syndrome
G-BA	Federal Joint Committee [Germany]
GDMT	goal-directed medical therapy
GORD	gastro-oesophageal reflux disease
GP	general practitioner
HCP	healthcare professional
HRQoL	health-related quality of life
IBD	inflammatory bowel disease
IBS	irritable bowel syndrome
ICD	implantable cardioverter–defibrillator
ICU	intensive care unit
IPDAS	International Patient Decision Aid Standards
iPROM	individualized patient reported outcome measure
IPU	integrated practice unit
IQTIG	Institute for Quality Assurance and Transparency in Health Care
LHS	learning health systems
LVAD	left ventricular assist device
MAGIC	Making Good Decisions in Collaboration
MCC	multiple chronic conditions
MM	multiple myeloma or multimorbidity
MS	multiple sclerosis
MSK	musculoskeletal
NCD	national coverage determination
NHS	National Health Service
NICE	National Institute for Health and Care Excellence
OPSCC	oropharyngeal squamous cell carcinoma
PCC-Net	International Network for Patient-Centered Care
PDSA	Plan–Do–Study–Act
PH	public health
PPIR	patient and public involvement in research
PREM	patient-reported experience measure
PROM	patient-reported outcome measure
PtDA	patient decision aid
PwKF	people with kidney failure
RMDs	rheumatic and musculoskeletal diseases
rUTI	recurrent urinary tract infection
SDM	shared decision making
SDM-Q-9	nine-item Shared Decision Making Questionnaire
SDM-Q-Doc	Shared Decision-Making Questionnaire—physician version
SHAIR	Shared decision making Adoption Implementation Resource
SMI	severe mental illness
SOC	standard of care
SUNDAE	Standards for Universal reporting of patient Decision Aid Evaluations
USPSTF	United States Preventive Services Task Force
VBHC	value-based healthcare

PART 1

Introduction

1

Enabling shared decision making in practice

Glyn Elwyn, Natalie Joseph-Williams, Karina Prévost, Adrian Edwards, and Christopher R. Jacobs

Introduction

We introduce this book by using a description of shared decision making (SDM) that we have heard from our patient co-author, Karina Prévost:

> Essentially, shared decision making happens when a healthcare professional takes your hand and walks together with you on your journey.

Yes, there are decisions to take along the way, but there is so much more to this description of involving people when they interact with healthcare services. The metaphor of a journey is apt, and illness makes any journey much more difficult. The route becomes more difficult, the work that has to be done is much harder, and the obstacles that come along are more challenging. There are decisions to be made, often with very little information to be found and more uncertainty than fact. Journeys are tough enough when we are confidently autonomous and can face the future with courage (Gulbrandsen et al., 2016). But being ill is an exercise in adaptation and finding solutions that do not make a tough situation even tougher to manage.

We'd all like a personal guide, and sometimes, we can work with a healthcare professional who can 'hold our hand' on an extended basis. More often than not, we increasingly rely on a team of professionals to tackle this work and, hopefully, tackle the complex, continuous work of coordinating and communicating with us as we progress along our illness trajectories. Increasingly, we observe that SDM is not only about single interactions but also requires the coordinated work of teams, families, microsystems, and organizations that occurs over illness journeys. Understanding the implications of that future will likely be the work of more editions.

We will return to the issue of definition and the implications of how SDM is understood and achieved. First, we want to explain what is new and different about this book.

The first edition of this book was called *Evidence-Based Patient Choice: Inevitable or Impossible?* and was published in 2001. Looking back, we were still determining whether or not the approach would find a life beyond the academic papers that had been published at the time. The second edition followed it in 2009—*Shared Decision Making in Health Care: Achieving Evidence-Based Patient Choice*. By this point, there was clear evidence that the approach had gained widespread recognition, many more peer-reviewed publications had appeared, and significant policy developments were appearing in several countries. We used the same title for the third edition in 2016. These three editions built on the increasing interest in the approach, and it was clear that health professionals worldwide had grasped the idea and advocated for it in their health systems. It was, therefore, a delight to hear that for the fourth edition, Oxford University Press wanted to change the status of the work so that it would become the *Oxford Textbook of Shared Decision Making in Healthcare*.

Changes in this fourth edition

We decided it was time to make two significant changes to the book.

The first was to ensure that every chapter included a patient's voice. This reflects not only the importance we attach to the contribution of patients, carers, and citizens using healthcare but also that a significant cohort of patients with lived experience of SDM related to their conditions has developed in recent years and now advocates powerfully for more change. Who better to learn from than those who have lived through these decisions?

The second was to create two entirely new sections where we invited clinicians from many clinical specialities and allied healthcare disciplines to lead a chapter and involve a patient or patients as they focused on developments in their fields. At first, we were still determining whether we could find sufficient clinician advocates. We should not have been concerned. As we searched for articles across the many disciplines, it soon became clear that we could find reviews, studies, and editorials in numerous clinical disciplines. It was also gratifying to experience the willingness of clinicians to review work in their discipline, summarize existing work, and consider future developments. This was strong evidence that SDM had become an established idea, not only across healthcare in academic circles, but was now being gradually adopted by many pioneers across the various clinical disciplines.

Overview of sections

We start by summarizing each section and providing an overview of the content.

Part 1: Introduction

This first chapter indicates the changes made from the first three editions and reflects on the challenge of enabling SDM in clinical practice. We include excerpts of work that has yet to be published in a peer-reviewed journal which enlisted International Shared Decision Making Society members. The work aimed to describe SDM in terms of the obstacles clinicians commonly meet and consider how those challenges might be handled.

Part 2: The theory of shared decision making

Is involving patients in decisions at every possible opportunity appropriate? Some advocate for this view, suggesting that it is ethical to do so and view SDM as a broadly humanistic approach to patient-centred care. They argue that there is no situation where SDM is inappropriate. The first chapter in this section takes a different view and proposes limits to SDM: situations where other factors, such as professional standards, constrain the offer of options. Other chapters consider ethical perspectives, the need for adaptations to support patients with diminished cognitive capabilities, the need to make cultural adaptations, and how SDM could support complex trade-offs during diagnostic processes. Two additional chapters delve into the interface between co-production, value-based healthcare, and SDM.

Part 3: Methods in shared decision making research

This section has three chapters on measuring SDM. The first is an overview, followed by chapters that focus on patient-reported measures and observational measures. An additional chapter summarizes developments in innovative research methods.

Part 4: Approaches to teaching and training

This section provides an overview of teaching frameworks and describes innovations in teaching SDM. It also describes an approach developed by Margaret 'Gretchen' Schwarze, a surgeon from the USA. She calls it the 'Best Case/Worst Case' because it lays out a method for surgeons to describe the outcomes of significant surgical procedures to patients so that they obtain a realistic view of their likely recovery process and decide whether to proceed with the operation.

Part 5: Implementation

This is one of the most significant sections of the textbook, which illustrates very well that efforts have shifted to putting SDM into practice, using teaching, interventions, quality improvement, and other methods. The section starts by providing an overview of progress at an international level, drawing on data from multiple sources. The next chapter focuses on the different implementation approaches in the field. Many implementation efforts have involved using patient decision aids. Three chapters provide an overview, drawing on the International Patient Decision Aids Standards Collaboration, of what makes a good patient decision aid, summarize the evidence of their impact, and discuss the challenge of keeping these tools up to date and accessible. Four chapters then provide more detailed case studies of implementation projects in Germany, the USA, Denmark, and the Netherlands. The final chapter in this section describes the use of quality improvement methods to implement SDM.

Part 6: The view from the clinical specialties

This is a new section where we have asked clinicians from 29 fields to summarize the role and impact of SDM. We were keen that these author lists should include a range of professional, improvement, or research perspectives. Importantly, each chapter includes a perspective of one or more patients as they have experienced SDM or its challenges in that domain. Future recommendations, priorities, and research are identified.

Part 7: The view from allied disciplines

SDM has also been actively adopted in allied healthcare fields. We include chapters in this section that cover midwifery, physiotherapy, advanced nursing, pharmacy, dentistry, and psychology. Again, patients' perspectives on the opportunities of SDM across these professional groups are insightful.

Part 8: The way forward

In this section, we look at where we are now, where we might see developments, and the role of legal changes in how services are regulated and managed. First, we consider the role of technological developments, including the potential role of generative artificial intelligence. However, it is difficult to predict the likely significant impact of large language models on many aspects of healthcare. The next chapter presents an evaluation of SDM from the perspective of patients, underlining the importance of autonomy in healthcare decisions. The rising cost of healthcare is an important concern in many economies, and we devote a chapter to this issue, which is particularly relevant in locations that do not provide universal coverage for their populations and often use provider systems that rely on income from commercial insurance companies. The rising cost of healthcare is frequently associated with stark inequities in access and quality. Therefore, we devote a chapter to considering how SDM could tackle this increasingly common problem. In the next chapter, recent developments in the law and SDM are covered. In the final chapter, we attempt to combine the many threads and summarize the remaining key challenges and priorities.

Latest developments in the theory, research methods, teaching, training, and implementation

Sections in this book describe the latest developments in SDM theory, methods of researching, teaching, training, and implementation. These also show significant progress in the field since the 2016 third edition of this book. We summarize key advances below (Table 1.1).

Table 1.1 Key advances since the third edition

Diversity	Chapter 6: Cultural adaptations of shared decision making and patient-centred care models
Adaptive SDM	Chapter 7: Is shared decision making appropriate for diagnostic decisions? Chapter 5: Patient capacity and shared decision making Chapter 14: Best Case/Worst Case: a framework to improve medical communication and decision making in high-risk and uncertainty situations Chapter 34: Shared decision making in care for older adults with multiple chronic conditions Chapter 6: Cultural adaptations of shared decision making and patient-centred care models Chapter 60: Shared decision making for people living with multimorbidity: perspectives from psychology, physiotherapy, occupational therapy and lived experience Chapter 53: Shared decision making in psychosomatic conditions Chapter 41: Shared decision making in public health: balancing individual choice with the common good Chapter 28: Shared decision making in paediatrics and child healthcare *See also various 'Clinical specialities' and 'Allied disciplines' chapters that acknowledge adaptation for disabilities*
Alignment with complementary healthcare initiatives	Chapter 4: Value-based healthcare and shared decision making Chapter 3: Co-production and learning health systems Chapter 25: How to improve shared decision making in your practice: using improvement methods to drive change *See also 'Implementation', 'Clinical specialities', and 'Allied disciplines' chapters*
Artificial intelligence and technology	Chapter 61: Technological innovations: use of artificial intelligence in shared decision making Chapter 12: Innovations in shared decision making measurement Chapter 15: Innovations in shared decision making teaching
Limits of SDM	Chapter 2: The limits of shared decision making

A common thread throughout the book is '*diversity*'. In this edition, we see a much-needed improvement in recognizing and appreciating differences between patient populations and individuals. Our authors have described adapted theories, models, and approaches to ensure a more diverse range of patients can be involved in healthcare decisions.

Linked to this is greater recognition of the *adaptive* nature of SDM. We always knew that one size did not fit all. However, the latest work highlights key areas where we need to adapt, rather than refine, SDM models and tools, including limited patient capacity, diagnostic and public health decisions, and multimorbidity.

Since the last edition, authors have focused more on the *alignment of SDM with complementary healthcare initiatives*, specifically, on how these can be leveraged to embed SDM in practice. We include specific chapters on value-based healthcare (Chapter 4), quality improvement (Chapter 25), and learning healthcare systems (Chapter 3), but the implementation, clinical specialities, and allied discipline chapters provide abundant further examples.

A new and exciting innovation for the fourth edition is the potential of *artificial intelligence*—across multiple chapters, authors summarize the role it could play in risk communication, measurement, developing sustainable evidence-based patient decision aids, and in personalized treatment plans that could streamline the SDM process (this is summarized in Chapter 61).

Finally, but not least, this edition includes an important discussion around the *limits of SDM*. With the increasing policy and practice interest in SDM, it is essential we recognize these limitations. By being honest about these situations, it ensures SDM is not too easily dismissed as an impossible ideal and that SDM is not forced in situations of profound distress and uncertainty that could negatively impact patients.

Enabling SDM: common challenges for clinicians

Despite our observation that most clinical disciplines have heard of and are actively considering the implications of involving patients in decisions, a recurring theme over the last three decades is that the increasing interest is not mirroring wide adoption in routine clinical practice settings. We see the emergence of clinical champions, but it is still true that most patients in most clinical settings are not offered significant involvement in decision making. Many studies have highlighted the barriers.

However, we also need to revisit how the process of sharing decisions has been described, pay attention to some key issues that make it difficult for clinicians to embrace this approach, and understand those circumstances in which patients may not welcome the approach. To tackle this goal, we include excerpts from a not-yet-published multi-author article. We invited members of the International Shared Decision Making Society to contribute ideas. We agreed that, even though over 50 years have passed since Veatch first described the concept of SDM (Veatch, 1972), clinicians lack a short explanatory introduction of what exactly is meant by the term SDM and how to overcome the typical reactions of patients to the offer of being involved in decisions. We saw this as putting together a short introduction to SDM that clinicians could follow. In summary, it is a 'primer' that considers the complexity of using the approach in clinical practice.

Numerous definitions and descriptions of SDM have been published, often led by social scientists (Charles et al., 1997; Makoul and Clayman, 2006; Bomhof-Roordink et al., 2019). Still, most of the definitions avoid the viewpoint of clinicians about the work involved, especially when communicating with people with limited resources, low expectations, or meagre prior experiences of agency. For example, a recent definition is based on the assumption that two, and only two, agents with full autonomy arrive at a mutually agreed decision (Chambers, 2023).

We disagree: these assumptions do not match the conditions observed in healthcare interactions. Achieving SDM needs a different approach when supporting a 35-year-old social worker with breast cancer striving to preserve her fertility versus a 77-year-old pensioner with limited literacy and numeracy facing a choice between surgery and radiotherapy for lung cancer. The researcher typically expects information and autonomy. The pensioner usually prefers guidance and declines decisional responsibility. Nevertheless, individuals vary considerably from these stereotypes, and clinicians are frequently surprised at someone's preference for involvement in decision making.

To be helpful, clinicians need a way to think about SDM that helps them navigate the inevitable range of personalities, contexts, and preferences (Elwyn et al., 2017). In addition, there is often uncertain or limited evidence coupled with the relentless time pressure of clinical schedules. Clinicians need practical ways to navigate the challenges of adapting to the diverse needs of people served in the clinic.

We highlight two critical barriers to SDM that clinicians have repeatedly expressed (Landmark et al., 2015). First, SDM rests on the ethical principle of respecting autonomy. However, people seeking healthcare are often in vulnerable emotional states and, as a result, are often far from being confidently autonomous (Gulbrandsen et al., 2016). Patients and clinicians may be at odds about the goals: while professionals might want to offer options and elicit reactions, their patients may want to decline decisional responsibility, preferring to seek guidance, at least initially. Second, SDM is particularly difficult in encounters where profound differences in power, knowledge, and lived experience exist, often manifesting as a strong deference to clinicians and experts (Mishler, 1984). Such asymmetry explains some people's preferences to decline a role in decision making and request guidance (Pilnick and Dingwall, 2011). Conversely, clinicians who, by their nature, assume control may exclude others who want a greater decision making role.

Shifting levels of agency and a preference for different roles will influence these interactions. Clinicians will want to respect people's wishes to decline decision making roles. Conversely, some people will put a higher value on a collaborative approach (Longo et al., 2006). A description of SDM that emphasizes the need for an empathic, flexible, context- and time-sensitive approach to SDM may be more readily embraced by clinicians.

Therefore, clinicians would benefit from a brief statement, a primer, describing tasks that would facilitate SDM. We invited members of the International Shared Decision-Making Society and, subsequently, a wider group of clinicians and patient representatives to co-produce the proposed statement. After several consultation rounds with patients and a wider group of clinicians in practice, the group of authors agreed on a short statement, which we called a primer (Box 1.1). We also added a commentary to expand on the short statements contained in Box 1.1.

Box 1.1 A primer on shared decision making

Definition SDM in healthcare is a collaboration between individuals that blends science, clinical experience, and people's preferences when comparing options or plans to determine decisions.

An explicit invitation People usually need to be invited and supported by clinicians to become aware of key decisions to be made, that options exist, and be encouraged to take part in the process of deciding.

Non-abandonment People should also understand that they do not have to take on the burden of decisions and that they will not be left (abandoned) to make difficult decisions on their own.

Many people, iterative process Relatives, friends, and multiple clinicians may be involved, and the process often occurs over more than one conversation.

Goal elicitation Eliciting a person's goals helps outline the best options, including the possibility of not taking action or making changes.

Trustworthy information A key task is to help people become aware of the possible range of options or actions and provide information to compare them carefully—information that is trustworthy, balanced, and easy to understand. Being open about uncertainty or the lack of good information is equally vital.

Deliberation: perspective elicitation and determination Arriving at, or deferring, a decision involves dialogue: listening and eliciting questions, views, emotions, fears, priorities, and preferences of the people involved. The aim is to co-produce, if possible, a preference for the option or plan that is considered best at the time while leaving it open to review.

Clarification of the primer elements

An explicit invitation

If the patient (and/or family) is not explicitly invited to participate, there is a significant risk that people will not realize that there are different expectations and that they have a role that might be new to them. There may also be a preparation phase: an orientation to the condition and what may be possible (Joseph-Williams et al., 2019). Without a careful explanation of motives, trust might be at risk: people may consider that such a clinician lacks knowledge, confidence, or both. They may think the clinician is absolving responsibility and may be unwilling in patients' eyes to undertake their expert role (Schneider, 1998). Patients should also understand that if asked, a health professional is willing to make recommendations but will do so only after becoming aware of personal perspectives and contexts.

Non-abandonment

People might fear being coerced into making a decision or being abandoned to face a difficult decision alone (Quill and Cassel, 1995). Non-abandonment means reassuring patients that they do not have to shoulder decisional responsibility alone and will be supported no matter how long or difficult the illness.

Many people

The process cannot be assumed to be a dyadic interaction. Other healthcare professionals will likely be part of the process at different levels of input and expertise. In this way, clinical teams also need to support this approach explicitly. Interdisciplinary teams often become actors in decisions, and the integration of patient preferences in clinical team discussions is frequently neglected (Heuser et al., 2023). To variable extents, relatives and others will be involved, usually supportive, but not always (Laidsaar-Powell et al., 2013). It becomes clear that deliberations about specific decisions or future actions will be distributed across various actors (Rapley, 2008).

Iterative process

Acknowledging that SDM may be 'distributed' across many interactions also means accepting that the process may take place across time, even in a dyadic situation. Typically, the more complex the decision or problem, the more time is required. Supporting people over an extended process demands very good record-keeping.

The range of options

Awareness that a choice of options exists is the cornerstone of SDM (Kunneman et al., 2018). Options cannot be considered if they are left unspecified. The option of taking no action, sometimes called watchful waiting, declining a test or treatment, or perhaps de-escalating an existing treatment, is often left unmentioned and sometimes viewed negatively by clinicians and patients. In some situations, it may be necessary to convey 'no action' or postponement as valid strategies that will not lead to a withdrawal of care but rather be respected.

Goal elicitation

When selecting options, eliciting individual goals, short and long term, will help achieve alignment on what is possible or desirable. Parsing goals into those that are symptom-based, functional, or fundamental could guide the selection of comparisons (Elwyn and Vermunt, 2020).

Trustworthy information

SDM brings together parallel developments in evidence-based medicine and patient-centred care (Barratt, 2008). These streams underpin the development of tools, often called patient decision aids, that help patients and healthcare professionals compare options (Stacey et al., 2024).

Deliberation: perspective elicitation

When goals and options are outlined and contextual information understood, the subsequent collaborative phases of SDM can proceed. Personal perspective elicitation is about checking views, emotions, concerns, priorities, and preferences related to the decision (Rake et al., 2022). An individual's values, beliefs, and experience with a condition will be influential.

Deliberation: determination

The next deliberation step is to determine which option is considered best (Elwyn and Miron-Shatz, 2009). While some determinations are irreversible, such as undergoing surgery, others are less so, as in the constant decisions involved in living with a long-term illness, so offering to revisit and review decisions will be highly valued.

Summary

The primer statement (Box 1.1) puts the work of explicitly eliciting and integrating patients' perspectives at the heart of clinical practice, informed by comprehensible science and clinical experience. It emphasizes that the ideal is not always possible: a clinician's best efforts to guide an anxious patient and *contextualize* decisions would be progress.

This primer also emphasizes the importance of a clear invitation and a careful justification when initiating a process that might be novel for many: patient involvement is voluntary, should not be mandated, and no one should be abandoned to face tough decisions alone. The primer reminds clinicians that mutual agreement, while welcome, is not the only goal of SDM. This textbook will further unpack the steps required to achieve this process and relate experiences of how it can be achieved across healthcare disciplines and settings.

REFERENCES

Barratt, A. 2008. Evidence based medicine and shared decision making: the challenge of getting both evidence and preferences into health care. *Patient Educ Couns*, **73**, 407–412.

Bomhof-Roordink, H., Gärtner, F. R., Stiggelbout, A. M., Pieterse, A. H. 2019. Key components of shared decision making models: a systematic review. *BMJ Open*, **9**, e031763.

Chambers, D. W. 2023. Toward an operational definition of shared decision making: a conceptual analysis. *J Eval Clin Pract*, **29**, 1061–1067.

Charles, C., Gafni, A., Whelan, T. 1997. Shared decision-making in the medical encounter: what does it mean? (Or it takes at least two to tango). *Soc Sci Med*, **44**, 681–692.

Elwyn, G., Durand, M. A., Song, J., et al. 2017. A three-talk model for shared decision making: multistage consultation process. *BMJ*, **359**, j4891.

Elwyn, G., Miron-Shatz, T. 2009. Deliberation before determination: the definition and evaluation of good decision making. *Health Expect*, **13**, 139–147.

Elwyn, G., Vermunt, N. P. C. A. 2020. Goal-based shared decision-making: developing an integrated model. *J Patient Exp*, **7**, 688–696.

Gulbrandsen, P., Clayman, M. L., Beach, M. C., et al. 2016. Shared decision-making as an existential journey: aiming for restored autonomous capacity. *Patient Educ Couns*, **99**, 1505–1510.

Heuser, C., Schellenberger, B., Ernstmann, N., et al. 2023. Shared-decision-making experiences in breast cancer care with and without patient participation in multidisciplinary tumor conferences: a mixed-methods-study. *J Multidiscip Healthc*, **16**, 397–409.

Joseph-Williams, N., Williams, D., Wood, F., et al. 2019. A descriptive model of shared decision making derived from routine implementation in clinical practice ('Implement-SDM'): qualitative study. *Patient Educ Couns*, **102**, 1774–1785.

Kunneman, M., Branda, M. E., Hargraves, I., Pieterse, A. H., Montori, V. M. 2018. Fostering choice awareness for shared decision making: a secondary analysis of video-recorded clinical encounters. *Mayo Clin Proc Innov Qual Outcomes*, **2**, 60–68.

Laidsaar-Powell, R. C., Butow, P. N., Bu, S., et al. 2013. Physician–patient–companion communication and decision-making: a systematic review of triadic medical consultations. *Patient Educ Couns*, **91**, 3–13.

Landmark, A. M. D., Gulbrandsen, P., Svennevig, J. 2015. Whose decision? Negotiating epistemic and deontic rights in medical treatment decisions. *J Pragmat*, **78**, 54–69.

Longo, M. F., Cohen, D. R., Hood, K., et al. 2006. Involving patients in primary care consultations: assessing preferences using discrete choice experiments. *Br J Gen Pract*, **56**, 35–42.

Makoul, G., Clayman, M.L. 2006. An integrative model of shared decision making in medical encounters. *Patient Educ Couns*, **60**, 301–312.

Mishler, E. G. 1984. *The Discourse of Medicine: Dialectics of Medical Interviews*. Greenwood Publishing Group.

Pilnick, A., Dingwall, R. 2011. On the remarkable persistence of asymmetry in doctor/patient interaction: a critical review. *Soc Sci Med*, **72**, 1374–1382.

Quill, T. E., Cassel, C. K. 1995. Nonabandonment: a central obligation for physicians. *Ann Internal Med*, **122**, 368–374.

Rake, E. A., Box, I. C. H., Dreesens, D., et al. 2022. Bringing personal perspective elicitation to the heart of shared decision-making: a scoping review. *Patient Educ Couns*, **105**, 2860–2870.

Rapley, T. 2008. Distributed decision making: the anatomy of decisions-in-action. *Sociol Health Illn*, **30**, 429–444.

Schneider, C. E. 1998. *The Practice of Autonomy: Patients, Doctors, and Medical Decisions*. Oxford University Press.

Stacey, D., Lewis, K., Smith, M., et al. 2024. Decision aids for people facing health treatment or screening decisions. *Cochrane Database Syst Rev*, **1**, CD001431.

Veatch, R. M. 1972. Models for ethical medicine in a revolutionary age. What physician–patient roles foster the most ethical relationship? *Hastings Cent Rep*, **2**, 5–7.

PART 2

The theory of shared decision making

2

The limits of shared decision making

Glyn Elwyn, Amy Price, Juan V.A. Franco, and Pål Gulbrandsen

Introduction

The foundation of shared decision making (SDM) is the view that people should be aware of relevant choices and that their personal views, priorities, and preferences are relevant factors when determining action. There is increasing interest in SDM, an ethical imperative, and supporting evidence that well-designed tools help people compare options and make more informed choices. We strongly advocate SDM and think the approach can be applied widely—perhaps more widely than many health professionals think possible (Fried, 2016; Hargraves et al., 2019).

Nevertheless, we have identified situations where we consider there to be clear limits to SDM, including where wider interests can override the priority given to individual preferences. While we think individual priorities and preferences should be respected where possible, there are situations where other factors determine the decisions (Thériault et al., 2020).

We feel it is essential to clarify these situations. SDM can be too easily dismissed as an impossible ideal if we do not acknowledge the limitations. Delineating exceptions will illustrate the demarcation between what can be considered the pinnacle of patient-centred care and situations where the approach is rightly constrained by ethical, professional, or societal factors (Hargraves et al., 2019).

First, let's agree that decisions come in different forms: some are conscious and episodic, as in 'Shall I have this procedure?' Some result from commitment decisions, such as agreeing to take medication for a long-term illness (Montori et al., 2006). Others go unnoticed in conversations, such as when a clinician suggests a solution which results in assumed acceptance. Such subtle decisions may occur because of deference to an expert or an unwillingness to disagree (Frosch et al., 2012). SDM makes the process of determining decisions more explicit (Elwyn and Miron-Shatz, 2009). In healthcare, the skills of supporting people to become aware, consciously deliberate, and arrive at better-considered decisions, whether for irreversible or continuous actions, are of utmost value.

It therefore follows that SDM can be applied to a wide range of situations. When there is no evidence that one management option is considered superior to another reasonable option, SDM could be seen as a *necessary* approach. This situation has been described as one where clinical equipoise exists (Elwyn et al., 2000). Indeed, it might be considered unethical not to provide information about alternatives in such situations (Schneider, 1998; Barry and Edgman-Levitan, 2012).

More common, however, is the situation where a range of options exist and where the extent of evidence, and its quality, varies considerably, exacerbating uncertainty (Han, 2021). Sometimes the evidence is sparse, poor, or points in different directions, yet there are reasonable options, including watchful waiting or taking no action. Sometimes there is good evidence supporting the positive effect of a treatment, yet there are important trade-offs to consider, including side effects, additional burdens, and costs. In these scenarios, individual preferences will contribute to assessing what action to take.

To the degree that it is reasonable to compare options, these situations also qualify as having clinical equipoise (Franco et al., 2020). SDM is necessary because there will always be a need to consider harms alongside benefits, and critically, the relative weighting of those factors will vary according to the priorities and preferences of people who will live with the consequences of decisions made and the trade-offs they are willing to make.

However, there are also situations where a shared approach to decisions may not be possible, although this does not rule out the need to provide empathetic care. There are limits to SDM, and the goal of this chapter is to be clear about the type of situations where SDM faces limits and where other strategies may need to be considered. We also consider how patients want to know about these limits (see Box 2.1 later in this chapter).

Limits on SDM will occur when:

- Wider interests override individual wishes
- Evidence of benefit is insufficient or absent
- Lowered decisional capacity is present
- Profound existential uncertainty exists.

Wider interests override individual preferences

One of the clearest situations that severely limits SDM is when an individual's preference overrules clinicians' responsibility for the safety of the individual or the broader population.

Antibiotics for self-limiting illness

A good example is when antibiotics are requested for self-limiting illness (Butler et al., 2001). This scenario may occur when a parent feels a child needs antibiotics for a viral illness. We can offer to negotiate, educate, and provide the option of watchful waiting pending more developments. We lack a good term for this respectful form of arbitration. However, there is no clinical equipoise in this situation: the clinician does not think antibiotics would improve the child's health. Giving antibiotics on demand increases antibiotic resistance in the child and others. Prescribing in this situation is not a safe, reasonable option.

Unscheduled opiate prescriptions

A similar wider set of responsibilities also exists when an individual addicted to drugs such as opiates requests additional medication outside an agreed schedule. A particularly difficult situation occurs when a person visits many clinics seeking opiate prescriptions. Such requests do not represent situations of clinical equipoise. As in the previous example, exploring context issues will be critical. What is motivating the demand? What are the risks of supplying the drugs compared to the benefits? Is prescribing likely to support crime? There are contingencies available to clinicians, such as negotiating an agreement or coming to a compromise, recognizing that point-blank refusal can lead to conflict and potential harm (Henry et al., 2019). Nevertheless, SDM cannot proceed in such fraught situations.

Vaccine hesitancy

Resistance to vaccines provides a complex example where public interest can be at odds with individual preferences. From a population perspective, the emergence of herd immunity, or the reduced spread of a harmful disease, is considered an argument for advocating vaccination. Offering financial incentives to clinicians to vaccinate a significant percentage of children or denying access to school or the right to continued employment are examples of persuasive vaccination efforts. SDM faces limits when strong public health arguments exist, at least from the perspective of health professionals who prioritize societal benefits. However, there are also arguments to support SDM when dealing with vaccine hesitancy. The provision of good information coupled with the development of trust in a longitudinal interaction can be an effective strategy (Scalia et al., 2022).

Absent or insufficient evidence of benefit

Scientific evidence supporting or opposing a course of action is a key determinant of how clinicians frame decisions in patient discussions, although the influence of peers and accepted norms is arguably just as important (Gabbay and le May, 2004). For various reasons, increased attention is frequently given to the absence of evidence of net benefit in some situations, especially when the evidence is of low quality or contradictory.

There are three common situations where this may be the case:

1. *When there is no evidence.* For many options, there is little to no research available to allow comparison. However, it is not unusual for patients to have strong prior beliefs about needing a specific treatment or a test. The clinician may need to become better informed or may already be aware that insufficient evidence exists or that there is likely harm. These scenarios require skilful negotiation to explain why the request for the option may be declined, especially if the option likely brings harm or unjustified use of resources. Such discussions are made more complex when patients are exposed to media that promote novel healthcare developments. Transparency may help, but a consensus is often difficult to achieve. This situation is often one where clinical equipoise does not exist and therefore places limits on SDM.
2. *Scientific evidence of inferiority.* Clinicians may also be *unwilling* to consider SDM when evidence exists in favour of some options compared to others or where situations have high stakes and the use of effective treatment is considered imperative or is widely viewed as a standard of care, even if individual patient preferences vary. Clinicians report a moral and professional obligation to recommend superior options in such situations (Grad et al., 2022). They experience the need to follow clinical guidelines and harbour concerns that they will be viewed as either incompetent or negligent for not adhering to professional norms. There is evidence that the willingness of clinicians to practise SDM varies, especially in the face of strong clinical practice recommendations (Grad et al., 2022).
3. *Cost-effectiveness and regulatory restraints.* Some countries restrict access to therapies that do not meet thresholds of cost-effectiveness or place restrictions on effective care on other grounds (i.e. abortion bans). Conversely, some forms of screening, such as newborn screening, may be mandated by the law. Moreover, people may be required to undergo medical screening to participate in sports or to access certain types of work activities. Decisions about whether to offer such alternatives to individuals are explicitly guided by system-level decisions. While clinicians may opt to become patient advocates, these decisions fall outside the scope of SDM.

Lowered decisional capacity

It is perhaps obvious that SDM is inappropriate when an individual has lost the capacity to make decisions (Lahey and Elwyn, 2020). This could be transient, as in loss of consciousness or the influence of drugs, or prolonged, as in dementia. Decisional capacity may vary over time, so clinicians must establish the threshold at which cognitive capacity remains appropriate (Lahey and Elwyn, 2020). It may well be that others can act as proxies.

These situations are special cases that deserve more detailed consideration elsewhere. Nevertheless, such cases should remind us that even for proxies, the quality and the simplicity of information are critical, along with the support needed to elicit proxy preferences—what things might matter to the individual who lacks capacity. Our capacity to process information can be severely compromised when stressed. Health professionals overestimate people's ability to process information, especially when it is complex and high volume.

Profound existential uncertainty

It is also clear that profound uncertainty and serious illness can lower decisional capacity and place limits on SDM. A pulmonologist describes her difficulty counselling people with incurable lung cancer. An increasing number of second-line treatment options are available that aim to delay cancer progression rather than offer a cure. But the response varies. Sometimes these treatments lead to remission, but more commonly, the treatments have severe, painful side effects and do not significantly delay progression. Nonetheless, despite the uncertainty and possible harm, optimism often leads to a trial of therapy, despite clinicians' strenuous efforts to provide balanced information about these complex agents.

At the same time, the inherent uncertainty makes it more difficult to confront the prognosis: death could be close (Hillen et al., 2017). Euphemistic language often amplifies optimism. Fear and emotion undermine rational comprehension, and so decisional capacity is severely compromised (Han, 2021; Larsen et al., 2022).

Clinicians tend to resort to guidelines, seeking professional norms. Landmark and colleagues describe this uncomfortable process as one of competing authority to decide (Landmark et al., 2015). Clinicians try to give very ill individuals deontological authority, whereas such individuals point to the clinicians' epistemological authority. Patients, in times of great need, often want to trust the expertise of others. Eagerly involving seriously ill people in difficult decisions can put their well-being at risk (Mol, 2008; Kristvik, 2011).

See Box 2.1 for our patient perspective.

Box 2.1 Patient perspective

If there are limits, explain, don't patronize me

While I understand there are situations where SDM in healthcare has limits, as a patient, I deeply value maintaining my voice and dignity. There are times when my individual preferences cannot be the sole deciding factor in my care. While I desire to make informed choices, I recognize there are wider considerations my healthcare providers must weigh.

If a treatment has little evidence of benefit yet clear risks of harm, I will not insist upon it just because it aligns with my preferences. I trust my care team will explain the lack of supporting evidence and potential dangers transparently and without demeaning me. Please allow variation from a guideline when other choices are available. I deeply value the opportunity to explore options further, provided we can do so safely and ethically.

When public health or societal interests take precedence over my intentions, and I seem resistant, remember I am facing my own mortality and fears. I desire autonomy, but I accept that clinicians may need to prioritize broader population outcomes at times. I only ask these situations be explained with evidence and empathy, not patronization.

If my ability to understand and decide on treatments becomes impaired, approach me with dignity. Involve me as my capacity allows, but also consider loved ones who know me best. Respect my cultural beliefs and traditions, and wish to have loved ones or even pets at my bedside. How you respond influences their healing too. Assuming I lack capacity entirely could dehumanize me.

If I have profound existential distress or uncertainty about my path forward, I need to know from your words and body language that you will not abandon me. Even if no further interventions are possible, the knowledge you will stand by and bear witness is immensely comforting. You cannot undo my anguish or my family's, but your reassuring presence comforts us through the darkness.

Possible solutions

Clinicians inevitably meet these situations, which are often compounded by concern, stress, and emotion at individual and family levels. There are no simple solutions. However, we advocate using approaches that build trust, preserve dignity, and bolster autonomy where possible. These approaches are summarized in Table 2.1.

Criticism of these proposed limits highlights that a traditional definition of a deliberative model for SDM may be the limiting factor in these situations (Montori and Kunneman, 2023). Alternatively, conceptualized forms of SDM focusing on clarifying positions and negotiating conflicts may prove useful in these scenarios (Hargraves et al., 2019).

Conclusion

Considering the historical underappreciation of the need for patient involvement in their own care, there is a need for more SDM. While evidence may help, it might not be enough. It is widely reported that many interventions in medicine do not have strong evidence of effectiveness (Ebell et al., 2017; Howick et al., 2020), and that more research to determine clinical effectiveness is required. In addition, evidence from randomized trials cannot be easily applied to individuals with different characteristics, and such evidence definitely lacks information about the context, priorities, and preferences of individuals (Sackett et al., 1996). We, therefore, contend that the need for SDM is *increasing* given the increasing complexity of therapeutic potential coupled with comorbidity.

Nevertheless, as we outline, there are situations that limit when decisions can or should be shared (Weiner, 2022). Clinicians have a duty of care to the people they advise and, in our view, should involve them carefully in decisions. They also have obligations to their profession, to society, and to science. It helps to be clear when those other obligations take precedence and, therefore, limit the use of SDM.

Acknowledgements

Some of the ideas in this paper were part of conversations with Professor Lyndal Trevena, and we wish to thank her for her insight into these issues in email discussions. A previous version of this article was published as a journal article (Elwyn et al., 2023).

Table 2.1 Suggested approaches when SDM is inappropriate or difficult

Exemplified scenarios (age in brackets)	Suggested approaches
Wider interests override individual preferences	
Vaccine hesitancy: Samira and Yael do not want their child (1) to receive a vaccine that is effective in reducing the severity of cases and transmission. They are vaccine hesitant	A possible approach close to SDM is to explore their concerns, listen, provide information, and take time to build trust over several meetings
Absent or insufficient evidence of benefit	
Absence of evidence: Samantha (37) wants to try a herbal preparation as a treatment for her severe depression, anxiety, and panic attacks. Her clinician finds no evidence supporting its use, albeit no report of serious harmful effects. At the same time, the clinician worries that Samantha will not agree to more effective therapy, and there are grounds to be concerned about suicide	Discussions would highlight the uncertainties surrounding the use of an herbal preparation with no evidence of benefit and voice a parallel concern that Samantha needs effective treatment. Clinicians may want to advocate for a combined approach by suggesting the addition, where feasible, of known effective therapy
Scientific evidence of inferiority: Michael (53) has a very high cardiovascular risk. According to guidelines, he should be taking active steps plus medications to reduce the risk of myocardial infarction and stroke. However, Michael is focused on his cholesterol levels and wants to try chia seeds, an approach where there is no evidence of effectiveness	Patients who wish to use treatment that is less effective than more effective alternatives place limits on SDM. As in other similar situations, a possible approach is to explore, listen, inform, and take time to build trust to guide Michael to take steps to lower his risk
Cost-effectiveness and regulatory restraints: María wants her son (2) to receive a new drug for his congenital condition, considered a rare disease. Her paediatrician informs her by letter that the novel drug is not covered by her health insurance due to cost-effectiveness issues. She has thought of going to a lawyer. Her primary care clinician is aware of the policy decision and, while willing to be her advocate, does not raise her hopes that she could reverse policy decisions of this nature	Declarations that novel therapies are not judged to be cost-effective are increasingly commonplace and set limits on SDM. Discussions at individual levels are helpful when they explain the scientific evidence and the deliberations and trade-offs that led to the policy-level decisions
Lowered decisional capacity	
Ramón (75) has deteriorating cognitive impairment. He has previously told his clinician of his preference to delay surgery for an expanding abdominal aneurysm. Now, the aneurysm has reached a diameter where surgery may be indicated, but the balance between the risk and the benefit from surgery is small. The surgeon fears that Ramón has lost the capacity to declare an informed preference	Lahey and Elwyn (2020) suggest a tailored approach based on assessing the decisional capacity and availability of a surrogate
Profound existential uncertainty	
Jane (63) has incurable lung cancer. Her clinician explains that there are additional second-line expensive treatments that may, for some people, lead to temporary remission, although more commonly, the treatments lead to severe, painful side effects that may lower her quality of life. Jane, already anxious, says that her priority is to spend her last days peacefully	Moving away from explicit decision-making to solace, support, and guidance may be more appropriate for Jane

Contributorship

GE initiated the article, and all authors contributed to the writing and revisions.

REFERENCES

Barry, M. J., Edgman-Levitan, S. 2012. Shared decision making—the pinnacle of patient-centered care. *N Engl J Med*, **366**, 780–781.

Butler, C. C., Kinnersley, P., Prout, H., Rollnick, S., Edwards, A., Elwyn, G. 2001. Antibiotics and shared decision-making in primary care. *J Antimicrob Chemother*, **48**, 435–440.

Ebell, M. H., Sokol, R., Lee, A., Simons, C., Early, J. 2017. How good is the evidence to support primary care practice? *Evid Based Med*, **22**, 88–92.

Elwyn, G., Edwards, A., Kinnersley, P., Grol, R. 2000. Shared decision making and the concept of equipoise: the competences of involving patients in healthcare choices. *Br J Gen Pract*, **50**, 892–899.

Elwyn, G., Miron-Shatz, T. 2009. Deliberation before determination: the definition and evaluation of good decision making. *Health Expect*, **13**, 139–147.

Elwyn, G., Price, A., Franco, J. V. A., Gulbrandsen, P. 2023. The limits of shared decision making. *BMJ Evid Based Med*, **28**, 218–221.

Franco, J. V. A., Riganti, P., Ruiz Yanzi, M. V., Kopitowski, K. 2020. Equipoise is preference sensitive. *Can Fam Physician*, **66**, 551–552.

Fried, T. R. 2016. Shared decision making—finding the sweet spot. *N Engl J Med*, **374**, 104–106.

Frosch, D. L., May, S. G., Rendle, K. A., Tietbohl, C., Elwyn, G. 2012. Authoritarian physicians and patients' fear of being labeled 'difficult' among key obstacles to shared decision making. *Health Aff (Millwood)*, **31**, 1030–1038.

Gabbay, J., le May, A. 2004. Evidence based guidelines or collectively constructed 'mindlines'? Ethnographic study of knowledge management in primary care. *BMJ*, **329**, 1013.

Grad, R., Sandhu, A., Ferrante, M., et al. 2022. Using incorpoRATE to examine clinician willingness to engage in shared decision making: a study of family medicine residents. *Patient Educ Couns*, **105**, 3529–3533.

Han, P. K. J. 2021. *Uncertainty in Medicine: A Framework for Tolerance*. Oxford University Press.

Hargraves, I. G., Montori, V. M., Brito, J. P., et al. 2019. Purposeful SDM: a problem-based approach to caring for patients with shared decision making. *Patient Educ Couns*, **102**, 1786–1792.

Henry, S. G., Paterniti, D. A., Feng, B., et al. 2019. Patients' experience with opioid tapering: a conceptual model with recommendations for clinicians. *J Pain,* **20,** 181–191.

Hillen, M. A., Gutheil, C. M., Strout, T. D., Smets, E. M. A., Han, P. K. J. 2017. Tolerance of uncertainty: conceptual analysis, integrative model, and implications for healthcare. *Soc Sci Med,* **180,** 62–75.

Howick, J., Koletsi, D., Pandis, N., et al. 2020. The quality of evidence for medical interventions does not improve or worsen: a metaepidemiological study of Cochrane reviews. *J Clin Epidemiol,* **126,** 154–159.

Kristvik, E. 2011. For whom and for what. Exploring the question of 'informed consent' in treatment decision making processes. *Med Antropol,* **23,** 9–43.

Lahey, T., Elwyn, G. 2020. Sliding-scale shared decision making for patients with reduced capacity. *AMA J Ethics,* **22,** E358–E364.

Landmark, A. M. D., Gulbrandsen, P. P., Svennevig, J. 2015. Whose decision? Negotiating epistemic and deontic rights in medical treatment decisions. *J Pragmat,* **78,** 54–69.

Larsen, B. H., Lundeby, T., Gerwing, J., Gulbrandsen, P., Førde, R. 2022. 'Eh—what type of cells are these—flourishing in the liver?' Cancer patients' disclosure of existential concerns in routine hospital consultations. *Patient Educ Couns,* **105,** 2019–2026.

Mol, A. 2008. *The Logic of Care: Health and the Problem of Patient Choice.* Routledge.

Montori, V., Kunneman, M. 2023. Caring without boundaries: delimiting shared decision-making. *BMJ Evid Based Med,* **28,** 226–227.

Montori, V. M., Gafni, A., Charles, C. 2006. A shared treatment decision-making approach between patients with chronic conditions and their clinicians: the case of diabetes. *Health Expect,* **9,** 25–36.

Sackett, D. L., Rosenberg, W. M., Gray, J. A., Haynes, R. B., Richardson, W. S. 1996. Evidence based medicine: what it is and what it isn't. *BMJ,* **312,** 71–72.

Scalia, P., Durand, M.-A., Elwyn, G. 2022. Shared decision-making interventions: an overview and a meta-analysis of their impact on vaccine uptake. *J Intern Med,* **291,** 408–425.

Schneider, C. E. 1998. *The Practice of Autonomy: Patients, Doctors, and Medical Decisions.* Oxford University Press.

Thériault, G., Grad, R., Dickinson, J. A., et al. 2020. To share or not to share: when is shared decision making the best option? *Can Fam Physician,* **66,** 327–331.

Weiner, S. J. 2022. Contextualizing care: an essential and measurable clinical competency. *Patient Educ Couns,* **105,** 594–598.

3

Co-production and learning health systems

Paul B. Batalden, E. Chandlee Bryan, Anna Edwards, and Eugene C. Nelson

Introduction

The focus of this book is on shared decision making (SDM), and this chapter provides an overview of two concepts that are closely aligned with SDM: first, co-production of health and healthcare, and second, learning health systems (LHS) for improving outcomes, value, and science. Our contributors with lived experience believe a degree of healthcare co-production must exist for SDM to take place, and view LHS as a key channel for feeding information to drive decisions, research, and individual and aggregate research outcomes. SDM, by its very nature, leverages co-production as it calls for engaging the patient and the clinician in the process of making good decisions—based on patient preferences and the evidence base—about the best 'next steps' in the patient's treatment plan. Likewise, SDM is also embedded in a key position in our LHS co-production model described later in this chapter.

Co-production of healthcare service

All services, at some level, are co-produced.

Paul B. Batalden

Thought trends: evolution of co-production of healthcare service

Co-production of healthcare services has been evolving from antiquity to modern times. A paper published in 2016 traces the evolution of co-production of healthcare services from the second century BC and Hippocrates' first aphorism, 'The physician must be ready, not only to do his duty himself, but also to secure the co-operation of the patient' (Miles, 2009), to the late twentieth century with the introduction of Wagner's chronic care model (Wagner et al., 2001) that features an informed, activated patient working with a prepared, proactive practice team and describes more key developments taking place in the first part of the twenty-first century (Batalden et al., 2016).

Co-production of healthcare service: definition and discussion of fundamental concepts

Many different words have been used to describe the interactions between people involved in designing and making the healthcare services they provide. By the 'co-production of healthcare service' we mean:

> The interactive work of users and professionals in the design, creation, development, delivery, assessment and improvement of the relationships and actions that contribute to the health of individuals and populations through mutual respect and partnership that notices and invites each participant's unique strengths and expertise. (Batalden et al., 2016)

People have used many other words to describe the nature, focus, or substance of these two parties' interactive work. Such terms as 'patient activation' or 'patient engagement' invite attention to helpful efforts that have an enabling contribution to the collaborative work. 'Patient-focused', 'person-centred', or 'therapeutic alliance' invite attention to the nature of the aim, the participants, and the process of the work. Patient-reported outcome and experience measures, 'PROMs' and 'PREMs', or patient satisfaction scales, invite attention to the work's measurement. Clarifying the working meaning of the terms in use is basic to a good, shared understanding.

Several types of knowledge and skills contribute to co-producing a healthcare service. They fit into four clusters, which are illustrated in Figure 3.1. The four clusters are:

1. Lived reality of the person sometimes known as a 'patient'
2. The journey to be navigated in the experience of creating the service
3. The various scientific epistemologies that inform the practice
4. Lived reality of the person sometimes known as a 'professional'.

These contributing streams of knowledge and skill come together and manifest in a healthcare service logic involving action tasks and kin relationships called out in Figure 3.1. The two persons (i.e. the patient-person and the professional-person) involved in healthcare service work involve people acting in different roles. They are fundamentally related, however, as persons, 'kin' to each other.

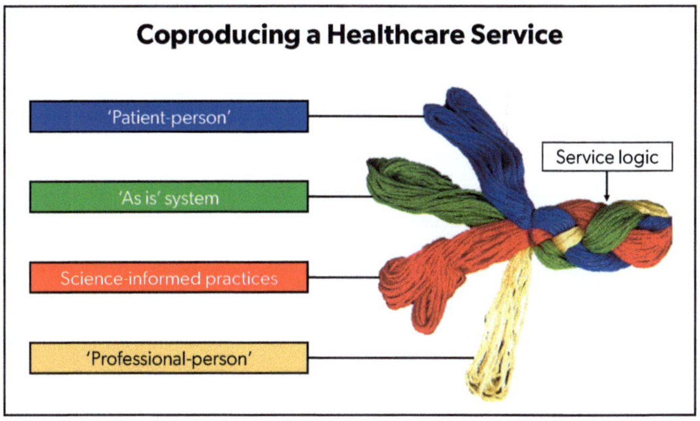

Figure 3.1 The four strands work together to co-produce a healthcare service.

© Paul Batalden. Source: data from Batalden, M., et al. 2016. Coproduction of healthcare service. *BMJ Qual Saf*, 25, 509–517.

Figure 3.1 calls attention to the work of at least two parties as they work together to co-create the service. 'User' is the role name of a person sometimes known as the 'patient' and 'professional' is the role name of the person sometimes known by the name of the discipline, such as 'physician'. A wide collection of illustrative 'work' activities is intentionally named. Key is the 'relationship' between the parties and the 'actions', which are usually co-created by the efforts of one or both of the parties. These 'actions' include the decision making involved in the shared work. This work may occur among individuals or within groups or populations. Fundamental is the respect and trust that the parties have for each other. Implied is the notion that a person (such as a patient) is the 'owner' of that person's health and that it is very difficult to 'outsource' or delegate that responsibility to another person in any lasting way.

Learning health systems

Evolution of LHS

The ideas on which LHS are based have evolved. In 1910, Codman developed his *End Results System* based on a surgical registry that tracked patient characteristics, treatments, and outcomes. Codman used his registry to promote transparency, learning, and improvement at his *End Results Hospital* (Nakayama, 2023). Codman's methods were rediscovered in the 1990s and inspired emerging LHS, including the Northern New England Cardiovascular Study Group, Dartmouth Spine Center, and Swedish Rheumatology Quality Register (Nelson et al., 2016). In 2007, the principles underlying LHS were clarified, disseminated, and popularized by the Institute of Medicine. The Institute of Medicine provided this definition:

> A learning health system … generates and applies the best evidence for the collaborative health care choices of each patient and provider … [and] drives the process of discovery as a natural outgrowth of patient care. (Olsen et al., 2007)

In 2019, the Agency for Healthcare Research and Quality published its own definition:

> A health system in which internal data and experience are systematically integrated with external evidence, and that knowledge is put into practice. As a result, patients get higher quality, safer, more efficient care, and health care delivery organizations become better places to work. (Agency for Healthcare Research and Quality, 2019)

LHS: places and principles

Today, LHS come in all shapes, sizes, and locations. Places that have implemented LHS range from clinical programmes serving a defined population such as the Palliative Care programme at Dartmouth Health (Tosteson et al., 2023), to large integrated health systems serving a regional population such as Geisinger Medical Center (Williams et al., 2018), to national networks such as the Cystic Fibrosis Foundation's Centers of Excellence (Van Citters et al., 2023). Some LHS are international: the Vermont Oxford Network's neonatal intensive care unit programme has over 9000 neonatal units worldwide (Edwards et al., 2019).

While LHS definitions vary, six principles support many of them:

1. *Assessment and care planning*: assessing the patient's health status, goals, and concerns based on patient-generated and clinical data and using these to co-create a treatment plan based on the best available evidence and the patient's preferences.
2. *Documentation and registry*: recording the patient's characteristics, health status, treatments, and outcomes over time and using these data to create a registry for a defined patient population.
3. *Analysis and reporting*: analysing registry data and providing longitudinal performance reports displaying variations in patient characteristics, treatments, and outcomes by type of patient for use by clinical teams and others for learning and improvement.
4. *Improvements and innovation*: using the registry data to instigate improvements and innovations that aim to enhance quality, outcomes, efficiency, and equity.
5. *Research*: using registry data to conduct retrospective research and to provide a foundation for prospective research.
6. *Patient and professional engagement*: encouraging active participation in all aspects of the LHS by patients, families, clinicians, health professionals, researchers, and others to foster person-centred care.

Co-production LHS: a special blend

The principles of co-production and LHS have been brought together in a model (Figure 3.2): a registry-based LHS for co-producing better health, healthcare value, and science.

Aim

The aim is to co-produce effective actions by patients, families, health professionals, and researchers to generate optimal health outcomes, high-value services, and research. The model includes four components that work together to achieve the overall aim.

1. *Partnership for co-production*: at the heart of the model is a partnership for healthcare co-production that engages patients and families working with clinicians and care teams to co-assess the current health status, co-decide the next steps in the care plan, co-design the care plan to fit the context, and co-deliver the needed services. The partnership is supported by patient-generated and clinical data displayed in 'feed-forward' dashboards.

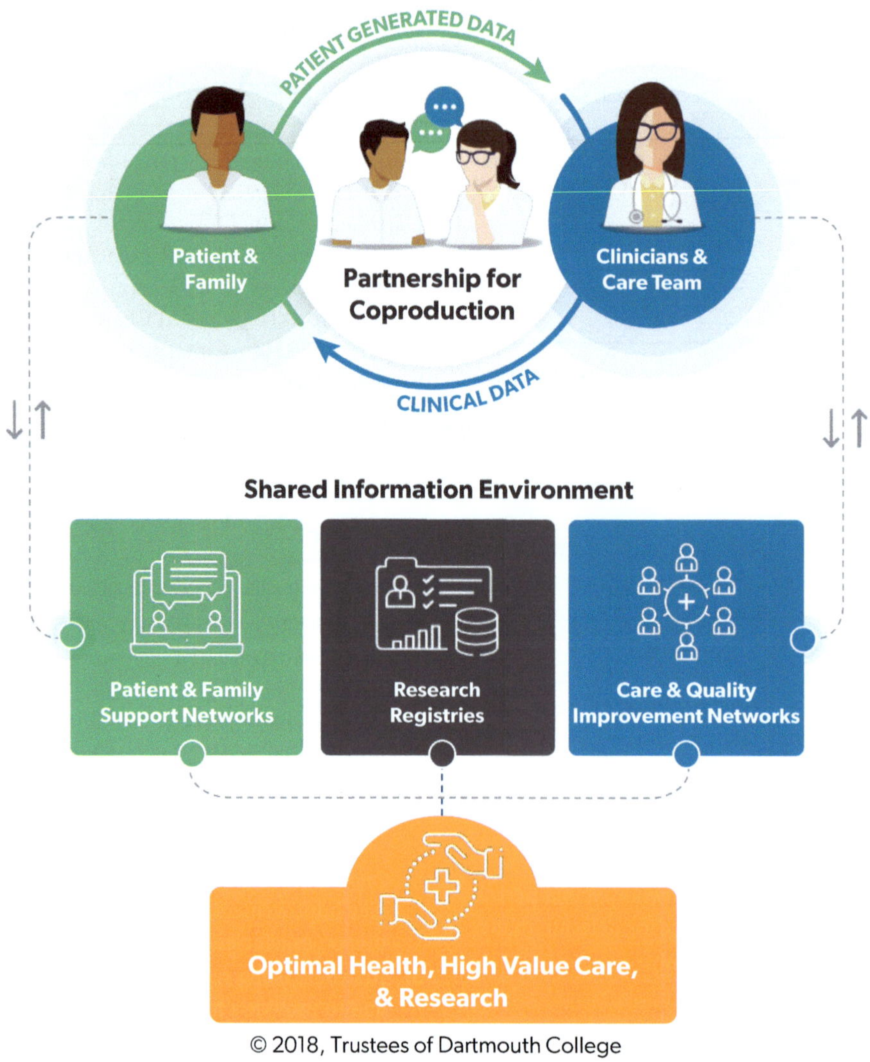

Figure 3.2 A LHS for co-producing optimal outcomes, experience, value, and science.

Reproduced from Dixon-Woods, M., Campbell, A., Chang, T., et al. 2020. A qualitative study of design stakeholders' views of developing and implementing a registry-based learning health system. *Implementation Sci*, 15, 16 under a Creative Commons Attribution 4.0 International License (https://creativecommons.org/licenses/by/4.0/).

2. *Registries for improvement and research*: key patient-generated and clinical data are fed forward and used at the point of care and flow directly into a registry and used to support self-management, improvement, and research.
3. *Quality improvement and research networks*: quality improvement and research networks use registry data for learning, improvement, and research. The registry data can be used to (a) provide comparative performance data for each participating clinical programme to support quality improvement; (b) support retrospective research on variations in treatments, outcomes, and costs of care for different types of patients; and (c) provide a platform to support prospective research and clinical trials.
4. *Patient and family support networks*: facilitated peer support networks are used to provide emotional support, practical advice, access to vetted health information, and navigation assistance to learn about relevant health, social, and community services. Peer support networks may use both traditional (in-person) meetings and/or virtual platforms.

Summary

These four components can be implemented simultaneously or one at a time to establish high-impact co-production LHS to provide person-centred care, innovations, improvements, and science.

The Improve Care Now learning health network model

The co-production LHS model described above provides insight into how the model of co-production might be integrated into the mainstream of healthcare and into learning health networks. This model offers specific advice for measuring and monitoring the work of co-designing, co-delivering, co-assessing, and co-deciding—opening the connection between co-producing of healthcare service and the organizational frame of a learning health network.

However, as Pomare and colleagues point out in a bibliometric review of the literature on LHS, the organizational and human factors necessary to facilitate these systems need deeper description (Pomare et al., 2022).

In support of that aim, the 'Improve Care Now' conceptual model was developed based on an exploratory case study of the nearly two decades of experience of the Improve Care Now LHS network organized and led by a team based at Cincinnati Children's Hospital and Medical Center (Fjeldstad et al., 2020).

This model (Figure 3.3) focuses on leading learning health networks to successfully conduct improvement, service, and research. It brings together actors who are co-producing improvements and creating a context that enables ongoing improvement in health outcomes. Special attention is paid to three facilitative leadership practices that contribute to positive results:

1. Building and sustaining community for co-production and improvement.
2. Enabling collaborative problem-solving.
3. Developing and using helpful structures.

Discussion

The patient perspective

We kick off our discussion with the patient perspective (Box 3.1). This offers a vital lens on co-production of health and healthcare and is based on the lived experiences of E. Chandlee Bryan and Anna Edwards, two people who have worked with many clinicians to help them deal with the challenges imposed by living with a serious chronic illness.

SDM and co-production of healthcare

Healthcare, by its very nature, is, for the most part, co-produced. Self-care is the dominant mode of care in the sense that the person and family live with and deal with their health issues every day of the year. But as life's journey unfolds, people have health events that bring them together with clinicians and health professionals who can help the individual prevent future health problems and treat existing health conditions. This is where co-production of healthcare and SDM come together.

As mentioned above, when people work with clinicians a four-part play unfolds:

1. Co-assess the problem.
2. Co-decide on the best next steps in the care plan.
3. Co-design how to execute these steps in a viable and affordable way.
4. Co-deliver the treatments that often involve a special blend of self/family care and professional care.

Step 2 in this flow, co-decide, is where SDM happens. And it is at the heart of this four-part play. Getting the correct diagnosis (based on the assessment) and arriving at the best, evidence-informed, patient-preferred decision about the treatment/s to be used are critical steps in the process. In this sense, SDM is at the heart of the co-production process.

It should be noted that people are different with respect to their willingness to participate in SDM. Some people want to decide about the next steps in their treatment on their own: 'Just give me the facts and options, and I will decide.' Some people really want to have a dialogue with their clinician and to make a shared decision that both patient and clinician think is the best choice given the facts, evidence, and context. Finally, some people are not confident or do not trust their own judgement about the best treatment decision and simply want their doctor or clinician to make the decision for them: 'Tell me what you would choose to do if it were you, and that's what I would like to do.'

Conclusion

We offer these approaches—co-production of healthcare service and LHS—in further support for the shared work of good healthcare service for person-centred care and optimal health outcomes. Like a tapestry, where each colour and thread are recognizable and yet part of a pattern that contributes to a greater 'whole', we believe

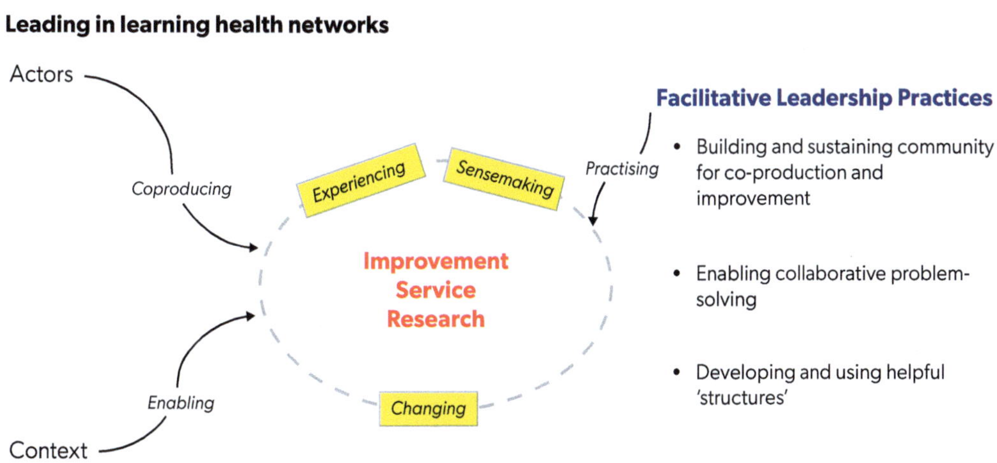

Figure 3.3 Model of the Improve Care Now LHS network developed by Cincinnati Children's Hospital and Medical Center.

 Source: data from Fjeldstad, Ø. D., Johnson, J. K., Margolis, P. A., Seid, M., Hoglund, P., Batalden, P. B. 2020. Networked health care: rethinking value creation in learning health care systems. *Learn Health Syst*, 4, e10212.

Box 3.1 Patient perspective

As individuals living with chronic illness, we'd like to delve into part of Paul's opening statement that 'All services, at some level, are co-produced'. We find the balance of participation between users and professionals to be complex, depending on the individual and where they are in the patient journey.

We have both lived with chronic illness for years, are educated to the graduate/postgraduate level, and work in our respective health systems. One might expect us to be experts at co-producing our patient journey, but we can readily identify times when this has not been the case. Chandlee recalls her first visit to a urologist following her diagnosis with multiple sclerosis (MS):

> My initial medical history was taken by a student. As I sat waiting, I overheard the student summarize my history to the urologist on the other side of the door.
>
> When they returned, the urologist said, 'I recommend a urodynamics exam to get a bladder functionality baseline and monitor MS progression. I've had MS patients faint during the exam. Bring someone to drive you home.'
>
> I felt informed but uncomfortable. I sought care from another practice and drove 60 miles for a urodynamics exam. During the procedure, the care team invited me to watch a monitor that enabled me to see how my bladder empties in real time. I felt empowered and confident. I didn't faint. I smiled as I drove myself home.

Anna lives with Crohn's disease 24/7/365:

> I have had multiple surgeries where my survival was not guaranteed. At my sickest, I couldn't always address immediate goals due to overwhelming existential considerations. However, at any given moment, I could recite my fundamental goals in terms of what matters to me and have been fortunate enough to be able to co-produce potential outcomes with my clinicians due to long held doctor–patient relationships.

We have found Arnstein's Ladder of Participation (Figure 3.4) a useful framework in managing this challenge as it can 'help practitioners and individuals consider where they are in their journey towards co-production' (EQUIL, 2015). Chandlee places her initial experience with the urologist at 'Educating' and 'Informing' and her later experience at 'Engagement'.

Given the complexity described here between different patients and the same patient at different stages on their journey, we believe that there's a need for better training and signposting for professionals/service users/families/advocates on the options available to co-produce healthcare. While all services 'can be' co-produced, the degree to which 'they are' co-produced should be one that is determined through an interactive discussion with all participants, including professionals and people living with their health condition/s. In this way, Arnstein's Ladder could be repurposed as a tool for SDM and education—a modern-day variation of the 'golden rule': it's not about treating others as you would want to be treated, part of kinship is about learning how others prefer to be interacted with first. One size does not fit all.

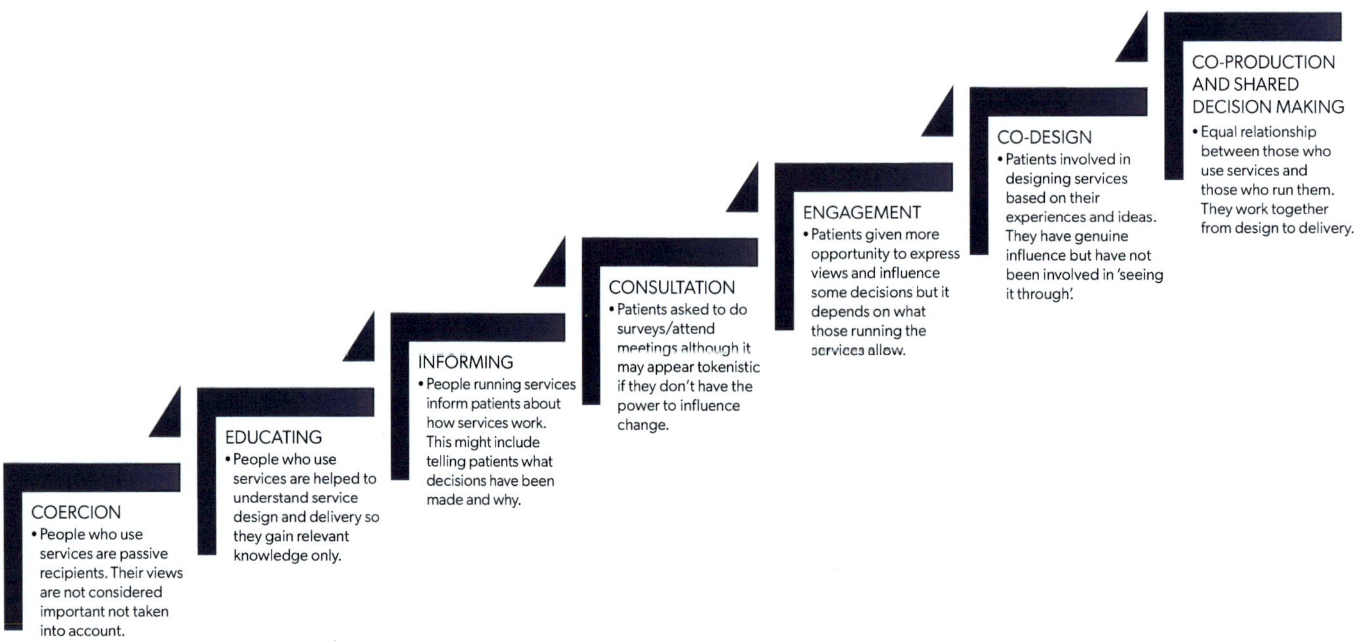

Figure 3.4 Arnstein's Ladder of Citizen Participation.

Adapted from ThinkLocalActPersonal (https://thinklocalactpersonal.org.uk/). Concept originally from Arnstein, S. R. 1969. A ladder of citizen participation. *Journal of the American Institute of Planners*, 35, 216–224.

these approaches can share a 'purpose' that transcends their words, and which involves accompanying behaviours, technologies, and actions.

Using these approaches requires 'space' in time and amid other priorities. Their synthesis can be described in many ways. Snowden suggests a 'mélange' of lenses through which complex systems like SDM, learning health networks, and the co-production of healthcare service may be viewed. This involves creating a clear awareness of the situation being faced, who is involved in making decisions, what is involved, and how and when decisions might be made, offering a sense of *agency*; an understanding of the circumstances, the contributing factors, the time, and the helpful capabilities which all contribute to a sense of the enabling ecosystem of *affordance* for the work; and by design, testing, assembly, and feedback the work of integration occurs, offering a sense of what is involved in the *assemblage* of the complex system (Snowden, 2022).

Taken together, these approaches invite emergent syntheses. Each approach offers new insights into the complex work of one person helping another. Such a synthesis can help *build a community* of innovation and ongoing learning and improvement. It can start with the simple, deep insight of Arthur Ashe who suggested that people should 'Start where you are. Use what you have. Do what you can.' (Roosevelt, 1913).

REFERENCES

Agency for Healthcare Research and Quality. 2019. *Learning Health Systems: Making the Case Against Business as Usual.* Agency for Healthcare Research and Quality.

Batalden, M., Batalden, P., Margolis, P., et al. 2016. Coproduction of healthcare service. *BMJ Qual Saf,* **25**, 509–517.

Edwards, E. M., Ehret, D. E. Y., Soll, R. F., Horbar, J. D. 2019. Vermont Oxford Network: a worldwide learning community. *Transl Pediatr,* **8**, 182–192.

EQUIL. 2015. *A Toolkit for Co-Production.* Mersey Care NHS Foundation Trust. Available at: https://cesie.org/media/IO4-En-Toolkit.pdf

Fjeldstad, Ø. D., Johnson, J. K., Margolis, P. A., Seid, M., Hoglund, P., Batalden, P. B. 2020. Networked health care: rethinking value creation in learning health care systems. *Learn Health Syst,* **4**, e10212.

Miles, S. H. 2009. Hippocrates and informed consent. *Lancet,* **374**, 1322–1323.

Nakayama, D. K. 2023. Ernest Amory Codman and the end result idea in surgical quality. *Am Surg,* **89**, 4237–4240.

Nelson, E. C., Dixon-Woods, M., Batalden, P. B., et al. 2016. Patient focused registries can improve health, care, and science. *BMJ,* **354**, i3319.

Olsen, L., Aisner, D., McGinnis, J. M. (Eds.) *The Learning Healthcare System: Workshop Summary* (Institute of Medicine Roundtable on Evidence-Based Medicine). The National Academies Press.

Pomare, C., Mahmoud, Z., Vedovi, A., et al. 2022. Learning health systems: a review of key topic areas and bibliometric trends. *Learn Health Syst,* **6**, e10265.

Roosevelt, T. 1913. *Theodore Roosevelt; An Autobiography.* The Macmillan Company.

Snowden, D. 2022. A mélange of potential, not a mindset. The Cynefin Company. Available at: https://thecynefin.co/a-melange-of-potential-not-a-mindset/

Tosteson, A. N. A., Kirkland, K. B., Holthoff, M. M., et al. 2023. Harnessing the collective expertise of patients, care partners, clinical teams, and researchers through a coproduction learning health system: a case study of the Dartmouth Health Promise Partnership. *J Ambul Care Manage,* **46**, 127–138.

Van Citters, A. D., Buus-Frank, M. E., King, J. R., et al. 2023. The Cystic Fibrosis Learning Network: a mixed methods evaluation of program goals, attributes, and impact. *Learn Health Syst,* **7**, e10356.

Wagner, E. H., Austin, B. T., Davis, C., Hindmarsh, M., Schaefer, J., Bonomi, A. 2001. Improving chronic illness care: translating evidence into action. *Health Aff (Millwood),* **20**, 64–78.

Williams, M. S., Buchanan, A. H., Davis, F. D., et al. 2018. Patient-centered precision health in a learning health care system: Geisinger's genomic medicine experience. *Health Aff (Millwood),* **37**, 757–764.

4

Value-based healthcare and shared decision making

Anne M. Stiggelbout, Willem Jan W. Bos, Lowri Smith, and Sally Lewis

Introduction

See Box 4.1 for a perspective from our patient representative.

The many faces of value-based healthcare

The 2006 book *Redefining Health Care: Creating Value-Based Competition on Results* accelerated the earlier idea to move from volume-driven healthcare to value-driven or value-based healthcare (VBHC) (Porter and Teisberg, 2006). Porter and Teisberg's approach focuses on achieving value for patients and society. Value is defined as outcomes relevant to patients achieved per monetary unit spent to achieve that value; or, in other words, how long a life expectancy and what quality of life do we obtain for each dollar or euro spent?

Therefore, VBHC promotes both *effective* care, or care that achieves relevant health outcomes, and *efficient* care delivery—achieving these goals with reasonable input of manpower and means. VBHC promotes the organization of care around patients with specific medical conditions (in so-called integrated practice units (IPUs)) to improve both effectiveness and efficiency and patient-centredness. Other elements of the VBHC strategic agenda proposed by Porter and Teisberg include the measurement of outcomes and costs, a move to quality-based reimbursement, the integration of care across facilities, geographic expansion, and an enabling information technology platform (Porter and Lee, 2013).

Shifting the focus away from 'costs' to 'outcomes in relation to costs' is one possible explanation for the enthusiasm among patient representatives, medical professionals, hospital administrators, insurers, and government towards the VBHC approach. Quality improvement initiatives appeal to the intrinsic motivation of care professionals to deliver high-quality care to their patients; whereas for government and insurers, the VBHC perspective is appealing due to the focus on more effective use of resources (adapted from Bos, 2019).

The concept of VBHC has been interpreted and implemented in different ways. In a recent overview, Steinmann et al. (2020) distinguish four views, each with their own perception regarding the main purpose of VBHC:

1. *Patient empowerment discourse*: strengthening the position of patients in medical decision making.
2. *Governance discourse*: viewing VBHC as a toolkit with incentives for providers.
3. *Professionalism discourse*: describing VBHC as a methodology for healthcare delivery.
4. *Critique discourse*: criticizing the dogma of manufacturability.

Not only do the ways in which VBHC is understood differ, but its implementation in clinical practice differs as much (van Staalduinen et al., 2022). Most healthcare organizations focus on the implementation of one or two items of the original strategic agenda—most often (1) 'measuring outcomes and costs for every patient' and (2) 'organizing care into IPUs'. In general, implementation in the USA focuses more often on quality-based reimbursement schemes. Implementation in the typically publicly funded healthcare systems in Europe focuses more often on quality improvement and promoting patient-centredness, as well as on achieving equitable outcomes sustainably (Hurst et al., 2019).

Despite variation in implementation, and while not specifically mentioned by Porter and Teisberg (2006) or Porter and Lee (2013), these different discourses on VBHC find common ground in shared decision making (SDM) as a key approach to achieve patient value (Steinmann et al., 2020). As van der Nat states in a proposal for an extension of the Porter and Teisberg model: 'Communication on value, and specifically on outcomes that matter to patients, is essential to a successful implementation of value-based healthcare' (van der Nat, 2022).

Elements of VBHC that support SDM

VBHC in its essence is about achieving the outcomes that matter to people at both the individual and population levels, while making best use of available resources (Hurst et al., 2019). At the micro level

Box 4.1 Patient perspective

Shared decision making and value-based healthcare

For decades, clinicians have been the decision makers and patients have refrained from questioning things. Slowly things are beginning to change. For a long time, clinicians talked at their patients and not to them. I think patients with complex health conditions are learning to become their own advocates. They are actively engaged in their own care. For example, I have been attending cardiac clinics my whole life and I want to be part of the discussion. My medical team understands that I will asking questions at every stage. They know that I will prepare a list of questions for each appointment that I expect to have answered during the appointment. I may have done my own research or spoken to other congenital heart patients which resulted in new questions. I will then go away and analyse the answers. They have been sending me copies of what was said at the appointment for over a decade, my general practitioner and I both receive a copy. I still remember a paediatric liver appointment back when I was around 15 years of age. I had never met the consultant before. The consultant had directed the entire conversation at me (the patient). My parents were in the room listening, impressed. But his focus was on me. There are occasionally times where I have had to use my patient experience and knowledge of my condition to alter the course of my treatment. This often occurs with clinicians who have limited experience of congenital heart conditions.

My congenital cardiac team are currently proposing two surgical procedures. I was told that these are not urgent procedures and that I could take my time in thinking about them. These procedures were first presented in May 2022. I have had several discussions with my team and I still haven't settled on a decision yet. They remain on the table. In my opinion, medical care should be a joint partnership which relies on trust and allows an open and honest discussion between all parties.

Value-based healthcare (VBHC) is about value to the patient, improving outcomes or reducing costs, or both. Redesigning care such that patients incur fewer (non-reimbursed) costs is valuable. For example, I am a warfarin patient and therefore need regular blood tests to manage my levels. I've spent many hours in waiting rooms simply to get a blood test. Usually there is no other reason for me being there. At the beginning of the pandemic, I was finally given my own self-testing machine which had previously been refused to me. This not only saves me time but also frees up appointments for other patients. This is a good example of value, not only to the patient but also to the larger system.

One very obvious example of VBHC is the video appointment. I have travelled to London for many years to receive specialist treatment, and costs were not always reimbursed. Since the pandemic all my London appointment have been online. This eliminates any expenses and travel time. I personally believe there should be a choice for face-to-face or online appointments.

of the individual patient, achieving the outcomes that matter to an individual requires healthcare to be person-centred, tailoring care to the needs, goals, and preferences of the individual. Otherwise, one may fall into the trap of making assumptions about a person's wishes, which could lead to interventions that do not enable that outcome to be achieved.

Therefore, SDM is ideally an essential component of VBHC. Goals and preferences for care should be elicited as part of every clinical consultation. Shared goal setting then becomes the start point for a shared decision on the best course of action. Further, if people are to achieve the best possible outcomes, they must also be supported to self-manage after they have made their treatment or management choices, in between visits to healthcare professionals. When patients succeed in effectively carrying out their self-management, this approach can enable a more flexible approach to communication with clinical teams. Care can thus move away from sometimes arbitrary, system-led touch points with the clinical team towards an environment where patients are much more directly involved with their care and can, to an extent, lead when they need to be seen. Besides being patient-centred, this can release clinical time so that patients in greater need can have more time, and those that are effectively self-managing need less.

However, and as reported in the other chapters of this book, there are common barriers to SDM, including lack of willingness from either the clinician or the person receiving care, lack of time, and lack of information. A VBHC approach could help to overcome these well-known and long-standing barriers to SDM through the implementation of patient-reported outcome measures (PROMs), improved digital tools and systems, and increased patient access to their own health information, such as tracking their own chronic disease indicators in between consultations.

Patient-reported outcome measures

PROMs can be seen as the modern form of quality-of-life questionnaires. Often, existing validated quality-of-life questionnaires are used as PROMs, including those used by the European Organisation on Research and Treatment of Cancer (e.g. the EORTC-QLQC30). They may be condition-specific, asking questions about symptom burden in a single disease, or they can be generic, enquiring about global quality-of-life indicators such as pain, sleep, and mobility. Aggregated PROM scores are used at the meso IPU level to benchmark and improve care. For benchmarking, or value-based competition (as proposed by Porter and Teisberg (2006)), it is important that different hospitals or systems use the same measures. For that reason, the International Consortium on Health Outcomes Measurement (see https://www.ichom.org/) was founded to support this standardization. It is hoped that growing PROMs databases will contribute to a body of real-world evidence that will allow more accurate predictions of outcome in support of more effective SDM ('patients-like-me' information).

PROMs are used at the individual patient level as a communication tool in the clinical consultation, or to monitor symptoms during self-management and follow-up (Damman et al., 2020; Kidanemariam et al., 2024), and can play a role in supporting SDM. First, the patient and doctor can focus on discussing the items for which a patient has indicated a less than optimal functioning, or those that are having the greatest impact on their lives. Second, if the PROM is filled out repeatedly, it can show improvement or deterioration in condition management or functioning and provide a focus for the shared discussion about the patient's goals, needs, and preferences and as the starting point for a shared decision about the best course of action (Basch et al., 2018; Damman et al., 2019). When used in the consultation they can highlight areas that are a priority for the patient at the outset, allowing the patient to play an active role in leading a discussion about what matters to them. They may also hint at issues which may not have been volunteered by the patient, such as mental health, allowing the clinician to open up new avenues of discussion (Kidanemariam et al., 2024). So far, most PROM use in SDM concerns chronic disease, where management based on PROMs puts the patient's perspective more central. A barrier to SDM may be that clinicians still prioritize clinical outcomes (e.g. survival) above PROMs and recommend treatments accordingly (Damman et al., 2020).

To achieve these aims, the PROMs chosen for a care path should measure what matters to patients. A drawback of many current PROMs is that they have generally been developed for use at the aggregate level, reflecting what the average patient (or the patient representative in the development group) considers important. Such a PROM may not be relevant for every individual patient or across different settings. For that reason, it is recommended to always ask patients who complete PROMs to be discussed in the clinical encounter, to also indicate any specific aspects they would like to discuss with their clinician that are not captured in the items; it might be that another symptom that was not in the PROM instrument is more bothersome and important to them. Further, it might be that they have indicated a certain symptom of disease or side effect of treatment because the PROM asked about it, but that it does not bother him or her at all. Therefore, PROMs should only be used as an adjunct to the conversation (Kidanemariam et al., 2024). The process of checking with patients what they want to discuss is essential to SDM and thereby VBHC.

Improved digital communication and systems

Successful and cost-effective PROM implementation requires improved digital communication with those patients who want and are able to interact with healthcare services in this way (Cronin et al., 2018). Improved digital communication with patients opens the way for more flexible interaction with healthcare teams, including patient-initiated follow-up (for an example, see Box 4.2). For a time-pressed workforce this can enable a scenario where patients are followed up only when necessary, releasing time for more meaningful face-to-face interactions when they are most needed, or for other patients most in need of these (see, e.g. Riis et al., 2020). For patients who experience multiple sequential appointments, this can also reduce the burden of care processes.

An area that has suffered a lack of attention and resource investment, outside of the research setting, is self-management support. Enabling people to fully participate in their care, particularly when they have a chronic long-term illness, is critical to maximize quality of life and reduce exacerbations leading to acute healthcare utilization (Cramm and Nieboer, 2015; Hodgkinson et al., 2020). Supported self-management is a high-value intervention. People need regular and easy access to information resources about their condition throughout their journey, not just at diagnosis. They should also have access to coaching on how to respond to a range of scenarios that might occur to them. With increased digitization, it is possible for patients to have greater access to their own health records, enabling them to be able to track their own blood results, for example (Scheckel et al., 2023). This enables far greater participation in healthcare, which gives people control and agency, and therefore supports meaningful SDM (Basch, 2017; Verweij et al., 2022). An example of such a patient-centred digital platform is 'CMyLife', for patients with chronic myeloid leukaemia (Ector et al., 2020).

VBHC encourages seamless integration of patient care across the whole pathway. In the original strategy by Porter and Teisberg, it was suggested that this should be achieved at the meso level through IPUs, where all healthcare professionals taking care of patients with a specific condition are co-located, aiming to make care more patient-centred, rather than organized in silos of medical specialties. In many healthcare systems it is possible, and often desirable, to integrate care through other means; where care is sustainably and effectively integrated across the pathway through close collaboration and digital integration between teams, for example (Box 4.3). The process of reorganizing care in this way can be a good opportunity to place greater emphasis on patient-centredness and SDM. First, by active patient participation, where the input from patient representatives is used at all levels to evaluate where patients experience hiccups in the process, to help select PROMs to be implemented, and to think along with the necessary digitization (e.g. van der Horst et al., 2022). Second, digital communication can be addressed in a structural way in the process of redesigning care. This way of redesigning pathways is a fundamental of the VBHC approach.

A promising tool for this redesign of care pathways to support SDM is 'Metro Mapping' (Stiggelbout et al., 2023). This is a service design method in which SDM is supported by redesigning the care

Box 4.2 Patient perspective

The use of digital technology to support person-centred care in the UK

The rapid access passport (called 'Care and Respond', see https://www.careandrespond.com/passport/) provides essential information for medical professionals and is particularly useful during an emergency hospital admission. Information may include suggested treatment or patient wishes for treatment, contact details for specialist teams, and helplines where further advice can be obtained if necessary. The hope is that this will save time, improve patient safety, and speed up decision making. The passport can be customized for each patient and their specific medical crisis. Patients themselves can authorize medical staff to access information on the app. Patients with long-term health conditions often have repeated admission to Emergency Departments and can use the passport to guide clinicians to important information, red flags, and specialist pathways.

It has been designed so that it can be used by patients who receive cross-border care from different hospitals or who travel abroad. It also allows for the patient to upload medical documents and test results. The data is owned by the patient avoiding any complex General Data Protection Regulation issues. The patient passport provides the patient with a greater level of autonomy.

We are also working with various ambulance services across the country meaning that the paramedics will have immediate access to essential medical information on scene.

Box 4.3 Patient perspective

Enhancing the value of care provided to patients in the UK

My cardiologist is trying to address this issue for some of her patients. Certain congenital heart patients also have liver problems. As a result, there is a joint cardiac/liver outpatient clinic in Liverpool. This reduces the need for multiple appointments and allows the consultants to work collaboratively for one day every month. This is something we should be aiming for across the NHS because it would save time and money. A congenital heart disease professor at the Royal Brompton emphasized the need to group all appointments/tests into one hospital visit. This is often more difficult than it needs to be. Pre-pandemic, I tried to organize three separate tests/scans during one admission. I pushed hard for this and made numerous calls to get this set up. It really shouldn't be up to be up to the patient to coordinate this. Again, it is due to poor communication.

pathway such that barriers to SDM are removed, and facilitators created. Barriers are often a lack of overview of the care path and thereby of the decision moments where patient input is relevant. Redesigning it using Metro Mapping should increase awareness on the side of the clinicians of where to involve patients. Barriers to patient participation stemming from the physical environment or complex medical devices may be addressed, but also those stemming from unclear division of tasks and responsibilities within the team. Patients and their caregivers or decision partners are empowered by the overview of the path as a Metro line, and by the accompanying information on the pathway with its decision moments and the team (see www.metromapping.org/en).

International implementation of VBHC

VBHC has been embraced in many health systems around the world, each with their own focus (van Staalduinen et al., 2022). A typical European best practice is described by the Santeon Hospitals in the Netherlands, which implemented VBHC to improve outcomes of care based on benchmarking of outcomes and costs between seven member hospitals and to stimulate patient participation based on outcome information (Engels et al., 2024).

NHS Wales provides a good example of a systems approach to VBHC, where good practice is described in the approach to chronic kidney disease and heart failure (NHS Wales, n.d.) Specifically, PROMs have been used to drive a patient-centred approach in these conditions.

In Australia, VBHC has been used as a vehicle to integrate care of providers attempting to reduce health inequalities in the remote population of North West Queensland through prevention and better organized chronic disease management, for example, in diabetes care (Queensland Government, 2022).

As noted previously, in the USA the focus of VBHC is on cost reduction and efficiency, and value-based competition is the main driver. By 2018, 48 states in the USA had implemented VBHC programmes to varying degrees and all 50 states were at least beginning to engage stakeholders to assist with implementation mostly in the form of accountable care organizations—patient-centred organizations in which a network of providers from different specialties delivers high-quality, coordinated care in a cost-effective manner (Harris and Le, 2022). An example of a VBHC approach in the USA in the elderly that is not so much focused on cost but on patient value is Patient Priorities Care (n.d.), an age-friendly, systematic approach for identifying patients' health priorities and aligning decision making and care to those priorities.

In Asia, healthcare systems are increasingly embracing VBHC as a strategy to maximize the value to patients and minimize costs (Cho et al., 2024). Singapore's Ministry of Health, for example, started a paradigm shift to VBHC, but value is expressed as clinical values per unity of costs, no PROMs or SDM are involved (Hoong et al., 2023).

Latin America is in the early stages of the movement towards more value-based organization of care (Makdisse et al., 2022). In 2017, a Value Management Office was created in Sao Paulo as a dedicated centre to support VBHC initiatives. VBHC rapidly gained attention by healthcare organizations throughout Brazil, VBHC implementation focuses mostly on new financing models, not so much on outcomes (Ramos et al., 2021).

In sub-Sahara Africa, PharmAccess is one of the first organizations to provide value-based care, with use of mHealth to collect patient data via the patient's mobile phone (see https://www.pharmaccess.org/stories/care-bundles/). Here, as in Asia and Latin America, SDM is (as of yet) not part of VBHC.

Further information on some example VBHC implementation and education initiatives is included in Table 4.1.

The future of SDM in a VBHC setting

The movement over the last decade towards VBHC has provided a strong impetus for the implementation of SDM, particularly in Europe. In the Netherlands, for example, SDM is seen as one of the major strategies to obtain value for the patient, either with or without PROMs. In the Netherlands and the UK, the VBHC agenda has strongly supported the implementation of SDM (Damman et al., 2020; Steinmann et al., 2020). Organizing care around the patient and the goal of making care truly patient-centred, should support care delivery that is adjusted to patient goals and preferences (which is the goal of SDM). PROMs are one of the most often implemented aspect of VBHC, together with organizing care around the patient (in IPUs) and measuring costs (van Staalduinen et al., 2022).

PROMs can act as a driver for and support the process of SDM, but caution is still needed. In the process of enthusiastically implementing PROMs, we must take care to ensure that the individual patient's needs and wishes are not sacrificed for the aim of standardization and benchmarking. Further, if clinicians use PROMs rigidly without the flexibility to adjust their conversations to explore what matters most to each individual patient (including those things that are not included in standardized PROMs), their

Table 4.1 Links to additional information on example VBHC initiatives worldwide

Implementation	
The Welsh Value in Health Centre	https://vbhc.nhs.wales/
Linnean—Dutch VBHC initiative	https://linnean.nl/home/default.aspx
Australian Healthcare and Hospitals Association	https://ahha.asn.au/
Education	
Erasmus VBHC courses	https://erasmus-vbhc-course.nl/
Value-Based Health and Care Academy	https://www.swansea.ac.uk/som/vbhc-academy/

use could come at the expense of patient-centred care. Research is needed to evaluate the impact of VBHC implementation on SDM, and on patient-centred care more broadly. Further, digitization is an important component of VBHC. However, current variation in hospital systems that are incompatible jeopardizes the organization of VBHC across hospital borders. In the current context of lack of funds and personnel, harmonization remains a challenge. However, when these issues of flexible use of PROMs and better integrated technology systems are addressed, VBHC offers an important and timely opportunity to integrate SDM in clinical practice and could be used as a stepping stone to more patient-centred care through the implementation of SDM.

REFERENCES

Basch, E. 2017. Patient-reported outcomes—harnessing patients' voices to improve clinical care. *N Engl J Med,* **376**, 105–108.

Basch, E., Barbera, L., Kerrigan, C. L., Velikova, G. 2018. Implementation of patient-reported outcomes in routine medical care. *Am Soc Clin Oncol Educ Book,* **38**, 122–134.

Bos, W. J. 2019. Gaining knowledge by asking the right questions: re-evaluation of outcomes of care. Inaugural lecture, Leiden University. Available at: https://www.isc.hbs.edu/Documents/pdf/Prof-Bos-VBHC-Lecture-Leiden-March-2019.pdf

Cho, J., Yoo, S., Lee, E. E., Lee, H. 2024. Impact of a nationwide medication history sharing program on the care process and end-user experience in a tertiary teaching hospital: cohort study and cross-sectional study. *JMIR Med Inform,* **12**, e53079.

Cramm, J. M., Nieboer, A. P. 2015. Disease management: the need for a focus on broader self-management abilities and quality of life. *Popul Health Manag,* **18**, 246–255.

Cronin, R. M., Conway, D., Condon, D., Jerome, R. N., Byrne, D. W., Harris, P. A. 2018. Patient and healthcare provider views on a patient-reported outcomes portal. *J Am Med Inform Assoc,* **25**, 1470–1480.

Damman, O. C., Jani, A., de Jong, B. A., et al. 2020. The use of PROMs and shared decision-making in medical encounters with patients: an opportunity to deliver value-based health care to patients. *J Eval Clin Pract,* **26**, 524–540.

Damman, O. C., Verbiest, M. E. A., Vonk, S. I. 2019. Using PROMs during routine medical consultations: the perspectives of people with Parkinson's disease and their health professionals. *Health Expect,* **22**, 939–951.

Ector, G. I., Westerweel, P. E., Hermens, R. P., et al. 2020. The development of a web-based, patient-centered intervention for patients with chronic myeloid leukemia (CMyLife): design thinking development approach. *J Med Internet Res,* **22**, e15895.

Engels, N., Bos, W. J., De Bruijn, A., et al. 2024. Santeon's lessons from a decade of implementing. *NEJM Catal,* **5**, 1.

Harris, A., Le, J. 2022. Value-based healthcare in the United States. Clinical Research Strategies. Available at: https://clinicalresearchstrategies.com/wp-content/uploads/crs-value-based-healthcare-in-the-united-states_112022-web.pdf

Hodkinson, A., Bower, P., Grigoroglou, C., et al. 2020. Self-management interventions to reduce healthcare use and improve quality of life among patients with asthma: systematic review and network meta-analysis. *BMJ,* **370**, m2521.

Hoong, J. M., Gibbons, B., Loh, B., et al. 2023. Impact of the value driven outcomes program among cataract surgery patients in Singapore: an interrupted time series analysis. *BMC Health Serv Res,* **23**, 486.

Hurst, L., Mahtani, K., Pluddemann, A., et al. 2019. Defining value-based healthcare in the NHS. CEBM report. Centre for Evidence-Based Medicine. Available at: https://www.cebm.ox.ac.uk/resources/reports/defining-value-based-healthcare-in-the-nhs

Kidanemariam, M., Neve, O. M., van den Heuvel, I., et al. 2024. Patient-reported outcome measures in value-based healthcare: a multiple methods study to assess patient-centredness. *Pat Educ Counsel,* **125**, 108243.

Kidanemariam, M., Allvin, T., Bos, W. J., et al. 2024. Value-based health care: managing the tensions with person-centred health care and population equity [Manuscript submitted for publication].

Makdisse, M., Ramos, P., Malheiro, D., et al. 2022. Value-based healthcare in Latin America: a survey of 70 healthcare provider organisations from Argentina, Brazil, Chile, Colombia and Mexico. *BMJ Open,* **12**, e058198.

NHS Wales. n.d. Patient reported outcome measures (PROMs) package. Available at: https://vbhc.nhs.wales/delivering-value/toolkits/education/patient-reported-outcome-measures-proms/

Patient Priorities Care. n.d. Homepage. Available at: https://patientprioritiescare.org/

Porter, M. E., Lee, T. H. 2013. The strategy that will fix health care. *Harv Bus Rev,* **91**, 24.

Porter, M. E., Teisberg, E. O. 2006. *Redefining Health Care: Creating Value-Based Competition on Results.* Harvard Business School Press.

Queensland Government. 2022. Allied health framework for value-based health care 2022. Available at: https://www.health.qld.gov.au/__data/assets/pdf_file/0026/1190267/Framework.pdf

Ramos, P., Savage, C., Thor, J., et al. 2021. It takes two to dance the VBHC tango: a multiple case study of the adoption of value-based strategies in Sweden and Brazil. *Soc Sci Med,* **282**, 114145.

Riis, C. L., Jensen, P. T., Bechmann, T., Möller, S., Coulter, A., Steffensen, K. D. 2020. Satisfaction with care and adherence to treatment when using patient reported outcomes to individualize follow-up care for women with early breast cancer—a pilot randomized controlled trial. *Acta Oncol,* **59**, 444–452.

Scheckel, B., Schmidt, K., Stock, S., Redaèlli, M. 2023. Patient portals as facilitators of engagement in patients with diabetes and chronic heart disease: scoping review of usage and usability. *J Med Internet Res,* **25**, e38447.

Steinmann, G., van de Bovenkamp, H., de Bont, A., Delnoij, D. 2020. Redefining value: a discourse analysis on value-based health care. *BMC Health Serv Res,* **20**, 862.

Stiggelbout, A., Griffioen, I., Brands, J., et al. 2023. Metro Mapping: development of an innovative methodology to co-design care paths to support shared decision making in oncology. *BMJ Evid Based Med,* **28**, 291–294.

Van der Horst, D. E. M., van Uden-Kraan, C. F., Parent, E., et al. 2022. Optimizing the use of patients' individual outcome information—development and usability tests of a Chronic Kidney Disease dashboard. *Int J Med Inform,* **166**, 104838.

Van der Nat, P. B. 2022. The new strategic agenda for value transformation. *Health Serv Manage Res,* **35**, 189–193.

Van Staalduinen, D. J., van den Bekerom, P., Groeneveld, S., Kidanemariam, M., Stiggelbout, A. M., van den Akker-van Marle, M. E. 2022. The implementation of value-based healthcare: a scoping review. *BMC Health Serv Res,* **22**, 270.

Verweij, L., Smit, Y., Blijlevens, N. M., Hermens, R. P. 2022. A comprehensive eHealth implementation guide constructed on a qualitative case study on barriers and facilitators of the digital care platform CMyLife. *BMC Health Serv Res,* **22**, 751.

5

Patient capacity and shared decision making

Tim Lahey, Angie Burke, and Glyn Elwyn

Introduction

Shared decision making (SDM) embodies the pre-eminent value in clinical ethics: respect for patient autonomy. In contrast to the paternalism of yesteryear, SDM positions the patient as an expert in their preferences and goals who is thus best seen as an equal partner with the medical experts who advise them (Emanuel and Emanuel, 1992).

SDM promotes more patient-centred conversations, improves the identification of patient preferences, enhances patient understanding of their own prognosis, and reduces patient decisional anxiety (Shay and Lafata, 2015; Clayman et al., 2016; Stacey et al., 2024). These impacts of SDM may, in turn, improve patient engagement in their own care, such as via increased adherence to treatments and satisfaction with the ongoing therapeutic alliance (Granados-Santiago et al., 2020). SDM may even cut healthcare costs via newly elicited patient refusal of preference-sensitive care options that are both expensive and typically undertaken by default (Oshima Lee and Emanuel, 2013; Walsh et al., 2014).

The stereotypic image of SDM involves respectful clinician advice given to an empowered and health-literate patient with intact decision making capacity. Yet, the benefits of SDM need not be earmarked exclusively for patients with fully intact decision making capacity. Rather, SDM can help achieve patient-centred care in patients with impaired decision making capacity as well.

Decision making capacity is non-binary, and can be partially impaired regarding some decisions, but not others, or wax and wane over time (Tunzi, 2001; Appelbaum, 2007). In patients with impaired decision making capacity, typically, the complexity of the decision being made determines their ability to make that decision unaided (Mellgard and Gligorov, 2022). Since SDM requires at least some degree of patient decision making capacity, it is, therefore, possible to engage in SDM when making the decisions a patient with impaired decision making capacity can make, at times they can make them (Mejia et al., 2019). Of course, patients who entirely lack decision making capacity cannot engage in SDM.

To conduct SDM in patients with partial impairment of decision making capacity, clinicians must identify which decisions the patient is capable of making at which times. A patient who prefers life-prolonging care, for instance, can be engaged around which activities give life meaning and indicate which forms of treatment might be unacceptably aversive even if they cannot logically weigh the nuanced differences between specific treatment options within those general trajectories of care. Alternatively, a patient with waxing and waning delirium may be fully capable of engaging in SDM in the morning but incapable later on the same day.

Structuring graded SDM to align to whatever decision making capacity the patient possesses enacts respect for patient autonomy better than assuming a patient with partially impaired decision making capacity cannot engage in SDM at all. Arguably, finding a way to respect the residual decision making capacity of patients with impaired decision making capacity helps ensure that the only autonomy threats faced by the patient result solely from whatever condition infringes on their decision making capacity rather than being compounded by inappropriate clinician assumptions of a lack of preferences or ability to engage decisions that reflect them.

Beyond the abstract act of respecting patient autonomy, and assuring that the care provided is the best possible match to their preferences, even the act of soliciting patient preferences and engaging them in decision making to the extent they are able can be a powerful communication of respect, as highlighted in Box 5.1 which describes a patient's perspective.

The mandate to honour the autonomy of patients with impaired decision making capacity requires adaptation of SDM to patient decision making capacity. Since decision making capacity can vary over time, Lahey and Elwyn have likened the adaptation of SDM to patient decision making capacity to the titration of insulin doses in hospitalized patients with labile blood sugar. They call SDM used in patients with impaired decision making capacity sliding-scale SDM (Lahey and Elwyn, 2020).

Figure 5.1 illustrates the sliding-scale adaptation of SDM to patient decision making by depicting three levels of SDM appropriate to three different degrees of decision making capacity. There are, of course, innumerable degrees of impairment in patient decision making capacity to which the SDM conversation can adapt. The steps in capacity-adjusted, sliding-scale SDM are outlined in Box 5.2.

Box 5.1 Patient perspective

SDM despite impaired decision making capacity

Angie Burke, RN, worked over 25 years as a bedside nurse in Ontario, Canada, before suffering a large stroke in 2013. The ensuing experience of medical care—including having to face challenging medical decisions while her own decision making capacity was impaired—led to important insights about SDM even when patient decision making capacity is partly impaired.

On multiple occasions, Ms Burke faced medical decisions while the stroke inhibited her ability to process medical information. Would she consent to this test or that treatment? She wrote, 'on a few occasions, I was forced to sign documents when my husband/caregiver was not with me. To this day, I have no idea what I signed.'

Ms Burke says she feels lucky to have a supportive husband who was able to help with medical decisions that Ms Burke was unable to handle on her own at that moment. When deciding about transition to a rehabilitation centre, she appreciated that documents were left with her and 'time was allotted for me to consult with my husband, and together we made the decision'. That approach enhanced trust and the sense that her agency was being respected.

Ms Burke felt grateful to clinicians and her family for 'recognizing and acknowledging that I had a decreased ability for decision making and pivoting their approach accordingly'. When they presented 'information slowly and concisely and in small segments'—and even repeatedly if needed—she felt more engaged and respected.

When asked about how clinicians could have supported her decision making better, Ms Burke wrote that the most important thing was 'allowing me the time to express myself and not speak for me'. She didn't want clinicians to 'expect me to make decisions quickly and on the spot', but instead wanted them to 'allow time for me to consult with my husband/caregiver'. When making allowances for her to process information slowly, or to incorporate input from her husband, it was important to Ms Burke that clinicians 'not speak to me in a manner that made me feel stupid or I was being treated like a child'.

Ms Burke wrote:

> This is my life ... it was my right to be included in the decision making process. Ultimately, I was the one that was going to have to live with the consequences. By being included, I felt as though I had control over any decisions. Even though I struggled, and it took longer for this process, I felt respected by clinicians. It would have been unfair and unjust for me not to be included.

As detailed in Box 5.2, the adaptation of SDM to patient decision making capacity requires repetition over time. Imagine a patient with mild cognitive impairment who is fully capable of indicating a desire to receive life-sustaining therapy and a willingness to undergo any necessary invasive procedures for a new diagnosis of breast cancer. Because she has difficulty remembering statistics regarding the incidence of postoperative tumour recurrence and complications of surgery, however, she may struggle to weigh the pros and cons of lumpectomy versus mastectomy. In such a situation, SDM is entirely appropriate when discussing whether the patient is interested in repeat surgery or even intensive care unit admission in the event of unforeseen operative complications but might need support from a surrogate decision maker to select a specific surgical approach.

The breast surgeon caring for the patient described above may keep decision making about intensive care unit transfer at a fairly simple level with the patient in the days after a surgical complication arises, but on re-exploration farther out from surgery, the surgeon may find that the patient is prepared to take on more sophisticated discussions without help.

Decision making capacity can wane progressively such that the patient loses the ability to make decisions irrevocably and altogether. Prior to that loss of decision making capacity, engagement in sliding-scale SDM is not wasted. Engaging surrogate decision makers in graded SDM in an increasingly supportive partnership with patients can help surrogate decision makers ease into the assumption of increasing decisional responsibility, perhaps with less ambivalence about the surrogate decision making role or their competence to fulfil it (Bolcic-Jankovic et al., 2014; Su et al., 2020). The process of providing partial support for patient SDM over time may also earn the trust of the patient and help them relinquish responsibility for decision making to the surrogate less ambivalently.

Decision aids can support surrogate decision makers who are supporting patients with impaired decision making capacity, and can even help surrogate decision makers become clearer about their responsibilities to the patient and decision making process (Einterz

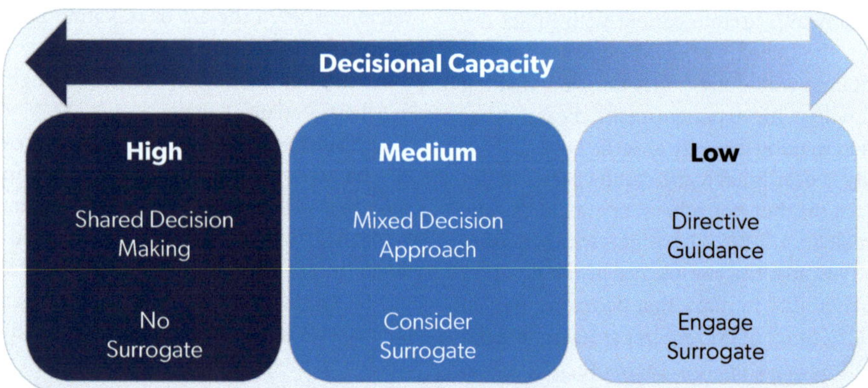

Figure 5.1 Sliding-scale surrogate decision making. SDM can be adapted to patient decision making capacity. Patients with high decisional capacity can engage in unrestricted SDM, and do not need a surrogate decision maker. Patients with partially impaired decision making capacity benefit from a mixed model of SDM in which they participate in some decisions, and their chosen surrogate decision maker supports more nuanced aspects of the SDM conversation. Patients with low decisional capacity may indicate the broadest of preferences (for cure-oriented or comfort-directed care, for instance) but require surrogate decision maker engagement in all aspects of SDM. There are, of course, many gradations of SDM between these general categories of patient decisional capacity.

Reproduced from Lahey, T., Elwyn, G. 2020. Sliding-scale shared decision making for patients with reduced capacity. *AMA J Ethics*, 22, E358–E364. *AMA Journal of Ethics*, The *AMA Journal of Ethics*® is a registered trademark of the American Medical Association.

Box 5.2 Steps in sliding-scale SDM

1. Assess the patient's decision making capacity and their openness to SDM in three stages we have called *team talk*, *option talk*, and *decision talk*.
   a. Explain that a decision is needed and that you, as a patient's clinician, will support the patient's decision making process. We call this *team talk*.
   b. Explain the options in terms that are clear, accessible, and relevant to the patient's goals. We call this *option talk*.
   c. Elicit patient preferences to the extent possible, which is critical to successful SDM. We call this *decision talk*.
2. Reflect on whether the steps above suggest that patient decision making capacity is impaired, and, if required, engage formal assessment by psychiatry of a patient's decision making capacity or formal consultation with ethics.
3. Tailor next steps to patient decision making capacity. When patient decision making capacity is impaired, take a more directive approach and engage surrogate decision makers more intensively.
4. Reassess both patient preferences and decision making capacity over time.
5. Close conversation with patient and any involved surrogate decision makers regarding how well the process of SDM worked for them and whether they have any questions about future conversations.

Reproduced from Lahey, T., Elwyn, G. 2020. Sliding-scale shared decision making for patients with reduced capacity. *AMA J Ethics,* 22, E358–E364. *AMA Journal of Ethics*,

et al., 2014; Shepherd et al., 2021). Thus, some of the tools often used solely to support patients can be brought to bear in sliding-scale SDM.

When a patient cannot engage in SDM regarding a particular decision at a specific time, the clinician should attempt to shift the SDM conversation to the patient's surrogate decision maker. This transition need not exclude the patient. In fact, gauging the patient's general response to the surrogate's more nuanced and particular decision making can involve the patient in decision making to the maximal extent possible, ratify the surrogate's ultimate determination on the patient's behalf, and maintain open lines of conversation between the patient and surrogate.

Different forms of impaired decision making capacity can benefit from different supports for SDM. Table 5.1 provides examples.

Surrogate decision makers are imperfect; one systematic review suggested they represent patient preferences inaccurately a third of the time (Shalowitz et al., 2006). Some degree of inaccuracy is unavoidable, and perhaps not categorically different from the imperfect decisions humans make for themselves on a regular basis. Yet, given the importance of respecting patient autonomy by engaging them in as many decisions (including SDM) as their capacity allows, SDM should be augmented by advanced care planning to the degree enabled by prior forethought. The combination of advance care planning and sliding-scale SDM can optimize the chances the patient's overall goals (expressed previously and at the present time) and current partially impaired thinking can be incorporated and augmented by a trusted surrogate (Rosca et al., 2023).

To enact the core bioethical value of respect for patient autonomy even in patients with impaired decision making capacity, clinicians and surrogate decision makers should engage in sliding-scale SDM in which patient goals and preferences are taken into account to the extent possible and then supplemented by a trusted surrogate if possible with a backdrop of advance care planning.

Table 5.1 Examples of ways to engage in sliding-scale SDM depending on the nature of the patient's partial impairment in decision making capacity

Nature of partial impairment in patient decision making capacity	Surrogate role in sliding-scale SDM	Practices and decision aids that clinicians can use to support sliding-scale SDM
Slowed cognitive processing time precluding real-time decision making but not engagement of the same decision on a slow timeline	Encourage clinicians to defer non-urgent decisions to allow independent surrogate review of the decision with the patient followed by later discussion with clinicians	Provide time and, where appropriate, written material to support slower decision making. Return to the conversation with patient and surrogate decision maker at a later time. Consider if the decision—such as regarding a multi-part treatment plan—can be made in increments
Ability to make simple not complex healthcare decisions, such as when risks and benefits are closely balanced or the differences between treatment options are subtle	Defer to the patient in simple healthcare decisions	Emphasize the patient's centrality to the conversation, and an understanding of their overall preferences
	When more complicated decisions arise, involve the patient in discussions, and solicit overall preferences for care, then suggest decision options with explicit linkages to the patient's overall goals of care for the patient's confirmation	Defer to the surrogate decision maker's determination regarding more complicated decisions, encouraging their involvement of the patient and references back to overall patient goals of care
Waxing and waning decision making capacity	Advocate for deferral of non-urgent decisions if patient is approached during times of relative impairment in decision making capacity	Accept safe deferrals in decision making. Provide asynchronous materials to review if appropriate, such as a website address or recording of a clinician conversation with a surrogate decision maker. Return in person—or via a clinical team member—at a later time to inquire if decision making has become more feasible

REFERENCES

Appelbaum, P. S. 2007. Assessment of patients' competence to consent to treatment. *N Engl J Med,* **357**, 1834–1840.

Bolcic-Jankovic, D., Clarridge, B. R., LeBlanc, J. L., Mahmood, R. S., Roman, A. M., Freeman, B. D. 2014. Exploring determinants of surrogate decision-maker confidence: an example from the ICU. *J Empir Res Hum Res Ethics,* **9**, 76–85.

Clayman, M. L., Bylund, C. L., Chewning, B., Makoul, G. 2016. The impact of patient participation in health decisions within medical encounters: a systematic review. *Med Decis Making,* **36**, 427–452.

Einterz, S. F., Gilliam, R., Chang Lin, F., McBride, J. M., Hanson, L. C. 2014. Development and testing of a decision aid on goals of care for advanced dementia. *J Am Med Dir Assoc,* **15**, 251–255.

Emanuel, E. J., Emanuel, L. L. 1992. Four models of the physician–patient relationship. *JAMA* **267**, 2221–2226.

Granados-Santiago, M., Valenza, M. C., López-López, L., Prados-Román, E., Rodríguez-Torres, J., Cabrera-Martos, I. 2020. Shared decision-making and patient engagement program during acute exacerbation of COPD hospitalization: a randomized control trial. *Patient Educ Couns,* **103**, 702–708.

Lahey, T., Elwyn, G. 2020. Sliding-scale shared decision making for patients with reduced capacity. *AMA J Ethics,* **22**, E358–E364.

Mejia, A. M., Smith, G. E., Wicklund, M., Armstrong, M. J. 2019. Shared decision making in mild cognitive impairment. *Neurol Clin Pract,* **9**, 160–164.

Mellgard, G., Gligorov, N. 2022. Complexity, not severity: reinterpreting the sliding scale of capacity. *Camb Q Healthc Ethics,* **31**, 506–517.

Oshima Lee, E., Emanuel, E. J. 2013. Shared decision making to improve care and reduce costs. *N Engl J Med,* **368**, 6–8.

Rosca, A., Karzig-Roduner, I., Kasper, J., Rogger, N., Drewniak, D., Krones, T. 2023. Shared decision making and advance care planning: a systematic literature review and novel decision-making model. *BMC Med Ethics,* **24**, 64.

Shalowitz, D. I., Garrett-Mayer, E., Wendler, D. 2006. The accuracy of surrogate decision makers: a systematic review. *Arch Intern Med,* **166**, 493–497.

Shay, L. A., Lafata, J. E. 2015. Where is the evidence? A systematic review of shared decision making and patient outcomes. *Med Decis Making,* **35**, 114–131.

Shepherd, V., Wood, F., Griffith, R., Sheehan, M., Hood, K. 2021. Development of a decision support intervention for family members of adults who lack capacity to consent to trials. *BMC Med Inform Decis Mak,* **21**, 30.

Stacey, D., Lewis, K., Smith, M., et al. 2024. Decision aids for people facing health treatment or screening decisions. *Cochrane Database Syst Rev,* **1**, CD001431.

Su, Y., Yuki, M., Hirayama, K. 2020. The experiences and perspectives of family surrogate decision-makers: a systematic review of qualitative studies. *Patient Educ Couns,* **103**, 1070–1081.

Tunzi, M. 2001. Can the patient decide? Evaluating patient capacity in practice. *Am Fam Physician,* **64**, 299–306.

Walsh, T., Barr, P. J., Thompson, R., Ozanne, E., O'Neill, C., Elwyn, G. 2014. Undetermined impact of patient decision support interventions on healthcare costs and savings: systematic review. *BMJ,* **348**, g188.

6

Cultural adaptation of shared decision making and patient-centred care models

Paulina Bravo, Eman Abukmail, Yuko Goto, Irma Vargas, Lyndal Trevena, and Martin Härter

Introduction

Worldwide, there is an increasing momentum towards patient-centred care (PCC), including the promotion of active involvement of patients in the clinical decision making process through shared decision making (SDM) (Bravo et al., 2022). Although the empirical evidence of the effectiveness of PCC and SDM continues to accrue, it is worth noting that most of this research and reported clinical experience has been conducted in high-income countries from the global north. This is not new to the scientific community, and there are drives for a more equitable production of knowledge that aims to eradicate historical inequalities (Castro Torres and Alburez-Gutierrez, 2022).

In the context of PCC and SDM, this becomes a critical challenge. Conceiving PCC and SDM, as derived from the global north, as benchmarking strategies could harm their ethos regarding spread and scale in other countries. Mere *importation* of internationally developed interventions for PCC and SDM may be fundamentally flawed if it does not address the contextual setting and cultural issues for adoption in the global south and other lower-income settings.

While there are different ways to define 'culture', it can broadly be considered as 'the ideas, customs, and social behaviour of a particular people or society' ('Culture', noun, 2023). These shared perspectives can influence cognition, mainly how we process information and learn (Gutchess and Rajaram, 2023). Since SDM involves understanding options and sharing values, it makes sense to consider cultural factors when developing tools and implementing SDM in practice.

Despite this apparent synergy, more research is needed on how cultural factors can best be incorporated into the SDM process. Some studies have explored this connection, cautioning against cultural stereotypes. Culture can impact peoples' desire for family involvement in health decisions and their preferred level of information and involvement in decisions, but this is often quite variable *within* cultures (Dolan et al., 2019). In other words, SDM models and tools should enable the inclusion of cultural factors to the level at which they are important to the individual.

This chapter describes the rationale behind the cultural and contextual adaptation of PCC and SDM models and interventions. Examples from different countries and cultures will show how adaptation has been successful.

The theoretical foundation of cultural adaptation of healthcare interventions

Irrespective of the ongoing discussions regarding the definitions of PCC and SDM, it remains crucial to consider the broader perspective of involving patients in the decision making process. The latest report about PCC and SDM adoption discussed the global trend of promoting patient involvement, showing variation in the use and implementation of PCC and SDM across countries (Bravo et al., 2022). The report presents an optimistic insight towards the future implementation of SDM, particularly the integration into professional training, education, and use of SDM tools across various countries and regions. However, it also highlights some of the main challenges facing SDM implementation in policymaking and adaptations to different specialities or specific groups. Moore et al. (2021) defined adaptation as:

> Intentional modification(s) of an evidence-informed intervention, to achieve a better fit between an intervention and a new context. Modification can include planned adaptations (changes made before introducing a new intervention) and responsive adaptations (changes made intentionally but in response to emerging contextual issues occurring during implementation). Adaptation of interventions is likely to be ongoing as context changes over time.

Replicating PCC and SDM interventions in different contexts without a proper adaptation process could risk failing to achieve the expected results, and ultimately impact the effectiveness of the intervention. A cultural adaptation process fosters a deeper understanding of contextual and cultural beliefs and values, facilitating greater acceptance and uptake of interventions within communities. Notably, it is most efficient in settings with restricted healthcare or health research funding, allowing them to leverage evidence-based interventions produced elsewhere (Moore et al., 2021).

Adapting healthcare interventions must entail a rigorous, auditable process to ensure that the quality of the intervention is maintained. This field of research is relatively new, with a growing number of frameworks offering guidelines for effective adaptation practices.

Once an intervention has been identified as pertinent to address the PCC or SDM challenge, some of the primary considerations for the adaptation process involve the following (Day et al., 2023):

1. *Content modification*: including precision/refinement of the target population and inclusion of culturally appropriate language.
2. *Contextual adjustment*: changes in the format, facilitators, length, and timing.
3. *Fidelity*: a review of outcomes and associations between variables.
4. *Stakeholders' engagement*: considering cultural facilitators and patient representatives.

Experiences of cultural adaptation of PCC and SDM

Working with Aboriginal communities in Australia

In Australia, the healthcare funding landscape is intricate, with various types of care funded by combinations of government and private health insurers. Consumers, patients, or individuals seeking healthcare services for themselves or those under their care often contribute financially where coverage is partial or non-existent. Despite this complexity, coupled with the rich cultural diversity, Australia is demonstrating progressive improvement in implementing PCC and SDM nationally. The Australian Commission on Safety and Quality in Health Care, responsible for the National Safety and Quality Healthcare Standards, is the leading authority in shaping the policy landscape of SDM nationally. These standards focused on consumer partnership, clinical governance integration, and tailored communication to diverse consumer needs, explicitly focusing on collaborating with First Nations communities to address their healthcare needs. The Australian Commission on Safety and Quality in Health Care mandates integrating these standards across all healthcare providers, including hospitals, day procedure providers, and dental care services, while extending improvements to primary and community healthcare and digital mental healthcare.

Australia thrives in implementing SDM on different levels, such as involving consumers in policymaking and research. For example, the Consumer Health Forum is a national representative body with increased research and healthcare policymaking engagement. It also shows great progress in developing patient decision tools and resources to support SDM and integrating them into diverse clinical practices and guidelines (Dimopoulos-Bick et al., 2023). Health information services such as 'Healthdirect' provide online health information and a symptom triage system to support patient engagement and empowerment (www.healthdirect.gov.au). These resources are intended to help patients make informed decisions about their healthcare and improve their health literacy. Other developments included the integration of patient decision aids into clinical practice and guidelines and the integration of SDM concepts into training and teaching for undergraduate and graduate students across universities (Albarqouni et al., 2018).

Some noteworthy examples of cultural adaptation emerging from the Australian experience deserve attention; one is the *expanded model of SDM*, which incorporated *health literacy concepts* (Muscat et al., 2021). This model promotes a *dual-level intervention approach*: facilitating SDM while enhancing patients' health literacy skills, equipping them to make well-informed decisions. It also enhances SDM by increasing communication targeting and fostering the development of transferable health literacy skills among individuals.

The second example is *Finding Your Way* (Dimopoulos-Bick et al., 2023), a culturally adapted model for Australian Aboriginal communities (First Nations) to support them in making decisions that align with their values. This model took inspiration from existing models but was underpinned by the *Aboriginal Eight Ways of Learning*, both in the co-design process with Aboriginal people and in the model itself. Finding Your Way was developed through a collaborative effort involving community, healthcare, research, and government-funded stakeholders. It also included aboriginal partners and leaders throughout the process to ensure cultural sensitivity and relevance. Rooted in the Indigenous understanding of interconnectedness and holistic health, the model embodies eight interconnected circles symbolizing the traditional learning pathways within Aboriginal culture where the core elements of SDM comprise the model's eight inner circles, highlighting the importance of 'process' rather than 'content' for many Aboriginal people. These include sharing stories, non-verbal cues, deconstruction and reconstruction, non-linear processes, community and land links, and learning maps.

Interestingly, unlike traditional linear models of SDM, which often depict decision making as a step-by-step progression from problem identification to a decision, Finding Your Way acknowledges the complexity and fluidity of decision making processes. By incorporating indigenous perspectives, cultural values, and holistic understandings of health, the model embraces decision making's dynamic and interconnected nature. It demonstrates that several factors influence decisions, including cultural beliefs, personal experiences, community dynamics, and social contexts. This non-linear approach allows for a more holistic and inclusive understanding of decision making, ensuring a culturally appropriate process, and is culturally safe and very acceptable (Dimopoulos-Bick et al., 2023).

A third example is the *People And ContExt (PACE) framework*, which outlines a method of cultural adaptation for patient decision aids. PACE has six stages (Dolan et al., 2022):

1. Selection and appraisal of the patient decision aid (searching for local and international resources and assessing against the International Patient Decision Aids Standards criteria and the European Centre for Disease Control framework).
2. Review by content experts (review content against local guidelines, policy and data, update resources).
3. Content validity and usability pre-testing (review by a small number of end-users, e.g. healthcare providers and targeted population).
4. Translation into the relevant language.

5. Decisional needs assessment (interviews and focus groups to assess unmet needs).
6. Acceptability, usability, and feasibility testing in real-world settings.

This framework was used to adapt a series of US-developed family planning patient decision aids for use with Chinese Australian women.

Challenges for the adaptation of PCC and SDM in Japan

Japan, culturally located in East Asia, has a solid family-oriented culture. A *Confucian culture of familism* still exists in East Asia today although its influence may have waned since 2000. Family-oriented cultures emphasize harmony, obedience, and respect for the elderly, while individualist cultures emphasize equal relationships. They have a substantial impact on attitudes regarding PCC and SDM as well as on the communication between patients and clinicians. Familism may differ slightly by region, with Japanese familism being characterized by an emphasis on parent–child and marital relationships regardless of whether they are related by blood.

A study from China (Yang et al., 2022) found that Confucian familism may weaken patient–clinician SDM in end-of-life care for advanced cancer patients. While it may be hard to believe from the perspective of individualistic cultures in the Western hemisphere, even today it is not uncommon that treatment and care decisions are made solely by family members (not the patient) and the healthcare, long-term care, and welfare providers. In addition, informed consent is thoroughly practised, but ensuring that the family understands the treatment and care, not the patient (Xu and Yuan, 2024).

However, in Japan, the Ministry of Health, Labour and Welfare has been working on two initiatives since 2018: first, it disseminates guidelines to promote the fact that decision making support should be provided to 'patients' rather than 'family members' (www.mhlw.go.jp). The second is a public awareness campaign to encourage patients to verbalize their values and discuss the kind of medical care they want to receive with their families. The ministry has created a nickname and logo, '*The Life Conference*', for the clinical situation of advanced care planning (www.med.kobe-u.ac.jp).

In addition to government initiatives, interest in PCC and SDM has grown recently, particularly among the nursing profession. Several decision support guidelines, including SDM as an overarching principle, have been disseminated by medical societies with the focus on long-term conditions and geriatrics, with various decision support training initiatives also advocated and conducted. Although the influence of the family-oriented culture is significant and behaviour change is challenging, steady progress has been made in disseminating PCC and developing SDM education (Goto and Miura, 2023). The implementation of SDM training in Japan has proven that patient-centred decision support can be practised with appropriate training, even in Japan, with its solidly family-oriented culture.

Based on this characteristic of Japanese culture, a PCC and SDM training programme has been developed. This includes a particular registration strategy that offers the training at the organization or community level rather than for individual participants. By doing this, the training programme takes a team-building approach pertinent for the healthcare sector. Otherwise, potential training participants risk becoming isolated when practising PCC and SDM in their organization. It is necessary to conduct training in multidisciplinary groups consisting of several health professionals. This allows the training participants to practise PCC and SDM after the training is completed, and in turn, their behavioural changes are more likely to occur and be sustained. There are clear lessons here for SDM training in all countries. In these trainings, newly developed Japanese versions of assessment tools, like the nine-item Shared Decision Making Questionnaire (SDM-Q-9) and the Shared Decision-Making Questionnaire—physician version (SDM-Q-Doc), were used to adapt international SDM and PCC concepts to Japanese practice.

The training content also includes critical aspects of Japanese culture. For example, the content allows training participants from various fields, organizations, and specialities to form groups and learn how to support an individual patient's decision making. Taking advantage of this strength, the concept of *group SDM* has been established. The training programme is designed to teach PCC and SDM and 'improve' the group's collective support, thus enabling participants to learn PCC and SDM with little resistance and to change their behaviours toward person-centred care (Goto and Miura, 2023). Again, there may be clear lessons here for SDM training in all countries.

Person-centred care as a public health policy in Chile

In recent years, a significant concern in public health in Chile revolves around the growing number of individuals living with *multimorbidity*, with more than 70% of the population affected by two or more long-term conditions. The ageing population, socioeconomic disparities, and increased life expectancy exacerbate this situation. This context underscores the urgent need for new forms of care based on the population's health needs and risks.

Chilean primary care faces the dual challenge of directing resources towards those most in need while simultaneously leading changes in the circumstances that determine population health. This challenge establishes comprehensive PCC as a public policy. Through the Division of Primary Care at the Ministry of Health, the country is implementing the *Strategy for Comprehensive Person-Centered Care in the Context of Multimorbidity* (ECICEP for its name in Spanish), aiming to reorganize care and service provision with a focus on individuals, SDM, and care continuity within the network.

This is a significant endeavour, considering the bio-medicalized and paternalistic approach that still shapes healthcare in the country. Aware of this, a group of Chilean and German researchers offered to collaborate with the Ministry of Health. The research group created the *International Network for Patient-Centered Care* (PCC NET—www.pcc-network.org). PCC NET aims to facilitate and promote professional exchange, networking, and discussion on PCC between researchers, educators, healthcare professionals, and patients. The work of PCC NET involves several strategies, including conceptualizing PCC in the Latin American region (Klimesch et al., 2023). This allowed the team to understand some fundamental cultural differences that needed to be considered in PCC and SDM (e.g. the family-centred approach). In addition, a qualitative study was conducted to understand the main barriers and facilitators that stakeholders considered necessary to implement PCC and SDM in the country. All this work was conducted in a culturally appropriate way, ensured by the close relationships established with public representatives at the Ministry of Health (Box 6.1). This allowed the team to

Box 6.1 Patient perspective

Irma Vargas

From the perspective of a patient and public representative, cultural adaptation in PCC and SDM interventions is of utmost importance. Cultural adaptation acknowledges the diverse values, beliefs, and contexts that shape individuals' healthcare preferences and decision making processes. It ensures that interventions resonate with and respect the cultural nuances of different populations, thereby enhancing their effectiveness and relevance.

Involving patients and the public in cultural adaptation is essential for several reasons:

- Interventions will genuinely reflect the needs and preferences of the individuals they are intended to serve, as the involvement process provides valuable insights into the unique cultural considerations that may influence healthcare decision making.
- When patients see their perspectives and experiences reflected in healthcare initiatives, they are more likely to engage with and benefit from them, fostering acceptance and trust in the adapted intervention. This promotes a sense of ownership and empowerment among patients, improving healthcare outcomes and patient satisfaction.
- This reflects the true spirit of PCC. Incorporating the knowledge, beliefs, and needs of those directly affected by the interventions into the care process helps build trust between patients and healthcare providers.

As a public representative, I advocate for meaningful patient involvement in all aspects of healthcare planning, implementation, and evaluation to ensure that interventions truly meet the needs of those they are intended to serve. The work conducted in Chile in collaboration with PCC NET is one key example. The alliance established between the Ministry of Health and PCC NET allowed us to ensure that all the strategies conducted by PCC NET were relevant to the Chilean system (for patients and health professionals) and that cultural specificities were considered. I was part of the organization's team that defined the training stream of the network, helping to identify the needs of health professionals, linking it to patient and professional organizations, and recruiting hundreds of health professionals across the country so they could access the training as part of their usual activities. This allowed all the country's health services to participate in the network's activities, with a successful conference streamed nationwide and reaching thousands of Chilean professionals.

set up a work plan that responded to the needs of the Chilean health professionals in their own language and included the unique characteristics of the local healthcare system.

Furthermore, a series of free online training sessions was offered nationwide to health professionals. These were facilitated by internationally known experts in the field of PCC and SDM, covering topics such as the theoretical aspects of PCC and SDM, health literacy, implementation sciences, patient decision aids, and risk communication. For the latter, it is worth noting that the language barrier must be addressed. In the experience of PCC NET, when online seminars were simultaneously translated, an average of 250 participants joined the training. To acknowledge the PCC work done in the country, the strategy included organizing the '1st Latin American Conference on Patient-Centred Care', which took place in January 2024 in Santiago, Chile.

Conclusion

Adapting PCC and SDM interventions to diverse cultural contexts is paramount for ensuring their effectiveness and relevance. While global trends promote patient involvement in decision making, challenges persist in implementing and adapting these approaches across different cultural settings. The experiences from Australia, Japan, and Chile underscore the importance of systematic and diverse adaptation processes that consider cultural nuances, values, and preferences. By embracing cultural diversity and employing tailored strategies, healthcare systems can enhance patient engagement, improve healthcare outcomes, and ultimately advance towards more equitable, respectful, and PCC practices globally.

REFERENCES

Albarqouni, L., Hoffmann, T., Straus, S., et al. 2018. Core competencies in evidence-based practice for health professionals: consensus statement based on a systematic review and Delphi survey. *JAMA Network Open*, **1**, e180281.

Bravo, P., Härter, M., McCaffery, K., Giguère, A., Hahlweg, P., Elwyn, G. 2022. Editorial: 20 years after the start of international shared decision-making activities: is it time to celebrate? Probably . . . . *Z Evid Fortbild Qual Gesundhwes*, **171**, 1–4.

Castro Torres, A. F., Alburez-Gutierrez, D. 2022. North and South: naming practices and the hidden dimension of global disparities in knowledge production. *Proc Natl Acad Sci U S A*, **119**, e2119373119.

'Culture', noun. 2023. In: *Oxford English Dictionary*, 3rd edition. Oxford University Press. Available at: https://doi.org/10.1093/OED/4985345143

Day, S., Laver, K., Jeon, Y.-H., Radford, K., Low, L.-F. 2023. Frameworks for cultural adaptation of psychosocial interventions: a systematic review with narrative synthesis. *Dementia*, **22**, 1921–1949.

Dimopoulos-Bick, T., Follent, D., Kostovski, C., et al. 2023. Finding Your Way—a shared decision making resource developed by and for Aboriginal people in Australia: perceived acceptability, usability, and feasibility. *Patient Educ Couns*, **115**, 107920.

Dolan, H., Alden, D. L., Friend, J. M., et al. 2019. Culture, self, and medical decision making in Australia and China: a structural model analysis. *MDM Policy Pract*, **4**, 238146831987101.

Dolan, H., Bateson, D., Li, M., et al. 2022. Acceptability and perceived feasibility of adapted encounter decision aids on contraceptive methods: an interview study with healthcare providers and Chinese migrant women. *PEC Innov*, **1**, 100031.

Goto, Y., Miura, H. 2023. Evaluation of an advanced care planning training program incorporating online skills in shared decision making: a preintervention and postintervention comparative study. *Healthcare*, **11**, 1356.

Gutchess, A., Rajaram, S. 2023. Consideration of culture in cognition: how we can enrich methodology and theory. *Psychon Bull Rev*, **30**, 914–931.

Klimesch, A., Martinez-Pereira, A., Topf, C., Härter, M., Scholl, I., Bravo, P. 2023. Conceptualization of patient-centered care in Latin America: a scoping review. *Health Expect*, **26**, 1820–1831.

Moore, G., Campbell, M., Copeland, L., et al. 2021. Adapting interventions to new contexts—the ADAPT guidance. *BMJ*, **374**, n1679.

Muscat, D. M., Shepherd, H. L., Nutbeam, D., Trevena, L., McCaffery, K. J. 2021. Health literacy and shared decision-making: exploring the relationship to enable meaningful patient engagement in healthcare. *J Gen Intern Med*, **36**, 521–524.

Xu, H., Yuan, M. 2024. Family roles in informed consent from the perspective of young Chinese doctors: a questionnaire study. *BMC Med Ethics*, **25**, 2.

Yang, Y., Qu, T., Yang, J., Ma, B., Leng, A. 2022. Confucian familism and shared decision making in end-of-life care for patients with advanced cancers. *Int J Environ Res Pub Health*, **19**, 10071.

7

Is shared decision making appropriate for diagnostic decisions?

Paul K.J. Han, Laura Zwaan, Désirée Hairwassers, and Glyn Elwyn

Introduction

Shared decision making (SDM) is grounded in the ethical principle of respect for patient autonomy. It aims to inform and empower individuals to make choices with their clinicians based on the best available evidence and what matters to each patient. SDM is indicated in cases of clinical equipoise, where there are multiple reasonable options. This could be due to scientific uncertainty of available interventions or personal uncertainty about an individual's values and preferences.

In principle, SDM applies to decisions about any medical intervention, diagnostic or therapeutic, but therapeutic interventions have received relatively more attention than diagnostic interventions (Berger et al., 2017; Bellolio et al., 2023). Disease screening interventions are a notable exception; a great deal of effort has been devoted to promoting SDM about screening decisions, for example, prostate-specific antigen testing for prostate cancer and low-dose computed tomography for lung cancer. However, the success of these efforts remains an open question. Furthermore, these efforts have focused primarily on questions about the benefits and harms of diagnostic tests themselves, as opposed to the knowledge that they yield. These limitations in the application of SDM to diagnostic decisions both reflect and reinforce a view that diagnostic knowledge is always beneficial for individuals. As our patient representative says: 'we are often not aware of the possible harms of tests' (Box 7.1).

We believe this view is simplistic and short-sighted; diagnostic knowledge is not always beneficial and may even be harmful for some individuals and situations. For these reasons, SDM is appropriate for at least some diagnostic decisions, and in this chapter we will defend this view.

We will analyse three key issues that raise the need for SDM:

- The harms of diagnostic testing.
- The harms of diagnostic knowledge and the benefits of diagnostic ignorance.
- Variation in individuals' preferences for diagnostic knowledge and the need to respect these preferences.

We will develop a conceptual framework to help clinicians determine when and how to engage patients in SDM about diagnostic testing, instead of simply ordering or foregoing such testing.

We do not intend to dismiss the value of all diagnostic tests. Instead, we advocate for a more balanced view that considers the potential harms of the knowledge produced by at least some tests, which should be acknowledged, communicated to patients, and mitigated by clinicians. As our patient author notes, awareness that the knowledge produced by tests has harms is often missing (Box 7.1). SDM is a useful and necessary strategy for accomplishing this task and ensures diagnostic testing is valuable for patients themselves.

The hidden harms of diagnostic testing

Textbooks and journal articles on evidence-based medicine are replete with discussions of the principles and pitfalls of diagnostic testing. All diagnostic tests are inaccurate to some degree and produce two types of error: false negatives and false positives. Tests may be highly specific (minimizing false positives) or highly sensitive (minimizing false negatives), but typically trade off one error for the other. Both types of error can produce harm to patients. False positives can result in emotional distress and additional diagnostic tests that can produce various iatrogenic harms, while false negatives can produce unfounded reassurance that prevents ill patients from seeking and receiving needed care. Most existing efforts to promote SDM for disease screening tests have focused on informing patients about these potential harms.

The harms of diagnostic knowledge

However, the harms of diagnostic testing extend beyond test inaccuracy and its direct downstream consequences to the harms of diagnostic knowledge itself, which has a two-sided nature. On the one hand, diagnostic knowledge is unquestionably beneficial and necessary. Knowledge of the true presence or absence of a disease often enables further preventative, therapeutic, or palliative medical interventions, reduces uncertainty, and enhances patient well-being. On the other hand, diagnostic knowledge sometimes results in no

Box 7.1 Patient perspective

'We are often not aware of the possible harms of tests'

Humans make decisions in their personal lives every day. Do I take my car or not? Do I want to do paragliding or not? Do I smoke or not? With every decision, they consider benefits and harm. Sometimes there is a lack of knowledge to make decisions. Sometimes information is ignored. Humans make good, bad, careful, risky, and even harmful decisions, with at least some degree of confidence.

However, as soon as we enter the door of the medical practice, our position changes. As patients, we are strangers in a new and unfamiliar medical world. We are visitors. Our medical journey is typically only a small part of our life. Our world is much larger, we have a role, a job, hobbies, social interactions, a place to stay, and people to care about.

We don't know the medical language. We don't know the medical code. We lack knowledge and know little about how the body works or how science and scientific evidence can be relevant.

We are brought up with well-known proverbs like 'prevention is better than to cure', a saying attributed to the Dutch philosopher Desiderius Erasmus around 1500. Nowadays, 'early detection' is often mentioned as a key concept in cancer care, but also in hypertension, diabetes, cardiology, and dementia.

Yet we are not aware that diagnostic tests can also come with harm. We are not aware that we might acquire knowledge about our health that we had preferred not to know. At least, not at that time. It requires a deliberate mental exercise to decide if one can live with not knowing. It is not, at first, an obvious good thing.

Journalist Peggy Orenstein, in a *New York Times* article called 'The wrong approach to breast cancer', criticizes the acceptance of preventive mastectomy of healthy breasts without medical need (in patients without hereditary predisposition to breast cancer) due to anticipated regret—choices being made out of fear of future remorse (Orenstein, 2014).

This concept is unfamiliar to us as patients. We make decisions out of fear of not having tried everything in our power to get better or to prevent future health issues. Anticipated regret might play an enormous role in agreeing with diagnostic tests, even if there is a huge risk the results will not contribute to the quality of our life and our goals and even cause harm. Healthcare professionals should know about benefits and harm, and they should understand this state of the patient's mind, and the risk of overreacting with anticipated regret.

You, physicians, are in the lead and have the critical role to guide the SDM process. You have to protect us from decisions driven by fear. It is your task to understand what is important in the life of your patient, what our personal goals are, and to make a good judgement on whether the knowledge acquired by diagnostic tests has a valuable contribution to us or not. Only then, healthcare professionals and patients can discuss the possible options of what to do, and what to leave alone, and share the decision. Let's not forget that the joy of living is far more important than the threat of a possible disease.

material change in medical management or health status, produces new uncertainties, and leads to harms that extend beyond false-negative and false-positive results.

The most obvious harms of diagnostic knowledge are the negative consequences of the follow-up actions it prompts. For example, knowledge of the presence of low-risk localized prostate cancer can lead to surgical intervention that results in iatrogenic harm, including sexual dysfunction and incontinence. But knowledge can also lead to other harms that are less obvious and rarely acknowledged:

- *Psychological harms*: the emotional distress caused by knowing that one has a serious illness, such as cancer, or that one is at risk for cancer or other feared outcomes due to a genetic predisposition.
- *Moral harms*: for example, the decisional burden of knowing that a fetus has a genetic anomaly identified through non-invasive prenatal testing or the guilt and regret of knowing that one's choices may have led to a bad health outcome, even if unintentional.
- *Existential harms*: for example, the despair (and resulting outcomes such as suicide), sense of meaninglessness, and threat to self-identity caused by knowing that one has a serious illness or disability. For many, to know about an increased risk of cancer is to become a different person—one who will, at the very least, feel less healthy, have greater concerns, and struggle to integrate this knowledge into one's daily life.

In these many ways, diagnostic testing can harm patients through the knowledge it imparts.

The benefits of diagnostic ignorance

Perhaps more overlooked than the harms of knowing are the benefits of *not knowing*:

- *Psychological benefits*: the most obvious is the absence of emotional distress, achieved by foregoing knowledge that one either has or is at elevated risk for a serious illness. This benefit motivates at least some presumably healthy persons to avoid cancer screening and persons with family histories of frontotemporal dementia and other degenerative neurological disorders to avoid genetic testing (Kolker, 2023).
- *Moral benefits*: not knowing one's own diagnosis or prognosis can free individuals from the burden of making decisions involving trade-offs that are morally distressing or unacceptable (e.g. between prolonging life and hastening death). Individuals can also accrue moral benefits of not knowing when the lack of knowledge involves other parties. For example, not knowing the diagnosis of a patient can promote just and equitable treatment by health, life, and disability insurers (e.g. genetic susceptibility to cancer or other diseases), and by clinicians who care for the patient (e.g. stigmatized conditions such as substance use or HIV/AIDS).
- *Existential benefits*: perhaps the most important benefit of not knowing is that not knowing one's diagnosis or prognosis can preserve the sense of self-integrity, freedom, and agency needed to pursue goals that give meaning and purpose to people's lives.

Diagnostic testing can harm patients by depriving them of these benefits of diagnostic ignorance.

Legitimizing preferences for not knowing in healthcare

Yet the harms of diagnostic knowledge and the benefits of diagnostic ignorance are often overlooked in clinical practice. One reason is the *foundational role* of diagnostic testing: it is the primary focus of the signature activities that clinicians undertake (e.g. obtaining a medical history and conducting a physical examination). Another reason is *clinical expediency*: it is much easier to suggest a test—and by doing so, to raise the strong expectation that the knowledge gained will be advantageous—than to explain the complexities of this knowledge. A final reason is *cultural*: the value of knowledge is so deeply embedded in the culture of Western society and medicine that the very idea of a person foregoing knowledge seems irrational, pathological, and perhaps even sinful. There is a powerful moral pressure to become knowledgeable whenever possible and to censure any rejection of knowledge—typically described using value-laden constructs such as 'denial', 'avoidant coping', 'unrealistic optimism', or 'wishful thinking' (Han, 2016). The very word 'ignorance' has pejorative connotations, and ignorance achieved through wilful action—which Gigerenzer and Garcia-Retamero have termed 'deliberate ignorance' (Gigerenzer and Garcia-Retamero, 2017)—even more so. A large body of behavioural research has reflected and reinforced a view of 'information avoidance' as 'bad' or maladaptive (Foust and Taber, 2025).

Yet there are both empirical and theoretical reasons to question this view. Past research suggests that preferences for health-related knowledge vary, and that many individuals prefer deliberate ignorance. Gigerenzer and Garcia-Retamero conducted public surveys in Germany and Spain that asked, 'Would you want to know today when you will die?' and 'Would you want to know today from what cause you will die?' Nearly 90% of participants responded 'No' to both questions, and older age was associated with a greater preference for ignorance (Gigerenzer and Garcia-Retamero, 2017). Individual preferences against health-related knowledge have also been documented in studies of patients with various conditions (Ziegler et al., 2001; Germeni and Schulz, 2014), including advanced cancer and other life-limiting illnesses (Fallowfield et al., 1995; Kutner et al., 1999; Hagerty et al., 2004). Individual variation in patient preferences for health-related knowledge challenges the view that such preferences are necessarily irrational, and supports the need to respect these preferences.

The critical questions regarding diagnostic testing, however, are not only empirical but normative: how much moral weight should be granted to the harms of knowing and benefits of not knowing? To what extent should an individual's preferences for *not knowing* be respected? The moral legitimacy of preferences for not knowing has been acknowledged in the bioethics literature in debates over the 'right not to know' (Berkman and Hull, 2014), which focused on conditions such as Huntington's disease—an inherited, high-penetrance neurodegenerative disease with no effective preventive or therapeutic interventions. Diagnostic knowledge of such conditions might conceivably benefit affected persons and family members, such as by enabling them to plan for the future; nevertheless, its value is unclear at best, and the right not to know affirms individuals' autonomy to avoid this knowledge (Berkman, 2017).

However, the right not to know has been controversial. Berkman has argued it is less applicable to conditions with effective medical interventions, and that individuals' preferences for or against knowing may be context-dependent, unstable, and difficult to ascertain, making it practically difficult to respect individuals' right not to know in real clinical contexts (Berkman, 2017). Yet, we believe these challenges do not justify ignoring these preferences. No matter what the potential benefits of diagnostic knowledge might be for any given individual or situation, the potential harms may matter just as much—or even more. Only individuals themselves, furthermore, can weigh these benefits and harms. We believe the practical difficulties of respecting patients' preferences for diagnostic knowledge versus ignorance call for a more nuanced, pragmatic approach that allows clinicians to act on assumed patient preferences when these states have a positive or negative value for most individuals but to actively elicit preferences when their value is unclear.

Leaving space for 'intentional unknowing': a way forward

Such an approach acknowledges that it is both impractical and ethically unnecessary to assess individual patient preferences for knowing versus not knowing for all possible conditions. The very act of seeking medical attention implies a patient's preference for obtaining at least some knowledge of their condition. In most situations, clinicians are justified in assuming this preference and pursuing diagnostic interventions. In some situations, however, patients do not know how they might be affected by the knowledge produced by these interventions. This is especially true for medical conditions that lack either accurate diagnostic tests or effective treatments. In these situations, both clinicians and patients need to be made aware of the potential harms of knowing and benefits of not knowing, and to be reassured that to *not know* is a medically reasonable option—an adaptive stance that promotes psychological, moral, and existential well-being. They need to understand that deciding *not to seek* a test can be a legitimate, informed, active choice based on weighing the harms and benefits of such knowledge.

The question is how to leave appropriate space for not knowing in decisions about diagnostic testing. We believe an important starting point is to change the language used to describe the choice not to know. Rather than the term 'deliberate ignorance', which has pejorative connotations, we propose the alternative term *intentional unknowing*. We believe this term frames the lack of knowledge less negatively and better captures the active and dynamic nature of this state. It helps legitimize the choice not to know.

However, respecting patient preferences for not knowing in diagnostic testing decisions requires more than words; it requires SDM. In the context of diagnostic testing, SDM leaves space for individual variation in patients' values and preferences—not only for diagnostic tests themselves but for knowing versus not knowing. Yet because diagnostic decisions have not been a major focus of SDM interventions, more empirical research is needed to determine when and how to respect individual patient preferences for intentional unknowing, which may vary not only for different patients but for different diagnostic tests and the medical conditions they detect. Until then, however, we propose a provisional conceptual model that attempts to clarify when and where SDM is more or less important in diagnostic test decisions and to identify useful directions for future research.

A conceptual model of SDM for diagnostic testing

Our three-dimensional model focuses on three main factors: (1) benefits of knowledge, (2) harms of knowledge, and (3) diagnostic test accuracy. The combination of these factors determines the need for SDM and the ethically appropriate 'default option' for clinicians and patients to undertake when considering diagnostic testing. Figure 7.1 presents a two-by-two table that illustrates these factor combinations and their associated default options.

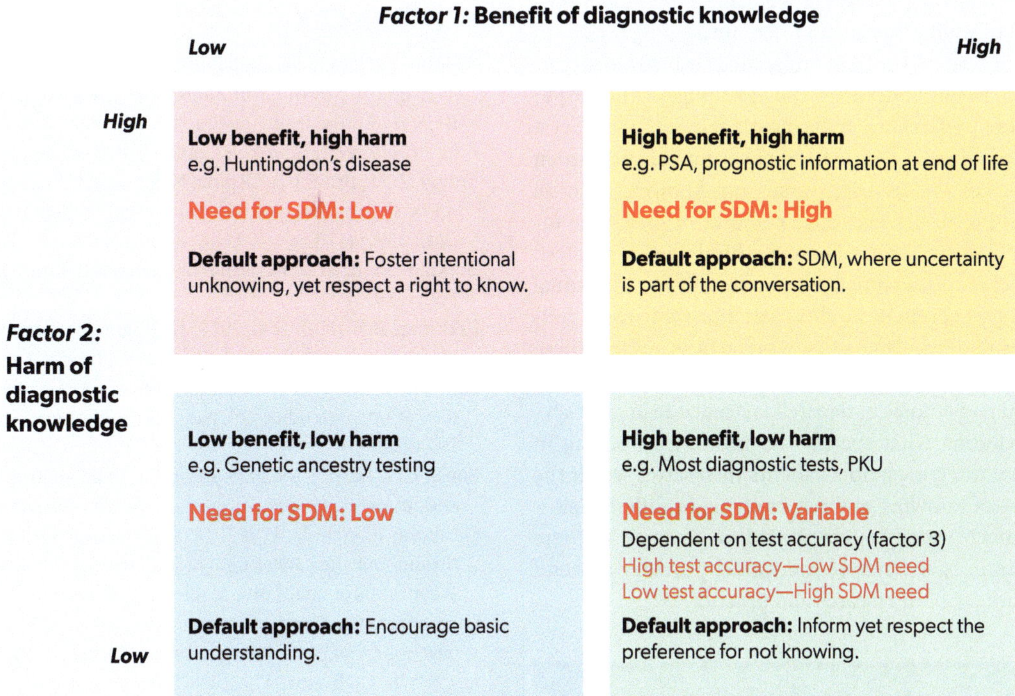

Figure 7.1 SDM for diagnostic testing: tabulating benefits by harms. PKU, phenylketonuria; PSA, prostate-specific antigen.

High need for SDM: high potential benefit, high potential harm

SDM is the clear default option for diagnostic tests that produce knowledge with both high potential benefit and harm (upper right quadrant). Clinicians must ensure that patients are informed about the full range of potential benefits and harms of *knowledge* (as opposed to the medical interventions per se) and weigh these benefits and harms according to their own values and preferences. Examples include prostate-specific antigen screening for prostate cancer and diagnostic tests that produce prognostic knowledge (e.g. genetic testing for cancer susceptibility).

Variable need for SDM: high potential benefit, low potential harm, variable test accuracy (diagnostic uncertainty)

Diagnostic tests that produce knowledge with high potential benefit and low potential harm (lower right quadrant) ordinarily involve a low need for SDM, and the default option is to simply order the test with little or no discussion of the benefits and harms of diagnostic knowledge. Most diagnostic tests in everyday clinical practice fall into this category; for these tests, we believe it is ethically appropriate for clinicians to assume a patient preference for knowledge and to simply be aware that occasional patients may prefer not to know. The exception are diagnostic tests that have low or unclear accuracy and thus substantial diagnostic uncertainty. Examples include low-dose computed tomography scanning for lung cancer screening, which involves a substantial false-positive rate. The diagnostic uncertainty produced by the limited accuracy of such tests is a third critical factor that raises the need to engage patients in SDM about the benefits and harms of diagnostic knowledge.

Low need for SDM: low potential benefit, low potential harm

At the opposite end of the SDM spectrum are diagnostic tests that produce knowledge with both low potential benefit and harm (lower left quadrant). For such tests, the need for SDM is low; clinicians have no or minimal obligation to inform patients about the potential benefits and harms of the knowledge these tests produce, and the default is to allow testing. Examples include genetic ancestry testing, which can be accessed by patients without any clinician involvement whatsoever.

Low need for SDM: low potential benefit, high potential harm

The final category of diagnostic tests produces knowledge with low potential benefit and high potential harm (upper left quadrant), where the default option is to forego testing without engaging patients in SDM. Examples include genetic testing for Huntington's disease or APOE-e4 testing for Alzheimer's dementia, both of which are therapeutically non-actionable. For these tests, we believe it is ethically appropriate for clinicians to assume patient preferences for intentional unknowing, and to simply be aware that occasional patients may prefer to know.

Challenges and promises of the conceptual model

Our model, like all conceptual models, simplifies reality and sidesteps important challenges. It imposes categorical distinctions upon phenomena that are continuous in nature and debatable in magnitude. It does not specify what 'minimal' patient counselling consists of and justifies information non-disclosure in some cases—which raises other ethical concerns. However, we believe the model provides a sound and useful foundation for integrating SDM in diagnostic testing. It gives the patient preference for intentional unknowing the ethical weight it deserves and encourages clinicians to make space for these preferences in diagnostic test decisions. Yet it also makes space for clinicians to be freed of the unrealistic burden of eliciting preferences for knowing versus not knowing with all diagnostic tests, and to direct the scarce resource of their time towards engaging patients in SDM when the ethical need is greatest. However, the model requires clinicians to be sensitive to individual variation in patient preferences in all situations, even when 'full-blown' SDM is not required, and to be motivated to respect these preferences.

More conceptual and empirical research is needed to answer several questions, including what specific diagnostic tests belong in different conceptual categories; how patients themselves weigh the benefits and harms of knowing and not knowing in different situations; and how much moral weight should be assigned to these states. In the meantime, we believe the model provides a useful orienting framework for both research and practice.

Conclusion

SDM is relevant for diagnostic interventions, not only for inherent test inaccuracy but because diagnostic knowledge itself has harms and benefits. For some patients and situations, diagnostic knowledge can be a worse state than diagnostic ignorance, as paradoxical as this might seem to clinicians or other patients. The direct harms and benefits of diagnostic knowledge, along with individual variation in patients' values and preferences for this knowledge, warrant greater attention in clinical care and a deliberative, collaborative approach. In at least some situations, SDM is needed to help clarify the benefits and harms of diagnostic knowledge, to elicit patients' values and preferences for such knowledge, and to ultimately create space for intentional unknowing as a reasonable medical option. Our conceptual model provides a way to achieve this in routine clinical practice.

REFERENCES

Bellolio, F., Hess, E. P., Carpenter, C. R. 2023. Shared decision-making in diagnostic testing. In: Pines, J. M., Bellolio, F., Carpenter, C. R., Raja, A. S. Eds. *Evidence-Based Emergency Care: Diagnostic Testing and Clinical Decision Rules*, pp. 664–677. Wiley.

Berger, Z. D., Brito, J. P., Ospina, N. S., et al. 2017. Patient centred diagnosis: sharing diagnostic decisions with patients in clinical practice. *BMJ*, **359**, j4218.

Berkman, B. E. 2017. Refuting the right not to know. *J Health Care Law Policy*, **19**, 1–72.

Berkman, B. E., Hull, S. C. 2014. The 'right not to know' in the genomic era: time to break from tradition? *Am J Bioeth*, **14**, 28–31.

Fallowfield, L., Ford, S., Lewis, S. 1995. No news is not good news: information preferences of patients with cancer. *Psychooncology*, **4**, 197–202.

Foust, J. L., Taber, J. M. 2025. Information avoidance: past perspectives and future directions. *Perspect Psychol Sci*, **20**, 241–263.

Germeni, E., Schulz, P. J. 2014. Information seeking and avoidance throughout the cancer patient journey: two sides of the same coin? A synthesis of qualitative studies. *Psychooncology*, **23**, 1373–1381.

Gigerenzer, G., Garcia-Retamero, R. 2017. Cassandra's regret: the psychology of not wanting to know. *Psychol Rev*, **124**, 179–196.

Hagerty, R. G., Butow, P. N., Ellis, P. M., et al. 2004. Cancer patient preferences for communication of prognosis in the metastatic setting. *J Clin Oncol*, **22**, 1721–1730.

Han, P. K. 2016. The need for uncertainty: a case for prognostic silence. *Perspect Biol Med*, **59**, 567–575.

Kolker, R. 2023. The vanishing family. *The New York Times*, 20 July 20. Available at: https://www.nytimes.com/2023/07/20/magazine/family-genetics-frontotemporal-dementia.html

Kutner, J. S., Steiner, J. F., Corbett, K. K., Jahnigen, D. W., Barton, P. L. 1999. Information needs in terminal illness. *Soc Sci Med*, **48**, 1341–1352.

Orenstein, P. 2014. Opinion: the wrong approach to breast cancer. *The New York Times*, 26 July 2014. Available at: https://www.nytimes.com/2014/07/27/opinion/sunday/the-wrong-approach-to-breast-cancer.html

Ziegler, D. K., Mosier, M. C., Buenaver, M., Okuyemi, K. 2001. How much information about adverse effects of medication do patients want from physicians? *Arch Intern Med*, **161**, 706–713.

8

The individual and social ethics of shared decision making

Critiques and responses

Zackary Berger and Angela Williams

Summary of the chapter's approach

In this chapter, we will begin with an overview and critique of the ethical claims made for shared decision making (SDM). We will organize these critiques considering the relationship of SDM to communities, institutions, and society. We will then consider the experience of patients with SDM as it is practised. Finally, we conclude with a consideration of SDM in historical context and some deliberation on potential alternatives to the approach.

Overview of the claims made for SDM

Claims made for SDM can be framed as normative in ethical terms or as descriptive claims regarding the desires of patients. Adherents of SDM often say that most people want to be involved in their own decision making, or at any rate, that 'many patients want more information and involvement in decisions about treatment, care or support than they currently experience' (Coulter and Collins, 2011). However, some people do not want to be involved in their healthcare decision making. For example, they might say that they would prefer that their doctor make decisions for them or that they have no preference:

> Many patients do not want to make decisions about their care. They prefer a more passive role (because they are ill, question their abilities, or fear the consequences of making the wrong choice) and ask the doctor to recommend what is best. (Woolf, 1997)

(Such cases can also be understood differently, as patients making a different sort of decision, deciding that they do not want to choose among the options given.) If not all patients want SDM, perhaps they should be convinced of its benefits.

Normative

Normative claims involve some version of the following statement: healthcare requires an intimate knowledge of a person's embodied life. Thus, healthcare that aims at the best interest of the patient, as the argument goes, is only possible when the patient is directly involved in decisions related to their own health.

Note that these claims do not depend on the claim that health outcomes are actually better if patients are involved in their decision making (Shay and Lafata, 2015). These claims could be grounded in several ways. One could, of course, take a deontological approach; possibilities include a Levinasian approach to the Other (i.e. the image of another human being makes irrefutable moral demands) (Burns, 2017) or a Buberian necessity of dialogue—an authentic meeting between two beings in their whole selves without any instrumentalizing of them (Abramovitch and Schwartz, 1996). The most obvious deontological grounding for the normative importance of SDM is autonomy as one of the ethical principles. (This assumes that SDM prioritizes autonomy; but, as will be seen in what follows, it might be a compromise with patients' autonomy limited by social structures.)

In general, normative approaches to SDM have been problematized by Jon Tilburt and others, who point out that the notion of the good in a multicultural society is not shared in general, and certainly not necessarily between doctor and patient (Tilburt, 2011).

Other possibilities include an approach via virtue ethics—one would want to be the kind of provider who treats patients as independent people who can make decisions about their own health (Pastura and Land, 2016). A practice of active listening is not just effective in carrying out patient-centred communication but in developing oneself into the kind of practitioner, the kind of human being, who listens well to people, patients included.

There are other potential approaches to a normative framing of SDM. These have to do with the contributions made by various countercultural or counterhegemonic philosophies of care, which question the assumptions underlying the treatment of patients by providers. Feminist and queer theory can construct alternative notions of autonomy which supplement the individualist and dyadic worldview that underlies SDM (Ahmed, 2020; Sarela, 2023).

Descriptive

Historical accounts of SDM often take a pre-existing paternalistic medical regimen as their point of departure (Taylor, 2009). Many social phenomena underwent considerable change in the 1970s, the decade when the first reference to SDM is found in the literature. The rise of SDM coincided with a decline in trust in institutions (Lipset and Schneider, 1983).

SDM as an idea emerged in the same era as the first patient bill of rights. This bill of rights was a response to the demonstration by the National Welfare Rights Organization at the meeting of the American Hospital Association in 1970 (D'Oronozio, 2001). It was an attempt to use the patient–provider dyad as a focus for response to unrest, contrary to what the National Welfare Rights Organization and other organizations tried to implement as changes in the societal relationship between the patient and healthcare institutions.

The weakness of the descriptivist ethical approach is its dependence on historical contingency. Understanding ethics as a product of historical phenomena leads to a relationship between patient and provider that can veer in various directions depending on the nature of healthcare institutions in the contemporary moment.

Critique of SDM as relevant to different realms of patient care (cf. the domains in the chronic care model)

Another way to approach the ethics of SDM is not from a descriptive or normative perspective but by understanding how SDM affects the various domains of the individuals, structures, and systems that participate in healthcare.

WIth regard to individuals

Critiques by Christian Munthe and collaborators are important in understanding the potential complications of SDM. They dissect the philosophical assumptions of SDM, considering how exactly SDM is operationalized in terms of the relationship between patient and provider choice (Sandman and Munthe, 2010). and, more relevantly to the relationship between SDM and ethics, understanding the precise relationship between SDM and patient autonomy (Sandman and Munthe, 2009). Munthe et al. (2012) point out that the actual implementation of SDM involves concrete assumptions about the desirability of prioritizing patients' sharing of personal narratives as a way of engaging in patient-centred care. If SDM is done this way, it would require patients' personal involvement in deliberative decision making and an openness to divulging personal information.

These objections have yet to lose their force over the intervening years. Currently, individual patients are not just participants in the healthcare systems, but also can be the raw material for the creation of algorithms (Murdoch, 2021) and the selling of healthcare data for the benefit of institutions (Kaplan, 2015). It is no wonder then that patients express mistrust associated with sharing their personal healthcare data.

With regard to communities and institutions

There are ways in which SDM might imply a change in communities and institutions to achieve a more ethical practice. If the status quo does not enable an ethical implementation of SDM in healthcare systems, healthcare systems should change to make that possible (Kerasidou et al., 2020). Some of these changes might include the following: care that considers the needs of patients without regard to their financial circumstances, documentation, or ability to pay; placing patient preferences at the centre of the visit without regard to what procedures or codes generate the most revenue; and, often cited as the greatest barrier to SDM, making it possible to spend uninterrupted time with a patient face to face. Whether SDM can claim these changes as ethical necessities depends on whether SDM can also demand far-reaching changes in the relationship between health, healthcare, and society.

With regard to society

SDM might provide a microcosm in which relations between patient and provider, as a dyad, reflect more far-reaching changes regarding a patient and the healthcare system. Such potentialities are likely constricted by SDM's general emphasis on the individual rather than the group, on the patient as a decision making individual. That is a large constraint to bear, and it could be that SDM, under that assumption, is a bridge too far for those looking for an organizing rubric for far-reaching systematic change. Those who might be at the bottom of the system, patients, might not be able to drive the system.

Munthe et al. (2012) also consider this possibility:

> A basic issue for ethicists to ponder is to what extent transfers of responsibility from caregivers to patients of the sort sketched here are desirable in their own right. [...] Handing over responsibilities may serve to empower patients in terms of decision competence and control. [...] [Here] lies a deeper issue about how such transfers would square with standard views on the professional responsibility of caregivers, the institutionalised version of this in terms of best treatment standards and the traditional notion of a duty of care.

Munthe et al. (2012) point out that how SDM might restructure patient care systems depends on how patient-led systems of care differ in terms of prioritization, cost, and the definition of best treatment standards.

The patient experience with actual existing SDM

The authors of this chapter work together frequently, trying to share decisions as doctor (ZB) and patient (AW). Angela Williams shares her experience with SDM in real life, see Box 8.1.

Healthcare out of reach of patients—is SDM a solution?

In the 1970s, SDM arose in the context of institutional responses to communal agitation for patient rights. Patient participation in

Box 8.1 Patient perspective

A patient's experience with SDM

Making decisions with my doctor can be emotional, fearful, hard, or happy. Most times I prepare to approach or question my doctor to change anything, I do extensive research, write out the pros and cons, and prepare for battle. My doctor is a higher authority to me. I'm always ready for him to say no. Fortunately, my doctor is full of surprises. No matter what I want, my doctor helps me see all available options. Together we talk openly. My doctor helps me see what is most important and not a band-aid decision. Other times my doctor has decided and won't hear me. That is when I am bravest. I question his stand. He is brave as well and tells me why he said no. For over 15 years, we have built a relationship on our shared trust. I tell him about my real-life situations. My doctor considers my situation. I have proven that I will not overdose or sell medicine which is a realistic problem in the area where I live. That alone helps me to be open and honest. Then he surprises me with his 'Let's look at the big picture' speech. We look together to see what can be most helpful. I'm grateful to have had outstanding interactions with the doctor I chose. I hope he sees that too.

decision making was presented as an individual response to communal agitation. Today, SDM, as a response to material inequities, faces the same conflict between individuals and societal contexts. Patients from whom revenue cannot be generated seek effective new pharmaceuticals that are out of their reach because the pharmaceutical companies, already effective profit-generating enterprises, can seek as much profit as they want. Nothing about SDM will make new biological medications priced within the range of more patients. The freedom in decision making imputed to individuals on the part of the philosophy of SDM appears ever more distant from the rooms and halls in which decisions are actually made (Mullan, 2006).

The percentage of clinicians who implement SDM behaviours, when observed and recorded using validated techniques, is less than perfect. The response is to advocate that measures can be taken to educate and incentivize SDM and de-incentivize the behaviours or philosophies that are at cross-purposes with SDM. However, another possibility is that there is something (or many large things) about the health system as currently constructed that militates against SDM (Galasiński et al., 2023).

Alternatives to SDM as an organizing concept

SDM is an ethically important concept because it confronts the contemporary practitioner with the knowledge that the principle of patient choice taken as understood in contemporary medical systems does not actually hold true in the typical patient–practitioner encounter, and to make it hold true, a mere change in habits of thought is not sufficient.

However, the changes in practice (communication, the selection, and framing of decision options) that are needed to operationalize SDM do not obviate the ethical difficulties inherent in the approach: that is, the assumption that it is individuals that can make decisions, over and above the constraints placed upon them by systems. An alternative would be to make all patients, in their social organizations, the owners of health systems so that they, as groups, can drive the distribution of resources, the selection of priorities, and the provision of treatments can be directed in a way that patients have control of.

Conclusion: a re-centred SDM responsive to these critiques

We group the above critiques into two categories. The first is that SDM does not consider the context that impinges upon the patient. This could be addressed by a process of receptive, appreciative inquiry into those contexts and modifying the process of SDM on that basis (e.g. through the patient deciding whether or not they are able to make a decision given their constraints and what constraints might need to be modified or dismantled to make a decision). The second category of reservations has to do not with systemic constraints as they apply to the patient making decisions, but the constraints themselves, and how they nullify the possibility of substantive patient decision making from the very start. Addressing the second type of reservation would demand a fundamental reorganization of patient care, beginning with enabling patients and their representatives to drive decisions regarding the distribution of resources and priorities of medical centres, medical research, teaching, and treatment. It would also demand a reorientation of representative political bodies and sources of capital that determine the resources used to address, or not address, social determinants of health. Only in a system that pursues equity can SDM be a concept that is implemented not just in the dyad but in all corners of a healthcare system.

REFERENCES

Abramovitch, H., Schwartz, E. 1996. Three stages of medical dialogue. *Theor Med*, **17**, 175–187.

Ahmed, S. 2020. *Queer Phenomenology: Orientations, Objects, Others*. Duke University Press.

Burns, L. 2017. What does the patient say? Levinas and medical ethics. J Med Philos, **42**, 214–235.

Coulter, A., Collins, A. 2011. *Making Shared Decision-Making a Reality*. King's Fund.

D'Oronozio, J. C. 2001. A human right to healthcare access: returning to the origins of the patients' rights movement. *Cam Q Healthc Ethics*, **10**, 285–298.

Galasiński, D., Ziółkowska, J., Elwyn, G. 2023. Epistemic justice is the basis of shared decision making. *Patient Educ Couns*, **111**, 107681.

Kaplan, B. 2015. Selling health data: de-identification, privacy, and speech. *Cam Q Healthc Ethics*, **24**, 256–271.

Kerasidou, A., Bærøe, K., Berger, Z., Brown, A. E. C. 2020. The need for empathetic healthcare systems. *J Med Ethics*, **47**, E27.

Lipset, S. M., Schneider, W. 1983. The decline of confidence in American institutions. *Polit Sci Q*, **98**, 379–402.

Mullan, F. 2006. *White Coat, Clenched Fist: The Political Education of an American Physician*. University of Michigan Press.

Munthe, C., Sandman, L., Cutas, D. 2012. Person centred care and shared decision making: implications for ethics, public health and research. *Health Care Anal*, **20**, 231–249.

Murdoch, B. 2021. Privacy and artificial intelligence: challenges for protecting health information in a new era. *BMC Med Ethics*, **22**, 1–5.

Pastura, P. S. V. C., Land, M. G. P. 2016. The perspective of virtue ethics regarding the process of medical decision-making. *Rev Bioét*, **24**, 243–249.

Sandman, L., Munthe, C. 2009. Shared decision-making and patient autonomy. *Theor Med Bioethics*, **30**, 289–310.

Sandman, L., Munthe, C. 2010. Shared decision making, paternalism and patient choice. *Health Care Anal*, **18**, 60–84.

Sarela, A. I. 2023. Using legal doctrine and feminist theory to move beyond shared decision making for the practice of consent. *Clin Ethics*, **18**, 361–367.

Shay, L. A., Lafata, J. E. 2015. Where is the evidence? A systematic review of shared decision making and patient outcomes. *Med Decis Making*, **35**, 114–131.

Taylor, K. 2009. Paternalism, participation and partnership—the evolution of patient centeredness in the consultation. *Patient Educ Couns*, **74**, 150–155.

Tilburt, J. 2011. Shared decision making after MacIntyre. *J Med Philos*, **36**, 148–169.

Woolf, S. H. 1997. Shared decision-making: the case for letting patients decide which choice is best. *J Fam Pract*, **45**, 205–208.

PART 3
Methods in shared decision making research

9

Measurement of shared decision making

Isabelle Scholl, Denitza Williams, Otmar Kodalle, and Marleen Kunneman

Introduction

In this chapter, we explain the significance of measurement in healthcare and explore its various purposes. We highlight the importance of precisely defining the concepts to be measured and provide an overview of measurable elements within the domain of shared decision making (SDM). Additionally, we present an overview of how different constructs related to SDM can be effectively measured, with detailed discussions available in subsequent chapters of this book (see chapters 10–12). The chapter concludes by addressing key challenges in measuring SDM, offering a perspective on the intricacies involved in assessing SDM in healthcare settings.

Purposes of measurement

Measurement of SDM serves multiple purposes, including relevance for research, practice, and education. In *research*, measurement provides a systematic approach for observational studies, clinical trials, and implementation studies to advance our understanding of patient–healthcare professional (HCP) collaboration, healthcare delivery, effective interventions, and how they can be implemented in routine practice. Such research not only has academic value, but also has clinical value as initiatives to improve SDM are translated into practice. In *clinical practice*, SDM measurement provides HCPs with valuable insights into perceived individual patient care and their own communication skills to conduct effective SDM consultations. These can be complemented by assessments of patient outcomes, experiences, and their ability to implement the care plan in real life (i.e. adherence).

An SDM approach can facilitate consideration of care plans and modifications to ensure they are preference-based and sustainable for individual patients. On a system level, quality assessment is considered essential for systematically enhancing the performance of healthcare systems (Burstin et al., 2016). It informs large quality improvement initiatives, enabling healthcare institutions to refine protocols and enhance service delivery. Examples of measurable indicators of effective healthcare provision include clinical processes (e.g. compliance with regulatory standards including guidelines recommending the use of SDM (National Institute for Health and Care Excellence, 2021)) and the efficiency of care delivery, but also patient outcomes (e.g. recovery rates, symptom improvement, and well-being), experiences, and satisfaction to gauge the extent to which services align with patient expectations. As our patient representative notes: the concept of SDM is increasingly accepted in society (Box 9.1).

Finally, all insights from measuring the occurrence and enhancement of SDM play a pivotal role in *healthcare education*, spanning from undergraduate education to professional development.

Box 9.1 Patient perspective

SDM is now widely accepted

In SDM, the doctor's obligation to provide information, elicit the patient's preferences, and ensure a preference-based decision plays a central role and is a key feature of the treatment decision to which both parties should agree. The informed consent discussion and the treatment decision are two essential components of the doctor–patient relationship and are fundamental to guaranteeing the patient's self-determination and the doctor's duty of care.

In Germany, comparable to health policy in other countries, the Law on Patients' Rights comprises the right to informed decisions based on providing comprehensive information on medical options, promoting SDM. The concept is now widely accepted, especially as the levels of information available to patients have risen considerably in the last decade thanks to the media options available to everyone. Doctors are encountering increasingly 'emancipated' patients who wish to participate in joint decision making processes.

Although the concept of SDM is undisputedly regarded as an essential feature of doctor–patient communication, studies on the implementation of SDM in routine clinical care have shown a very mixed picture. SDM is not yet widespread in German hospitals due to the implementation complexity. This primarily concerns the training of medical professionals in communication. Furthermore, experience has shown that patients are not yet provided with sufficient information on treatment options as evidence-based decision making aids and are not supported enough to make preference-based decisions.

When selecting measurement methods for the implementation of SDM, the focus should be on process quality, with the aim of capturing the patient's experience from the patient's perspective. In addition, the quality of outcomes should also be measured to assess patient satisfaction with decision making. Therefore, it is necessary to combine different measurement methods to assess the implementation of SDM.

A broad range of assessment methods exist in education, such as written exercises, assessments by supervising HCPs, clinical simulations, and multisource assessments. Different domains can be assessed, including knowledge, clinical skills, and SDM communication skills, for example, through objective structured clinical examinations (Cömert et al., 2016; Durand et al., 2018). Assessment can be conducted for formative, summative, and professional development purposes (Epstein, 2007).

What can we measure?

SDM has been described as a key element and one of many facets of the broad construct of patient care (Barry and Edgman-Levitan, 2012; Scholl et al., 2014; Zill et al., 2015). Yet, the measurement of SDM is a complex endeavour in itself, especially as the construct of SDM has been described in different ways. Informed by initial conceptual work (e.g. Charles et al., 1997), one common definition describes SDM as a collaborative process wherein HCPs and patients jointly determine the optimal course of action by evaluating available evidence, assessing benefits and risks, and incorporating patient preferences (Elwyn et al., 2010). A systematic review analysed 40 distinct SDM models, highlighting conceptual heterogeneity and a lack of consensus regarding the definition of SDM (Bomhof-Roordink et al., 2019). Nevertheless, many models and definitions agree that certain components are key to SDM: (1) fostering choice awareness, (2) discussing viable options and their respective pros and cons, (3) eliciting patient views and preferences, and (4) making the final decision based on patient preferences (Kunneman et al., 2019a). This stresses the importance of choosing an SDM measure that aligns with the definition of the concept to be measured for each situation. For example, if you were to measure SDM in a clinical research study, a measure that focuses on assessing information provision about treatment options might be appropriate. The measure might show high scores in general; however, it is important to acknowledge that the high score is limited to this particular element of SDM (information provision) (Kunneman et al., 2019a). Previous studies show that different tools exhibit different conclusions about the effectiveness of SDM interventions due to the way different SDM constructs are measured (Stacey et al., 2024).

A systematic review of SDM measurement (Scholl et al., 2011) described the need for an SDM measurement framework. It introduced a tentative classification of SDM measures in three broad categories: decision antecedents, decision process, and decision outcomes. This classification has been built upon in subsequent work on SDM measurement (Sepucha and Scholl, 2014) and has been tested empirically (Chen et al., 2022). Table 9.1 offers an overview of the categorized constructs of SDM measurement. To summarize, for any measurement purpose described above, the first step is clearly defining *what* you want to measure.

How can we measure?

Currently, there is no standardized way to capture the different constructs of SDM, that is, antecedents, decision process, and decision outcomes. Diverse sets of measurement approaches have been developed to date. However, assessing the extent to which SDM occurs can be challenging because the nature of decision making varies (van der Horst et al., 2023). For example, more complex decisions are often distributed across different healthcare consultations and professionals over time (Williams et al., 2019), while other more acute decisions can be made within one appointment. The degree of SDM is mainly measured quantitatively with three primary approaches: patient-reported measures, clinician-reported measures, and observational measures, each offering unique insights and facing specific challenges. Qualitative assessment is also possible but much less common.

Patient-reported SDM measures rely on the self-assessment of individuals involved in the decision making process. This approach captures the subjective experience of patients, offering valuable insights into their perception of SDM. Direct access to the patient's perspective allows an understanding of their perceived involvement in decision making. However, it may be influenced by recall bias or social desirability, and patients might interpret and recall experiences differently. Also, these subjective measures are prone to ceiling effects (high scores without much variance) and halo effects (difficulty in disentangling the evaluation of SDM from the evaluation of other aspects of care or their overall satisfaction with care) (Kunneman et al., 2019b; Williams et al., 2019). Frequently used patient-reported measures include the nine-item Shared Decision Making Questionnaire (SDM-Q-9) (Kriston et al., 2010), CollaboRATE (Barr et al., 2014), and the SDM Process scale (Valentine et al., 2021). Also, an adapted version of the Control Preferences Scale is often used as a measure to evaluate patients' perceived degree of involvement (Degner et al., 1997).

SDM can also be assessed by a HCP's self-report of perceived SDM within a consultation. This method provides an insight into

Table 9.1 Constructs of SDM measurement

Category	Description	Examples
Antecedents	Features of the patient, HCP, or institution influencing the decision making process	Patient preference for participation, health literacy, HCPs' skills and attitudes, availability of decision aids, time allocated to consultations
Decision process	Behaviours of HCPs, patients, and family members during medical consultations or in between consultations	Level of patient engagement, topics discussed, use of patient decision aids, amount of deliberation
Decision outcomes	Proximal and distal results of the decision making process	Decision quality, decision regret, decisional conflict, satisfaction, health outcomes

Adapted with permission from Scholl, I. et al. 2011. Measurement of shared decision making—a review of instruments. *Z Evid Fortbild Qual Gesundhwes*, 105, 313–324, and Sepucha, K. R., Scholl, I. 2014. Measuring shared decision making: a review of constructs, measures, and opportunities for cardiovascular care. *Circ Cardiovasc Qual Outcomes*, 7, 620–626.

Table 9.2 Checklist for measurement selection

Criterion	Description/definition
1. Relevance to study	Does the instrument assess a construct relevant to the research questions of the study?
2. Rigorous development process	Was there a well-structured development process for item generation? Were explicit connections made to pertinent decision making theories or conceptual frameworks? Was cognitive testing conducted to ensure respondents interpret items and responses as intended? Was there pilot testing in the intended sample or setting?
3. Robust psychometric properties	
Reliability	Does the measure consistently yield similar results under comparable conditions?
Validity	How well does the measure assess the intended construct?
Objectivity	To what extent is the administration, scoring, and interpretation of the measure independent of the person who is in charge of these tasks?
4. Clinical meaningfulness	
Responsiveness	Can the measure identify changes of importance to patients and HCPs, such as those resulting from interventions?
Interpretability	Is there evidence that the scores are meaningful to both HCPs and patients?
5. Practicality	
Acceptability	Is the length and content of the measure acceptable to respondents, as evidenced by low missing data and high response rates?
Feasibility	Is the measure easy to administer, score, and interpret?

Adapted with permission from Sepucha, K. R., Scholl, I. 2014. Measuring shared decision making: a review of constructs, measures, and opportunities for cardiovascular care. *Circ Cardiovasc Qual Outcomes*, 7, 620–626.

the HCP's perceived involvement in SDM and it can offer valuable information on the HCP's commitment to SDM in clinical practice. However, it may be subject to different forms of cognitive biases, including social desirability bias and the strive to reduce cognitive dissonance, leading to HCPs overestimating their efforts to involve patients or reporting what is considered ideal rather than their actual practice. A commonly used clinician-reported measure is the physician version of the SDM-Q-9 (SDM-Q-Doc) (Scholl et al., 2012).

Observational SDM measures involve external observers evaluating interactions between HCPs and patients. This method offers a more objective assessment of behaviours, communication patterns, and decision making dynamics within a consultation. It provides a perspective on the actual occurrence of SDM that is less prone to bias. Observer-based measures are the most robust for assessing the presence and quality of SDM (National Institute for Health and Care Excellence, 2021). However, they are time- and resource-intensive and are less feasible for use in routine clinical practice. Furthermore, the presence of an observer or the use of audio/video recording may alter the interaction, leading to potential bias. Among the most prominent observer measures are the Observer OPTION-12 and the Observer OPTION-5 scales (Elwyn et al., 2005; Barr et al., 2015), which have been used to assess both video- and audio-recorded consultations, as well as verbatim transcripts of consultations.

Besides these quantitative forms of assessing SDM, qualitative methods, such as participant observation, detailed transcript analyses, interviews, and field notes, can assess the richness of decision making processes. By providing researchers with more data about the context of healthcare interactions, these methods have a greater ability to capture nuances, unspoken cues, and contextual factors influencing SDM. While providing in-depth insights, qualitative approaches are time-consuming and rely on the researcher's interpretation of the data.

Quality criteria should guide the selection of the right SDM measure (Sepucha and Scholl, 2014). Table 9.2 gives an overview of commonly recommended criteria.

In summary, there is no gold standard method of measuring SDM and each measurement approach has its strengths and limitations. Defining the concept to be measured is crucial, and combining multiple methods can provide a more comprehensive understanding of the complexity of SDM and a more robust evaluation of SDM. Still, a range of studies have shown that there is a lack of correlation between the assessments of patients, HCPs, and observers (Scholl et al., 2015). This finding warrants caution about how to interpret different measurement methods. One measure that attempts to integrate all three perspectives is MAPPIN'SDM (Forner et al., 2022). Also, a recent study using a skills network approach has shown that it was possible to accurately predict observer-rated SDM competence of HCPs from patient-reported assessments of the HCP's SDM skills (Kriston et al., 2023), an innovative statistical approach that needs more research.

Challenges in SDM measurement

For research purposes, we face several challenges in the realm of SDM measurement. When evaluating the effectiveness of an intervention, selecting appropriate end points is crucial. This involves establishing clear reasons and methods for anticipating how the intervention will impact specific outcomes, such as health-related quality of life in patient decision aid effectiveness trials (Rutherford et al., 2019). Most measures are designed for one-off decision making encounters where decision making is initiated and completed in one discrete consultation (e.g. surgical options for early-stage breast cancer). This limits the relevance of existing measures for situations where decisions may be distributed over many encounters, such as in long-term conditions, or across multiple HCPs, such as during collaborations between different clinicians who work in teams. SDM in these situations requires either longitudinal measurement methods or different interpretations as scores vary across different interactions, where decision making intensity is not uniform. Further, some healthcare consultations are 'planning' in nature and do not result in a definitive 'decision' at a clear time point. Tailored SDM measurement timing within a patient care pathway is crucial, as is avoiding a rigid data capture time point plan that misses the key deliberation points.

Performing meta-analyses and clinical benchmarking of SDM competency across different studies is challenging. The lack of a 'gold standard' patient-reported measure results in significant variability in the measures used and the data obtained in different clinical contexts and cultures. This limits our ability to achieve meaningful comparison and benchmarking.

In addition, a general challenge in quality measurement is the lack of alignment in the use of measures and evidence-based improvement strategies (Burstin et al., 2016). For SDM this means that excellent measures are not enough. We also need effective interventions, such as effective training for health professionals, that can be implemented in healthcare settings.

Conclusion

In conclusion, there is no one-size-fits-all recommendation on how to measure SDM. It is important to define the purpose of measurement, to choose one or several SDM constructs fitting this purpose, as well as the perspective to be measured. As each existing measure has advantages and disadvantages, the quality criteria—relevance, rigorous development process, robust psychometric properties, clinical meaningfulness, and practicability—can be helpful in deciding which measure to use for a specific intent.

REFERENCES

Barr, P. J., O'Malley, A. J., Tsulukidze, M., Gionfriddo, M. R., Montori, V., Elwyn, G. 2015. The psychometric properties of Observer OPTION(5), an observer measure of shared decision making. *Patient Educ Couns,* **98,** 970–976.

Barr, P. J., Thompson, R., Walsh, T., Grande, S. W., Ozanne, E. M., Elwyn, G. 2014. The psychometric properties of CollaboRATE: a fast and frugal patient-reported measure of the shared decision-making process. *J Med Internet Res,* **16,** e2.

Barry, M. J., Edgman-Levitan, S. 2012. Shared decision making—pinnacle of patient-centered care. *N Engl J Med,* **366,** 780–781.

Bomhof-Roordink, H., Gartner, F. R., Stiggelbout, A. M., Pieterse, A. H. 2019. Key components of shared decision making models: a systematic review. *BMJ Open,* **9,** e031763.

Burstin, H., Leatherman, S., Goldmann, D. 2016. The evolution of healthcare quality measurement in the United States. *J Intern Med,* **279,** 154–159.

Charles, C., Gafni, A., Whelan, T. 1997. Shared decision-making in the medical encounter: what does it mean? (Or it takes at least two to tango). *Soc Sci Med,* **44,** 681–692.

Chen, C. H., Chuang, H. Y., Lee, Y., Elwyn, G., Hou, W. H., Kuo, K. N. 2022. Relationships among antecedents, processes, and outcomes for shared decision making: a cross-sectional survey of patients with lumbar degenerative disease. *Med Decis Making,* **42,** 352–363.

Cömert, M., Zill, J. M., Christalle, E., Dirmaier, J., Harter, M., Scholl, I. 2016. Assessing communication skills of medical students in objective structured clinical examinations (OSCE)—a systematic review of rating scales. *PLoS One,* **11,** e0152717.

Degner, L. F., Sloan, J. A., Venkatesh, P. 1997. The Control Preferences Scale. *Can J Nurs Res,* **29,** 21–43.

Durand, M. A., Dimilia, P. R., Song, J., Yen, R. W., Barr, P. J. 2018. Shared decision making embedded in the undergraduate medical curriculum: a scoping review. *PLoS One,* **13,** e0207012.

Elwyn, G., Hutchings, H., Edwards, A., et al. 2005. The OPTION scale: measuring the extent that clinicians involve patients in decision-making tasks. *Health Expect,* **8,** 34–42.

Elwyn, G., Laitner, S., Coulter, A., Walker, E., Watson, P., Thomson, R. 2010. Implementing shared decision making in the NHS. *BMJ,* **341,** c5146.

Epstein, R. M. 2007. Assessment in medical education. *N Engl J Med,* **356,** 387–396.

Forner, D., Noel, C. W., Boland, L., Pieterse, A. H., Borkhoff, C. M., Hong, P. 2022. The multifocal approach to sharing in shared decision making: a critical appraisal of the MAPPIN'SDM. *Med Decis Making,* **42,** 114–124.

Kriston, L., Scholl, I., Holzel, L., Simon, D., Loh, A., Harter, M. 2010. The 9-item Shared Decision Making Questionnaire (SDM-Q-9). Development and psychometric properties in a primary care sample. *Patient Educ Couns,* **80,** 94–99.

Kriston, L., Schumacher, L., Hahlweg, P., Harter, M., Scholl, I. 2023. Application of the skills network approach to measure physician competence in shared decision making based on self-assessment. *PLoS One,* **18,** e0282283.

Kunneman, M., Henselmans, I., Gartner, F. R., Bomhof-Roordink, H., Pieterse, A. H. 2019a. Do shared decision-making measures reflect key elements of shared decision making? A content review of coding schemes. *Med Decis Making,* **39,** 886–893.

Kunneman, M., Lavecchia, C. M., Singh Ospina, N., et al. 2019b. Reflecting on shared decision making: a reflection-quantification study. *Health Expect,* **22,** 1165–1172.

National Institute for Health and Care Excellence. 2021. *Evidence Review for Interventions to Support Effective Shared Decision Making: Shared Decision Making: Evidence Review B.* National Institute for Health and Care Excellence.

Rutherford, C., King, M. T., Butow, P., et al. 2019. Is quality of life a suitable measure of patient decision aid effectiveness? Sub-analysis of a Cochrane systematic review. *Qual Life Res,* **28,** 593–607.

Scholl, I., Koelewijn-Van Loon, M., Sepucha, K., et al. 2011. Measurement of shared decision making—a review of instruments. *Z Evid Fortbild Qual Gesundhwes,* **105,** 313–324.

Scholl, I., Kriston, L., Dirmaier, J., Buchholz, A., Harter, M. 2012. Development and psychometric properties of the Shared Decision Making Questionnaire—physician version (SDM-Q-Doc). *Patient Educ Couns,* **88,** 284–290.

Scholl, I., Kriston, L., Dirmaier, J., Harter, M. 2015. Comparing the nine-item Shared Decision-Making Questionnaire to the OPTION Scale—an attempt to establish convergent validity. *Health Expect,* **18,** 137–150.

Scholl, I., Zill, J. M., Harter, M., Dirmaier, J. 2014. An integrative model of patient-centeredness—a systematic review and concept analysis. *PLoS One,* **9,** e107828.

Sepucha, K. R., Scholl, I. 2014. Measuring shared decision making: a review of constructs, measures, and opportunities for cardiovascular care. *Circ Cardiovasc Qual Outcomes,* **7,** 620–626.

Stacey, D., Lewis, K., Smith, M., et al. 2024. Decision aids for people facing health treatment or screening decisions. *Cochrane Database Syst Rev*, **1**, CD001431.

Valentine, K. D., Vo, H., Fowler, F. J., Jr., Brodney, S., Barry, M. J., Sepucha, K. R. 2021. Development and evaluation of the Shared Decision Making Process scale: a short patient-reported measure. *Med Decis Making*, **41**, 108–119.

Van der Horst, D. E. M., Garvelink, M. M., Bos, W. J. W., Stiggelbout, A. M., Pieterse, A. H. 2023. For which decisions is shared decision making considered appropriate?—a systematic review. *Patient Educ Couns*, **106**, 3–16.

Williams, D., Edwards, A., Wood, F., et al. 2019. Ability of observer and self-report measures to capture shared decision-making in clinical practice in the UK: a mixed-methods study. *BMJ Open*, **9**, e029485.

Zill, J. M., Scholl, I., Harter, M., Dirmaier, J. 2015. Which dimensions of patient-centeredness matter?—results of a web-based expert Delphi survey. *PLoS One*, **10**, e0141978.

10

Patient-reported measurement in shared decision making

K.D. Valentine, Rachel C. Forcino, E. Chandlee Bryan, and Karen R. Sepucha

Introduction

Why measure shared decision making?

Patient-centeredness is recognized as a core component of healthcare quality (Institute of Medicine Committee on Quality of Health Care in America, 2001), and measuring shared decision making (SDM) has become an important way to identify, understand, improve, and incentivize/reward patient-centred care (NEJM Catalyst, 2017). Purposes for SDM measurement in routine clinical care range from audit and feedback for individual clinicians on their SDM skill development, to system-level efforts to improve service delivery within learning health systems (Nelson et al., 2016).

Policy initiatives further promote SDM. These initiatives require reliable measurement to facilitate accountability. For example, the Centers for Medicare and Medicaid Services in the USA have required SDM in three clinical decision contexts: lung cancer screening, left atrial appendage closure procedures, and implantable cardioverter–defibrillator placement (Elwyn et al., 2023). However, without reliable measures in place, there is a risk that SDM policy requirements add substantial clinician documentation burden or simply become 'one more box to tick'—thus losing the substance of SDM behind the requirements (Montori et al., 2023).

High-quality measures of SDM also help us understand what interventions work to improve SDM research efforts to evaluate interventions aiming to improve SDM and patient-centred care benefit from valid and reliable measures.

Why measure SDM from the patient's perspective?

Patient-reported measurement invites and welcomes patients' feedback, providing explicit opportunities for patients to have direct input into health service improvement. While more research is needed on the effectiveness of patient-reported measures in improving health outcomes (Boyce and Browne, 2013), patient-reported measurement—when used in ways that matter to patients—may contribute to empowerment and participation in care processes as well as enhancing our models and understanding of patient experiences.

Patient-reported measures are also generally more efficient and pragmatic to collect than observer measures (see Chapter 11 for detail on observer measures). While observing clinical encounters requires a significant time commitment to both collect data and have trained analysts conduct detailed rating and analysis, brief patient-reported measures can be collected efficiently both at the point of care and in the community through a variety of survey modalities. Additionally, it is worth noting that research suggests that patient and observer measures of the same conversation often disagree on the level of SDM that occurred (Kasper et al., 2011). Thus, it is important to clearly identify which perspective is being prioritized for measurement so the appropriate measure can be used.

Key constructs for SDM measures

SDM measures are designed to describe either the process of SDM itself or the impact of SDM on health-related outcomes.

The decision-making process—how SDM is done

Core components of the SDM process include (1) defining or explaining the problem; (2) presenting options; (3) discussing pros and cons; (4) discussing the patient's values and preferences; (5) discussing the clinician's knowledge and/or recommendations; (6) checking understanding; (7) making or explicitly deferring a decision; and (8) arranging follow-up (Charles et al., 1999; Makoul and Clayman, 2006; Sepucha and Mulley, 2009; Elwyn et al., 2017; Bomhof-Roordink et al., 2019).

Although a recent systematic review of SDM conceptual models identified 24 components of SDM (Bomhof-Roordink et al., 2019), most patient-reported measures cover a subset of these components or consolidate components into categories to reduce response burden.

Decision-making outcomes—the impact of SDM

In addition to measures of the SDM process, key outcomes of SDM that are captured include: (1) knowledge of health condition, and available treatment/management options; (2) realistic expectations of treatment/management options; and (3) alignment between treatment/management choice and the patient's personal values and informed preferences.

We would like to note that in prior versions of this chapter (Barr et al., 2016), authors chose to highlight not only patient-reported measures of SDM process and outcomes, but also measures of decision antecedents (e.g. role preference) and decision outcomes (e.g. regret). While we agree these are important measures to discuss, we chose to focus on measures of preference for SDM involvement and SDM experience.

Choosing existing measures for your project

When choosing a measure of patient-reported SDM, it is important to ensure the measure meets your specific project's needs and has strong psychometrics. Two commonly reported psychometrics properties are reliability (e.g. Cronbach alpha for internal reliability or intraclass correlation coefficient for retest reliability) and validity (e.g. content and construct validity). These and several other properties are important for SDM measures including responsiveness, accuracy, acceptability, and feasibility (see, e.g. Table 1 in Sepucha et al., 2014).

To determine whether a measure meets your project's needs, you need to clarify the specific purpose of the study or project. For example:

1. Are you interested in patients reporting on their preference for involvement in SDM, or their experience of SDM?
2. If you are interested in the experience of SDM, are you more interested in the role the patient played in the conversation or the role the clinician played?
3. Are you interested in how the patient experiences SDM in general at this hospital or with this clinician, or do you want to hone in on how one specific decision or visit included SDM?

Example patient-reported SDM measures

Several measures of patient-reported SDM exist, have been reported on in various prior publications (Barr et al., 2016; Clayman et al., 2016; Gärtner et al., 2018), are used in studies included in the Cochrane review of decision aids for people facing health treatment or screening decisions (Stacey et al., 2024), and are highlighted by the Ottawa Hospital patient decision aid evaluation measures (Ottawa Hospital Research Institute, 2023).

For the purpose of making this chapter most useful, we will now focus on providing examples of patient-reported measures of SDM across a few distinct categories:

- Measures of SDM that focus on either the patient's *preference* for SDM versus their *experience* of SDM.
- Measures that place the *impetus* of SDM on the *healthcare provider* (e.g. 'My healthcare provider asked about …') or on the *patient* (e.g. 'I asked about …'), or *both*.
- Measures that seek to understand the SDM *experience more generally* (e.g. 'My doctor usually …') or if the experience was *focused on a specific decision or visit* (e.g. 'At my last visit I … ').

In Table 10.1, you will find examples of measures that have been shown to be psychometrically sound (e.g. measures which have shown at least good reliability and validity), including details on what items look like, and what type of projects might best fit a given

Table 10.1 Example SDM measures and potential applications

Measure name (number of items)	Scale citation (psychometric citations)	Perspective	Example of items	Project applications
Control Preferences Scale (1 item)	Degner et al., 1997 (Clayman et al., 2016; Gärtner et al., 2018)	Assesses general preference for decision making with the impetus on the patient's perspective	'I prefer that my doctor and I share responsibility for deciding which treatment is best for me'	Brief assessment of patient preference for participation in the decision making process. Good for assessing how an individual wants to be involved in the decision making process
9-item SDM Questionnaire (SDM-Q-9) (9 items)	Kriston et al., 2010 (Barr et al., 2016; Clayman et al., 2016; Gärtner et al., 2018)	Assesses specific experiences with decision making with the impetus on the healthcare provider's perspective	'My doctor wanted to know exactly how I want to be involved in making the decision'	Assessment of patient experience of SDM in a specific encounter. The impetus of SDM is on the provider. May be a bit long for use in routine clinical care but provides sufficient detail for testing impact of decision support interventions
MAPPIN'SDM (15 items)	Kasper et al., 2012 (Barr et al., 2016; Clayman et al., 2016)	Assesses specific experiences with decision making with the impetus on the patient's perspective	'My expectations and fears about how to manage the concrete problem were discussed'	Broad assessment of patient experience from the patient's perspective; can be applied to quality improvement or other research studies to understand what aspects of SDM are occurring in detail
Shared Decision Making Process Scale (4 items)	Valentine et al., 2021 (Gärtner et al., 2018)	Assesses specific experiences with decision making with the impetus on the healthcare provider's perspective	'Did the healthcare provider explain there were choices in what you could do to treat your [condition]?'	4-item, Partnership for Quality Measurement-endorsed scale highlights healthcare provider's actions; this focus may be useful for projects involving audit and feedback on SDM performance. Can be applied to any clinical context
CollaboRATE (3 items)	Elwyn et al., 2013 (Barr et al., 2016; Gärtner et al., 2018)	Assesses specific experiences with decision making with the impetus from a broader 'others' perspective	'How much effort was made to listen to the things that matter most to you about your health issues?'	3-item, Partnership for Quality Measurement-endorsed scale captures a broad sense of whether SDM took place; may therefore be useful in routine healthcare practice as an SDM screening measure

scale. It is important to note that we only include a few select examples in Table 10.1, but many other measures exist and can be found via the following studies: Barr et al. (2016), Clayman et al. (2016), and Gärtner et al. (2018).

When deciding if a measure suits your study needs, consider the following:

- Does the scale ask about the *concept* I'm interested in (e.g. preference for involvement versus experience)?
- Does the scale ask about the *frame* I am interested in (e.g. timing and impetus of SDM)?
- Does the scale have good *psychometric* properties (e.g. is there evidence of good reliability, validity)?
- What *trade-offs* are needed for my study (e.g. short scales may be better suited for use in routine clinical care but may not provide the variability necessary to indicate the efficacy of a new intervention)?
- Is the scale *endorsed* by key organizations (e.g. Partnership for Quality Measurement)?

Strengths and challenges of patient-reported SDM measures

There are several key strengths to patient-reported measures of SDM

First, as patient experience fundamentally underpins patient-centred care, we need to be most concerned with how the patient is interpreting the care experience. Further, measures that focus on the perspective of the clinicians may not provide the most accurate representation of the process; numerous studies have indicated that patients and physicians often have discordant views of the same conversations, and physicians are often incorrect when identifying what is important to patients or what treatment they prefer (Valentine and Scherer, 2022). In addition, if an objective outside observer using an observer-based SDM measure indicates that SDM is occurring, but the patient does not report experiencing SDM, this indicates an important gap that needs to be filled in their care. Only by having the patient report on their experience using high-quality measures can we truly identify those areas where we are meeting or falling short of the SDM ideal.

Second, patient care can be complex, involving multiple clinicians and multiple visits. The patient is the only one consistently present to identify the care they have received. Asking the patient about their care journey is the only way to get a complete image of the continuity of care they have experienced. Third, patient-reported surveys can be quick, inexpensive, and straightforward ways to understand if basic elements of SDM are occurring. As illustrated in Table 10.1, several patient-reported measures, with evidence of good validity and reliability, are available for use.

However, challenges to patient-reported SDM measurement exist as well

First, those wishing to measure patient-reported SDM will need to identify the appropriate timing of measurement given their interests. If a clinician has not had a chance to have an SDM conversation about a topic or the patient has not yet met with all members of their care team to participate fully in SDM, then measurement at these times may lead to an invalid or incomplete picture of SDM. Second, the measure needs to be framed appropriately—should the patient be rating a single visit, or a set of visits with a clinician; or a set of interactions across all healthcare providers who participated in the decision making process? Having clarity in the goal of measurement is essential.

Third, rapid patient-reported measures may be relatively limited measures of patient experience as compared to more time-intensive measures such as observational coding. As such, users should be cognizant of the limitations of the patient-reported measure they choose to use, as well as the potential strengths described above. Such limitations include the number of SDM elements covered by a given measure, and the depth of information provided about each element. For example, in the 'SDM Process scale' (Valentine et al., 2021), patients may report on how much clinicians spoke about reasons not to have a procedure, but we do not know explicitly what those risks or downsides were.

Fourth, patients may not even recognize that a decision needs to be, or indeed was, made. Most measures assume a certain level of knowledge about SDM, or even that a decision has been made—both of which are not reached for some patients. This may lead to inaccurate descriptions of the decision experience. And finally, implementing patient-reported measures into routine data collection takes time and effort. It is important to ensure that clinicians and clinical staff understand the value of collecting the information from patients, as well as ensuring patients understand the reason these items are being asked and how they will be used to improve care moving forward.

See Box 10.1 for our patient perspective.

Box 10.1 Patient perspective

I strongly agree with my fellow authors' comment: 'patient-reported measurement—when used in ways that matter to patients—may contribute to empowerment and participation in care processes.'

I was diagnosed with multiple sclerosis (MS) at 42. As the daughter of a clinician, I arrived at my first neurology appointment equipped with my dad's version of an option grid—dad wanted to ensure all treatment options were considered. Weighing risks and medication efficacy, my neurologist and I came to a shared decision on a medication that continues to work for me. Everyone was satisfied with the outcome.

While a shared decision on medication was perhaps the most important task for my neurologist, I needed help with what wasn't covered—learning to live with MS symptoms. MS is a chronic, progressive disease and people with MS experience unique symptoms depending on the area and severity of myelin damage in the brain and spine.

When I visit my neurology practice, my symptoms are assessed through questions on the Multiple Sclerosis Impact Scale (MSIS-29), a measure that assesses quality of life and functional status by asking about the impact of MS on day-to-day life during the past 2 weeks (Hobart et al., 2001).

There are no qualitative or open-ended questions—and sometimes the symptoms I need to address (balance issues, fatigue) haven't been experienced in a fortnight but are still important.

Unless I ask, MSIS-29 results aren't discussed in appointments. The patient side of my electronic medical record displays a single aggregate MSIS-29 score for each assessment administration. The score gives no indication of the areas where my functional or psychological status is improving or worsening. Gathering but not sharing the full results is a missed opportunity for patients and providers to have a conversation on what's working and what's not working, particularly as I have learned that there is a simple strategy to get good healthcare for MS: coordinated care with a team of providers! My neurologist prescribes disease-modifying therapy; my primary care provider and other specialists help me address and live with symptoms.

While the MSIS-29 likely serves a purpose for my clinician, I'd like to recommend that neurologists treating MS consider replacing or supplementing the MSIS-29 with the Multiple Sclerosis Self-Management Scale—Revised (MSSM-R) (Ghahari et al., 2014). In addition to measuring patient-provider communication, the MSSM-R measures five dimensions of self-management and behaviour in people with MS including:

- Healthcare provider relationship and communication
- Treatment adherence/barriers
- Social/family support
- MS knowledge
- Health maintenance/behaviour.

For individuals facing chronic illness, measures like the MSSM-R offer the best of both worlds—providing space for clinicians and those receiving treatment to have conversations not only on their clinic experience and shared decisions, but also on the steps taken outside the clinic to manage and care for themselves. This can contribute to identifying opportunities for improvement in both provider care and self-care, leading to a greater sense of self-efficacy and empowerment for individuals. It is important not only to measure the current state of well-being, but also the levels of knowledge and support one has available to address the condition.

Conclusion

Patient-reported measures of SDM are important to assess the quality of medical decisions, to evaluate the impact of interventions such as patient decision aids, and to promote improvements in patient-centred care. Several SDM measures that have demonstrated strong psychometric properties are available.

Key takeaways:

- Measuring SDM from the patient perspective allows us a better understanding of how patients are experiencing their care journey.
- Several well-validated patient-reported measures of SDM already exist.
- Choosing an appropriate patient-reported measure of SDM requires a thoughtful understanding of what aspects of SDM are of interest, the context of that decision, the goal of measuring SDM, and who will be using the results of those measures.

REFERENCES

Barr, P. J., Scholl, I., de Silva, D. 2016. Patient-reported measures of shared decision making. In: Elwyn, G., Edwards, A., Thompson, R. Eds. *Shared Decision Making in Health Care: Achieving Evidence-Based Patient Choice*, 3rd edition, pp. 168–175. Oxford University Press.

Bomhof-Roordink, H., Gärtner, F. R., Stiggelbout, A. M., Pieterse, A. H. 2019. Key components of shared decision making models: a systematic review. *BMJ Open,* **9**, e031763.

Boyce, M. B., Browne, J. P. 2013. Does providing feedback on patient-reported outcomes to healthcare professionals result in better outcomes for patients? A systematic review. *Qual Life Res,* **22**, 2265–2278.

Charles, C., Gafni, A., Whelan, T. 1999. Decision-making in the physician-patient encounter: revisiting the shared treatment decision-making model. *Soc Sci Med,* **49**, 651–661.

Clayman, M. L., Bylund, C. L., Chewning, B., Makoul, G. 2016. The impact of patient participation in health decisions within medical encounters: a systematic review. *Med Decis Making,* **36**, 427–452.

Degner, L. F., Sloan, J. A., Venkatesh, P. 1997. The control preferences scale. *Can J Nurs Res,* **29**, 21–43.

Elwyn, G., Barr, P. J., Grande, S. W., Thompson, R., Walsh, T., Ozanne, E. M. 2013. Developing CollaboRATE: a fast and frugal patient-reported measure of shared decision making in clinical encounters. *Patient Educ Couns,* **93**, 102–107.

Elwyn, G., Durand, M. A., Song, J., et al. 2017. A three-talk model for shared decision making: multistage consultation process. *BMJ,* **359**, j4891.

Elwyn, G., Sierpe, A., Forcino, R. 2023. Do payment programs incentivize shared decision making in US healthcare? *Patient Educ Couns,* **113**, 107798.

Gärtner, F. R., Bomhof-Roordink, H., Smith, I. P., Scholl, I., Stiggelbout, A. M., Pieterse, A. H. 2018. The quality of instruments to assess the process of shared decision making: a systematic review. *PLoS One,* **13**, e0191747.

Ghahari, S., Khoshbin, L. S., and Forwell, S. J. 2014. The multiple sclerosis self-management scale: clinicometric testing. *Int J MS Care,* **16**, 61–67.

Hobart, J., Lamping, D., Fitzpatrick, R., Riazi, A., Thompson, A. 2001. The Multiple Sclerosis Impact Scale (MSIS-29): a new patient-based outcome measure. *Brain,* **124**, 962–973.

Institute of Medicine Committee on Quality of Health Care in America. 2001. *Crossing the Quality Chasm: A New Health System for the 21st Century*. National Academies Press.

Kasper, J., Hoffmann, F., Heesen, C., Köpke, S., Geiger, F. 2012. MAPPIN'SDM—the multifocal approach to sharing in shared decision making. *PLoS One,* **7**, e34849.

Kasper, J., Heesen, C., Köpke, S., Fulcher, G., Geiger, F. 2011. Patients' and observers' perceptions of involvement differ. Validation study on inter-relating measures for shared decision making. *PLoS One,* **6**, e26255.

Kriston, L., Scholl, I., Hölzel, L., Simon, D., Loh, A., Härter, M. 2010. The 9-item Shared Decision Making Questionnaire (SDM-Q-9). Development and psychometric properties in a primary care sample. *Patient Educ Couns,* **80**, 94–99.

Makoul, G., Clayman, M. L. 2006. An integrative model of shared decision making in medical encounters. *Patient Educ Couns,* **60**, 301–312.

Montori, V. M., Ruissen, M. M., Hargraves, I. G., Brito, J. P., Kunneman, M. 2023. Shared decision-making as a method of care. *BMJ Evid Based Med,* **28**, 213–217.

NEJM Catalyst. 2017. What is patient-centered care? *NEJM Catalyst.* Available at: https://doi.org/10.1056/CAT.17.0559.

Nelson, E. C., Dixon-Woods, M., Batalden, P. B., et al. 2016. Patient focused registries can improve health, care, and science. *BMJ,* **354**, i3319.

Ottawa Hospital Research Institute. 2023. Patient decision aid evaluation measures. Available at: https://decisionaid.ohri.ca/eval.html

Sepucha, K. R., Matlock, D. D., Wills, C. E., et al. 2014. 'It's valid and reliable' is not enough: critical appraisal of reporting of measures in trials evaluating patient decision aids. *Med Decis Making,* **34**, 560–566.

Sepucha, K., Mulley, A. G., Jr. 2009. A perspective on the patient's role in treatment decisions. *Med Care Res Rev,* **66**, 53S–74S.

Stacey, D., Lewis, K. B., Smith, M., et al. 2024. Decision aids for people facing health treatment or screening decisions. *Cochrane Database Syst Rev*, **1**, CD001431.

Valentine, K. D., Scherer, L. D. 2022. Interpersonal (mis)perceptions and (mis)predictions in patient–clinician interactions. *Curr Opin Psychol*, **43**, 244–248.

Valentine, K. D., Vo, H., Fowler, F. J., Jr., Brodney, S., Barry, M. J., Sepucha, K. R. 2021. Development and evaluation of the shared decision making process scale: a short patient-reported measure. *Med Decis Making*, **41**, 108–119.

11

Observational measurement of shared decision making

Anik Giguere, Marleen Kunneman, and Karina Prévost

Introduction

In this chapter, we examine observational instruments (OIs), also known as 'coding schemes', used to evaluate the construct 'shared decision making (SDM) process'. SDM processes encompass the decision making behaviours of both the clinician and the patient in clinical consultations. OIs provide insights into SDM processes from an observer's perspective, in contrast to self-report questionnaires, which capture these processes from the patient's or clinician's perspective. In this chapter, we will describe the OIs, their strengths and limitations, measurement properties, and applications, and identify opportunities for future development.

Description

OIs are used by two or more independent and trained assessors to code SDM processes either in real time or through the analysis of audio or video recordings of consultations. This approach is meant to be objective because it limits potential biases associated with self-reporting, such as social desirability, recall bias, or interpretation bias (Warden, 2021). Twelve OIs have been validated to evaluate SDM processes (Table 11.1). While there is no consensus among SDM model authors on which behaviours are required for effective SDM, there is general agreement on the importance of certain elements, such as creating choice awareness, describing treatment options, discussing patient preferences, and making a decision (Bomhof-Roordink et al., 2019). However, a review of available OIs found that only five OIs assess all four of these SDM elements (Table 11.1) (Kunneman et al., 2019b).

SDM models and OIs do not cover all dimensions of the SDM process. Research suggests that OIs complement patient self-report instruments by providing different insights into the assessment of SDM processes. For instance, patient self-report instruments are more associated with affective–cognitive health outcomes such as understanding and satisfaction, whereas OIs correlate more with behavioural outcomes such as treatment choice and adoption of health behaviours (Shay and Lafata, 2015).

On the one hand, OIs allow for a thorough examination of *information exchange*, an essential aspect of SDM that sets it apart from patient-centred care. OIs break down conversations into their fundamental elements, such as discussing options or patient preferences. This task-oriented approach associates technical and focused discussion with enhanced decision making (Siebinga et al., 2022), filling a gap left by patient self-report instruments, which struggle to capture these specific SDM practices due to a discrepancy between patients' perceptions of SDM and its academic definition (Entwistle et al., 2008). On the other hand, OIs have not been designed to assess *relationship-building* behaviours to develop the quality of the patient–clinician relationship (Box 11.1). A systematic review of several SDM-related measures found a limited number of items assessing the quality of the patient–clinician relationship in the six OIs examined (Table 11.1) (Kunneman et al., 2019a).

Relationship building and information exchange are both crucial and complementary dimensions of the SDM process. Research has shown that patients associate their involvement in decision making with various features within these two dimensions, as illustrated in Figure 11.1.

Strengths and limitations

OIs are less susceptible to ceiling and halo effects than patient self-report questionnaires, making them more sensitive to change (Ubbink et al., 2022). Conversely, OIs often focus on the clinician's behaviour and neglect the patient's contribution to the interaction. This omission limits the ability of OIs to capture important aspects of the interaction (Shay and Lafata, 2014). Additional strengths and limitations of OIs are listed in Table 11.2.

Measurement properties

There is a significant gap in knowledge about the measurement properties of SDM OIs, due to either unassessed properties or inadequate methodologies (Gärtner et al., 2018; Ahmad et al., 2020).

Table 11.1 OIs for measuring shared decision-making processes

OI name (reference to the initial validation study*)	No. items					
	Total	Focus on (Kunneman et al., 2019b)**				Focus on humanistic communication (Kunneman et al., 2019a)
		Fostering choice awareness	Discussing options	Discussing patient preferences	Making a decision	
OPTION-12 (Elwyn et al., 2003)	12	2	2	2	3	1
OPTION-5 (Elwyn et al., 2013; Barr et al., 2015)	5	2	1	1	1	0
MAPPIN'SDM, observational version (Kasper et al., 2012a, 2012b; Kienlin et al., 2017)	15	2	3	1	4	1
Decision Support Analysis Tool (DSAT) (Guimond et al., 2003)	22	1	3	3	6	n.a.
DSAT-10 (Stacey et al., 2008)	11	0	3	2	5	n.a.
Rochester Participatory Decision-Making Scale (RPAD) (Shields et al., 2005)	9	0	0	0	2	n.a.
Elements of Informed Decision Making (IDM) (Braddock et al., 1999)	7	0	3	0	2	0
Decision Analysis System for Oncology (DAS-O) (Brown et al., 2011)	70	8	26	3	6	2
Parental Engagement Scale (PES) (Kearney and Byrne, 2011)	3	0	0	0	0	n.a.
Detail of Essential Elements and Participants in Shared Decision Making (DEEP-SDM) (Clayman et al., 2012)	10	0	4	2	1	n.a.
Shared Decision Making Rating Scale (SDMRS) (Salyers et al., 2012)	10	0	4	1	3	2
Shared Decision Making Scale (SDM-Scale) (Singh et al., 2010)	20	0	8	1	3	n.a.

n.a., not assessed.

* For more information on additional validation studies, see Appendix A in Kunneman et al. (2019a).

** Number of items per element of SDM does not necessarily add up to 100% of the total number of items, since items may assess other aspects than the four core SDM elements.

Box 11.1 Patient perspective

As someone living with a degenerative genetic disease, I have had several difficult discussions with various clinicians over the past 20 years. I've had great encounters, but I have also faced empty rooms with a brochure in my hand. These conversations were not always easy or successful, but when SDM was part of the process, I was always amazed at how beneficial it was to me. Engaging in SDM has empowered me, providing a sense of regained autonomy over my life. The difference it has made for me is immeasurable.

In hindsight, I realize that the success of my SDM conversations depended on the quality of the therapeutic relationship between my clinicians and myself. The depth and quality of these relationships have been the foundation for navigating my health challenges. I have always needed to feel supported, as if someone were holding my hand, but also to be involved in all decisions affecting my health. For me, SDM represents a blend of teamwork and balance, a perfect synergy between the patient and the clinician. It takes work and effective communication to flourish.

I was therefore really surprised when I realized that the OIs do not take our perspective as patients into account, and that we were not involved in their development. How can measurement claim to fully capture patient experiences without our direct contribution? How can it ascertain a positive impact without first consulting us on what such impact entails for us? The absence of the patient voice in the development of OIs is a huge gap for me. Our lived experiences, values and needs can only be fully understood and valued if we are actively involved in matters that directly and significantly impact the quality of our care.

Consequently, I emphasize the conclusions in this chapter that we need ways to measure the true connection and collaboration between a patient and their clinician. While the existing tools undoubtedly rest on sound science and strive for fairness, I believe they also miss essential elements of successful SDM. Trust, empathy, and the essence of a genuine person-to-person conversation are fundamental elements that are currently not adequately captured.

The introduction of the DAS-O marks a significant shift, as patients were involved in its development. This is a good start, but I believe that our involvement should go beyond simply creating new instruments. Truly incorporating our voices, experiences, and perspectives is critical to adding depth to the conversation.

In conclusion, while OIs are fundamental to the assessment of SDM processes, I strongly believe that a deeper transformation is needed to fully capture the entire patient journey, in co-construction with patients and for the benefit of all stakeholders. This, in my view, is crucial to accurately and fully evaluate SDM practices.

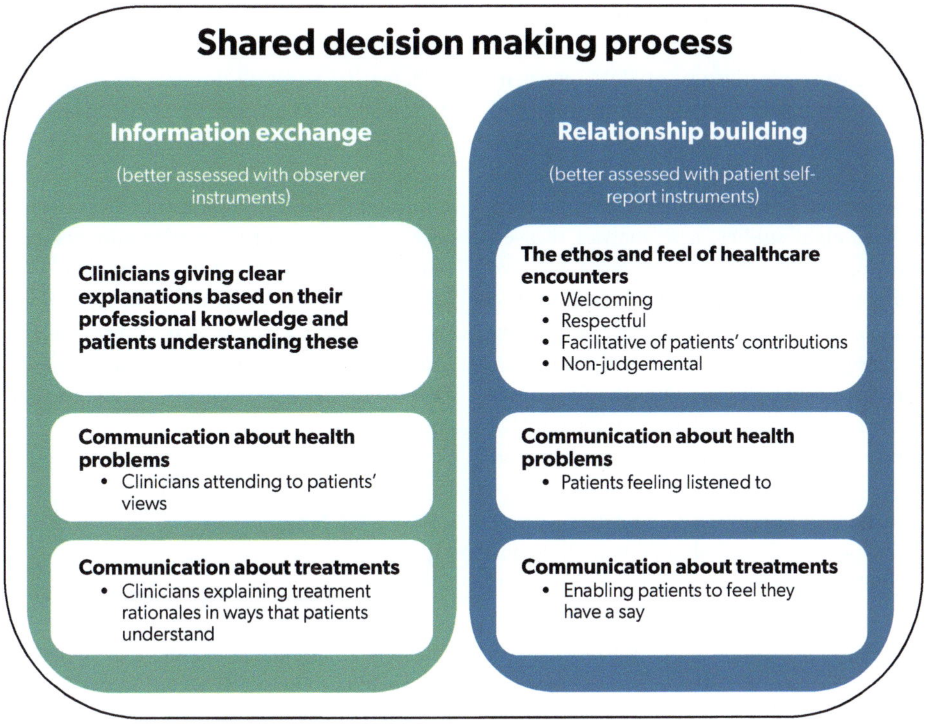

Figure 11.1 A new interpretation of the construct 'SDM Process' with the complementary dimensions 'Information exchange' and 'Relationship building', incorporating key features from Entwistle et al. (2008).

Source: data from Entwistle, V., Prior, M., Skea, Z. C., Francis, J. J. 2008. Involvement in treatment decision-making: its meaning to people with diabetes and implications for conceptualization. *Soc Sci Med*, 66, 362–375.

Nonetheless, and considering their methodological advantages, OIs are commonly used in SDM-oriented research. Therefore, it is crucial to critically evaluate studies based on OIs, by examining the constructs being measured (see 'Description'), and the available evidence concerning their measurement properties.

Content validity is a particularly important measurement property for OIs. Development work with target groups and experts seeks to ensure content validity, in which all items are relevant and comprehensive (Terwee et al., 2018). A review highlighted that among 12 OIs, only the DAS-O demonstrated content validity, supported by moderate evidence (Gärtner et al., 2018). The items were developed based on consultation audio analysis, and subsequent refinement by experts in ethics, cancer medicine, cancer survivors, and patient advocates, to ensure relevance and comprehensiveness (Brown et al., 2011). However, none of the other OIs reviewed reported patient involvement in item generation (Gärtner et al., 2018), highlighting a gap in incorporating patient perspectives in OI development.

Table 11.2 Strengths and limitations of OIs in assessing SDM processes

Strengths	Limitations
• More objective compared to self-report questionnaires • Less prone to ceiling and halo effects than patient self-report questionnaires • Can be used without restrictions/adaptations for consultation with patients with lower literacy skills	• Time and resource intensive and less convenient for assessors • Tend to focus exclusively on the clinician's behaviour, not on the patient's behaviour • OIs only assess the current consultation. This may lead to an underestimation of the quality of the SDM process by the OI and cause inconsistencies with self-report instruments where patients have experienced SDM across multiple consultations • Patients or clinicians may have privacy concerns about their personal data being recorded • Patients may feel uncomfortable being recorded in conversations with their clinicians

Inter-rater reliability is another important measurement property that assesses whether different observers produce consistent results on the same occasion (Mokkink et al., 2010). Inter-rater reliability is assessed whenever OIs are used, because the objective nature of OIs requires two or more observers to independently assess the consultation and reach a consensus. Many of the inter-rater reliability assessments of OIs are not satisfactory (Gärtner et al., 2018). Observer training and consensus-building discussions during the coding process can improve inter-rater reliability within a given study (Gärtner et al., 2018).

Applications

Originally, OIs were developed for research purposes. The knowledge gained during the development and evaluation of SDM interventions then fed into a growing number of projects focusing on the implementation of SDM in routine clinical practice (Bravo et al., 2022). As we move from research to implementation, OIs may also become useful for continuing professional development, quality improvement activities, and learning health systems.

Studies using OIs to evaluate the effectiveness of SDM interventions are summarized in two systematic reviews. The first focused on decision aids for people facing decisions about health treatments or screening (Stacey et al., 2024) (see also Chapter 19). Of the 209 studies included in this review, only ten used OIs, eight of which used OPTION-12. For those eight studies, a re-analysis showed that decision aids used during the consultation were more effective than usual care in improving patient–clinician communication. The second systematic review concerned interventions for increasing the use of SDM by healthcare professionals (Légaré et al., 2018). Of the 87 studies included in this review, 28 used OIs. The OPTION-12 scale was most often used (15 studies), followed by OPTION-5 (two studies). In addition, 14 other scales or subscales were used once each.

OIs can also be used in quality improvement activities. A systematic review of studies using OPTION-12 showed that clinicians exhibited low levels of patient-involvement behaviours (mean score = 23 ± 14 on a scale of 0–100, with higher scores indicating more involvement) (Couet et al., 2015). It is challenging for learners to reflect on their own behaviours (Dickson et al., 2012; Back et al., 2019) but systematic assessment using OIs could potentially be incorporated into SDM training to provide feedback to learners (Ospina et al., 2020). Targeted practice followed by feedback is a key learning strategy for communication skills development (Berkhof et al., 2011; Ospina et al., 2020). However, to be implemented for formative purposes, OIs need to be validated against additional criteria: interpretability, acceptability, and feasibility of interpretation (Trenaman et al., 2021).

On a larger scale, OIs could also be used in a learning health system capacity.

Opportunities for future development

As illuminated in Box 11.1, instruments need to be co-created with patients for measurements to be relevant and valid. This collaborative approach could extend to engaging patient partners as observers in the assessment, to capture their perspective on the validity of the OI, with the added value of offering feedback directly from their invaluable perspective. Involving patient partners in such a role also requires some adaptations to the OIs. Prior work on adapting OIs for patient use found that several adaptations were required in terms of clarity, brevity, and grammatical consistency to ensure that items were interpreted by patients in a way that was consistent with the core constructs of SDM (Melbourne et al., 2011).

Conclusion

In their reflection on the distinctions between OIs and patient self-report measures in assessing SDM processes, Scholl and colleagues emphasized that 'the confounding of perspective and construct is likely to be one of the central issues in research on SDM in general' (Scholl et al., 2015, p. 147). Almost a decade later, in the wake of several studies on the specifics of each type of SDM process measure, OIs still play an important role in assessing the information exchange activities that take place in the SDM process. However, the currently available OIs, by themselves, are not sufficient to assess all dimensions of the SDM process, since they do not allow for assessment of the 'ethos and feel' (Entwistle et al., 2008) of consultations that are required for patients to feel that a decision was 'mutually agreed upon' (Shay and Lafata, 2014). The solution may be to complement OI assessment with patient-centred care assessments, or to develop and evaluate new OIs that incorporate relationship-building items that are also central to SDM. Where any new OI is created, content validation will require cognitive interviewing with patients trained in SDM concepts. Given the progress in patient-oriented research (Oliver et al., 2008), 'patient experts' or 'patient partners' are now invaluable collaborators who could offer this perspective.

REFERENCES

Ahmad, M., Abu Tabar, N., Othman, E. H., Abdelrahim, Z. 2020. Shared decision-making measures: a systematic review. *Qual Manag Health Care*, **29**, 54–66.

Back, A. L., Fromme, E. K., Meier, D. E. 2019. Training clinicians with communication skills needed to match medical treatments to patient values. *J Am Geriatri Soc*, **67**, S435–S441.

Barr, P. J., O'Malley, A. J., Tsulukidze, M., Gionfriddo, M. R., Montori, V., Elwyn, G. 2015. The psychometric properties of Observer OPTION(5), an observer measure of shared decision making. *Patient Educ Couns*, **98**, 970–976.

Berkhof, M., van Rijssen, H. J., Schellart, A. J., Anema, J. R., van der Beek, A. J. 2011. Effective training strategies for teaching communication skills to physicians: an overview of systematic reviews. *Patient Educ Couns*, **84**, 152–162.

Bomhof-Roordink, H., Gärtner, F. R., Stiggelbout, A. M., Pieterse, A. H. 2019. Key components of shared decision making models: a systematic review. *BMJ Open*, **9**, e031763.

Braddock, C. H., 3rd, Edwards, K. A., Hasenberg, N. M., Laidley, T. L., Levinson, W. 1999. Informed decision making in outpatient practice: time to get back to basics. *JAMA*, **282**, 2313–20.

Bravo, P., Härter, M., McCaffery, K., Giguère, A., Hahlweg, P., Elwyn, G. 2022. 20 years after the start of international shared decision-making activities: is it time to celebrate? Probably.... *Z Evid Fortbild Qual Gesundhwes*, **171**, 1–4.

Brown, R. F., Butow, P. N., Juraskova, I., et al. 2011. Sharing decisions in breast cancer care: development of the Decision Analysis System for Oncology (DAS-O) to identify shared decision making during treatment consultations. *Health Expect*, **14**, 29–37.

Clayman, M. L., Makoul, G., Harper, M. M., Koby, D. G., Williams, A. R. 2012. Development of a shared decision making coding system for analysis of patient–healthcare provider encounters. *Patient Educ Couns*, **88**, 367–372.

Couet, N., Desroches, S., Robitaille, H., et al. 2015. Assessments of the extent to which health-care providers involve patients in decision making: a systematic review of studies using the OPTION instrument. *Health Expect*, **18**, 542–61.

Dickson, R. P., Engelberg, R. A., Back, A. L., Ford, D. W., Curtis, J. R. 2012. Internal medicine trainee self-assessments of end-of-life communication skills do not predict assessments of patients, families, or clinician-evaluators. *J Palliat Med*, **15**, 418–426.

Elwyn, G., Edwards, A., Wensing, M., Hood, K., Atwell, C., Grol, R. 2003. Shared decision making: developing the OPTION scale for measuring patient involvement. *Qual Saf Health Care*, **12**, 93–99.

Elwyn, G., Tsulukidze, M., Edwards, A., Légaré, F., Newcombe, R. 2013. Using a 'talk' model of shared decision making to propose an observation-based measure: observer OPTION 5 Item. *Patient Educ Couns,* **93**, 265–271.

Entwistle, V., Prior, M., Skea, Z. C., Francis, J. J. 2008. Involvement in treatment decision-making: its meaning to people with diabetes and implications for conceptualisation. *Soc Sci Med,* **66**, 362–375.

Gärtner, F. R., Bomhof-Roordink, H., Smith, I. P., Scholl, I., Stiggelbout, A. M., Pieterse, A. H. 2018. The quality of instruments to assess the process of shared decision making: a systematic review. *PLoS One,* **13**, e0191747.

Guimond, P., Bunn, H., O'Connor, A. M., et al. 2003. Validation of a tool to assess health practitioners' decision support and communication skills. *Patient Educ Couns,* **50**, 235–245.

Kasper, J., Hoffmann, F., Heesen, C., Köpke, S., Geiger, F. 2012a. Completing the third person's perspective on patients' involvement in medical decision-making: approaching the full picture. *Z Evid Fortbild Qual Gesundhwes,* **106**, 275–283.

Kasper, J., Hoffmann, F., Heesen, C., Köpke, S., Geiger, F. 2012b. MAPPIN'SDM—the multifocal approach to sharing in shared decision making. *PLoS One,* **7**, e34849.

Kearney, J. A., Byrne, M. W. 2011. Planning with parents for seriously ill children: preliminary results on the development of the parental engagement scale. *Palliat Support Care,* **9**, 367–376.

Kienlin, S., Kristiansen, M., Ofstad, E., et al. 2017. Validation of the Norwegian version of MAPPIN'SDM, an observation-based instrument to measure shared decision-making in clinical encounters. *Patient Educ Couns,* **100**, 534–541.

Kunneman, M., Gionfriddo, M. R., Toloza, F. J. K., et al. 2019a. Humanistic communication in the evaluation of shared decision making: a systematic review. *Patient Educ Couns,* **102**, 452–466.

Kunneman, M., Henselmans, I., Gärtner, F. R., et al. 2019b. Do shared decision-making measures reflect key elements of shared decision making? A content review of coding schemes. *Med Decis Making,* **39**, 886–893.

Légaré, F., Adekpedjou, R., Stacey, D., et al. 2018. Interventions for increasing the use of shared decision making by healthcare professionals. *Cochrane Database Syst Rev,* **7**, CD006732.

Melbourne, E., Roberts, S., Durand, M.-A., Newcombe, R., Légaré, F., Elwyn, G. 2011. Dyadic OPTION: measuring perceptions of shared decision-making in practice. *Patient Educ Couns,* **83**, 55–57.

Mokkink, L. B., Terwee, C. B., Patrick, D. L., et al. 2010. The COSMIN study reached international consensus on taxonomy, terminology, and definitions of measurement properties for health-related patient-reported outcomes. *J Clin Epidemiol,* **63**, 737–745.

Oliver, S. R., Rees, R. W., Clarke-Jones, L., et al. 2008. A multidimensional conceptual framework for analysing public involvement in health services research. *Health Expect,* **11**, 72–84.

Salyers, M. P., Matthias, M. S., Fukui, S., et al. 2012. A coding system to measure elements of shared decision making during psychiatric visits. *Psychiatr Serv,* **63**, 779–784.

Scholl, I., Kriston, L., Dirmaier, J., Härter, M. 2015. Comparing the nine-item Shared Decision-Making Questionnaire to the OPTION Scale—an attempt to establish convergent validity. *Health Expect,* **18**, 137–150.

Shay, L. A., Lafata, J. E. 2014. Understanding patient perceptions of shared decision making. *Patient Educ Couns,* **96**, 295–301.

Shay, L. A., Lafata, J. E. 2015. Where is the evidence? A systematic review of shared decision making and patient outcomes. *Med Decis Making,* **35**, 114–131.

Shields, C. G., Franks, P., Fiscella, K., Meldrum, S., Epstein, R. M. 2005. Rochester participatory decision-making scale (RPAD): reliability and validity. *Ann Fam Med,* **3**, 436–442.

Siebinga, V. Y., Driever, E. M., Stiggelbout, A. M., Brand, P. L. P. 2022. Shared decision making, patient-centered communication and patient satisfaction—a cross-sectional analysis. *Patient Educ Couns,* **105**, 2145–2150.

Singh, S., Butow, P., Charles, M., Tattersall, M. H. N. 2010. Shared decision making in oncology: assessing oncologist behaviour in consultations in which adjuvant therapy is considered after primary surgical treatment. *Health Expect,* **13**, 244–257.

Singh Ospina, N., Toloza, F. J. K., Barrera, F., Bylund, C. L., Erwin, P. J., Montori, V. 2020. Educational programs to teach shared decision making to medical trainees: a systematic review. *Patient Educ Couns,* **103**, 1082–1094.

Stacey, D., Lewis, K. B., Smith, M., et al. 2024. Decision aids for people facing health treatment or screening decisions. *Cochrane Database Syst Rev,* **1**, CD001431.

Stacey, D., Taljaard, M., Drake, E. R., O'Connor, A. M. 2008. Audit and feedback using the brief Decision Support Analysis Tool (DSAT-10) to evaluate nurse-standardized patient encounters. *Patient Educ Couns,* **73**, 519–525.

Terwee, C. B., Prinsen, C. A. C., Chiarotto, A., et al. 2018. COSMIN methodology for evaluating the content validity of patient-reported outcome measures: a Delphi study. *Qual Life Res,* **27**, 1159–1170.

Trenaman, L., Jansen, J., Blumenthal-Barby, J., et al. 2021. Are we improving? Update and critical appraisal of the reporting of decision process and quality measures in trials evaluating patient decision aids. *Med Decis Making,* **41**, 954–959.

Ubbink, D. T., van Asbeck, E. V., Aarts, J. W. M., et al. 2022. Comparison of the CollaboRATE and SDM-Q-9 questionnaires to appreciate the patient-reported level of shared decision-making. *Patient Educ Couns,* **105**, 2475–2479.

Warden, G. 2021. Definitions of bias in clinical research. In: Parfrey, P. S., Barrett, B. J. Eds. *Clinical Epidemiology: Methods in Molecular Biology*, vol. **2249**, pp. 35–52. Humana.

12

Innovations in shared decision making assessment

Marleen Kunneman, Matthijs Graner-Baars, and Isabelle Scholl

Introduction

The term 'sharing of decision making' was first used in scientific literature by Veatch in 1972 (Veatch, 1972). Yet, it was not until the mid-1990s, around Charles and colleagues' landmark paper, that shared decision making (SDM) gained momentum (Charles et al., 1997). After decades of research and an increasing number of policy initiatives, SDM is more widely seen as ethically desirable and practically feasible, and as the pinnacle of patient-centred care (Barry and Edgman-Levitan, 2012). Given the strong ethical justification for SDM—respecting patients' autonomy, their right to know, and their right to participate in decisions about their own body and health—and the absence of evidence of harm (Kunneman, 2024), the current body of evidence may be sufficient to justify efforts to implement SDM as a routinely used method of care in situations that warrant its use (usually termed 'preference-sensitive').

At the same time, these decades of research have shown variable levels of SDM, and variable effects of SDM interventions (Kunneman, 2024). In this chapter, we reflect on the current state of SDM assessment and on innovations in current and future initiatives to improve the impact and relevance of SDM assessments for science and clinical practice. We relate these debates to an individual person's perspective that illustrates powerfully what a patient may want from SDM and how a holistic understanding of their goals for managing their condition should shape what we seek to measure. Ultimately, innovating SDM methods and measurements to create a stronger evidence base that reflects patients' wants and goals in real life (and clinicians in their practice) may strengthen the drive to make SDM a common experience in routine healthcare.

See Box 12.1 for our patient perspective.

Box 12.1 Patient perspective

In today's society, people are increasingly in charge of their own bodies and minds. This is no different in the world of diabetes. Although a small proportion of people with diabetes are still fine with the doctor determining the treatment plan, there is an ever-growing group that likes to have a say in this. This is especially true in the target group of young adults. My experience as founder of the ééndiabetes foundation (https://eendiabetes.nl/)—a foundation for young adults (ages 18–35) with type 1 diabetes—is that young adults want to be in control. For them, being involved and in charge of managing their diabetes is essential. SDM makes the person with diabetes feel that there is an equal relationship between doctor and patient because the doctor tries to empathize with the daily life of the person across the desk from them. A person with diabetes whose physician understands (or makes an effort to understand) the person's perspective on life and the way they cope with diabetes is more likely to engage with the physician about the treatment plan and follow their physician's advice. This also creates a safe environment where the person with diabetes is more likely to discuss difficult topics.

As discussed in this chapter, SDM might be more than just fostering choice awareness and providing information, etc. There may be other approaches to collaboration, such as when a person with diabetes takes charge in the conversation and determines what topics are discussed. It is important that doctors are open-minded about techniques that they may not be familiar with or recommend (Do-It-Yourself Closed Loop by the #wearenotwaiting community, for example) and are open to discussing topics for which—in the experience of the person with type 1 diabetes—there is often a taboo among doctors, because they advise against its use (smoking, drug and alcohol abuse) or of which the person may be ashamed (problems during sex).

A real-life example: many young adults like to go to festivals. Some of those with diabetes also like to use a drug while partying. Most avoid talking about this with their doctor because they fear a negative reaction. Others do not shy away from such a conversation. Remember that the person with diabetes takes the initiative here and makes themselves vulnerable to the physician. Practice shows that doctors react differently to such conversations. Some respond disapprovingly and advise the person with diabetes against using drugs, with the possible result that this person will not bring up the subject again in the future. What's more, the question is whether this person will indeed stop using drugs. Another group of physicians responds in an understanding manner. Although they can still point out that drugs can be dangerous, they consider how this person can use the drug in the safest way possible. For example, advice is given that those around the person with diabetes are

Innovation in assessment of decision outcomes: the achievements of SDM

SDM trials to date have had a strong focus on affective–cognitive outcomes such as understanding of information, knowledge, aware of the diabetes and that a sober person keeps an eye on them. Such conversations contribute to making care fit into the lives of people with diabetes.

Personally, I am convinced that when physicians openly engage in the conversation, with the person with diabetes leading the discussion on topics to be addressed, SDM is achieved more effectively. Treatment will be better suited to the person's life and quality of life will improve significantly as a result. It is therefore highly desirable to find new ways that give both physician and patient tools to facilitate this.

satisfaction (e.g. with their clinician, consultation, and the art or technical aspects of care), and trust in clinicians. Indeed, studies evaluating the effectiveness of SDM-related interventions—like pre-encounter patient decision aids or within-encounter conversation tools—produced moderate to high certainty of evidence of improved patient knowledge, accuracy of risk perceptions, decisional comfort, and clarity about their own values (see also Chapter 19). At the same time, these studies have produced inconsistent effects on behavioural outcomes (adherence, health behaviours), health outcomes (symptom reduction, quality of life), but also on healthcare use, litigation, and costs, strongly suggesting a 'regression to the mean' when a procedure is over- or underused at baseline (Shay and Lafata, 2015; Kunneman, 2024) (see also Chapter 19). Only a few studies have assessed the effects of SDM on improving clinician outcomes, generally finding that using SDM interventions promoted clinician satisfaction with decision making and with the clinical encounter (Dobler et al., 2019).

In determining whether these outcomes, and the methods used to assess these outcomes, are comprehensive and holistic for SDM (Cribb and Entwistle, 2011), we need to reflect on what SDM is trying to achieve. The outcomes used in current research seem to imply that the objective of SDM is to increase patient knowledge, to make them adhere better to care plans, or to contribute to solving problems in healthcare like high costs and over- or underuse of care. All these aspects may be considered proxies for SDM 'done well', yet these objectives are often left implicit. In future research, these objectives should be made more explicit, to be transparent about exactly for which problem SDM is intended to be the solution. It will then be possible to review the extent to which such assessment is indeed holistic for the goals of SDM.

A holistic approach should include seeing SDM as a method of care with the objective of designing care plans that fit well for each person (Kunneman, 2024). In line with this approach, the assessment of SDM outcomes may focus on the extent to which SDM contributes to the coherence of care plans, and to our commitment to achieve high-quality patient-centred care for each person. For this, we may assess the rational, emotional, and practical sense of care plans: whether (and why) we understand that the care plan makes sense, feels right, and can be implemented in daily life by the individual patient. This evaluation is fundamentally a subjective judgement, best aided by narrative evaluations (Kunneman et al., 2022).

Innovation in assessment of decision processes: what SDM looks like

Assuming SDM describes any collaborative approach between a patient and a clinician to design a care plan (Ruissen et al., 2023), SDM clearly emerges as a core clinical activity taking place in patient–clinician conversations. Evaluating whether SDM happened should therefore evaluate, ideally directly, behaviours of SDM during the clinical encounter. Over the years, both observational coding tools and patient-reported tools have been developed and validated for this purpose (see Chapters 10 and 11). These measures can provide insight into the extent to which behaviours supportive of SDM took place and were perceived to have taken place, but at the same time measures of SDM typically quantify these behaviours out of the context of their relevance for that particular situation and conversation. For example, in longitudinal care, behaviours supportive of SDM may be distributed over numerous encounters that patients have with a multidisciplinary team and over a period of time. Longitudinal care, such as in long-term conditions, is an ongoing and iterative process in which care plans are continuously re-evaluated and modified, especially when the patient's medical or personal situation changes. Single SDM measurements will not capture this.

This needs a reconsideration of how to interpret and place a value on such quantitative assessment of decision processes, as lower scores may be acceptable for encounters isolated from the care trajectory. Yet, supportive guidelines on this interpretation in longitudinal care are largely missing. One observer rating measure, the OPTION-5 scale, describes how the measure can be used to rate a deliberative process that takes place across multiple clinical encounters (Elwyn et al., 2013). However, when seeing SDM more broadly as a collaborative approach of designing care plans, we may also need to design or adjust quantitative assessment tools that specifically align with this objective. While existing measures operationalize SDM through a particular set of behaviours—including fostering choice awareness, providing information, discussing patient preferences, and making a final decision—there may be other approaches to operationalize collaboration when designing care plans and which instruments need to be able to capture. A study based on direct observations of clinical encounters in diabetes care suggested that SDM may actually be highly prevalent in practice, if SDM were to describe any collaborative design of care plans between a patient and a clinician (Ruissen et al., 2023). Current measures have more narrowly focused on evaluating how different care options are weighed against patient preferences, and may be less sensitive to capturing other collaborative approaches (Hartasanchez et al., 2022).

Importantly, assessment of SDM processes should reach further than merely the content of patient–clinician collaboration. As conversations are tailored to the needs, abilities, and situation, relationships are being built and maintained. SDM should be embedded in conversations based on mutual respect, willingness to accept each other's contributions, empathy, humanity, and dignity. We need to combine the assessment of SDM processes with evaluations of the extent and quality of humanistic communicative approaches, such as interpersonal skills, relational empathy, and the extent to which conversations allow unhurried collaborations (Kunneman et al., 2019). For this, either psychometrically sound patient-reported experience measures or qualitative methods can be used. An example of a recently developed patient-reported experience measure is the Experienced Patient-Centeredness Questionnaire (EPAT). It is a condition-generic tool based on the integrative model of patient-centredness comprising 16 dimensions (Scholl et al., 2014; Christalle et al., 2018). It was developed in a multi-step process ensuring content validity and showed good psychometric properties in a large sample of adults undergoing treatment for cancer, cardiovascular diseases, musculoskeletal disorders, and mental disorders in inpatient or outpatient settings (Christalle et al., 2022).

Innovation in the assessment of contextual factors

While SDM takes place in—and around—clinical encounters, each clinical encounter is embedded in a specific organizational or health system with specific characteristics influencing this encounter (Scholl et al., 2018; Hower et al., 2019). Future research should focus on evaluating whether and how appropriate contexts for SDM are created and on thoroughly assessing the impact and interaction of organizational- and system-level characteristics on SDM implementation (Scholl et al., 2018). This includes research into the extent to which guidelines and other policy initiatives support, or at the very minimum allow, SDM to occur. Time, usually the duration of an encounter, is an often-reported barrier to SDM, and although most studies show no increase in encounter duration when using SDM (Veenendaal et al., 2023), the influence of policies and restrictions on actual or perceived time for SDM should be evaluated more thoroughly. To this end, a measure to assess the unhurriedness of conversations was recently developed and validated (Mandhana et al., 2024).

In addition, the culture of medicine and the organization of healthcare may also inadvertently and variably stand as barriers or facilitators to the adoption of SDM in practice. This includes national or local reimbursement policies (e.g. fee for service or pay for performance) and the extent to which clinicians consider patients as expert assessors of the usefulness, feasibility, and desirability of their care plan. Cultural norms may contribute to patients' and clinicians' views and behaviours. Even before becoming patients or clinicians, people may develop preconceptions about how patients and clinicians should communicate, collaborate, and design care plans. These may be shaped by examples they see or hear, for example, in their personal networks or in popular medical drama series. Indeed, recent research showed that such drama series consistently portray limited patient–clinician conversations and patient involvement (Kunneman et al., 2024). At individual levels, little is known about some phenomena that influence interpersonal behaviour in general and which could also impact decision making processes in medical encounters, such as personality characteristics or implicit attitudes (Weller et al., 2018).

More research is needed to determine how these contextual and individual factors contribute to the use of SDM in clinical practice, and how SDM can reach its full potential. Alternatively, such research may help us calibrate our expectations of what SDM may achieve given current healthcare systems and the context in which patient–clinician conversations take place.

Large-scale evaluation

In the last few decades, real-life observations of patient–clinician SDM conversations in clinical practice—either through direct observation or through observing recordings of encounters—was a time- and resource-consuming activity. These complex large-scale evaluations on the occurrence of SDM and the effects of interventions to enhance SDM motivated, among other reasons, the use of subjective patient-reported measures to evaluate the degree of SDM. With recent developments, automated and systematic recording, transcribing, and analysis of conversations are feasible with the use of artificial intelligence (see Chapter 61). This offers opportunities for larger scale studies and assessment, which may help to build high-quality and high-certainty evidence on the potential effects of SDM. At the same time, though, we need to be careful to count what counts, not just what can be counted.

In future research we need to incorporate more bespoke approaches to SDM studies and their methods of evaluation. For example, choosing what an appropriate process or outcome of SDM is, and therefore should be evaluated, may depend on each patient's own situation. Such flexible research designs with individualized measures may complicate the interpretation and comparability of data generated through these studies—perhaps less in large-scale studies—but it may also help minimize the work and burden of research participation for patients and clinical teams by not having to offer them an extensive battery of measures to make sure we assess all outcomes that may be relevant across the study population. Indeed, in general we need to be cautious of the work SDM and SDM studies pose to patients. Future evaluations of SDM could strengthen and broaden the body of evidence by also focusing on the possible work, workload, and burden of SDM—for example, cognitive, emotional, temporal, social, logistical, or financial—on patients, clinicians, and health systems.

Conclusion

Innovation in SDM assessment should fundamentally come from reflections on the holistic objective of SDM and identifying to which problem SDM is intended to be the solution. To this end, we need to consider the rational, emotional, and practical sense of care plans; how SDM is positioned in longitudinal care; and how contextual and cultural factors stimulate, or allow, SDM. To uncover SDM's true value to high-quality care, SDM assessments need to be combined with assessments of humanistic communicative approaches, patient-reported experience measures, and qualitative methods. While recent developments in artificial intelligence pave the way for larger-scale studies, determining the appropriate SDM approach and measures needs to depend on each individual patient and their situation.

REFERENCES

Barry, M. J., Edgman-Levitan, S. 2012. Shared decision making—pinnacle of patient-centered care. *N Engl J Med*, **366**, 780–781.

Charles, C., Gafni, A., Whelan, T. 1997. Shared decision-making in the medical encounter: what does it mean? (Or it takes at least two to tango). *Soc Sci Med*, **44**, 681–692.

Christalle, E., Zeh, S., Hahlweg, P., Kriston, L., Harter, M., Scholl, I. 2018. Assessment of patient centredness through patient-reported experience measures (ASPIRED): protocol of a mixed-methods study. *BMJ Open*, **8**, e025896.

Christalle, E., Zeh, S., Hahlweg, P., et al. 2022. Development and content validity of the Experienced Patient-Centeredness Questionnaire (EPAT)—a best practice example for generating patient-reported measures from qualitative data. *Health Expect*, **25**, 1529–1538.

Cribb, A., Entwistle, V. A. 2011. Shared decision making: trade-offs between narrower and broader conceptions. *Health Expect,* **14**, 210–9.

Dobler, C. C., Sanchez, M., Gionfriddo, M. R., et al. 2019. Impact of decision aids used during clinical encounters on clinician outcomes and consultation length: a systematic review. *BMJ Qual Saf,* **28**, 499–510.

Elwyn, G., Tsulukidze, M., Edwards, A., Légaré, F., Newcombe, R. 2013. Using a 'talk' model of shared decision making to propose an observation-based measure: observer OPTION 5 item. *Patient Educ Couns,* **93**, 265–271.

Hartasanchez, S. A., Grande, S. W., Montori, V. M., et al. 2022. Shared decision making process measures and patient problems. *Patient Educ Couns,* **105**, 2457–2465.

Hower, K. I., Vennedey, V., Hillen, H. A., et al. 2019. Implementation of patient-centred care: which organisational determinants matter from decision maker's perspective? Results from a qualitative interview study across various health and social care organisations. *BMJ Open,* **9**, e027591.

Kunneman, M. 2024. Shared decision-making to design care that fits for each patient. *Nat Rev Dis Primers,* **10**, 32.

Kunneman, M., Gionfriddo, M. R., Toloza, F. J. K., et al. 2019. Humanistic communication in the evaluation of shared -decision making: a systematic review. *Patient Educ Couns,* **102**, 452–466.

Kunneman, M., Hargraves, I. G., Sivly, A. L., et al. 2022. Co-creating sensible care plans using shared decision making: patients' reflections and observations of encounters. *Patient Educ Couns,* **105**, 1539–1544.

Kunneman, M., Poort, E. V. D., Zeeman, A., et al. 2024. 136 Setting the example? A videographic analysis of patient involvement in medical drama series. *BMJ Evid Based Med,* **29**, A61–A62.

Mandhana, D. M., Jacome, C. S., Ballard, D. I., et al. 2024. Developing and validating the Unhurried Conversations Assessment Tool (UCAT). *Patient Educ Couns,* **123**, 108237.

Ruissen, M. M., Montori, V. M., Hargraves, I. G., et al. 2023. Problem-based shared decision-making in diabetes care: a secondary analysis of video-recorded encounters. *BMJ Evid Based Med,* **28**, 157–163.

Scholl, I., Larussa, A., Hahlweg, P., Kobrin, S., Elwyn, G. 2018. Organizational- and system-level characteristics that influence implementation of shared decision-making and strategies to address them—a scoping review. *Implement Sci,* **13**, 40.

Scholl, I., Zill, J. M., Harter, M., Dirmaier, J. 2014. An integrative model of patient-centeredness—a systematic review and concept analysis. *PLoS One,* **9**, e107828.

Shay, L. A., Lafata, J. E. 2015. Where is the evidence? A systematic review of shared decision making and patient outcomes. *Med Decis Making,* **35**, 114–131.

Veatch, R. M. 1972. Models for ethical medicine in a revolutionary age. What physician–patient roles foster the most ethical relationship? *Hastings Cent Rep,* **2**, 5–7.

Veenendaal, H. V., Chernova, G., Bouman, C. M., Etten-Jamaludin, F. S. V., Dieren, S. V., Ubbink, D. T. 2023. Shared decision-making and the duration of medical consultations: a systematic review and meta-analysis. *Patient Educ Couns,* **107**, 107561.

Weller, J., Ceschi, A., Hirsch, L., Sartori, R., Costantini, A. 2018. Accounting for individual differences in decision-making competence: personality and gender differences. *Front Psychol,* **9**, 2258.

PART 4
Approaches to teaching and training

13 Shared decision making teaching frameworks

Tammy C. Hoffmann, Mina Bakhit, and Anna Waters

The importance of teaching shared decision making

Shared decision making (SDM) skills are not intuitive for most clinicians. Despite their clinical expertise, clinicians can find it difficult to communicate complex information comprehensibly, elicit patients' preferences and values, and foster collaborative decision making (Légaré et al., 2008). Patients often receive inadequate information and experience difficulty comprehending medical information, assessing risks, and articulating their preferences (Joseph-Williams et al., 2014). The mismatch between a collaborative decision making experience and what patients often experience highlights the need for explicitly training clinicians and student clinicians in SDM. The patient perspective box, later in this chapter (Box 13.1), contains reflections from a simulated patient with many years of involvement in helping student clinicians to develop skills in SDM.

It is worth noting that SDM skills are unlikely to be exhibited unless clinicians agree with the underpinning ethical principles of SDM, have a positive attitude towards it, and a willingness to learn them (Joseph-Williams et al., 2017). At its core, SDM is underpinned by the principles of good clinical practice, patients' right to know, and health decisions that should be based on patients' evidence-informed preferences and values (Elwyn et al., 2013; Hoffmann et al., 2014c). Many of the barriers to SDM uptake arise from clinicians' poor attitude to it and misperceptions about it, including the view that patients do not want to be involved in decisions or lack the capacity to be involved (Joseph-Williams et al., 2017), despite these misperceptions being refuted by research into patients' desires and capacity (Hoffmann et al., 2014a; Légaré et al., 2018). Therefore, SDM teaching must be more than skills; a core part is advocating for its uptake, addressing misperceptions, and facilitating learners' attitude towards its underlying rationale.

SDM relies on clinicians bringing together their skills in evidence-based practice and skills in patient communication (Hoffmann et al., 2014c). While SDM can be taught as a standalone subject, for student clinicians it is typically integrated into evidence-based practice or communication skills curricula (Hoffmann et al., 2014c; Simons et al., 2022). Ideally, SDM should be an integral component of undergraduate clinician training across all health disciplines, including medicine, nursing, and allied health. This early exposure is essential for ingraining SDM skills as habitual and integral aspects of clinical practice from the outset of a clinicians' career and has a positive impact on their SDM skills, confidence, and attitudes (Durand et al., 2018). Not all undergraduate health programmes include explicit SDM training and many clinicians will have graduated prior to SDM being incorporated into curricula, hence offering SDM training via postgraduate and continuing professional development opportunities is imperative to fostering a commitment to providing patient-centred decision making.

Overview of existing SDM teaching frameworks

Various frameworks have been developed to guide SDM teaching and practice. This chapter will overview some of the more widely used frameworks. Although there are some differences between the frameworks, all contain similar SDM fundamental principles and core elements. These include:

- Describing the options
- Discussing the benefits and harms of each option
- Learning about the patient and considering the patient's values and preferences
- Making or explicitly deferring individualized decisions.

The frameworks differ in their granularity of the steps and explicit inclusion of certain aspects of SDM.

The three-talk model

This model was developed to facilitate the training of clinicians in SDM (Elwyn et al., 2017). It divides the interaction between clinicians and patients into three types of 'talk' (Figure 13.1), with acknowledgement that the process is not always linear and conversations about decisions can be complex and recursive.

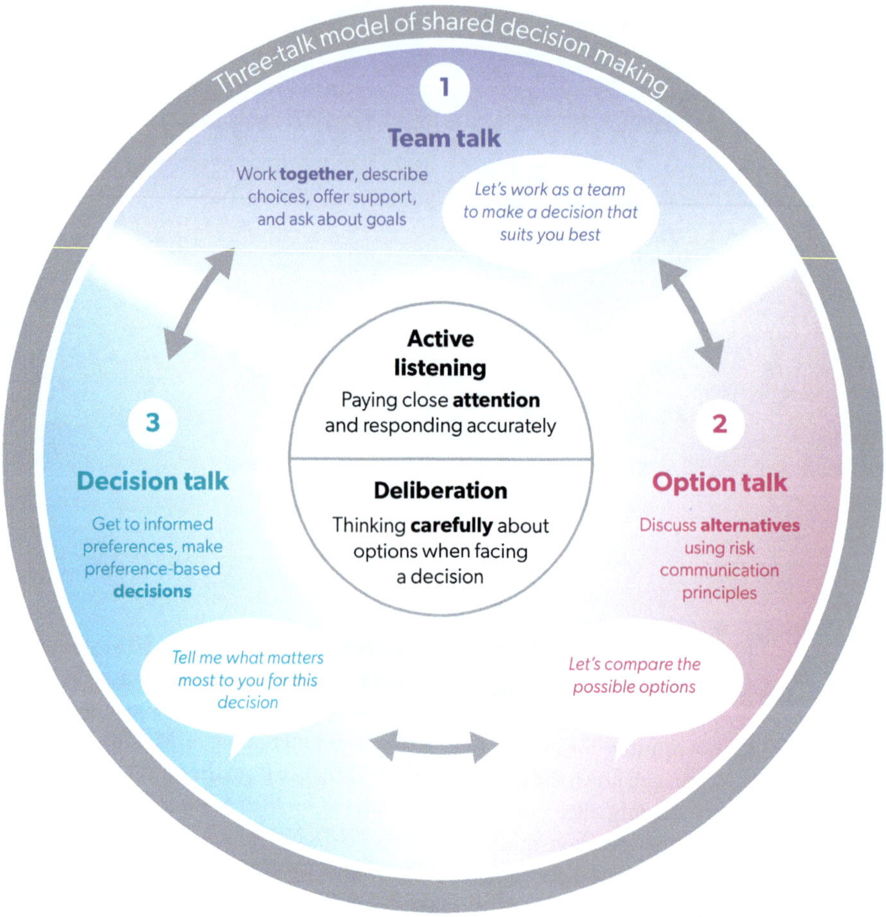

Figure 13.1 Three-talk model of SDM.

Reproduced with permission from Elwyn, G., Durand, M., Song, J., et al. 2017. A three-talk model for shared decision making: multistage consultation process. *BMJ*, 359, j4891.

Team talk serves as an initial and critical step in the process. It focuses on establishing a collaborative environment between the clinician and patient, emphasizing the importance of building a supportive partnership. Within this step, the clinician aims to make the patient aware of the available choices, provide necessary support, and identify the patient's health goals.

Option talk involves a detailed discussion about the available options. It includes effective communication of the potential harms and benefits of each option and aims to facilitate the patient's comprehension of the alternatives and aid in the decision making process.

Decision talk focuses on assisting the patient in making an informed decision based on their preferences and priorities and encourages patients to express what matters most to them in their healthcare journey. It emphasizes active listening and understanding the patient's unique circumstances and values, ultimately leading to a mutually agreed-upon decision that aligns with their goals and needs.

The Stiggelbout four-step framework

This framework distinguishes four steps in the SDM process, explicitly including a step where the clinician and patient discuss the patient's decisional role preference (Stiggelbout et al., 2015).

Step 1. Clinician informs the patient that a decision is to be made and that the patient's opinion is important

In this step, the clinician recognizes that options may lack clear, evidence-based solutions or involve options with differing outcomes. This creates a situation called 'equipoise', where the decision becomes preference-sensitive. The clinician explicitly informs the patient the decision depends on their personal values, emphasizing the need for the patient's input into decision making.

Step 2. Clinician explains the options and the pros and cons of each

Here, the clinician neutrally explains the available options, detailing their benefits and harms. Key considerations highlighted include the relevance and completeness of the information, the patient's prior knowledge, including how information about the risk is communicated (such as with percentages or natural frequencies), and ensuring, through stress-free communication checks, that the patient has understood the information conveyed.

Step 3. The discussion of patient preferences and supporting of deliberation

This step combines preference elicitation and deliberation, where patients form preferences via a deliberative process with the clinician.

The clinician explores the relevance of outcomes to the patient, using open questions and an explorative stance.

Step 4. Discussing the patient's wish to make the decision, making the decision, and discussing follow-up

The focus here is on the actual decision making phase. The patient's preferences for involvement in the decision making process are considered and the decision is made through a summary of the discussion and seeking the patient's opinion or confirmation. If needed, another appointment is scheduled; otherwise, both clinician and patient agree on the next steps, such as treatment, referrals, or follow-up consultations.

The SHARE approach

The SHARE approach (Seek, Help, Assess, Reach, Evaluate) is a five-step SDM process that involves comparing the available options and exploring the benefits and harms of each through a patient preference-centred dialogue (Agency for Healthcare Research and Quality, 2020).

Step 1. Seek your patient's participation

In this step, clinicians clearly communicate the existence of options to their patients and invite them to participate actively in the decision making process. The clinician needs to describe the problem clearly for the patient to understand that a decision needs to be made, emphasize the importance of their input, encourage questions, and facilitate discussion. The clinician should ask the patient to consider involving other family members or caregivers and reinforce the collaborative nature of the decision making process.

Step 2. Help your patient explore and compare treatment options

In Step 2, clinicians are advised to explore what their patients already know or understand about their condition or the available treatment options. Clinicians need to tell their patients about all available options, including watchful waiting, using plain language with clear differentiation between the specific options, the benefits and harms of each option, and highlighting the limitations of what is known and unknown about the options. This step can be facilitated by using evidence-based decision aids and other decision resources, which can be sent to the patient in advance, discussed with the patient during their visit, or given to the patient to review at home.

Step 3. Assess your patient's values and preferences

Clinicians should assess patient values and preferences by encouraging patients to discuss how the options might impact their lives. Clinicians should listen actively, utilize open-ended questions and show empathy. Acknowledging and paraphrasing patient values, aiming to agree on what matters most to the patient, fosters a collaborative decision making process.

Step 4. Reach a decision with your patient

Clinicians need to acknowledge that, especially for complex and irreversible options like surgery, patients may require time to identify their preferred option and may wish to consult with family, friends, or caregivers before deciding. To facilitate the decision making process, clinicians should check if the patient is ready to decide, offer additional information tools, and confirm decisions when the patient is ready to decide. Clinicians also need to verify the next steps needed, including communicating relevant timepoints and scheduling follow-up appointments.

Step 5. Evaluate your patient's decision

In this step, clinicians need to plan for future decision reviews after the decision has been made. They should remind patients that changes to the decision can be made if needed. It is important to monitor the implementation of decisions, assist patients in overcoming barriers, and, where relevant, provide access to self-management support programmes. Regularly revisiting decisions with the patient ensures ongoing support and helps determine the need for adjustments as necessary.

Five questions approach (as described by Hoffmann and colleagues)

Five questions can be used to guide clinicians through the process of learning SDM. The questions were initially developed for use by patients (Irwig et al., 2008), but the question wording and explanations were amended to provide clinicians with an easy-to-remember sequence of prompts for training clinicians in SDM (Hoffmann et al., 2014b). This approach emphasizes the importance of communicating the benefit and harm evidence for each option and explicitly articulates that the option of 'wait and watch' is often appropriate to present to patients.

Question 1. What will happen if the patient waits and watches?

Clinicians can begin by briefly explaining the process, clearly conveying there are choices to be made, that you (the clinician) will support them to make a decision collaboratively with you if they would like to, and by reassuring patients who may feel overwhelmed with decision making. In cases where the problem or diagnosis is clear, it is often relevant and important to provide information about the condition's natural history—that is, what is likely to happen without any intervention ('watch and wait'). Additionally, discussing the patient's expectations and experiences, including concerns and previously tried treatments is important. This allows for open discussion and correcting any misconceptions, either during this stage or later in the decision making process.

Question 2. What are the test or treatment options?

This question initiates a conversation about the available options (including the option of 'watching and seeing'—that is, not actively treating or testing if that is a reasonable option) and identifying patient-preferred options.

Question 3. What are the benefits and harms of each option?

This question facilitates a discussion about the benefits and harms of each option, including the likelihood or size of the benefit/s and harm/s of the options, based on evidence.

Question 4. How do the benefits and harms weigh up for the patient?

This question encourages clinicians and patients to weigh up the benefits and harms of the options, taking into account the patient's preferences, values, and circumstances.

Question 5. Does the patient have enough information to make a choice?

This encourages exploration of whether the patient is prepared to decide then or if they would like additional information, time, or the involvement of others before making a choice.

The importance of including patient perspectives in SDM teaching and approaches for doing so

Where possible, patient perspectives should be incorporated into SDM curriculum design and teaching to help learners consider SDM from this perspective and to foster an authentic patient-centred approach to decision making. There are various ways this can be done, depending on the teaching context and resources available.

Simulated patients, also known as simulated participants or standardized patients, are individuals tasked with representing various roles (e.g. patient, carer, or family member) in the context of educating and evaluating health professionals and students (Pritchard et al., 2020). Interactive teaching, when each learner has the chance to practise SDM skills with simulated patients (or ideally, but less likely to occur, patients), offers a unique opportunity for learners to receive helpful feedback from not only the academic/teaching staff, but also the 'patient'. This feedback loop aids learners in developing and refining crucial communication and SDM skills and provides insights into patient engagement intricacies (Cleland et al., 2009). Importantly, it allows learners to receive constructive feedback from the simulated patient—this can include feedback on what was communicated, how it was communicated, how the interaction made the patient feel, and improvements that could be made. This feedback is an invaluable element of SDM teaching as direct patient feedback on SDM processes in routine clinical situations is unlikely.

Some teaching programmes structure this learning activity so that a peer/another learner also observes the consultation between the learner and simulated patient and provides feedback. The opportunity to self-reflect and receive constructive feedback from a peer can help both the student who participated in the consultation and the student who observed it. Although using simulated patients can be resource intensive, the learners and simulated patients often comment on the value of this interactive experience in the development of SDM skills (Ritter et al., 2019)—see Box 13.1.

When developing and providing patient-centred SDM teaching, actively involving patients in the curriculum development and revision process is valuable. This collaborative engagement should ideally commence during the creation of courses/teaching materials and continue during periodic revisions of the curriculum, including the assessment tasks, to ensure the content remains current and aligned with patients' evolving needs (Jha et al., 2009).

Integrating patient narratives, testimonials, and video interviews into teaching can provide learners with authentic and nuanced perspectives on diverse patient journeys (Socal, 2020), which can foster a deeper understanding of the patient side of the consultation and illness journey. Inviting patients and caregivers to share their experiences and insights through panel discussions or guest lectures enables students to hear first-hand accounts of experiences with the healthcare system and decision making and provides the opportunity to ask questions. For example, genuine anonymized case studies can be useful in illuminating the complexity of health scenarios as they can illustrate clinicians' actual behaviour in a clinical situation and highlight the importance of considering patients' values and preferences (Dresselhaus et al., 2004).

Box 13.1 Patient perspective

Insights and reflection from a simulated patient of being involved with SDM teaching

For 14 years, I have been dedicated to my role as a simulated participant at two universities, contributing to training in multiple disciplines such as medicine, dietetics, physiotherapy, occupational therapy, and pharmacy.

Reflecting on my experience, I have identified several challenges that students commonly face during SDM sessions. Firstly, some struggle with using the decision aids appropriately, often encountering them for the first time. It is important that they are taught how to use them effectively and that the patient can understand what is being pointed out. Secondly, pinpointing patient needs can prove challenging for some, hindering their ability to identify the motivating factors that are crucial for informed decision making. Thirdly, the first student in an SDM learning group faces a disadvantage, lacking the insights gained from observing their peers in previous SDM sessions. Fourthly, students' beliefs and previous experiences are sometimes apparent and can influence students towards supporting certain decisions during their discussion with patients. Although they are taught the importance of putting aside their own beliefs and preferences, it is during encounters like this that the reality of doing so becomes apparent, often for the first time. Finally, some students default to authoritative roles rather than actively involving the patient in decision making and some prefer to solve the problem themselves rather than fostering genuine patient involvement.

Despite these challenges, engaging in multiple SDM sessions with students reveals a discernible improvement in their skills over time and often a positive shift in their attitude, highlighting the absolute value of this experiential learning approach.

Speaking as a patient, being actively involved in decision making is crucial, as is being viewed as an individual rather than a mere diagnostic case. Building rapport and understanding the nuances of a patient's life are key factors in facilitating SDM. When patients or their family members are included in the decision making process, they gain a sense of ownership and control over their situation. This is particularly advantageous when aiming to change behaviours, as people are more receptive when they feel involved in the decision making and are not just told what to do.

SDM teaching challenges and areas for future research

Most SDM approaches focus on the interaction between a patient and a clinician and do not cover specific principles to guide decision making in other situations, such as when an interdisciplinary team is involved or when more parties than only an individual patient and clinician are involved (Stacey et al., 2010). This focus on dyadic clinical encounters tends to be reflected in most SDM teaching. In many clinical situations, the involvement of an interdisciplinary team is crucial and while the optimal approach to prepare students for this collaborative process remains uncertain, some recent studies of SDM teaching have evaluated an interprofessional teaching approach with positive evaluations (e.g. Kienlin et al., 2022). It has also been suggested that an interprofessional approach to SDM teaching may reduce some barriers to SDM uptake by clinicians post-training (Boland et al., 2019). Similarly, teaching SDM skills for situations where it extends beyond a dyadic relationship, such as involving a child–parent–clinician or patient–caregiver–clinician triad (Bracher et al., 2020), remains an underexplored area. Having SDM skills for such consultations is important as consultations for children form a large part of clinical practice, and in some cultures, family-centred health decision making is prevalent.

There is much diversity in SDM teaching, including the combination of topics that are taught, the conceptual models used, and the delivery (e.g. face-to-face role-playing, group-based discussion, online platforms) (Légaré et al., 2012; Coates and Clerke, 2020; Lehane et al., 2023). Core competencies, which are the minimal set of a combination of attributes, such as applied knowledge, skills, and attitudes, that enable an individual to perform a set of tasks to an appropriate standard efficiently and effectively are often used in health education to ensure clarity and a shared language about the essential skills needed for the optimal performance of a behaviour. While SDM has been included within the core competencies needed to perform evidence-based practice (Albarqouni et al., 2018), consensus on a detailed set of SDM core competencies does not yet exist (Légaré et al., 2013). Even if agreement is attained, SDM teaching should be tailored according to the target learners' needs and experience as there will be distinct needs at different levels of clinical experience (such as undergraduate versus experienced clinicians (Baghus et al., 2021)) and across various disciplines (e.g. some health professions have a need to explain diagnostic options and the relevant evidence and this can require tailored training (Driever et al., 2022)).

While face-to-face teaching has proven effective in enhancing confidence and knowledge among undergraduate students in SDM (Durand et al., 2018), its accessibility poses a significant obstacle for postgraduate students and continuing professional development offerings. There is an urgent need to explore, and evaluate, alternative methods for delivering SDM teaching, including online, virtual, and self-directed learning approaches to address this limitation (Hoffmann et al., 2021). While these alternative teaching formats offer convenience for busy clinicians, one of the difficulties with online teaching is that it lacks the interactive communication and immediacy of feedback on the learner's performance. While it is possible to have students type the text that they would say, this method falls short in replicating the dynamic interactions that occur between a learner and a simulated patient during face-to-face activities. Potential resolution to this challenge may be possible using artificial intelligence and virtual patients (e.g. solutions like the Keele Virtual Patient: https://www.keelevp.com/virtual-patient/shared-decision-making). Technological advancements hold promise for providing opportunities for practical skill development, particularly for online interactive teaching.

When alternate teaching formats are used, they are rarely evaluated and their effectiveness is unknown. However, challenges also exist for assessing face-to-face teaching, with variation in how SDM teaching is assessed, ranging from self-assessment to objective structured clinical examinations. Evaluating the effectiveness and impact of SDM teaching requires a careful approach to selecting appropriate metrics and assessment tools, which are lacking (Singh Ospina et al., 2020). SDM's multifaceted nature demands a comprehensive evaluation strategy. Metrics should encompass traditional measures of knowledge acquisition and factors such as communication skills and patient satisfaction (Singh Ospina et al., 2020). Assessment tools must be sensitive to the dynamic and context-dependent nature of SDM, capturing nuances in evidence communication, empathy, and the use of decision aids (Brouwers et al., 2017). A balanced combination of qualitative and quantitative methods may offer a more holistic understanding of whether intended educational outcomes were achieved.

Summary

This chapter has addressed the importance of SDM teaching and overviewed four of the possible frameworks that can be used to help teach it. It also explored the value of incorporating patient perspectives into SDM teaching and some of the ways this can be done, such as with simulated patients. The chapter concluded by discussing some of the challenges in SDM teaching and where additional research is needed to guide SDM teaching.

REFERENCES

Agency for Healthcare Research and Quality. 2020. *The SHARE Approach: A model for shared decision-making-fact sheet.* Agency for Healthcare Research and Quality.

Albarqouni, L., Hoffmann, T., Straus, S., et al. 2018. Core competencies in evidence-based practice for health professionals: consensus statement based on a systematic review and Delphi survey. *JAMA Netw Open,* **1**, e180281.

Baghus, A., Giroldi, E., Muris, J., et al. 2021. Identifying entrustable professional activities for shared decision making in postgraduate medical education: a national Delphi study. *Acad Med,* **96**, 126–133.

Boland, L., Lawson, M., Graham, I., et al. 2019. Post-training shared decision making barriers and facilitators for pediatric healthcare providers: a mixed-methods study. *Acad Pediatr,* **19**, 118–129.

Bracher, M., Stewart, S., Reidy, C., Allen, C., Townsend, K., Brindle, L. 2020. Partner involvement in treatment-related decision making in triadic clinical consultations—a systematic review of qualitative and quantitative studies. *Patient Educ Couns,* **103**, 245–253.

Brouwers, M., Rasenberg, E., Van Weel, C., Laan, R., Van Weel-Baumgarten, E. 2017. Assessing patient-centred communication in teaching: a systematic review of instruments. *Med Educ,* **51**, 1103–1117.

Cleland, J., Abe, K., Rethans, J. 2009. The use of simulated patients in medical education: AMEE Guide No 42. *Med Teach,* **31**, 477–486.

Coates, D., Clerke, T. 2020. Training interventions to equip healthcare professionals with shared decision-making skills: a systematic scoping review. *J Contin Educ Health Prof,* **40**, 100–119.

Dresselhaus, T., Peabody, J., Luck, J., Bertenthal, D. 2004. An evaluation of vignettes for predicting variation in the quality of preventive care. *J Gen Intern Med,* **19**, 1013–1018.

Driever, E., Stiggelbout, A., Brand, P. 2022. Shared decision-making in different types of decisions in medical specialist consultations. *J Gen Intern Med,* **37**, 2966–2972.

Durand, M. A., Dimilia, P. R., Song, J., Yen, R. W., Barr, P. J. 2018. Shared decision making embedded in the undergraduate medical curriculum: a scoping review. *PLoS One,* **13**, e0207012.

Elwyn, G., Durand, M., Song, J., et al. 2017. A three-talk model for shared decision making: multistage consultation process. *BMJ,* **359**, j4891.

Elwyn, G., Tilburt, J., Montori, V. 2013. The ethical imperative for shared decision-making. *Eur J Pers Cent Healthc,* **1**, 129–131.

Hoffmann, T., Bennett, S., Tomsett, C., Del Mar, C. 2014a. Brief training of student clinicians in shared decision making: a single-blind randomized controlled trial. *J Gen Intern Med,* **29**, 844–849.

Hoffmann, T., Del Mar, C., Santhirapala, R., Freeman, A. 2021. Teaching clinicians shared decision making and risk communication online: an evaluation study. *BMJ Evid Based Med,* **26**, 253.

Hoffmann, T., Légaré, F., Simmons, M., et al. 2014b. Shared decision making: what do clinicians need to know and why should they bother? *Med J Aust,* **201**, 35–39.

Hoffmann, T., Montori, V., Del Mar, C. 2014c. The connection between evidence-based medicine and shared decision making. *JAMA,* **312**, 1295–1296.

Irwig, L., Irwig, J., Trevena, L., Sweet, M. 2008. *Smart Health Choices: Making Sense of Health Advice.* Hammersmith Press.

Jha, V., Quinton, N., Bekker, H., Roberts, T. 2009. Strategies and interventions for the involvement of real patients in medical education: a systematic review. *Med Educ,* **43**, 10–20.

Joseph-Williams, N., Elwyn, G., Edwards, A. 2014. Knowledge is not power for patients: a systematic review and thematic synthesis of patient-reported barriers and facilitators to shared decision making. *Patient Educ Couns,* **94**, 291–309.

Joseph-Williams, N., Lloyd, A., Edwards, A., et al. 2017. Implementing shared decision making in the NHS: lessons from the MAGIC programme. *BMJ,* **357**, j1744.

Kienlin, S., Stacey, D., Nytrøen, K., Grafe, A., Kasper, J. 2022. Ready for SDM-evaluation of an interprofessional training module in shared decision-making: a cluster randomized trial. *Patient Educ Couns,* **105**, 2307–2314.

Légaré, F., Adekpedjou, R., Stacey, D., et al. 2018. Interventions for increasing the use of shared decision making by healthcare professionals. *Cochrane Database Syst Rev,* **7**, CD006732.

Légaré, F., Moumjid-Ferdjaoui, N., Drolet, R., et al. 2013. Core competencies for shared decision making training programs: insights from an international, interdisciplinary working group. *J Contin Educ Health Prof,* **33**, 267–273.

Légaré, F., Politi, M. C., Drolet, R., Desroches, S., Stacey, D., Bekker, H. 2012. Training health professionals in shared decision-making: an international environmental scan. *Patient Educ Couns,* **88**, 159–169.

Légaré, F., Ratté, S., Gravel, K., Graham, I. 2008. Barriers and facilitators to implementing shared decision-making in clinical practice: update of a systematic review of health professionals' perceptions. *Patient Educ Couns,* **73**, 526–535.

Lehane, E., Curtin, C., Corrigan, M. 2023. Teaching strategies for shared decision-making within the context of evidence-based healthcare practice: a scoping review. *Patient Educ Couns,* **109**, 107630.

Pritchard, S., Denning, T., Keating, J., Blackstock, F., Nestel, D. 2020. 'It's not an acting job. Don't underestimate what a simulated patient does': a qualitative study exploring the perspectives of simulated patients in health professions education. *Simul Healthc,* **15**, 21–29.

Ritter, S., Stirnemann, J., Breckwoldt, J., et al. 2019. Shared decision-making training in internal medicine: a multisite intervention study. *J Grad Med Educ,* **11**, 146–151.

Simons, M., Rapport, F., Zurynski, Y., Stoodley, M., Cullis, J., Davidson, A. 2022. Links between evidence-based medicine and shared decision-making in courses for doctors in training: a scoping review. *BMJ Open,* **12**, e057335.

Singh Ospina, N., Toloza, F., Barrera, F., Bylund, C., Erwin, P., Montori, V. 2020. Educational programs to teach shared decision making to medical trainees: a systematic review. *Patient Educ Couns,* **103**, 1082–1094.

Socal, M. 2020. Patient narratives: a tool for people-centered health systems education. *Med Sci Educ,* **30**, 1437–1443.

Stacey, D., Légaré, F., Pouliot, S., Kryworuchko, J., Dunn, S. 2010. Shared decision making models to inform an interprofessional perspective on decision making: a theory analysis. *Patient Educ Couns,* **80**, 164–172.

Stiggelbout, A., Pieterse, A., De Haes, J. 2015. Shared decision making: concepts, evidence, and practice. *Patient Educ Couns,* **98**, 1172–1179.

14

Best Case/Worst Case

A framework to improve medical communication and decision making in high-risk and uncertainty situations

Melanie Fritz, Amy Zelenski, Margaret Schwarze, and Kathy Kastner

Introduction

We introduce our Best Case/Worst Case (BC/WC) tool by using a case study to indicate the need for such an intervention (Box 14.1).

What went wrong? The surgeon followed principles of both informed consent and shared decision making, offering alternatives, and describing risk. Yet, standard-practice risk prediction fails to help patients and families imagine the experience of major surgery. Families interpret an 80% chance of dying, having kidney failure, or respiratory failure as meaning there is a 20% chance of surgery returning them swiftly to their previous level of function. However, clinicians know that this is not the full story and that any major surgery has significant consequences for well-being and can come with serious complications. Ms Moore and her family were facing decisions under conditions that they had not previously experienced. Although the consequences of surgery are frequently described as a series of numerically conveyed risks, this did not help Ms Moore or her family envision how her choices might play out over the next days, weeks, or months.

Box 14.1 Case study: a life-threatening aortic aneurysm

Ms Moore is a 78-year-old woman who has chronic renal insufficiency, chronic obstructive pulmonary disease requiring 2 litres of home oxygen, and limited mobility due to arthritis. She arrived at the hospital with a tender thoracoabdominal aneurysm—an aneurysm that would lead to her death within a short time.

The attending vascular surgeon had a long conversation with the patient and her family to discuss surgery, noting important statistics such as a 50% chance of dying from surgery, a 60% chance of being on lifelong dialysis following surgery, and an 80% chance of being on a ventilator for a prolonged period. The surgeon also offered an alternative, comfort-focused palliative care. After considering these options, the patient and her family decided to move forward with surgery.

The patient then had a 10-hour operation through an incision across her chest and abdomen, followed by transfer to the intensive care unit (ICU), intubated, for routine postoperative monitoring and resuscitation. Rounding the following day, the surgical team found she was doing as well as they might have hoped for after this major urgent operation: passing urine, not requiring blood products, and on minimal vasopressors. Her family arrived later and saw their loved one with tubes coming out of her nose, mouth, chest, abdomen, and bladder, and with swollen arms and legs. She was unable to interact with them. They were horrified. They told the surgical team that this was not what she would have wanted and asked the team to withdraw all her life-supporting treatments.

Ms Moore's case is not unique; evidence suggests that many older adults in the USA receive high-intensity treatments at the end of life that may be inconsistent with their preferences and treatment goals (Fried et al., 2002). The BC/WC communication tool was initially developed for challenging treatment decisions for frail older adults. Yet it applies to other settings with high uncertainty and treatment burdens. It can help patients with serious illness understand prognosis and treatment options, weigh trade-offs, and articulate what they would and would not be willing to tolerate. In the patient perspective box (Box 14.2), Kathy Kastner, a noted patient advocate, describes how BC/WC benefits patients and families.

What is BC/WC?

The BC/WC communication tool uses scenario planning and a graphic aid to help patients and their loved ones make decisions when there are two reasonable options, high uncertainty, and high burdens of treatment. It is designed to help manage uncertainty, as the clinician describes a plausible story about each treatment option, including the best-case, worst-case, and most likely scenarios. It has two components: (1) a graphic aid and (2) the use of scenario planning to support decision making.

Graphic aid

The graphic aid is a simple diagram (Figure 14.1) that illustrates two options (Schwarze et al., 2013). Each line represents a possible

Box 14.2 Patient perspective

BC/WC as a communication tool

BC/WC is a communication tool for patients and families. It uses scenario planning to illustrate treatment options, acknowledge uncertainty, and clearly convey critical information about longer-term prognosis.

Patients and their families are often focused on the immediate medical procedure or intervention and are ill-equipped to understand the long-term possible consequences of difficult decisions. This can be a barrier to shared decision making.

BC/WC helps patients imagine what it is like to actually have (and recover from) surgery. This chapter explains how telling a story helps patients imagine an unfamiliar and complex experience, thus preparing for decisions based on what matters to them. The goal is to combine knowledge about the patient's overall health and medical condition to give patients and families your best estimate of what is most likely to happen. BC/WC walks patients and their loved ones through the after-intervention outcomes, helping patients and families know that even with treatment or intervention on this problem, things will not be the same as they were before.

treatment. The star at the top of each line represents the best-case scenario, the box at the bottom represents the worst-case scenario, and the oval in the middle represents the most likely scenario. The visual representation helps patients follow along in the moment and supports recall and future deliberation.

Scenario planning: a plausible story about the best, worst, and most likely scenarios

Scenario planning is a strategy for navigating uncertainty and supporting decision making. Initially developed for military planning, and subsequently used in the field of economics, scenario planning converts a series of probabilities into narratives to describe a range of plausible futures (Wack 1985a, 1985b; Schwarze and Taylor, 2017). Narratives encourage decision makers to imagine a variety of outcomes and how these outcomes respond to forces that drive change. Critically, for clinical decision making, scenario planning acknowledges uncertainty by allowing clinicians to say, 'While I cannot predict the future, if all goes well, this is what is likely to follow, and if things go poorly, this is what we can expect'. Best- and worst-case narratives connect events (e.g. surgery) to underlying medical conditions (e.g. chronic pulmonary disease) while elucidating the unknown (e.g. how a patient responds to treatment) and allow decision makers to envision a range of outcomes.

What is the best-case scenario for Ms Moore?

With surgery, the best-case scenario is that she has a 10-hour surgery and then goes to the ICU. If things go well, the breathing tube will be removed within a few days. She will stay in the ICU with lots of tubes and catheters connected to her body for about a week. When she leaves the ICU, she will need more time in the hospital to recover from this big operation. Even in the best case, she will be much weaker than before, and lose a fair amount of her functional

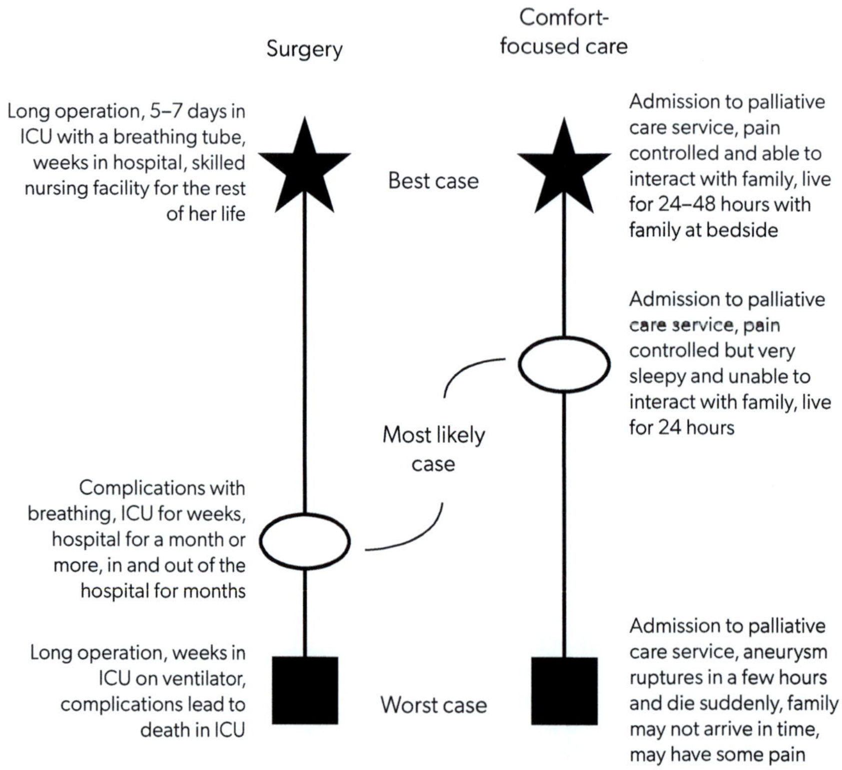

Figure 14.1 Example of the graphic aid component of the BC/WC tool for Ms Moore, who is facing a life-threatening aneurysm. The star represents the best case, the box represents the worst case, and the oval designates the most likely scenario. The location of the oval indicates where the most likely scenario is in relationship to the best case or the worst case. The clinician writes notes to document key parts of each story.

Adapted with permission from Schwarze, M. L., Kehler, J. M., Campbell, T. C. 2013. Navigating high-risk procedures with more than just a street map. *J Palliat Med*, 16, 1169–1171.

status. Given she was barely making it at home before surgery, it is hard to imagine her going home after surgery, so she will either need a nursing home or round-the-clock care at home for the remainder of her life, which is maybe a few years given her other medical problems.

What is the worst-case scenario?

The worst-case scenario with surgery is that she has a very long operation and goes to the ICU. Afterwards, there are complications, for example, kidney failure. She then has complication after complication, and her clinicians are unable to remove the breathing tube safely. The complications add up, and after weeks in the ICU it is clear she is not going to get off the ventilator. Her family, together with her clinicians, decides to withdraw life-sustaining treatment, and she dies.

What is the most likely scenario?

The most likely scenario, given her underlying kidney disease, lung disease, and arthritis, is probably closer to the worst case than the best. Although she gets off the ventilator in the ICU after a week, she still has multiple complications during her hospital course and is in the hospital for weeks to months. She leaves the hospital but still needs a lot of support in another institution. She is in and out of the hospital for months and then dies within a few months of surgery from complications and her other health problems.

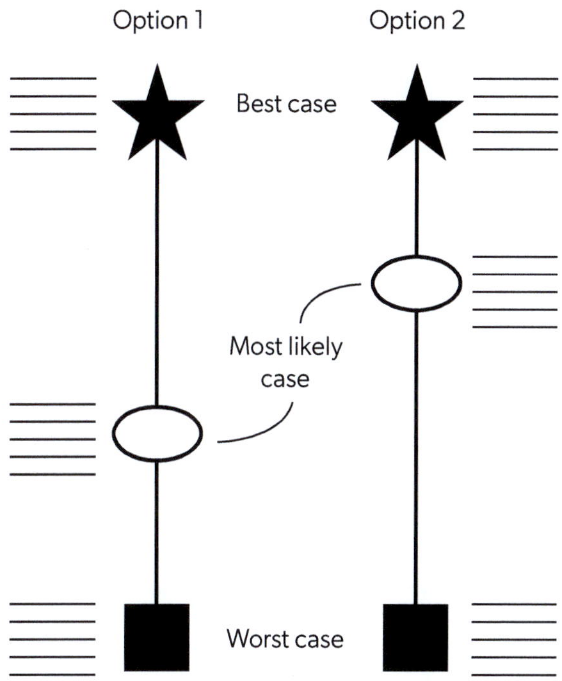

Figure 14.2 Example of the graphic aid template for BC/WC. There is space next to the best case (star), worst case (square), and most likely scenario (oval) to write key elements about the story.

Adapted with permission from Schwarze, M. L., Kehler, J. M., Campbell, T. C. 2013. Navigating high-risk procedures with more than just a street map. *J Palliat Med*, 16, 1169–1171.

Steps for using BC/WC

1. *Break bad news*: since these conversations often occur in the setting of very serious illness, patients and their loved ones need space to recognize the gravity of the situation. Presenting a choice between surgery or hospice may be difficult to hear for patients who have been living well, even with serious chronic illness, before an acute event. You might say, 'This is bad news. It's going to change her life. I worry she could die, even with surgery'. Using a headline like this one places the current clinical issue in the context of a patient's larger health picture, helping patients and their loved ones understand that things will be different than before.
2. *Draw the graphic aid*: the graphic aid (Figure 14.2) is best generated prior to talking with the patient to gather your thoughts, or it can be created in the moment. For each option, draw a star at the top, and a box at the bottom, connected by a vertical line. The most likely outcome is located somewhere along this line. It might be close to the best-case or worst-case scenario, or it might be in the middle. The strategy is to combine your knowledge about the patient's overall health to give patients and families your best estimate of what is most likely to happen. Make note of the key elements of the stories you tell about each scenario on the graphic aid next to best case, worst case, and most likely case.
3. *Tell a story*: translate the statistics you know into stories about how the patient might experience these possibilities. Tell a story with a beginning, middle, and end. Include details about short- and long-term recovery, tangible long-term outcomes including functional status, and how the treatment option affects the larger context of the patient's overall health.
4. *Elicit preferences*: to understand how patients and families feel about what you have just described with BC/WC, ask questions like, 'How are you thinking about this?' or 'What is important to you now?' If the patient is too ill to speak for themself, you might prompt their surrogate by asking, 'What would your loved one say about this?'

   This step is difficult because clinicians are used to asking for treatment preferences rather than learning more about how patients feel about what might happen under the conditions described. Telling stories helps patients understand the limits of what is possible and gives them words to articulate their feelings about events like prolonged intubation or loss of independence.

   If a patient says, 'I want to live', this is not enough information—it is a statement about emotion, not a statement about priorities or preferences. After empathically attending to this emotion, invite the patient to share more about their preferences for life after treatment. In the case of Ms Moore, we can imagine that prompting her, 'Say more about your feelings about being on a breathing machine after surgery', would have revealed that prolonged intubation was not in line with her preferences, which could have guided decision making.

   You might also ask, 'Tell me what you hope life looks like after treatment'. If a patient's response to this prompt aligns with the scenarios you have described, you can feel confident that moving forward with treatment is consistent with their values. If their response does not align, you can share your concern that surgery will not achieve what they hoped for and ask them to consider what is important to them now.

5. *Make a recommendation*: some believe autonomy requires that patients choose from the treatment options provided. Yet, this can engender feelings of abandonment. Rather than asking patients to choose to support their autonomy, clinicians might consider a relational autonomy approach. We all expect that the professionals in our lives will use their expertise to help us make a decision that is right for us. Similarly, patients have expectations that clinicians will use their expertise to support their navigation of a new and often confusing health problem (Quill 1996; Mackenzie, 2008). Use the knowledge you gain about what is valuable to them to explain which treatment option is likely to support their priorities.

   To make a recommendation, explain how what you've learned from them has helped you arrive at this recommendation. You might say, 'I'm hearing that she was fiercely protective of her independence. I'm worried that, even in the best case with surgery, she would spend several months in a nursing home and die there. Given what I know about her, I recommend we focus on her comfort now.' Using language like, 'This is how I am thinking about this; tell me if it fits with what's important to you', allows space for patients and families to disagree and extend the conversation, so you can be sure that your final plan is valuable to them (Fried, 2016). In the patient perspective box (Box 14.3), Kathy Kastner notes how BC/WC can help navigate power differentials in the clinical setting.

Evidence for BC/WC

BC/WC uses Elwyn's three-talk model (Elwyn, 2017) as a conceptual model to support deliberation in the context of life-threatening illness. It was initially evaluated and refined through focus groups with older adults and surgeons from private and academic medical practices in Wisconsin, USA (Kruser et al., 2015; The Patient Preferences Project, 2016). Focus group participants noted the tool was flexible enough to support a range of priorities and health states, and it would facilitate deliberation.

At the University of Wisconsin, we taught BC/WC to 25 surgeons and conducted a pre- and post-intervention analysis of decision making conversations with adults over 65 with acute surgical problems. Qualitative analysis of transcribed conversations demonstrated a marked shift in conversation structure with BC/WC, and median Observer OPTION-5 scores were significantly higher with less variation. This pilot study was not designed or powered to show efficacy (Kruser et al., 2017; Taylor et al., 2017).

Blumenthaler et al. (2023) compared, in video simulation, BC/WC to a traditional risk/benefit framework for discussing surgery for advanced cancer with acute gastrointestinal obstruction. This study found no preference for BC/WC in comparison to a risk/benefit model, although patients reported that BC/WC inspired higher confidence in surgeon trustworthiness than the risk/benefit video. Additionally, patients who preferred BC/WC had lower reported rates of trust in the medical profession than those who preferred the risk/benefit framework or had no preference (Blumenthaler et al., 2023).

Box 14.3 Patient perspective

Best- and worst-case narratives connect events

Best- and worst-case narratives connect events (e.g. surgery) to underlying medical conditions (e.g. chronic lung disease) while clarifying the unknown (e.g. how a patient responds to treatment) and allow decision makers to envision a range of outcomes.

With the power imbalance of highly trained and experienced doctors, and vulnerable patients and families, BC/WC helps promote mutually respectful shared decision making. Clinicians who may worry that making a recommendation is a setup for conflict if patients disagree, there is suggested language: 'This is how I think about this, so tell me if it fits with what's important to you' allows space for patients and families to disagree while preserving the clinician–patient relationship.

Applications outside acute care surgery

BC/WC has been adapted to support discussions in other settings. Our group has adapted BC/WC for nephrologists to support discussions about dialysis initiation with older frail patients with end-stage kidney disease (The Patient Preferences Project, 2019). This adaptation encourages nephrologists to share two possible paths with patients: life with and without dialysis. BC/WC in this setting describes patients' health trajectories with and without dialysis, conveys information about prognosis, and acknowledges uncertainty. This adaptation is currently under evaluation as part of a multisite randomized clinical trial (Zimmermann et al., 2020; Haug et al., 2022).

Similar challenges confront hepatologists who are discussing treatment with patients who have advanced liver disease. These conversations may inadvertently invoke a false binary: that liver transplant listing is a pathway to cure and life without transplant represents certain impending death. The adaptation of the BC/WC tool for this patient population describes the best- and worst-case scenarios for life with transplant listing and life without transplant listing (Ufere et al., 2023).

BC/WC has also been adapted for older adults with cancer. Stakeholder focus groups noted how BC/WC would support patient understanding of available treatment options, consider trade-offs, and deliberate. For patients who proceed with one treatment path but encounter toxic side effects or cancer recurrence, the initial BC/WC aid can provide context for discussing new options (Wong et al., 2022).

We have also adapted BC/WC for the trauma ICU (BC/WC-ICU). Instead of comparing discrete treatment options, BC/WC-ICU combines scenario planning with a daily description of the relationship between major events and prognosis to illustrate uncertainty and possible long-term trajectories (The Patient Preferences Project, 2020). Sharing prognostic information throughout the patient's ICU course provides context for subsequent treatment decisions, such as additional surgery or long-term ventilatory support. Discussing this information routinely facilitates families' awareness of the life-limiting nature of serious injury, providing space to consider whether comfort-focused care is more aligned with the patient's goals. This adaptation is currently being evaluated through a randomized clinical trial at eight major trauma centres (Zimmermann et al., 2021).

Summary

In summary, BC/WC uses scenario planning and a graphic aid to support shared decision making so that patients and families can understand the limits of what is possible, anticipate and prepare for the experience of treatment, and navigate the uncertainty that is so common and stressful in the setting of life-limiting illness.

It takes practice and intention to change the strategies clinicians have traditionally used to approach decision making. Our group has developed a curriculum for surgical residents focused on communication skills and decision making, including BC/WC, and we are in the process of disseminating and testing the impact of these educational tools. A series of videos about BC/WC are publicly available to support anyone seeking to learn more or practice using this new approach (The Patient Preferences Project 2016).

Acknowledgements

The writing of this book chapter was supported by the National Cancer Institute of Health under Award T32CA090217. The content is solely the responsibility of the authors and does not necessarily represent the official views of the National Institutes of Health.

REFERENCES

Blumenthaler, A. N., Robinson, K. A., Hodge, C., et al. 2023. Communication frameworks for palliative surgical consultations: a randomized study of advanced cancer patients. *Ann Surg*, **278**, e1110–e1117.

Elwyn G., Durand, M. A., Song, J., et al. 2017. A three-talk model for shared decision making: multistage consultation process. *BMJ*, **359**, j4891.

Fried, T. R. 2016. Shared decision making—finding the sweet spot. *N Engl J Med*, **374**, 104–106.

Fried, T. R., Bradley, E. H., Towle, V. R., Allore, H. 2002. Understanding the treatment preferences of seriously ill patients. *N Engl J Med*, **346**, 1061–1066.

Haug, K., Buffington, A., Zelenski, A., et al. 2022. Best Case/Worst Case: protocol for a multisite randomised clinical trial of a scenario planning intervention for patients with kidney failure. *BMJ Open*, **12**, e067258.

Kruser, J. M., Nabozny, M. J., Steffens, N. M., et al. 2015. 'Best Case/Worst Case': qualitative evaluation of a novel communication tool for difficult in-the-moment surgical decisions. *J Am Geriatr Soc*, **63**, 1805–1811.

Kruser, J. M., Taylor, L. J., Campbell, T. C., et al. 2017. 'Best Case/Worst Case': training surgeons to use a novel communication tool for high-risk acute surgical problems. *J Pain Symptom Manage*, **53**, 711–719. e5.

Mackenzie, C. 2008. Relational autonomy, normative authority and perfectionism. *J Soc Philos*, **39**, 512–533.

Quill, T. E. 1996. Physician recommendations and patient autonomy: finding a balance between physician power and patient choice. *Ann Intern Med*, **125**, 763–769.

Schwarze, M. L., Kehler, J. M., Campbell, T. C. 2013. Navigating high risk procedures with more than just a street map. *J Palliat Med*, **16**, 1169–1171.

Schwarze, M. L., Taylor, L. J. 2017. Managing uncertainty—harnessing the power of scenario planning. *N Engl J Med*, **377**, 206–208.

Taylor, L. J., Nabozny, M. J., Steffens, N. M., et al. 2017. A framework to improve surgeon communication in high-stakes surgical decisions: Best Case/Worst Case. *JAMA Surg*, **152**, 531–538.

The Patient Preferences Project. 2016. Best Case/Worst Case (BC/WC) surgeon communication tool—whiteboard video. 29 March. Available at: https://www.youtube.com/watch?v=FnS3K44sbu0&t=107s

The Patient Preferences Project. 2019. Best Case/Worst Case (BC/WC) nephrologist communication tool—whiteboard video. 5 August. Available at: https://youtu.be/oXfXr7koz_A?si=RsTr6PGqvFfWQ97Q

The Patient Preferences Project. 2020. Best Case/Worst Case (BC/WC) intensive care communication tool—whiteboard video. 19 October. Available at: https://youtu.be/31pv2Rlp6R4?si=Bsf2kuMCmPnAtGYa

Ufere, N. N., El-Jawahri, A., Ritchie, C., Lai, J. C., Schwarze, M. L. 2023. Promoting prognostic understanding and health equity for patients with advanced liver disease: using 'Best Case/Worst Case'. *Gastroenterology*, **164**, 171–176.

Wack, P. 1985a. Shooting the rapids. *Harv Bus Rev*, November. Available at: https://hbr.org/1985/11/scenariosshooting-the-rapids

Wack, P. 1985b. Uncharted waters ahead. *Harv Bus Rev*, September. Available at: https://hbr.org/1985/09/scenarios-uncharted-waters-ahead

Wong, M. L., Nicosia, F. M., Smith, A. K., et al. 2022. 'You have to be sure that the patient has the full picture': adaptation of the Best Case/Worst Case communication tool for geriatric oncology. *J Geriatr Oncol*, **13**, 606–613.

Zimmermann, C. J., Jhagroo, R. A., Wakeen, M., et al. 2020. Opportunities to improve shared decision making in dialysis decisions for older adults with life-limiting kidney disease: a pilot study. *J Palliat Med*, **23**, 627–634.

Zimmermann, C. J., Zelenski, A. B., Buffington, A., et al. 2021. Best Case/Worst Case for the trauma ICU: development and pilot testing of a communication tool for older adults with traumatic injury. *J Trauma Acute Care Surg*, **91**, 542–551.

15

Innovations in shared decision making teaching

Pål Gulbrandsen, Arwen H. Pieterse, and Arne Lein

Introduction

Shared decision making (SDM) emerged as a concept in 1972 (Veatch, 1972) and has been promoted as an integral part of patient-centred care for more than 40 years (Charles et al., 1997). SDM frequently requires discussions with relatives and others important to the patient; however, for simplicity, we only use the term patients in this text. The core principles of SDM align well with important values in modern societies, such as respect for autonomy, fairness, and dignity. Still, it has not gained much ground in clinical work (Joseph-Williams et al., 2017). A change in the teaching of SDM should start by understanding why this is so.

Doctors in the making

Few go through childhood without knowing what a doctor is. A doctor is associated with important knowledge and abilities, and perceived as benevolent, providing comfort and hope. The role carries an air of prestige and admiration. Many people will feel respect for doctors; some aspire to see their offspring as future doctors. In the modern era based on science, the status of doctors is based foremost on the advances in biomedicine over the last 150 years. This has formed a modern medical culture where mastery of interactions with others has not become a highly valued part of doctors' identity (apart from normal courtesy—their 'bedside manner'). Yet many patients still trust doctors (Box 15.1).

As the science era led to a shift towards more educated populations, people wanted to know more: expectations were rising, and so did interest in the quality of medical practice. The knowledge base in biomedicine grew rapidly and made it impossible for individual doctors to keep up with developments in their field. We saw the birth of the evidence-based medicine movement and, in turn, SDM. While evidence-based medicine gained traction relatively quickly, given its roots in the natural sciences, SDM, with its roots in the social sciences and the ethical principle of respect for autonomy, met much more resistance. Medical students were drilled to search for and follow guidelines, but less so in how to curate information for use by patients (Clayman et al., 2017).

Box 15.1 Patient perspective

Assigned ancient roles

I think the patient must be at the centre. How can training of the doctor help put the patient at the centre, and is the patient willing to be at the centre?

Terms signal how we think. The word 'patient' means 'one who suffers'. The term 'doctor', also from Latin, means one who 'teaches'. The roles are assigned: the words suggest an active role that meets the passive role of the person in need. That has been the relationship between doctor and patient for ages. Throughout history, these roles were assigned to people, partly by language and partly by tradition. The doctor was supposed to fix what was wrong. But times have changed. Until recently, there were few other than doctors, theologians, and lawyers who had the benefit of an academic education. Today, education of similar length is much more common in society. In addition, information is far more accessible than it was just a few years ago. Many patients look up health information on their own, admittedly of varying quality, but they know much more than before. We cannot therefore expect these roles to remain static.

Lack of integration

Gaining biomedical knowledge is critical to becoming a doctor, and the amount to assimilate is overwhelming. Students learn how to take an illness history from a patient. However, they soon experience that patients' representation of symptoms and signs rarely fit with what they have learned from texts, which leads to complexity and cognitive overload—a significant barrier to smooth communication. Students find it difficult to listen carefully to the patient while juggling what biomedical history questions to ask and, simultaneously trying to remember the importance of exploring the patient's perspective. Initiating a discussion about treatment options is even more challenging; few medical students feel they have sufficient knowledge to discuss the pros and cons of options. SDM is not easy for students during the early part of their learning: SDM must be taught stepwise at pre- and postgraduate phases.

However, teaching SDM as short courses with a prescriptive format is now common practice, and needs to be more integrated with the biomedical curriculum. The extent to which patients or clinically active doctors are teachers varies. Mandatory courses after graduation are uncommon. New doctors keep their heads above water by imitating more experienced doctors. If students are not told what SDM entails and how difficult SDM is from early on, they will likely fail, dismiss it, and not respect its importance before they meet more senior colleagues who master and endorse it.

Biomedicine builds on studies that show effective interventions. Deep insights into the use of language and the impact of social interactions from other academic fields are unfamiliar and do not convince doctors. An early introduction to these sciences concurrently with anatomy and physiology might create curiosity about communication in the medical student and even prevent later dismissal of its importance (Gulbrandsen et al., 2022).

Deference and demand

Doctors who have tried to implement SDM in their practice often experience patients resisting their right to be part of decision making (Landmark et al., 2015); some patients become bewildered or even suspicious. Patients have different reasons for not wanting to be involved in decisions: many have not ever experienced being masters in their own lives, were not raised to be independent, carry traumas, harbour distrust, or have a general feeling that they cannot handle complex information (Joseph-Williams, 2014). Others find consolation in just being in the hands of a doctor, who they find trustworthy because of their responsible role (Keij et al., 2024). The doctor may abandon SDM. Conversely, some patients are comfortable asking questions. These patients are likely to welcome SDM, although their approach does not necessarily make it easier. When wider interests override individual preferences or there is absence or insufficient evidence of benefit, the doctor may not consider what the patient prefers to be a relevant option (Elwyn et al., 2023; van der Horst et al., 2023). There is a risk of consumerism in these processes.

Teachers and doctors are taught in universities and colleges in a belief system where discussion, even debate, is the expected norm. While, ideally, SDM is described as a balanced discussion between two experts, truly balanced discussions about options and decisions are rare. Deliberation strategies cover a whole spectrum from non-controlling to controlling behaviour, with informing as the least controlling, followed by recommending, convincing, persuading, and manipulating, regardless of benevolent intentions (Fleisje, 2023). A doctor must be aware of and reflect upon these diverse deliberation methods (Box 15.2).

Box 15.2 Patient perspective

SDM changes the doctor–patient relationship

In Norway, patients have become more central through user participation over the past 20 years. However, patients need to be guided by doctors. Doctors know more about medicine and have experience of other patients to draw on. User participation must never mean the patient can insist on, or 'order' their treatment. If doctors accept that, they are failing to meet their professional role in relationship to the patient.

Recent societal changes have an impact on patients' expectations of doctors and conversations with them. If doctors do not understand these changes, they will not respond adequately to their patients' expectations. SDM is an important method for the doctor to meet the patient where the patient is, meaning to become aware of 'what the patient expects' and what might be possible. Consequently, SDM will change the doctor–patient relationship.

Uncertainty and mishaps

Looming behind the need to discuss options is the ubiquitous presence of uncertainty in medicine. At best, evidence is probabilistic and can be described in numbers. We know that framing probabilities as chances or risks changes understanding and decisions. In addition, many people struggle with innumeracy (Gigerenzer and Edwards, 2003). Further, evidence is sometimes conflicting and, therefore, ambiguous. To complete the picture, uncertainty frequently involves many factors and is complex and hard to decipher (Han, 2021). There is no obvious best option. This affects both the doctor and the patient. Many doctors tend to downplay uncertainty. For many patients, meeting uncertainty about diagnosis or treatment is a maiden voyage that elicits indecisiveness and anxiety. Anxiety may raise awareness and focus on important information though, above a certain level, it will tend to introduce a feeling of chaos and may lead to withdrawal. Even if the problem is not life-threatening, it may have serious implications. Such feelings and thoughts must be recognized and explored by the doctor. Seeing SDM as a pure, rational exchange of information between experts may introduce a feeling of abandonment (Pilnick, 2022).

Doctors add experience from clinical work to their knowledge, and what they consider to be the best options will tend to be formed by insight based on the diversity of patients they have met, treatments they have provided, and subsequent effects they have observed. Anticipated effects reinforce decisions made; unexpected effects may easily introduce bias, particularly if negative. Doctors are diverse in their propensity to avoid or accept uncertainty (Hoffmann and Del Mar, 2017). The professional environment is crucial to foster balanced judgement, interest in the diversity of needs and preferences of patients, and the ability to handle medical mishaps.

Curating information

The same way a curator in a museum selects what and how to present the museum's artefacts to create interest and spark visitors' memory, the doctor must consider carefully what to inform the patient about and how to do it (Clayman et al., 2017). Ironically, 'curate', 'cure', and 'care' have the same Latin root; they all signify 'looking after'. This common etymology is a bridge between the natural and social sciences, a reminder to doctors how important information is as a critical part of healing.

Time available needs to be considered when initiating SDM. Perceived time constraints may lead doctors to hurry. Information, however, like food, needs to be digested. Hence, doctors need to provide pauses, ideally between every sentence, sufficient to observe the patient is listening and to allow a response. A pause where the gaze is diverted from the other person's face does not work. Information is not just about the exchange of facts and opinions; no, understanding is created in the dynamic moments between two (or more) persons interacting using speech and body language. Note, however, that regular nodding from the patient while a doctor provides information is not necessarily evidence of understanding. The doctor must check whether recipients understand the main messages (Clark, 1996; Nordfalk et al., 2022) (Box 15.3).

Box 15.3 Patient perspective

Listen to, and treat people, not patients

Two steps can help SDM merge scientific evidence-based medicine and the traditional roles of doctors and patients.

First, through the active use of SDM, the doctor will appear more as an advisor. Patients receive advice on their own healing process from a counsellor, yet one who obviously knows more about the medical situation. Perhaps we could also proceed further along this path if we did not stick to terms such as patients that initially have created divisions. Maybe the doctor will no longer treat patients but guide people! The described teaching innovations seem to foster and emphasize equality between the doctors and the people they meet.

Second, active listening is essential. It is more than just hearing. It requires focused questions about what was said, with the intention to make sure that the recipient understands what the sender means. Active listening requires a great deal of attention. Notably, active listening is not just the responsibility of the doctor—it is also the responsibility of the person sitting with the doctor. The description of the curating process in this chapter tells us how doctors need to attend to details in this process.

Integration

To accomplish effective SDM, doctors must understand that communication is an integral part of care and cure. This means training must include an understanding of basic social science insights about what happens in interactions (such as pauses, gaze, prosody, sighs, and question types). Furthermore, understand that power asymmetry, cognitive overload, uncertainty, and vulnerability affect doctors just as much as they affect patients. Building on these insights, the rationale of the standard steps in patient-centred communication and SDM will seem obvious. Below we describe two initiatives to facilitate these steps, one that occurs during pre-graduate education in the Netherlands and one that occurs during postgraduate education in Norway.

A pre-graduate example

At the Leiden University Medical Centre, the Netherlands, medical students complete a 3-year bachelor's degree followed by a 3-year master's degree. SDM is taught in mandatory courses, integrated with clinical teaching, and taught by teachers with either a medical or a non-medical background. In year 3 of the bachelor's degree, basic topics on SDM (what, why, when, how to do SDM, and evidence on effects of SDM) are covered using an e-learning module and during a lecture (Figure 15.1). The e-learning showcases high-quality SDM interactions to allow role modelling. During their master's degree, we provide three SDM workshops spread over the students' clinical specialty rotations. In workshop 1, students' opinions about SDM, and perceived barriers and facilitators are discussed. Further, they consider the words they would use with a patient to introduce a choice of treatment options and to describe the treatment options. In workshop 2, students enact the role of resident and execute SDM steps one and two or three and four of the four-step model by Stiggelbout et al. (2015). They may use any material they wish to have to hand (e.g. description of the clinical case, own notes) to limit cognitive load. Next, tips are collected on how to address interactional challenges. The students prepare for workshop 3 by collecting a recording of their own consultation and getting feedback on it. Brief fragments of the recordings most relevant to SDM are discussed during the workshop. Students are invited to consider (1) what to do when they lack (medical) knowledge, (2) how to prioritize information and how to share information

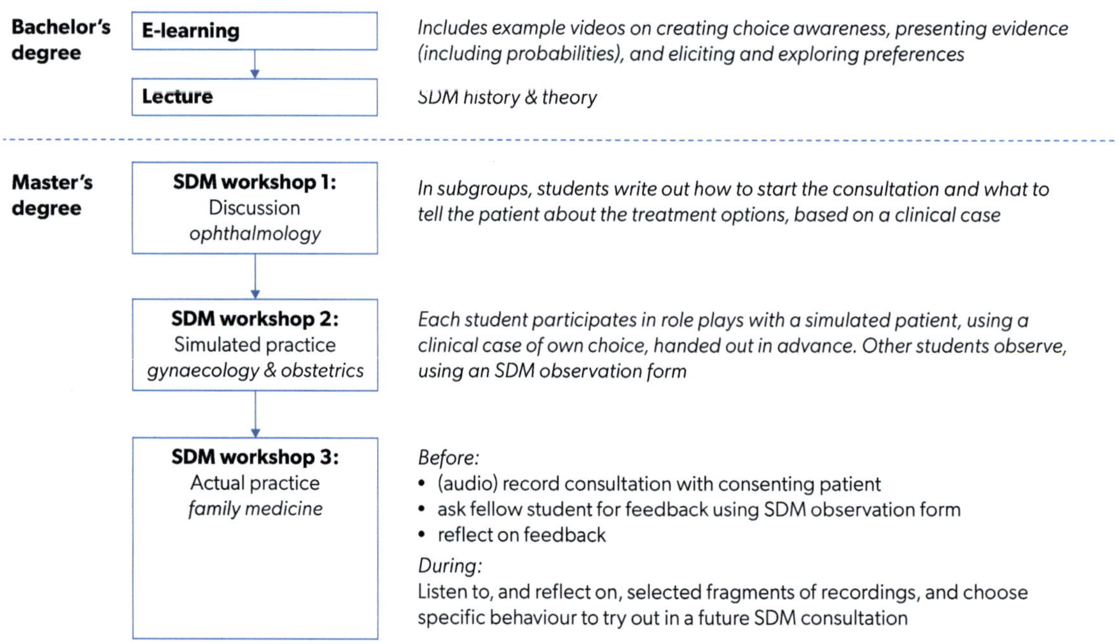

Figure 15.1 The structure of the pre-graduate SDM teaching programme at Leiden University Medical Center.

clearly with patients, and (3) how to handle situations in which patients find it hard to make a choice.

A postgraduate example

In Norway, Kaiser Permanente's communication skills course 'Four Habits', which includes SDM, was tested and found to change the behaviour of hospital doctors (Gulbrandsen et al., 2013). Participants who had prior communication skills training in medical school did not perform better before they attended the course than those who had not. However, the effect of the course was stronger for those with prior training, suggesting that postgraduate training is necessary to *reinforce* pre-graduate learning (Fossli Jensen et al., 2011). To reduce doctors' lack of comfort with role play and to deepen self-reflection, an initial section on doctor identity formation, normalizing vulnerability, uncertainty, insecurity, guilt, and shame, was added to the Four Habits.

In 2017, the Norwegian Directorate of Health introduced new legislation to improve the quality of supervision of trainee doctors. We viewed this as an opportunity to transpose the communication skills course to a different setting—to senior doctors who supervise and coach junior colleagues. By supervision, we mean the observation and feedback that junior doctors obtain during their time in training roles. Coaching describes an established system in Norway where all juniors in specialist training have one senior doctor who meets their assigned juniors in one-to-one meetings every 2 months to discuss challenges, difficulties, and progress.

Based on an understanding of the power of social learning (Bandura, 1969), we felt that we might be able to kill two birds with one stone by blending communication and supervision/coaching skills development. It could (1) reduce variation and improve the quality and efficiency of supervision and coaching, and (2) achieve quicker adaptation of good communication skills if senior doctors use such skills in interaction with junior colleagues. Using a SDM model represents less of a challenge in doctor–doctor interactions than in doctor–patient interactions. Additionally, it is particularly relevant for coaching. Junior doctors are in a vulnerable position when supervised. If the supervisor uses an SDM approach and makes the junior explicitly aware of this approach, both parties become aware of the processes involved, which is likely to amplify social learning.

The blending process required integrating the communication course with elements from the teaching of technical skills such as endoscopy training and harmonized with the principles in competency-based medical education. The aim is to prioritize excellent interaction skills to become the essential core of medical culture. To scale up the training, a regional programme was launched in which selected and motivated doctors were recruited from other hospitals to learn the principles and teach them locally. Learner-centred communication was deliberately and explicitly used throughout the programme (Figure 15.2).

In the programme, learners from all regional hospitals convene four times in one year. First, they are exposed to and learn general communication principles before focusing on applying skills in challenging situations, like providing formative feedback after a poor performance or informing junior doctors that they are not suited for their selected specialization. The third course is about how to apply the principles in teaching and facilitation. Finally, the learners conduct a course for doctors in their own hospital, supervised by one of the teachers in the regional programme.

Summary

SDM is an empowering tool. As such, it challenges power structures in general ways, not just in medicine. Despite the ideal formulated in the first article of the Universal Declaration of Human Rights, 'All humans are born free and equal in dignity and rights', a large proportion of the world's population is encultured to show deference, even subservience, to people in power. The medical culture, with its benevolent intentions, is a good place to foster freedom and dignity. However, even the medical culture is anchored in ancient roles that form the basis of the assumed doctor–patient relationship, providing a major barrier to SDM. To change this, people in power must understand what *not* being in power does to a person. Hence, SDM must permeate all interactions in healthcare, particularly in master–apprentice (supervisor–learner) relationships. Group reflections and feedback in pre-graduate teaching, such as occurs in the Leiden example, is necessary to create fertile ground for power shifts. Regular explicit exposure to SDM techniques during supervision and coaching during postgraduate training will reinforce doctors' understanding during specialization and foster learner- and patient-centred communication.

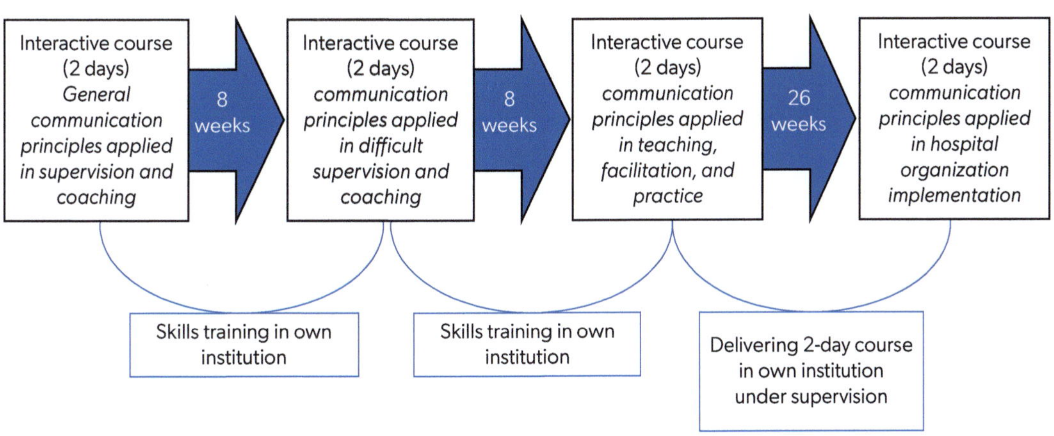

Figure 15.2 The structure of a postgraduate programme building communication skills and SDM into supervision and coaching of trainee doctors in two Norwegian healthcare regions.

REFERENCES

Bandura, A. 1969. Social-learning theory of identificatory processes. In: Goslin, D. A., Ed. *Handbook of Socialization Theory and Research*, pp. 213–262. Rand McNally.

Charles, C., Gafni, A., Whelan, T. 1997. Shared decision making in the medical encounter: what does it mean? (Or it takes at least two to tango). *Soc Sci Med*, **44**, 681–692.

Clark, H. H. 1996. *Using Language*. Cambridge University Press.

Clayman, M., Gulbrandsen, P., Morris, M. A. 2017. A patient in the clinic; a person in the world. Why shared decision making needs to center on the person rather than the medical encounter. *Patient Educ Couns*, **100**, 600–604.

Elwyn, G., Price, A., Franco, J. V. A., et al. 2023. The limits of shared decision making. *BMJ Evid Based Med*, **28**, 218–221.

Fleisje, A. 2023. Paternalistic persuasion: are doctors paternalistic when persuading patients, and how does persuasion differ from convincing and recommending? *Med Health Care Philos*, **26**, 257–269.

Fossli Jensen, B., Gulbrandsen, P., Dahl, F. A., et al. 2011. Effectiveness of a short course in clinical communication skills for hospital doctors: results of a crossover randomized controlled trial (ISRCTN22153332). *Patient Educ Couns*, **84**, 163–169.

Gigerenzer, G., Edwards, A. 2003. Simple tools for understanding risks: from innumeracy to insight. *BMJ*, **327**, 741–744.

Gulbrandsen, P., Fossli Jensen, B., Finset, A., et al. 2013. Long-term effect of communication training on the relationship between physicians' self-efficacy and performance. *Patient Educ Couns*, **91**, 180–185.

Gulbrandsen, P., Gerwing, J., Landmark, A. M. 2022. Time to advance the educational model of clinical communication in medicine. *Patient Educ Couns*, **105**, 1351–1352.

Han, P. K. J. 2021. *Uncertainty in Medicine. A Framework for Tolerance*. Oxford University Press.

Hoffmann, T., Del Mar, C. 2017. Clinicians' expectations of the benefits and harms of treatments, screening, and tests. A systematic review. *JAMA Intern Med*, **177**, 407–419.

Joseph-Williams, N., Abhyankar, P., Boland, L., et al. 2014. What works in implementing patient decision aids in routine clinical settings? A rapid realist review and update from the International Patient Decision Aid Standards Collaboration. *Med Decis Making*, **41**, 907–937.

Joseph-Williams, N., Lloyd, A., Edwards, A., et al. 2017. Implementing shared decision making in the NHS: lessons from the MAGIC program. *BMJ*, **357**, 1744–1749.

Keij, S.M., Stiggelbout, A. M., Pieterse, A. H. 2024. Patient readiness for shared decision making about treatment: conceptualisation and development of the ReadySDM. *Health Expect*, **27**, e13995.

Landmark, A. M. D., Gulbrandsen, P., Svennevig, J. 2015. Whose decision? Negotiating epistemic and deontic rights in medical treatment decisions. *J Pragmat*, **78**, 54–69.

Nordfalk, J. M., Menichetti, J., Thomas, O., et al. 2022. Three strategies when physicians provide complex information in interactions with patients: how to recognize and measure them. *Patient Educ Couns*, **105**, 1552–1560.

Pilnick, A. 2022. *Reconsidering Patient-Centred Care: Between Autonomy and Abandonment*. Emerald Publishing.

Stiggelbout, A. M., Pieterse, A. H., De Haes, J. C. 2015. Shared decision making: concepts, evidence, and practice. *Patient Educ Couns*, **98**, 1172–1179.

Van der Horst, D. E. M., Garvelink, M. M., Bos, W. J. W., et al. 2023. For which decisions is shared decision making considered appropriate?—a systematic review. *Patient Educ Couns*, **106**, 3–16.

Veatch, R. M. 1972. Models for ethical medicine in a revolutionary age. *Hastings Cent Rep*, **2**, 5–7.

PART 5
Implementation

16

Where are we now?

An overview of international progress in shared decision making implementation

Natalie Joseph-Williams, Adrian Edwards, Julie Kenealy, and Glyn Elwyn

Background

There is increasing global interest in person-centred healthcare services and the routine use of shared decision making (SDM). Efforts to implement SDM have grown in pace, scale, and reach. This may be supported by legislation promoting rights for informed care (e.g. The Supreme Court, 2013), national healthcare policies promoting person-centred approaches (e.g. National Institute for Health and Care Excellence, 2021), and widespread support for 'patients as partners', actively co-producing both research and service delivery (UK Research and Innovation, 2024). International implementation efforts continue to increase—but key barriers remain, and different countries report different levels of SDM implementation success or maturity.

In this chapter, we bring together international experience and progress in SDM implementation. We seek to (1) describe what has been reported to help or delay country-level SDM implementation, (2) present a preliminary model of SDM implementation maturity, and (3) use this model to assess the level of SDM implementation maturity self-reported by each country. This chapter presents a combined summary version of previously published country reports—we encourage readers to view the original papers for detailed descriptions of implementation at the country level. Importantly, the absence of countries in this update does not mean SDM efforts do not exist in those countries (these are indicated in grey in Figure 16.1).

Summary of countries reporting SDM implementation

We draw particularly on a special issue of *Zeitschrift fur Evidenz, Fortbildung und Qualitat im Gesundheitswesen* [*The Journal of Evidence and Quality in Health Care*] (volume 171, June 2022), which published updates on the state of SDM implementation in 21 countries worldwide (Bravo et al., 2022). These updates cover multiple geographical regions (Figure 16.1) including Europe (n = 10), East Asia and Pacific (n = 3), Latin America (n = 3), Northern America (n = 2), Middle East (n = 2), and the African Nations (n = 1). Most are from high-income countries, but upper middle-income (Argentina, Malaysia, Mexico) and lower middle-income (Iran) countries are included. With a couple of exceptions (e.g. Libya and Botswana), the African Nations update includes middle, lower-middle, and low-income countries. Country populations range in size from 6 million in Denmark to 331 million in the USA. A range of healthcare systems is described including those based on universal government-funded systems (n = 8), universal public–private insurance (n = 4), universal public insurance (n = 4), universal private health insurance (n = 3), and non-universal insurance (n = 1). The African Nations update reports several systems, but all are largely characterized by budgetary, resource, and leadership constraints.

Things that help country-level implementation

Nine broad categories of factors that help SDM implementation have emerged (Table 16.1), including policy and leadership; legislation; training/education; tools; measurement; coordination and networks; incentives; alignment; and adaptation.

The full list of factors reported as helping implementation are included in Table 16.1.

The top six factors that helped implementation were:

1. Access to high-quality patient decision support tools (e.g. patient decision aids, checklists, counselling, question prompts)
2. Legal mandate for SDM/person-centred care/informed consent
3. Professional bodies supporting SDM (guidance/accreditation/standards)
4. Patient organizations promoting SDM
5. Accessible learning/training packages for healthcare professionals
6. Policy support.

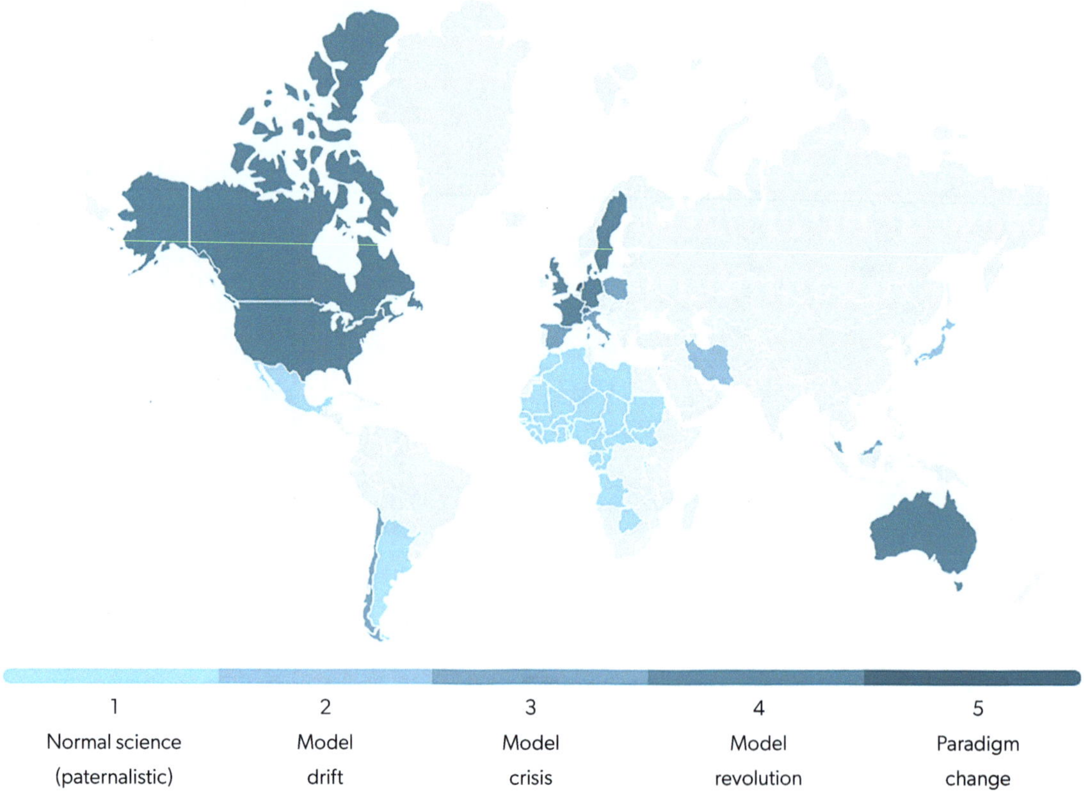

Figure 16.1 Geographical locations and level of SDM implementation maturity in regions/countries reporting 2022 updates.

Clinician- or patient-targeted interventions such as SDM tools and training feature internationally as two of the top six factors that help routine SDM implementation. The remaining four factors focus on top-down approaches, such as policy and legislative mandates, and support from professional or patient organizations. Increasingly, countries are reporting the importance of 'adaptation', or having tools that 'fit'. In such countries, which are typically non-Western and less advanced in SDM implementation (e.g. Iran), the cultural adaptation of existing tools, models, and measures is seen as a key driver for implementation.

Things that delay country-level implementation

Seven broad categories of factors that delay SDM implementation also emerged (Table 16.2), including policy and leadership; coordination; attitudes, knowledge, and beliefs; tools/education; resource and system capacity; incentives; and population characteristics/cultural considerations.

All countries reported the negative impact of the COVID-19 pandemic on SDM implementation. The full list of other factors reported as delaying implementation is included in Table 16.2.

The top six factors that delayed implementation were:

1. No national/centralized strategy for SDM training/education
2. No national/centralized strategy for SDM implementation
3. Lack of policy support
4. Support for paternalistic model in country
5. Lack of time/workforce pressures
6. No national/centralized strategy for developing/updating/implementing patient decision aids.

A key issue linking most of these factors that delay implementation is lack of country-level coordination. The absence of government policies that promote SDM, and support among healthcare professionals, and sometimes patients, for the dominant paternalistic model of care were also key barriers. Each country reported a lack of time due to increasing workforce pressures as an important delay factor. With increasing population sizes and prevalence of multimorbidity, healthcare workforce retention and recruitment issues, and financial restraints on service provision, it is unsurprising in the current climate that this is a limiting factor for successful SDM implementation.

Model of SDM implementation maturity

Using self-reported SDM implementation progress and factors described by each country as helping or delaying implementation (Bravo et al., 2022), our previous publications on SDM implementation (Elwyn et al., 2013; Joseph-Williams et al., 2017, 2021), and Kuhn's paradigm change cycle (Kuhn, 1962), we propose a new model of SDM implementation maturity (Figure 16.2). This model describes six key levels in moving from a country-level dominant paternalistic healthcare model to a dominant SDM model, and the key activities, barriers, and facilitators associated with each level (Figure 16.2).

Table 16.1 Things that help SDM implementation (countries ordered by level of SDM implementation maturity)

	Central Africa	North Africa	West Africa	ARG	MEX	IRA	ISR	JPN	MYS	CHL	ESP	ITA	POL	AUS	CAN	DEN	FRA	GER	NED	SWE	SUI	UK	USA
Level of SDM maturity (Figures 16.1 and 16.2)	1	1	1	1	1	2	2	2	3	3	3	3	3	4	4	4	4	4	4	4	4	4	4
Policy and leadership																							
Policy support								X		X				X	X	X	X	X	X	X		X	X
Professional body supporting SDM (guidance/accreditation/standards)		X		X			X	X	X					X		X	X	X	X	X	X	X	X
Patient organizations promoting SDM						X	X					X	X	X	X	X	X	X	X	X		X	
Healthcare organization-level leadership									X	X			X			X						X	
Legislation																							
Legal mandate for SDM/person-centred care/informed consent						X	X	X	X	X	X	X	X	X	X	X	X	X	X	X		X	X
Training/education																							
Accessible healthcare professional learning/training packages				X			X	X		X	X		X	X		X			X	X	X	X	
Inclusion in medical/healthcare education				X			X				X	X		X				X	X	X	X	X	
Patient education											X		X					X	X				
Tools																							
Access to high-quality patient decision support tools (e.g. patient decision aids, checklists, counselling, question prompts)	X			X		X		X		X	X		X	X	X	X	X	X	X	X	X	X	X
Patient decision aid standards/accreditation														X	X				X			X	X
Measurement																							
Measuring patients SDM experiences/outcomes								X			X	X					X			X		X	X
Learning healthcare systems																	X		X	X	X		X
Coordination and networks																							
Centralized coordination (funding/SDM initiatives)							X							X		X		X	X			X	
SDM networks/communities of practice				X				X			X			X		X	X	X	X	X			
Incentives																							
Financial incentives/health insurance renumeration											X								X				
Alignment																							
Alignment to other initiatives*							X					X	X				X			X	X	X	
Integration in clinical guidelines											X			X		X			X			X	X
Adaptation																							
Models and tools that fit—cultural adaptation						X	X	X	X					X		X							

* For example, health literacy, self-empowerment community engagement and activation, learning health systems, co-production.

ARG, Argentina; AUS, Australia; CAN, Canada; CHL, Chile; DEN, Denmark; FRA, France; GER, Germany; ESP, Spain; IRA, Iran; ISR, Israel; ITA, Italy; JPN, Japan; MEX, Mexico; MYS, Malaysia; NED, Netherlands; POL, Poland; SUI, Switzerland; SWE, Sweden; UK, United Kingdom; USA, United States of America.

Table 16.2 Things that delay SDM implementation (countries ordered by level of SDM implementation maturity)

	Central Africa	North Africa	West Africa	ARG	MEX	IRA	ISR	JPN	MYS	CHL	ESP	ITA	POL	AUS	CAN	DEN	FRA	GER	NED	SWE	SUI	UK	USA
Level of SDM maturity (Figures 16.1 and 16.2)	1	1	1	1	1	2	2	2	3	3	3	3	3	4	4	4	4	4	4	4	4	4	4
Policy and leadership																							
Lack of policy support	X	X	X	X	X	X	X				X	X	X										
Lack of integration into clinical guidelines					X								X			X	X						X
Coordination																							
No national/centralized strategy for SDM implementation	X	X	X			X				X	X				X	X				X	X	X	X
No national/centralized developing/updating/implementing of patient decision aids						X					X							X	X	X	X	X	X
No national/centralized strategy for SDM training/education					X	X	X	X			X	X	X		X	X	X			X	X	X	X
No national/centralized strategy for measuring SDM implementation											X			X								X	X
Attitudes, knowledge, beliefs																							
Predominant support for paternalistic model	X	X	X		X	X	X		X				X					X					
Lack of consensus on/understanding of SDM definition/purpose						X	X	X					X			X	X		X				
Patients feel they lack knowledge/skills		X					X			X			X										
Tools/education																							
Lack of tools	X	X	X																				
Lack of education in communication skills	X	X	X																				
Resource and system capacity																							
Lack dedicated SDM funding				X	X					X	X			X			X						
Lack of time	X			X	X		X		X				X		X		X						X
Limited access to care*	X				X		X			X					X		X	X					
Incentives																							
Lack of incentives (financial)	X												X				X						X
Population characteristics/cultural considerations																							
Low levels of health literacy				X		X			X								X		X				
Low literacy	X	X	X																				
Culturally specific factors**	X		X			X	X		X														
Tools/models that do not fit the population						X									X			X	X				
Underfunding of healthcare system	X	X	X																				

* For example, long wait times, appointment availability, migrant populations not accessing care, healthcare systems overburdened.

** Family involvement, paternalistic cultures, gender role in culture, need to 'protect' patients, religion.

ARG, Argentina; AUS, Australia; CAN, Canada; CHL, Chile; DEN, Denmark; FRA, France; GER, Germany; ESP, Spain; IRA, Iran; ISR, Israel; ITA, Italy; JPN, Japan; MEX, Mexico; MYS, Malaysia; NED, Netherlands; POL, Poland; SUI, Switzerland; SWE, Sweden; UK, United Kingdom; USA, United States of America.

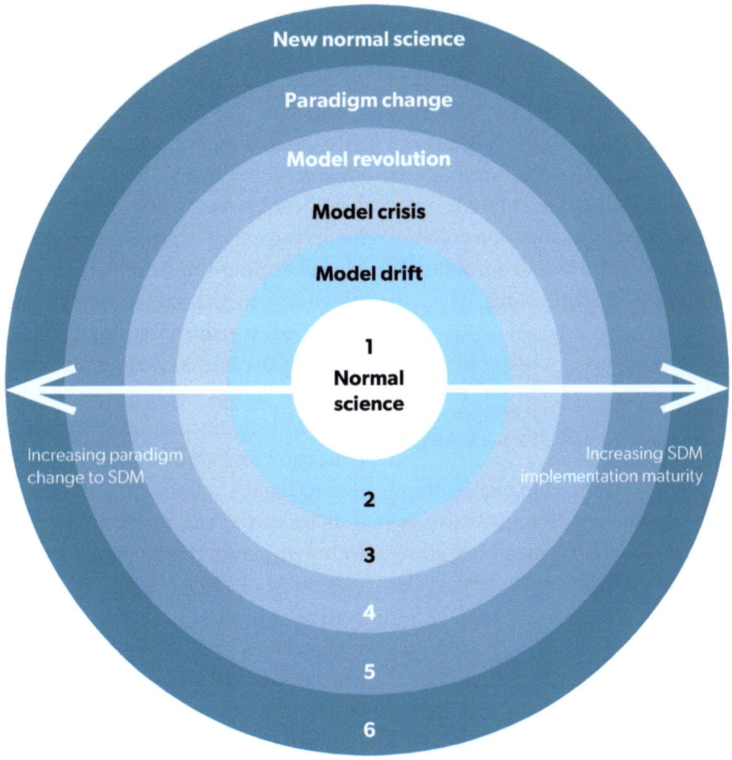

1	**Normal science**	Widespread consensus, acceptance, and implementation of dominant paternalistic approach in healthcare.	No SDM related activities reported.
2	**Model drift**	Anomalies/weaknesses of paternalism in healthcare arise, people question value of approach and alternative ideas put forward.	Largely academically driven. Interest in tool/model development/adaptation. Small-scale localized projects.
3	**Model crisis**	Paternalism grows increasingly weak and increasing time/resource investment in constructing new SDM models/solutions.	Increasing research interest (multiple centres, settings, patient populations); projects increase in scale, spread, and reach. Early adopters implementing into in practice. Large focus on attitudinal change and buy-in.
4	**Model revolution**	Rejection of paternalism, healthy debate & collaborative exploration on how to embed SDM in routine practice.	SDM champions driving change in local practice. Increasing availability of tools. Inclusion in training/education (undergraduate, postgraduate, and continuing professional development). Increasing awareness of benefits. Enduring commitment to change. Building networks/communities of practice. Move to top down approaches, including legislation.
5	**Paradigm change**	SDM model accepted and increasing in scale & spread. Healthcare systems sustainably transitioning away from paternalism across.	Embedded in education, political, and research agenda. Sustainable policy support and inclusion in guidelines/accreditation/standards. Demonstration sites. Intergrated with learning health care system (evidence of effectiveness). Alignment to other PCC initiatives. Increasing resource/funding. Focus on inclusive tools/models—adapting for different populations.
6	**New normal science**	Widespread consensus, acceptance, and collaborative coordination and integration of dominant SDM approach in healthcare.	Collaborative coordination and integration of SDM initiatives. Centralized strategies for implementation/training/measurement. Inclusive SDM. Widespread reach. Dedicated and sustained resource/funding.

Figure 16.2 Model of SDM Implementation Maturity.

In short, the six levels are (1) 'normal science' (dominant paternalistic approach), (2) 'model drift', (3) 'model crisis', (4) 'model revolution', (5) 'paradigm change', and (6) 'new normal science' (dominant SDM approach). The further towards the outside and higher level of the circular model, the more 'mature' SDM implementation is in that country.

Typically, as countries develop SDM implementation maturity, factors reported to help or delay implementation (Tables 16.1 and 16.2) evolve from micro (e.g. gaining clinical team buy-in to SDM), to meso (e.g. hospital policy to deliver SDM training to all staff), to macro (e.g. national healthcare policies or legislation aligned with SDM) levels (Figure 16.2). Thus, we see the increasing importance of top-down levers as countries and healthcare systems progress implementation efforts.

Our circular model conveys that at each level of maturity, the key activities and areas of focus build on, rather than replace, the previous. So ongoing 'buy-in' activities and upskilling of the healthcare workforce will remain even when national policies and coordinated SDM strategies are in place. Further, as SDM implementation maturity progresses in a country, there is an increasing focus on collaborative integration and coordination at the macro level, coordinated by governments and national health and care organizations.

SDM implementation maturity—where are the countries at?

We mapped the 21 countries to our model of SDM implementation maturity (Figure 16.2). Importantly, implementation maturity is not universal within a country, and variation is reported between regions, clinical areas, and patient populations. At a country level, there is a range in SDM implementation maturity (Figure 16.1; Tables 16.1 and 16.2), from level 1 'model drift' (n = 5) to level 4 'model revolution' (n = 10). The darker the shade in Figure 16.1, the higher the level of self-reported SDM implementation maturity in that country. Almost half of the countries are at maturity level 4 (n = 10), where paternalism is increasingly rejected and there is collaborative exploration of how to embed SDM in routine practice.

Five countries are at maturity level 1, where widespread consensus, acceptance, and implementation of paternalistic approaches remain. However, the fact that the countries at the earlier levels of implementation are reporting an update demonstrates early signs of 'model drift', where people are questioning the value of the paternalistic approach and proposing alternatives. No country is at maturity level 5 (paradigm change), where healthcare systems are sustainably transitioning away from paternalism, or level 6 (new normal science), where SDM is the dominant paradigm and fully embedded into routine clinical practice.

Macro-level coordination—the key to 'new normal science' and making SDM the norm?

Based on what has been reported in the country updates, almost half of the 21 countries are at maturity level 4, with some moving towards level 5 (paradigm change). Despite legislative mandates, policy support, increasing patient and professional buy-in, and accessible high-quality tools and training, many of these countries have been teetering at this tipping point from level 4 to level 5 for some time (up to 5–10 years). Based on international progress to date, the phase of 'new normal science' where SDM is the dominant accepted paradigm and fully embedded into routine practice is likely many decades away.

What will it take for these countries to move beyond this tipping point to a 'paradigm change' (level 5) and beyond that, to SDM becoming the 'new normal science'? When examining barriers reported by these level 4 countries alone, a consistent factor is the *lack of macro-level coordination*.

Most of these countries report that integrating SDM principles into legislation, licensure, policy, and guidelines is critical to driving change. Situating SDM implementation attempts within learning healthcare systems is another important driver, as are senior-level leadership and champions to drive the local improvement plans. Underpinning implementation efforts with collaborative communities of practice and the principles of co-production and adaptive SDM, which enable flexibility to adapt SDM models, tools, and training, are also key. However, these countries report that, despite all these things being place, the lack of macro-level *coordination* of SDM implementation, measurement, raising patient awareness, education and training, and decision support tool development is impacting their ability to progress.

Is improved macro-level coordination of these key tasks the key to moving over this tipping point to a paradigm change, or level 5 (Figure 16.3)? The evidence is that coordination could help to overcome duplication observed when SDM champions work in organization silos, increase efficiencies in financial and time investment, promote shared learning across healthcare systems, offer a coherent standard of practice (with room for adaptation) via agreed education and training programmes, assist benchmarking of SDM quality and outcomes, and support the development of sustainable SDM resources.

See Box 16.1 for our patient perspective.

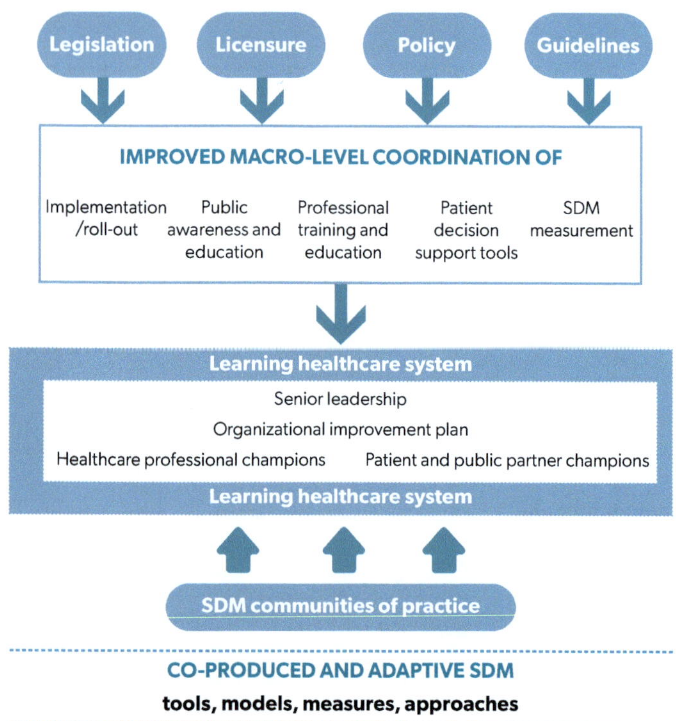

Figure 16.3 Improved macro level coordination of implementation, measurement, training, education, and patient decision support tools—the key to progressing to a 'paradigm change'?

Box 16.1 Patient perspective

From the information provided by each country, SDM has made steady progress. When you consider how long paternalistic medicine has been practised, this progress has been made in a relatively short space of time. It is interesting to see how uptake of SDM has been most frequent in higher-income countries then lower-income countries. We need to better explore the specific barriers in these lower-income countries. Could this be down to finance and resources, training and education, or other factors? Do these countries have other priorities, and so are currently only able to provide a basic provision of healthcare?

From my personal experience of having different types of major surgery, I have witnessed change. While surgical options were not feasible, I was still offered options around anaesthesia, level of painkiller medication and rehabilitation physiotherapy. It was really positive to be given these choices and it made a huge difference to be listened to. It meant I could adjust my medication, instead of taking the higher level of painkiller medication all the time, which I disliked. It also helped me to plan better for my recovery—I knew what to expect. Being given choices by healthcare professionals is positive; however, some responsibility must lie with the patient to take on board the information about the options and promote their own recovery.

Although I have experienced changes in healthcare over the years and have been offered choices, I was not aware of SDM before contributing to this book. If I had not been offered options during my appointments, I would not have known that I should have been. I think to really drive SDM implementation forward, one of the most important tasks is to improve public awareness and understanding of SDM. If the public don't know what it is or that they should expect this approach when making decisions about healthcare, we can't truly understand if it happens or not, or expect patients to feel able to take part. Public awareness campaigns, including advertisements and leaflets, will play a key role in informing patients that they can take part in making healthcare decisions and changing their expectations. Appointment letters should state that they would like patients to take part in SDM. Primary and secondary school pastoral programmes should also be promoting active involvement in healthcare, including decision making.

In addition, we need a clear strategy for SDM with secure legislation in place, so that healthcare professionals are supported with SDM and can be confident to discuss options with the patient, without fear of being held criminally liable (e.g. paperwork agreed between parties). I think that the amount of time allocated for appointments also needs to be considered—when people are given time, they feel like other people care. If healthcare teams are serious about involving patients, they need to rethink their care pathways to ensure enough time for both the healthcare professional and patient to be confident that the patient is fully informed about the choices they make. This may be difficult with current pressures and demands.

Thinking ahead, I don't think the speed of progress and spread is the most important thing—it is more important to make sure SDM is done well. A gradual transition to SDM allows time for people to work out how it can work best in their setting, and importantly, make sure everyone has an opportunity to be involved.

Summary and looking forward

Significant progress has been made in SDM implementation, and global interest in person-centred care continues to grow. Almost half of the countries reporting 2022 updates are at maturity level 4, where paternalism is increasingly rejected and there is collaborative exploration of how to embed SDM in routine practice. Most of these countries report that legislation, licensure, policy, and guidelines are critical. Learning healthcare systems, senior-level leadership, SDM champions, collaborative communities of practice, co-production and flexibility to adapt SDM models, tools, and training are also key. However, a key driver for further international progress in SDM becoming the norm is improved macro-level *coordination* of SDM implementation efforts, patient awareness and education, professional education and training, decision support tool development, and measurement.

REFERENCES

Bravo, P., Härter, M., McCaffery, K., Giguère, A., Hahlweg, P., Elwyn, G. 2022. Editorial: 20 years after the start of international shared decision making activities: is it time to celebrate? Probably .... *Z Evid Fortbild Qual Gesundhwes,* **171**, 1–4. [The 21 country updates are published in this special issue of the journal (Vol. 171).]

Elwyn, G., Scholl, I., Tietbohl, C., et al. 2013. 'Many miles to go ...': a systematic review of the implementation of patient decision support interventions into routine clinical practice. *BMC Med Inform Med Decis Mak,* **13**, S14.

Joseph-Williams, N., Abhyankar, P., Boland, L., et al. 2021. What works in implementing patient decision aids in routine clinical settings: a rapid realist review and update from the International Patient Decision Aids Standards Collaboration. *Med Decis Making,* **41**, 907–937.

Joseph-Williams, N., Lloyd, A., Edwards, A., et al. 2017. Implementing shared decision making in routine NHS settings—lessons from the MAGIC Programme. *BMJ,* **357**, j1744.

Kuhn, T. S. 1962. *The Structure of Scientific Revolutions.* University of Chicago Press.

National Institute for Health and Care Excellence. 2021. Shared decision making. NICE guideline [NG197]. Available at: https://www.nice.org.uk/guidance/ng197

The Supreme Court. 2013. Montgomery (Appellant) v Lanarkshire Health Board (Respondent) (Scotland). Available at: https://www.supremecourt.uk/cases/uksc-2013-0136

UK Research and Innovation. How UKRI supports public involvement in research and innovation. Available at: https://www.ukri.org/what-we-do/public-engagement/how-ukri-supports-public-involvement-in-research-and-innovation/

17

Overview of shared decision making implementation

Rachel C. Forcino, Danielle Schubbe, and Myrtle Mitchell

The current state of shared decision making implementation

Since its introduction into medical literature in the 1980s, the idea of shared decision making (SDM) in clinical care has gradually gained momentum. SDM no longer tends to spark debate among clinical teams about the merit of sharing treatment and management decisions with patients. Instead, the conversation has shifted to the mechanics of how to implement the approach among busy clinical teams, who face unprecedented pressures on their time and resources, and in systems that too often incentivize and reward high-volume over high-quality health services that effectively fit patients' needs and preferences.

The SDM literature includes both direct efforts to implement SDM (e.g. by changing clinicians' communication patterns), as well as efforts to implement interventions as mechanisms that enable these communication changes and facilitate SDM. Direct SDM implementation efforts often focus on some combination of the following clinician behaviours: (1) informing the patient of the decision to be made and inviting the patient's participation; (2) explaining the options, including their benefits and harms; (3) discussing the patient's preferences and deliberating together; and (4) making, deferring, and/or operationalizing the shared decision (Stiggelbout et al., 2015). Other interventions implemented to facilitate SDM include the use of patient decision aids and the provision of written notes to patients summarizing key aspects of their visits (Table 17.1).

The evidence in support of patient decision aids to promote and facilitate SDM has grown, and the methodological rigour of studies evaluating their effectiveness has also improved. It is currently well recognized that patient decision aids promote SDM, and there is substantial evidence that SDM improves the cognitive–affective outcomes that patients experience—like improved knowledge, more accurate risk perceptions, less decisional conflict, and more clarity about personal values (Shay and Lafata, 2015; Stacey et al., 2024). SDM can also benefit clinicians, who regard SDM highly despite limited training in its use (Forcino et al., 2018), and healthcare systems, who may benefit from reduced legal liability where SDM is implemented well (Lindor et al., 2016).

In light of these benefits, recent policy initiatives have promoted SDM across international contexts. However, widespread efforts to ensure adequate and effective implementation have lagged. For example, in the USA, federally administered health insurance programmes require SDM for three tests and procedures: (1) lung cancer screening, given specific age and smoking history criteria; (2) left atrial appendage closure to prevent stroke risk in people with atrial fibrillation; and (3) placement of an implantable cardioverter–defibrillator in some people at risk for an irregular heartbeat. Despite mandating SDM as a prerequisite for payment for these procedures, enforcement remains patchy (Elwyn et al., 2023). Similarly, in 2020, the Netherlands legislature began explicitly requiring SDM in discussions between physicians and patients; however, evaluation and quality assurance remain limited (van der Weijden et al., 2022).

Despite the strong evidence behind SDM and initial policy efforts in support of SDM implementation, its effective and sustained use in clinical practice remains limited. To make access to SDM in healthcare service more widespread and more equitable, we must tackle the question of how to implement SDM in widespread, sustainable ways with the same rigour that established its usefulness in the first place.

Table 17.1 Examples of SDM interventions and implementation strategies

SDM intervention examples	Implementation strategy examples
• Patient decision aids • Question-generation and/or values clarification worksheets • Evidence summaries • Clinic visit audio-recording and/or note-taking services • Advance care planning tools • SDM broadly defined by clinician communication patterns	• Training clinical teams and/or patients in use of the SDM intervention • Conducting small, iterative tests using the SDM intervention (e.g. PDSA cycles) • Revising roles to redistribute clinical team workloads • Practice facilitation or coaching of clinical team members • Audit and feedback on clinical teams' use of the SDM intervention

To address this issue, this chapter presents the following:

- Core principles of implementation science.
- Review of existing evidence on SDM implementation.
- Case studies of SDM implementation efforts in varied clinical contexts.

Implementation science—an approach to support SDM implementation

Moving evidence-based healthcare practices and interventions like SDM and patient decision aids from research into practice requires behaviour change, with a focus on clinical teams, service users, healthcare organizations, and the contexts in which they operate. Implementation science is a field focused on developing and testing 'methods to promote the systematic uptake of research findings and other evidence-based practices into routine practice ... to improve the quality and effectiveness of health services' (Eccles and Mittman, 2006). Use of the key implementation science principles described below strengthens SDM implementation efforts.

Implementation *strategies* are 'systematic and planned processes and actions that are designed to help integrate [evidence-based healthcare interventions] into practice settings' (Baumann and Cabassa, 2020) (see Table 17.1 for examples). Six key categories of implementation *processes* that the strategies seek to address include 'planning, educating, financing, restructuring, managing quality, and attending to the policy context' (Powell et al., 2012). Powell and colleagues worked with an expert panel to compile a list of 73 implementation strategies, which we recommend selecting from to support the design and reporting of SDM implementation efforts (Powell et al., 2015).

Implementation *theoretical frameworks* can enable the identification of implementation barriers and facilitators (also called implementation determinants), inform data collection, and guide the selection and roll-out of implementation strategies (Birken et al., 2017). Implementation science frameworks often used by SDM researchers include the Consolidated Framework for Implementation Research (CFIR) (Damschroder et al., 2022), Theoretical Domains Framework (TDF) (Michie et al., 2005), Diffusion of Innovations (Dearing and Cox, 2018), and the Reach, Effectiveness, Adoption, Implementation, and Maintenance (RE-AIM) framework (Glasgow et al., 2019). As implementation science frameworks focus on different parts of the process (e.g. identifying implementation determinants, evaluating the implementation programme), the selection of a guiding implementation science theoretical framework should be motivated by the specific problem or question being addressed.

What works for implementing SDM?

A recent literature review identified five strategies associated with successful implementation of patient decision aids in routine clinical settings to support SDM (Joseph-Williams et al., 2021). These include (1) co-production and/or local adaptation of decision aid content and processes; (2) training the entire clinical team; (3) preparing and prompting patients to engage in SDM; (4) leadership buy-in from senior levels of the healthcare organization; and (5) measuring progress towards SDM implementation. This review focused on one specific intervention (patient decision aids), representing one avenue towards achieving SDM in routine practice.

To expand our understanding beyond patient decision aids, we reviewed the published literature reporting broader SDM implementation efforts across multiple contexts—including routine health services, research, and quality improvement. We noted the clinical context, the implementation strategies used, and the involvement of patients and/or caregivers in implementation efforts. Of the 33 articles we identified, 21 reported implementation efforts within research studies, four reported implementation efforts in routine health services, and eight reported implementation efforts within quality improvement projects or initiatives. The SDM interventions being implemented were primarily decision aids, with others including care planning, audio recording, note-taking, and SDM broadly, characterized by changes in clinicians' communication patterns (Stiggelbout et al., 2015).

What strategies have been tried?

Common implementation strategies across articles, which reported varied levels of success, included clinician and/or clinical team training (with some 'train the trainer' programmes), improvement networks or learning collaboratives, Plan–Do–Study–Act (PDSA) cycles and other cyclical small tests of change (which allow clinical team members to serially trial the intervention on a small scale and adapt it as needed to suit the context), audit and feedback, outer-setting policy changes, practice facilitation, flexibility in implementation and use of the clinical intervention, and reconfiguring workflows and revising roles to assign SDM-related tasks to staff with spare bandwidth to contribute. However, fewer than half of these articles reported moderate to high levels of implementation success.

Most of the successful and/or sustained implementation efforts used bundles of multiple implementation strategies, summarized in Table 17.2. Of the 33 total articles, seven described involvement of patients and/or caregivers in the implementation process.

Case study 1: the Shared decision making Adoption Implementation Resource Collaborative for breast cancer care teams

The Shared decision making Adoption Implementation Resource (SHAIR) Collaborative is a recent SDM implementation project example: an online learning collaborative focused on implementing SDM with patients experiencing early-stage breast cancer (Schubbe et al., 2023).

SHAIR Collaborative member sites are actively implementing a text-based and picture-enhanced conversation aid for early-stage breast cancer treatment options that effectively increased SDM and other outcomes in a clinical trial. The SHAIR Collaborative has provided free and direct access to these conversation aids, which are continuously updated and available in perpetuity online. Before SHAIR sites started using the conversation aids in clinical practice, they watched five brief instructional videos (approximately 2 minutes each) and engaged with the SHAIR Collaborative project team in a 'site initiation visit' to discuss training and configure a tailored, context-sensitive implementation approach. SHAIR sites provide monthly data regarding patient reach, and there is also an optional patient survey to generate feedback to clinical teams. A feedback

Table 17.2 Summary of successful SDM implementation efforts

	Implementation in the context of a single or isolated decision	Implementation in the context of chronic care
Clinical contexts	• Device implementation for advanced heart failure • Breast cancer care—e.g. radiation, systemic therapy, surgery (see 'Case study 1') • Cancer care (across cancer types) • Colorectal cancer screening • Isolated decisions in primary care	• Asthma—ongoing management (see 'Case study 2') • Diabetes and coronary heart disease
Successful implementation strategies included across studies **See Powell et al. (2015) for further details on each strategy**	• Standard operating procedures operationalizing implementation • Practice facilitation, i.e. coaching of clinical team members • Changes to record systems (electronic health record documentation) • Training clinical team members (single instance) • Access to ongoing training for clinical team members • Audit and feedback, i.e. measuring implementation progress and feeding data back to clinical team members • Revising clinical team members' roles to redistribute workloads • Participation of patient representatives in implementation efforts • Site-level adaptability of the intervention to allow context-sensitive implementation • Clinical champions promoting implementation • Cyclical small tests of change (i.e. PDSA cycles) • Leadership support for implementation	• Participation in a learning collaborative or other network • Clinical champions promoting implementation • Site-level adaptability of the intervention to allow context-sensitive implementation • Training the whole clinical team • Co-design of workflows with clinical staff • Practice facilitation, i.e. coaching of clinical team members
Example of a successful implementation strategy bundle	• Introductory presentation; training of clinical team; ongoing access to training materials; flexible delivery and use of the SDM intervention (Matlock et al., 2020)	• Participation in a practice-based research network; practice facilitation/coaching; cyclical small tests of change (i.e. PDSA cycles) (Shade et al., 2020)
Methods of patient and/or caregiver involvement	• Patient-directed ordering of decision aids • Patient representative paired with each clinical team to participate in design, implementation, and evaluation of implementation programme—including training and designing feedback to clinicians	• Patient and caregiver representation on advisory board

dashboard is provided to SHAIR sites, visualizing patient reach and patient-reported outcomes from the patient survey. Other SHAIR Collaborative offerings include webinars with SHAIR sites and guidance for integrating the conversation aid into sites' electronic medical records.

The SHAIR Collaborative began with five pilot sites implementing the conversation aids. The Collaborative then expanded by adding another ten sites to implement the conversation aids in 2022. Since then, across all sites, the conversation aids have reached over 86% of eligible patients (n = 1771 as of February 2024). The SHAIR Collaborative has partnered with the American Society of Breast Surgeons to provide continuous access to the conversation aids and to SDM training for all of its members. Across participating sites, strong clinical championship and leadership buy-in contributed to implementation success.

Case study 2: asthma management in primary care

An example of an SDM implementation project in the chronic care context is a multi-site primary care implementation study (Shade et al., 2020). This study promoted implementation of a decision aid about asthma management through practice facilitation and cyclical small tests of change led by embedded nurses within practice-based research networks (Shade et al., 2020). To understand how to improve uptake of an SDM intervention, the study team compared the practice facilitation approach to a standalone 'lunch-and-learn' training approach.

The study team found that practice facilitation was associated with both higher uptake of the SDM toolkit intervention, higher levels of SDM, and fewer emergency department visits among patients receiving the SDM intervention in the practice facilitation arm. In addition to ongoing, structured coaching, the practice facilitator supported adaptation of the SDM toolkit to fit the local clinical context and provided feedback on the implementation process. The SDM toolkit was ultimately successfully implemented within four practice-based research networks, and all ten sites using a practice facilitation approach continued to be engaged with their facilitator beyond the study period.

See Box 17.1 for a reflection from our patient partner.

What gaps remain?

The literature surrounding SDM implementation is growing and becoming increasingly informative about which approaches best yield and embed SDM, including using tools like patient decision aids, and in which clinical contexts. However, as Powell and colleagues noted over a decade ago (Powell et al., 2012), implementation strategies are often not described in adequate detail to ensure clarity about what approaches were undertaken in each implementation effort. There is a trend in the SDM literature towards more comprehensive descriptions of implementation strategy bundles (as in Scholl et al., 2018); continued progress on this front will be valuable for the field.

Box 17.1 Patient perspective

Reflection from a patient partner

Efforts by providers and health systems to share the decision process with the client are often therapeutic from the client's perspective. In that emotion-filled space after receiving a major diagnosis, to be given a path forward in one's care is significant. It contributes to the quality, treatment, and well-being of the clients who are given the opportunity to participate in their care. SDM happens when providers, practices, and health systems are intentional about incorporating SDM.

SDM has been an integral part of my personal cancer care journey. This included SDM at the point of diagnosis, on the subsequent path to surgery, chemotherapy, and radiation, and throughout continued management which included lymphoedema therapy.

SDM, by its definition, involves clients, providers, healthcare facilities, and support systems. SDM in breast cancer care has elevated the treatment process because clients who may have historically been left out, marginalized, mismanaged, or taken advantage of are encouraged to engage as active participants in their care. SDM builds trust between patients and providers. So, another benefit of SDM is having trusted voices giving credibility in conversations around care plans in the aftermath of a cancer diagnosis.

SDM is still evolving as a universal practice. Health systems where SDM has been implemented now report important outcomes like less decision conflict and more satisfaction with the decision making process. However, the broader healthcare system is not unified in delivery practices, so there are still roadblocks and disparities. Resources of providers, finance, and supportive relationships are sometimes diminished, leading to differences in whether patients experience SDM in different health systems.

As a patient partner in SDM research, I have been able to experience first hand the impact of SDM implementation in the care of clients with breast cancer. Clients had a positive response to the patient decision aid their providers used to explain information about treatment options and help make a shared treatment decision.

Incorporating clients in the planning stages is helpful in establishing some of the guidelines to ensure their positive participation in SDM. To further encourage the use of SDM, it is important to acknowledge all the participants in the process. In collaboration with several of my patient partner colleagues, we have identified two focus areas for SDM implementation. One is retraining of providers in an affirming way, incorporating their skillset and knowledge and rewarding them when SDM improves care. The other is increasing the use of nurse patient navigators to bridge the gap between clients and providers, encouraging them to ask questions and be informed about the resources and treatment options available to them.

SDM is now an important part in the toolbox of breast cancer care. With increasing success in its implementation, SDM will eventually become the standard of care.

Despite the role of patient preparation and prompting as a key facilitator of SDM implementation efforts (Joseph-Williams et al., 2021), most of the articles we identified (26 of 33) did not report on patient involvement. Increased attention to the value of patient engagement and improved consistency in its reporting will further enhance our understanding of SDM implementation.

Finally, sustained and widespread access to evidence-based, up-to-date, effective decision aids continues to be a challenge to SDM implementation. The Ottawa Hospital Research Institute's A to Z Inventory of Decision Aids (https://decisionaid.ohri.ca/AZinvent.php) is a valuable resource for identifying and accessing various decision aids across a wide variety of clinical conditions. However, many existing patient decision aids have not been updated or reviewed for several years and/or are now behind a paywall designed for health system subscribers, as it is costly to maintain a high-quality product over time. In an environment where many healthcare organizations face increasing financial pressures and struggle to adequately staff their services, SDM is too often deprioritized. The incremental policy changes we have seen to date have not yet had a substantial impact on SDM implementation.

Summary

Implementation science improves the success of SDM implementation efforts through systematic identification of barriers and facilitators and by applying evidence-based implementation strategies. Successful strategies used to implement SDM include practice facilitation and coaching, revising clinical team members' roles to redistribute workloads, training of the clinical team, and cyclical small tests of change. Continued progress in SDM implementation will require clear and comprehensive reporting of implementation strategies in reports and publications, attention to patients as parties to SDM implementation efforts, and improved availability of evidence-based tools that support SDM.

REFERENCES

Baumann, A. A., Cabassa, L. J. 2020. Reframing implementation science to address inequities in healthcare delivery. *BMC Health Serv Res,* **20**, 190.

Birken, S. A., Powell, B. J., Shea, C. M., et al. 2017. Criteria for selecting implementation science theories and frameworks: results from an international survey. *Implement Sci,* **12**, 124.

Damschroder, L. J., Reardon, C. M., Widerquist, M. A. O., Lowery, J. 2022. The updated Consolidated Framework for Implementation Research based on user feedback. *Implement Sci,* **17**, 75.

Dearing, J. W., Cox, J. G. 2018. Diffusion of innovations theory, principles, and practice. *Health Aff,* **37**, 183–190.

Eccles, M. P., Mittman, B. S. 2006. Welcome to implementation science. *Implement Sci,* **1**, 1.

Elwyn, G., Sierpe, A., Forcino, R. 2023. Do payment programs incentivize shared decision making in US healthcare? *Patient Educ Couns,* **113**, 107798.

Forcino, R. C., Yen, R. W., Aboumrad, M., et al. 2018. US-based cross-sectional survey of clinicians' knowledge and attitudes about shared decision-making across healthcare professions and specialties. *BMJ Open,* **8**, e022730.

Glasgow, R. E., Harden, S. M., Gaglio, B., et al. 2019. RE-AIM Planning and Evaluation Framework: adapting to new science and practice with a 20-year review. *Front Public Health,* **7**, 64.

Joseph-Williams, N., Abhyankar, P., Boland, L., et al. 2021. What works in implementing patient decision aids in routine clinical settings? A rapid realist review and update from the International Patient Decision Aid Standards Collaboration. *Med Decis Making,* **41**, 907–937.

Lindor, R. A., Kunneman, M., Hanzel, M., et al. 2016. Liability and informed consent in the context of shared decision making. *Acad Emerg Med,* **23**, 1428–1433.

Matlock, D. D., McIlvennan, C. K., Thompson, J. S., et al. 2020. Decision aid implementation among left ventricular assist device programs participating in the DECIDE-LVAD Stepped-Wedge Trial. *Med Decis Making,* **40**, 289–301.

Michie, S., Johnston, M., Abraham, C., et al. 2005. Making psychological theory useful for implementing evidence based practice: a consensus approach. *Qual Saf Health Care,* **14**, 26–33.

Powell, B. J., McMillen, J. C., Proctor, E. K., et al. 2012. A compilation of strategies for implementing clinical innovations in health and mental health. *Med Care Res Rev,* **69**, 123–157.

Powell, B. J., Waltz, T. J., Chinman, M. J., et al. 2015. A refined compilation of implementation strategies: results from the Expert Recommendations for Implementing Change (ERIC) project. *Implement Sci,* **10**, 21.

Scholl, I., Hahlweg, P., Lindig, A., et al. 2018. Evaluation of a program for routine implementation of shared decision-making in cancer care: study protocol of a stepped wedge cluster randomized trial. *Implement Sci,* **13**, 51.

Schubbe, D., Yen, R. W., Leavitt, H., et al. 2023. Implementing shared decision making for early-stage breast cancer treatment using a coproduction learning collaborative: the SHAIR Collaborative protocol. *Implement Sci Commun,* **4**, 79.

Shade, L., Reeves, K., Rees, J., et al. 2020. Research nurses as practice facilitators to disseminate an asthma shared decision making intervention. *BMC Nurs,* **19**, 40.

Shay, L. A., Lafata, J. E. 2015. Where is the evidence? A systematic review of shared decision making and patient outcomes. *Med Decis Making,* **35**, 114–131.

Stacey, D., Lewis, K. B., Smith, M., et al. 2024. Decision aids for people facing health treatment or screening decisions. *Cochrane Database Syst Rev,* **1**, CD001431.

Stiggelbout, A. M., Pieterse, A. H., De Haes, J. C. J. M. 2015. Shared decision making: concepts, evidence, and practice. *Patient Educ Couns,* **98**, 1172–1179.

Van der Weijden, T., van der Kraan, J., Brand, P. L. P., et al. 2022. Shared decision-making in the Netherlands: progress is made, but not for all. Time to become inclusive to patients. *Z Evid Fortbild Qual Gesundhwes,* **171**, 98–104.

18

The International Patient Decision Aid Standards Collaboration

Evolution and current status

Robert J. Volk, Krystina B. Lewis, Maureen Smith, and Dawn Stacey

Introduction

In 2005, the International Patient Decision Aid Standards (IPDAS) Collaboration established the first set of standards about how to judge and appraise the quality of patient decision aids (PtDAs) (Elwyn et al., 2006). PtDAs are tools designed to support patients in the process of making decisions about their health (Stacey et al., 2024). In this chapter, we provide an overview of the genesis and evolution of the IPDAS Collaboration, describe the current domains and related standards, and highlight current efforts towards updating the standards. An update is occurring in 2024 in response to the IPDAS Evidence Update 2.0 (Stacey et al., 2021b) and the 2024 update of the Cochrane systematic review of PtDAs (Stacey et al., 2024).

The genesis of IPDAS and why standards matter

The IPDAS Collaboration is a volunteer, international organization of PtDA developers and researchers who share a common mission of improving the quality of patient decision making through a shared-evidence framework for the development, content, evaluation, and reporting of PtDAs (Stacey et al., 2021b). Launched in 2003, the IPDAS Collaboration was established as PtDAs were becoming increasingly common and were recognized as having the potential to dramatically impact the decisions people make.

In the absence of standards, the use of poor-quality PtDAs can lead to biased decisions with potential harms to patients. For example, a well-known bias when presenting probabilities involves the use of relative risk in the absence of absolute risk (i.e. the actual probability of an outcome happening), which can lead to an overestimation of the magnitude of risk or benefit to the patient. There are concerns about how conflicts of interest might impact development of PtDAs, especially when developers or funders of PtDAs stand to benefit or lose from the decisions people make.

Versions of the IPDAS criteria

The IPDAS criteria have gone through one previous revision and are currently in the process of its second update. Figure 18.1 shows the history of the Collaboration, including versions of the IPDAS criteria and updates of the evidence that informed them.

The original IPDAS checklist and IPDAS instrument

The Collaboration sought to develop guidance for developers and users of PtDAs that reflected the initial standards for high-quality PtDAs within 12 broad domains of a high-quality PtDA. A Delphi consensus process was used, where more than 100 individuals from 14 countries proposed criteria to reflect the quality domains (Elwyn et al., 2006). The original IPDAS checklist released in 2005 included 74 items from 11 domains (excluding patient narratives because of conflicting and minimal evidence). The IPDAS instrument assesses the quality of a PtDA by rating 47 items from the checklist on a 4-point scale, thus providing a more precise and reliable estimate of a PtDA's quality.

Minimum standards for PtDAs

In response to increasing calls for certification of PtDAs from policy-makers, the IPDAS Collaboration identified (in 2013) a set of criteria that represented essential or 'must-have' items (Joseph-Williams et al., 2014). The goal of this effort was to identify minimum criteria that could be used to inform certification of PtDAs. A Delphi consensus process was launched with input from 127 participants with PtDA experience from 16 countries. The two-stage voting process was to identity criteria that would reduce potential bias and harm to patients who used a PtDA. An expert panel of PtDA developers and researchers grouped the criteria as necessary to qualify as a decision aid, needed to be certified as a decision aid, and additional criteria that could enhance the quality of a decision aid (see Table 18.1 for qualifying and certifying criteria).

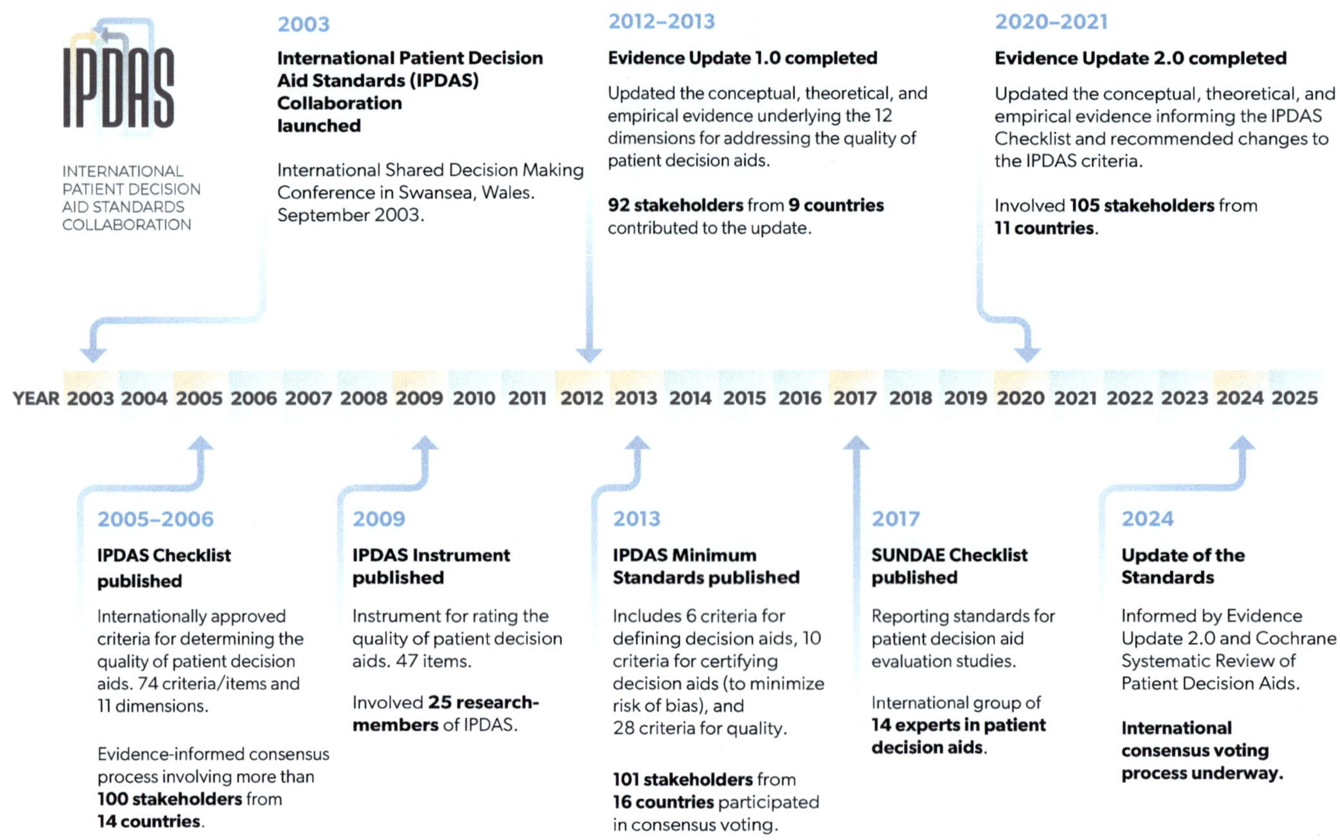

Figure 18.1 History of the IPDAS Collaboration.
Reproduced courtesy of Robert J. Volk and Dawn Stacey. © 2024 IPDAS Collaboration. Available at: https://decisionaid.ohri.ca/IPDAS/

Table 18.1 IPDAS qualifying criteria and criteria for minimizing risk of biased decisions

Qualifying criteria
Criteria to qualify as a patient decision aid. The patient decision aid . . .
1. Describes the health condition for which the index decision is required
2. Explicitly states decision to be considered
3. Describes the options available for the index decision
4. Describes positive features of options (benefits)
5. Describes negative features of options (harms)
6. Helps patients clarify their values for outcomes of options by asking people to think about which positive and negative features of the options matter most to them (explicit) and/or describing each option to help patients imagine the physical, social, and/or psychological effect (implicit)
Certification criteria
Criteria to lower the risk of making a biased decision. The patient decision aid . . .
1. Shows the negative and positive features of the options with equal detail (e.g. using similar fonts, sequence, presentation of statistical information)
2. Provides information about the levels of uncertainty around event or outcome probabilities (e.g. by giving a range or by using phrases such as 'our best estimate is')
3. Provides a production or publication date
4. Provides information about the funding source used for development
5. Provides citations for scientific evidence selected
6. Provides information about the update policy
Additional criteria for screening tests. The patient decision aid . . .
1. Describes what the screening test is designed to measure
2. Describes the next steps typically taken if the screening test detects the condition or problem
3. Describes the next steps if the condition or problem is not detected with the screening test
4. Has information about detection and treatment of disease that would not have caused problems if screening had not been done

Adapted from Joseph-Williams N, Newcombe R, Politi M, et al. 2014. Toward minimum standards for certifying patient decision aids: a modified Delphi consensus process. *Med Decis Making*, 34, 699–710.

Updating the IPDAS criteria

Building on new evidence from Evidence Update 2.0 and the 2024 Cochrane systematic review of PtDAs, the IPDAS Collaboration is now updating the standards. Domain teams were asked to propose changes to the standards, including revision of existing criteria, new criteria, and removal of criteria. A Delphi voting process (spring 2024) is being used to reach consensus on the qualifying criteria, essential criteria to reduce potential biased decisions, and additional criteria for improving the quality of a PtDA.

The IPDAS domains and supporting evidence: Evidence Update 2.0

A second update (2.0) of the evidence informing the standards involved 105 stakeholders from 11 countries and was published as a special issue of *Medical Decision Making* in 2021 (Stacey et al., 2021b). The following briefly describes each domain and summarizes the updated Evidence Update 2.0. Although the IPDAS standards were initially organized around 12 broad domains, the domains about presenting balanced information and presenting information about options were merged, and the domain about delivering PtDAs on the internet was included in considerations about implementation.

Systematic development

Evidence Update 2.0 emphasized a user-centred development process that involves careful assessment of users' decision making needs, development and refinement of prototypes, and assessment with various end users (Witteman et al., 2021a). Central to the development process is a series of iterations or cycles, where PtDAs are tested with users, modified, and retested, until it is acceptable for the target audience. A clear connection is made between user-centred design and implementation of PtDAs, recognizing that successful uptake of these tools requires significant input of users from the start. The team noted problems with under-reporting of development processes and encouraged publication of PtDA development to complement their evaluations.

The COVID-19 pandemic presented a challenge for PtDA developers where new tools needed to be produced rapidly to meet needs of the public. Stacey and colleagues used a rapid development strategy that streamlined creation of two new PtDAs to urgently meet COVID-19 decisional needs (Stacey et al., 2021a). In this example, user testing had to be limited to the development team which consisted of experienced PtDA developers and relevant stakeholders including physicians, nurses, a social worker, and a physiotherapist. This group was highly experienced in PtDAs and used an established framework (i.e. Ottawa Decision Support Framework) that had been previously evaluated in 24 randomized controlled trials, and a recent evidence synthesis on the topic to guide rapid development.

Conflicts of interest

A conflict of interest can occur when funders, developers, and/or distributors of PtDAs stand to gain or lose from the choices patients make. Users of PtDAs often come from the lay public and may not always be able to detect and evaluate the influence of potential conflicts of interest on PtDA content. Moreover, PtDAs may be developed and disseminated for use without the benefit of scrutiny by independent peer reviewers or an editor. The current standards require that sources of funding for a PtDA be disclosed, and acknowledgement about whether the developers and their affiliations stand to gain or lose based on patients' choices. There is ongoing discussion about establishing higher standards for addressing conflicts, such as requiring that *no sources of funding* for development come from a funder who stands to gain or lose by choices patients make about their options (Thompson et al., 2021).

Basing information on comprehensive, critically appraised, and up-to-date synthesis of scientific evidence

For PtDAs to be trustworthy, they must include information that is based on the best available evidence (Hoffmann et al., 2014). Sources of evidence can include systematic reviews, with assessments of study quality, description of consistency of findings, assessments of the appropriateness of study populations included in research studies, and clinical practice guidelines. At a minimum, PtDAs should provide complete citations to evidence sources, describe how the evidence was selected and synthesized, and provide a publication date. Assessment of the quality of the evidence, such as using the Grading of Recommendations, Assessment, Development, and Evaluations (GRADE) approach, is strongly suggested.

Presenting balanced information about options and outcomes

To make informed decisions patients need facts about the positive and negative features of the different options for testing or treating a health problem. This information may include what the procedure involves; possible benefits and advantages; and possible harms, side effects, or disadvantages. Information should be complete, relevant, transparent, and unbiased in how it is presented to users (Martin et al., 2021). Some ways to ensure the balance of positive compared to negative features are to use (1) a consistent format for options in written material (font, spacing, layout), (2) a consistent format for options in digital material (volume of sound, speed, amount of airtime), and (3) consistent framing of the options in terms of adjectives used and the display of numbers and statistics. There is debate about requiring side-by-side presentation of benefits and harms, and whether PtDAs should be required to include a 'wait-and-see' option, if relevant to the decision.

Presenting probabilities

A 'probability' is the chance or likelihood that something will happen. It could mean the chance of a disease, benefit, harm, or side effect of an intervention or healthcare option. Probabilities are often presented numerically or visually using figures and diagrams. In Evidence Update 2.0, the domain team suggested that numbers be presented over a specified period of time with a clear denominator, and use consistent formats with interpretation of the numbers for users (Bonner et al., 2021). In addition, the team continued to reinforce the use of independent event rates and incremental absolute risk differences and simple visual formats (Trevena et al., 2021). Evidence to support the use of personalized or interactive risk estimates is limited.

Clarifying values

PtDAs can help patients clarify their values by facilitating deliberation about different benefits, harms, and features of options, and encouraging patients to communicate their personal importance of them with others. The goal for the patient is to make a decision that aligns with their values (Witteman et al., 2021b). Ways of helping patients clarify and express their values include both implicit and explicit approaches. Implicit approaches include describing features of options in ways that help patients imagine what it is like to experience them and to live with the physical, emotional, and social consequences. Explicit values clarification approaches involve exercises to help patients rate or trade off different features of the options.

Using personal stories

Personal stories describe the experiences of other people who have faced the decision. Stories may include experiences of living with the condition, going through the steps of decision making, or living with the consequences of their choice. Stories are viewed as highly impactful in decision making, and there is concern about their potential biased effect on the healthcare choices selected. Evidence supporting the use of patient stories in PtDAs remains lacking (Shaffer et al., 2021), but important theoretical work has provided greater clarity about their types and roles.

Health literacy

The way in which health information is presented in PtDAs can promote understanding and improve readability for all audiences. Strategies that reduce cognitive demand include the choice of words, the structure or format used, the use of plain language (verified with readability formulas), and co-development with patients. Most PtDAs reviewed for Evidence Update 2.0 were not developed to address the needs of patients with low health literacy or from other underserved groups (Muscat et al., 2021). This team highlighted the importance of reporting reading levels, involving patients from lower-literacy groups in development of PtDAs, based on principles to enhance health communication.

Guidance and decision coaching

Guidance and decision coaching provide patients with a non-directive, structured way of thinking about their options and discussing them with a healthcare professional. Guidance is 'an explicit element embedded within the decision support materials' that promotes self-directed decision making (Rahn et al., 2021). Guidance can be accomplished using strategies such as a list of steps for making a decision, questions to ask a healthcare professional, and summaries of patients' priorities to view with a clinician, decision coach, or others. Decision coaching, used alongside PtDAs, is provided by a trained individual who is supportive but non-directive. It can be provided in person, or virtually, before, during, or after using a PtDA. When used alongside PtDAs, decision coaching is associated with improved patient knowledge.

Measuring effectiveness

This domain addresses the quality of the decision making process and quality of the decision. It also includes the measures used to establish the effectiveness of PtDAs. In the Evidence Update 2.0, few randomized trials of PtDAs included information about the properties of the outcome measures used to evaluate them (Trenaman et al., 2021). The team advocated for use of the Standards for Universal reporting of patient Decision Aid Evaluations (SUNDAE) (Sepucha et al., 2018) checklist to address these concerns (see below).

Ongoing challenges for developers, evaluators, and users

Reporting PtDA development and evaluation: the SUNDAE checklist

As the field of PtDAs has advanced, there has been a need to provide guidance on how their development and evaluation are reported. Incomplete reporting of PtDA studies poses challenges for clinicians and researchers needing to identify PtDA content to use in clinical practice and/or future research. The SUNDAE reporting guidelines include 26 items and is part of the Equator Network (https://www.equator-network.org/) (Sepucha et al., 2018).

Implementing PtDAs

Stacey and colleagues found that about one-quarter of PtDAs evaluated in randomized trials continued to be used after the trial (Stacey et al., 2019). For Evidence Update 2.0, Joseph-Williams and colleagues conducted a rapid realist review to identify articles that could contribute to theory about PtDA implementation (Joseph-Williams et al., 2021). The group made five recommendations: (1) co-produce PtDAs with end users for content and processes for use; (2) ensure the entire team is trained to use the PtDA; (3) engage patients by prompting them to use the PtDA; (4) ensure buy-in of senior leaders; and (5) continue to improve the PtDA and processes. Many of these issues are relevant for the development of PtDAs and involvement of users in the process.

Promoting equity in PtDAs

Equity-enhancing PtDAs reflect an understanding of the underlying causes of disparities, promote fairness across groups by making information appropriate and accessible, and support patients as partners in their healthcare. For PtDAs to meet the needs of various populations, evidence-based methods to engage, adapt, tailor, and implement high-quality, person-centred PtDAs are needed. While IPDAS provides guidance about the use of plain language when developing PtDAs, the standards are largely silent about processes for adapting current PtDAs across diverse populations and contexts. New criteria have been proposed that address the importance of involving populations with limited health literacy in co-design of PtDAs, use of gender-neutral pronouns, and cultural adaptation of existing PtDAs across languages and cultures.

Conclusion

The IPDAS Collaboration provides the only guidance on developing, evaluating, implementing, and reporting on quality PtDAs. Since 2003, the fully voluntary IPDAS Collaboration continues to provide evidence updates and key guidance for developers, researchers, and users of PtDAs. As evidence continues to accumulate about the impact of PtDAs on a variety of patient outcomes, the standards will be further refined.

See Box 18.1 for our patient perspective.

Box 18.1 Patient perspective

PtDAs are valuable tools for patients, caregivers, and members of the public to become involved in shared decision making processes about their healthcare. As a patient and caregiver who has used PtDAs, it is of utmost importance to me that they are of high quality. Determining what is high quality is not an easy task for a patient, caregiver, or member of the public, so I therefore rely on the standards established by the IPDAS Collaboration. The consequences of making healthcare decisions based on information presented in poor-quality PtDAs can be grave.

My involvement as a consumer on the updated systematic review of PtDAs and the ensuing update to the IPDAS checklist has afforded me an opportunity to reflect on how the healthcare world has changed since the first set of IPDAS standards were published in 2005. The paternalistic 'doctor knows best' approach is slowly being replaced by patient involvement in their healthcare, often in the form of shared decision making. PtDAs have emerged for numerous healthcare decisions such as screening and choosing interventions. Key to shared decision making is the necessity to understand all the options and align decisions with what is important to us (the consumers). A second issue that has emerged due to the COVID-19 pandemic is the proliferation of misinformation and disinformation and the harms that have occurred when decisions are not evidence-based. PtDAs are not immune to this challenge. These two realities make it obvious to me that the IPDAS Collaboration must do a better job of collaborating with patients, caregivers, and the public in the changes to its standards and in disseminating them in plain language.

A Delphi voting process (spring 2024) is being used to reach consensus on criteria needed to qualify as a PtDA, criteria that are essential for a PtDA to reduce potential biased decisions, and criteria that might enhance the quality of PtDAs. I'm proud to have played a role in ensuring that patients, caregivers, and the public will have the opportunity to share their perspectives on the criteria that are important to them, through a process that has been designed to be in plain language. As an end user of PtDAs I am concerned with several aspects, such as how risks are interpreted, biases in presenting the benefits or overstating these benefits, and potential conflicts of interest. Do the developers and their affiliations stand to gain or lose based on the choice patients make?

Updating the IPDAS standards with patient, caregiver, and public involvement will surely result in standards that consider what is important to PtDAs users and a greater understanding of what goes into developing high-quality PtDAs that we can trust.

REFERENCES

Bonner, C., Trevena, L. J., Gaissmaier, W., et al. 2021. Current best practice for presenting probabilities in patient decision aids: fundamental principles. *Med Decis Making,* **41**, 821–833.

Elwyn, G., O'Connor, A., Stacey, D., et al. 2006. Developing a quality criteria framework for patient decision aids: online international Delphi consensus process. *BMJ,* **333**, 417.

Hoffmann, T. C., Glasziou, P. P., Boutron, I., et al.2014. Better reporting of interventions: template for intervention description and replication (TIDieR) checklist and guide. *BMJ,* **348**, g1687.

Joseph-Williams, N., Abhyankar, P., Boland, L., et al. 2021. What works in implementing patient decision aids in routine clinical settings? A rapid realist review and update from the International Patient Decision Aid Standards Collaboration. *Med Decis Making,* **41**, 907–937.

Joseph-Williams, N., Newcombe, R., Politi, M., et al. 2014. Minimum standards for certifying patient decision aids: a modified Delphi consensus process. *Med Decis Making,* **34**, 699–710.

Martin, R. W., Brogård Andersen, S., O'Brien, M. A., et al. 2021. Providing balanced information about options in patient decision aids: an update from the International Patient Decision Aid Standards. *Med Decis Making,* **41**, 780–800.

Muscat, D. M., Smith, J., Mac, O., et al. 2021. Addressing health literacy in patient decision aids: an update from the International Patient Decision Aid Standards. *Med Decis Making,* **41**, 848–869.

Rahn, A. C., Jull, J., Boland, L., et al. 2021. Guidance and/or decision coaching with patient decision aids: scoping reviews to inform the International Patient Decision Aid Standards (IPDAS). *Med Decis Making,* **41**, 938–953.

Sepucha, K. R., Abhyankar, P., Hoffman, A. S., et al. 2018. Standards for UNiversal reporting of patient Decision Aid Evaluation studies: the development of SUNDAE Checklist. *BMJ Qual Saf,* **27**, 380–388.

Shaffer, V. A., Brodney, S., Gavaruzzi, T., et al. 2021. Do personal stories make patient decision aids more effective? An update from the International Patient Decision Aids Standards. *Med Decis Making,* **41**, 897–906.

Stacey, D., Lewis, K. B., Smith, M., et al. 2024. Decision aids for people facing health treatment or screening decisions. *Cochrane Database Syst Rev,* **1**, CD001431.

Stacey, D., Ludwig, C., Archambault, P., et al. 2021. Feasibility of rapidly developing and widely disseminating patient decision aids to respond to urgent decisional needs due to the COVID-19 pandemic. *Med Decis Making,* **41**, 233–239.

Stacey, D., Suwalska, V., Boland, L., Lewis, K. B., Presseau, J., Thomson, R. 2019. Are patient decision aids used in clinical practice after rigorous evaluation? A survey of trial authors. *Med Decis Making,* **39**, 805–815.

Stacey, D., Volk, R. J., Leads, I. E. U. 2021. The International Patient Decision Aid Standards (IPDAS) Collaboration: Evidence Update 2.0. *Med Decis Making,* **41**, 729–733.

Thompson, R., Paskins, Z., Main, B. G., et al. 2021. Addressing conflicts of interest in health and medicine: current evidence and implications for patient decision aid development. *Med Decis Making,* **41**, 768–779.

Trenaman, L., Jansen, J., Blumenthal-Barby, J., et al. 2021. Are we improving? Update and critical appraisal of the reporting of decision process and quality measures in trials evaluating patient decision aids. *Med Decis Making,* **41**, 954–959.

Trevena, L. J., Bonner, C., Okan, Y., et al. 2021. Current challenges when using numbers in patient decision aids: advanced concepts. *Med Decis Making,* **41**, 834–847.

Witteman, H. O., Maki, K. G., Vaisson, G., et al. 2021. Systematic development of patient decision aids: an update from the IPDAS Collaboration. *Med Decis Making,* **41**, 736–754.

Witteman, H. O., Ndjaboue, R., Vaisson, G., et al. 2021. Clarifying values: an updated and expanded systematic review and meta-analysis. *Med Decis Making,* **41**, 801–820.

19

Patient decision aids

Characteristics and evidence of effectiveness

Dawn Stacey, Krystina B. Lewis, Maureen Smith, and Robert J. Volk

Introduction

To achieve high-quality healthcare decisions, patients need to be informed by best available evidence and choose an option that is consistent with their values for the features and outcomes among the options available. However, current approaches to involve patients and their families in making healthcare decisions are inadequate and do not support them to achieve quality decisions. Often clinicians present patients with a single option when multiple options are available, and they are poor judges of their patients' values and preferences. Patients then proceed with the option recommended by the clinician, resulting in unrealistic expectations. This can lead to dissatisfaction with the decision making process and the selected option.

Patients report many barriers that interfere with their involvement in making quality healthcare decisions. These include inadequate knowledge of options, unclear values, power imbalances with clinicians, and feeling vulnerable or unable to advocate for themselves (Joseph-Williams et al., 2014). Common decisional needs among 2857 patients from 45 studies included feeling uninformed about benefits, harms, and other features of the options (64% studies); lack of access to information about the health condition, options, benefits, risks and scientific uncertainties (64%); feeling unclear about what is important to them (44%); feeling unsure about which option to choose (39%); and feeling unsupported in decision making (33%) (Hoefel et al., 2020). Patient decision aids (PtDAs) are well-established, effective, evidence-based interventions to help overcome these barriers and address patients' decision making needs (Stacey et al., 2017). Given the emphasis on providing patient- and family-centred care, many clinical practice guidelines recommend using PtDAs.

The purpose of this chapter is to summarize characteristics and evidence on PtDAs. The main systematic review that informed this chapter was the Cochrane review of PtDAs that was originally published in 1999 with updates in 2003, 2007, 2011, 2014, 2017, and 2024. The 2024 update reported on 209 randomized controlled trials involving 107,698 participants randomized to a PtDA or to usual care (Stacey et al., 2024). Those who received usual care may have received general information, a risk assessment, clinical practice guideline summary for health consumers, no information, or a placebo intervention (e.g. information on another topic).

Characteristics of PtDAs

PtDAs provide evidence-based information on options, benefits, and harms for a specific healthcare decision in a target population (Stacey et al., 2024). They also help patients clarify their values for features and outcomes of options in order to determine their preferred option. Some PtDAs have other elements to assist patients with decision making such as (1) probabilities or the chances of outcomes of options occurring, (2) patient narratives or stories describing their experiences making the decision, and/or (3) guidance in decision making by structuring the information in a series of steps or providing worksheets (Table 19.1). Information in PtDAs can also be used by 'decision coaches' when discussing options with patients to prepare them for consultation with their clinician (Stacey and Volk, 2021). Common PtDA formats include printed

Table 19.1 Elements in PtDAs to support the decision making process

Elements	Total N = 209
Information on options, benefits, and harms plus implicit or explicit values clarification*	100%
Information on the clinical condition	92%
Probabilities of benefits and harms	88%
Explicit values clarification exercise	67%
Guidance in the steps of decision making	73%
Patient stories or narratives describing decision making experiences and/or outcomes	37%

* Required for PtDAs.

resources, computer or tablet desk-top displays, or online resources such as PDFs, videos, or interactive programmes. Formats evaluated in earlier studies were decision boards, videocassettes, DVDs, and audiocassettes with booklets.

When and where have PtDAs been used?

PtDAs are indicated when there are two or more health or social care options that patients may value differently. One of the options, if appropriate, should be the option of wait and see (or not making a change). Example decision making contexts include prenatal screening or no screening; starting a new diabetes medication or continuing with current medications; and prostate cancer treatment with surgery, radiation, or active surveillance. The most common screening or treatment topics in PtDA evaluation studies are about cancer, cardiovascular disease, mental health, and pregnancy (Table 19.2). PtDAs are designed to be used independently of a consultation with a clinician, in preparation for a consultation, or by patients and clinicians together during the consultation.

International interest in PtDAs has grown dramatically over the past decade. Authors who have evaluated PtDAs in a randomized controlled trial are from a total of 19 countries on four continents (Figure 19.1). The most frequent countries where PtDAs were evaluated are Australia, Canada, the UK, and the USA.

The effects of PtDAs on patient, clinician, and health system outcomes

Patient-level outcomes

PtDAs are effective, evidence-based interventions for improving the quality of the decision and the quality of the decision making process. Compared to usual care, patients who use PtDAs have 75% higher quality decisions (informed and based on patients' values), 12% better knowledge, 94% more realistic expectations when probabilities are used, and 10% fewer patients felt uninformed. As well, 8% fewer patients report unclear values and 32% less undecided. There were 28% fewer patients allowing clinician-controlled decisions; patients prepared with PtDAs take on a more active role in decision making. When appraised using the Grading of Recommendations, Assessment, Development, and Evaluations (GRADE) approach (Andrews et al., 2013), all of these primary outcomes have high certainty/confidence in the evidence except for decision quality which has moderate certainty/confidence in the evidence.

No adverse effects

There were no reported harms associated with use of PtDAs. Compared to usual care, there was no difference in decision regret for those who used PtDAs. Of five studies that measured emotional distress, four showed no difference and one study reported less cancer-related distress for women testing positive for a breast cancer gene.

Patient and clinician-level outcomes

When patients used PtDAs ahead of consultations, they were more likely to discuss the topic with their clinician and be more satisfied with the decision making process. Evidence for shared decision making or patient–clinician communication depends on the measurement tool used. Eight studies that used OPTION-12 (Elwyn et al., 2005) to measure shared decision making showed a 12% improvement compared to usual care. But studies that used other instruments showed no difference.

Health system outcomes

For health system outcomes, there was no difference in consultation time between usual care and use of PtDAs in preparation for

Table 19.2 Examples of healthcare decisions addressed by PtDAs

Health conditions	Screening versus no screening	Treatment-related decisions		
		Medications for	Surgery	Other
Cancer	Colorectal, prostate, breast, cervical, lung	Breast chemoprevention	Breast, prostate	Prostate radiation; watchful waiting
Cardiovascular	Cardiovascular	Cardiovascular; atrial fibrillation	Left ventricular assist device, bypass	
Dental			Molars	
Diabetes	Glucose testing	Diabetes		
Kidney disease				Dialysis versus no dialysis
Mental health		Depression; anxiety; post-traumatic stress disorder; schizophrenia		Cognitive behavioural therapy
Pregnancy/gynaecology	Prenatal diagnostic testing		Hysterectomy; embryo transfer	Birth options post caesarean; post-partum care
Rheumatology/orthopaedics		Osteoporosis	Hip/knee replacement; spinal stenosis; herniated disc	
Vaccinations				Flu; rotavirus; measles, mumps, rubella; hepatitis B; COVID-19
Other	Brain injury	Sleep apnoea		Continuous positive airway pressure for sleep apnoea; blood transfusion; location of care

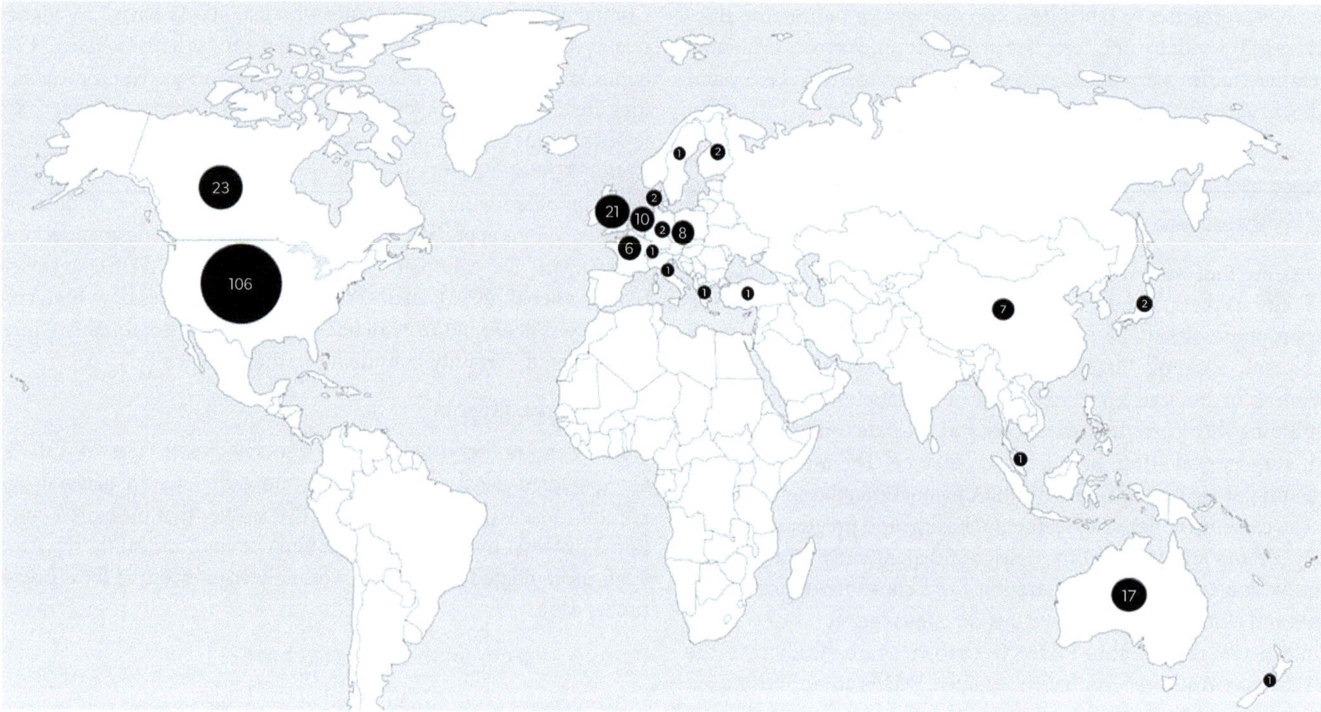

Figure 19.1 Map of countries where PtDAs were evaluated in randomized controlled trials.

the consultation. When the PtDA was used in the consultation, the consultation was on average 1.5 minutes longer compared to usual care. Of eight studies that measured healthcare resource use, seven showed no difference and one reduced the length of stay in the emergency department compared to usual care. For eight studies that measured associated costs or cost-effectiveness, there was no difference for five studies and three reported financial savings. Overall, few of the 209 studies measured health system outcomes.

Confidence in evidence supporting PtDAs over time

The original Cochrane review in 1999 and the 2014 update included randomized controlled trials evaluating PtDAs compared to usual care, as well as simple versus more detailed PtDAs (Table 19.3). The 2017 and 2024 updates only included randomized controlled trials that compared any PtDA to usual care. In 2024 compared to the previous update in 2017, the number of included studies nearly doubled with findings showing the same direction of effect. The main change over time for primary outcomes was a strengthening of the certainty/confidence in the evidence. For secondary outcomes, we had more studies measuring the same outcomes to facilitate meta-analysis for length of consultation time, patient–clinician communication, decision regret, and satisfaction with the decision making process.

Implementation of PtDAs following rigorous effectiveness studies

Although there is strong evidence of the effectiveness of PtDAs, few are implemented following the randomized controlled trials. We contacted the 106 authors of the 133 studies included in the previous Cochrane reviews of PtDAs to determine subsequent PtDA use in clinical practice following their trial (Stacey et al., 2019). Findings from the 98 authors who responded (93%) revealed 29 (28%) PtDAs were implemented, nine (9%) were disseminated to target users, and seven (7%) were diffused through various mechanisms. Author-reported barriers to use in clinical practice were lack of a post-study plan by the researcher team, outdated PtDAs, clinicians disagreed with their use, and lack of infrastructure or funding.

Suggestions for enhancing their use in clinical practice were co-designing PtDAs with users to ensure fit in clinical practice, online delivery of PtDAs, having an implementation plan, and endorsement by professional organizations, charities, and/or healthcare governments. These findings are consistent with a recent realist review focused on implementation of PtDAs (Joseph-Williams et al., 2021). This review recommended co-producing or co-adapting PtDAs with users including patients or health consumers, providing training in use of PtDAs, prompting patients to use PtDAs and discussing their perspectives on the decision, having PtDA use endorsed by senior leaders in the healthcare organization, and measuring outcomes for quality improvement.

To facilitate access to publicly available PtDAs, the Ottawa PtDAs Research Group at the Ottawa Hospital Research Institute established and maintains an international inventory of over 300 PtDAs (https://decisionaid.ohri.ca). Developers can submit their own PtDAs for inclusion in the inventory. To be eligible to be included, the resource needs to satisfy the definition of a PtDA (Table 19.1), be created, or updated with evidence that has been published within 5 years (fewer for rapidly emerging evidence), provide references to scientific evidence, and be freely accessible. The inventory provides a brief description of the PtDA, findings when it was appraised against the International Patient Decision Aid Standards, and a link to

Table 19.3 Effects of PtDAs compared to usual care on outcomes

Primary outcomes	1999 (N = 17)		2014 (N = 115)		2017 (N = 105)		2024 (N = 209)	
	Number of trials	Effect	Number of trials	Effect	Number of trials	Effect	Number of trials	Effect
Decision quality—informed values-based choice	0	-	13	+51% ⊕⊕⊖⊖	10	+106% ⊕⊕⊖⊖	21	+75% ⊕⊕⊕⊖
Knowledge of options, benefits, harms	4	+20%	42	+13% ⊕⊕⊕⊕	52	+13% ⊕⊕⊕⊕	107	+12% ⊕⊕⊕⊕
Realistic expectations of outcomes	1	n/s	19	+82% ⊕⊕⊕⊖	17	+110% ⊕⊕⊕⊖	25	+94% ⊕⊕⊕⊕
Feeling uninformed (decisional conflict subscale)	2	2+	22	−7% ⊕⊕⊕⊕	27	−9% ⊕⊕⊕⊕	58	−10% ⊕⊕⊕⊕
Feeling unclear values (decisional conflict subscale)	2	1 of 2+	18	−6% ⊕⊕⊕⊕	23	−9% ⊕⊕⊕⊕	55	−8% ⊕⊕⊕⊕
Undecided about which option	0	-	18	−41%	22	−36%	42	−32%
Clinician-controlled decision making	2	n/s	14	−34% ⊕⊕⊕⊖	16	−32% ⊕⊕⊕⊖	21	−28% ⊕⊕⊕⊕

GRADE certainty ratings: ⊕⊕⊕⊕ high; ⊕⊕⊕⊖ moderate; ⊕⊕⊖⊖ low; ⊕⊖⊖⊖ very low for 2014 to 2024.
n/s, not statistically significant.

access the PtDA. In 2016, Washington State Health Care Authority in the USA started certifying PtDAs using criteria based on these international standards. Certified PtDAs are listed on their website.

Role of patients and health consumers in PtDA research

Partnering with patients and health consumers as members of the research team enhances the relevance of the research for people who will use the findings (Bowen and Graham, 2013). Involvement of patient and health consumers has been strongly influenced by research funders in Australia, Canada, the UK, and the USA.

The teams conducting the Cochrane review of PtDAs and updates have included a patient or health consumer since the first publication in 1999 (O'Connor et al., 1999). The 2024 update included three patients/health consumers from Canada and Denmark who participated on the executive and steering committee teams (Stacey et al., 2024). Although the systematic review methods had to follow the *Cochrane Handbook for Systematic Reviews of Interventions* (https://training.cochrane.org/handbook), patients/health consumers participated in decisions about reducing the number of outcomes reported in this update, edited the plain language summary, and helped disseminate the findings. During this systematic review, we evaluated the extent to which team members, including patients/health consumers, felt meaningfully engaged. At baseline, we asked about their preferences for involvement in each of the 13 systematic review steps (e.g. 'keep me up to date' or 'invite to participate') and invited them to participate in the steps based on their preferences. Using the Patient Engagement in Research Scale (Hamilton et al., 2021), the responses of 13 team members indicated extremely meaningful engagement throughout the review process (including all three patients/health consumers). Two other team members reported being very meaningfully engaged, and two others moderately meaningfully engaged. At the end of the study, team members reported being satisfied with their level of involvement in the systematic review and believed it was a co-produced effort (Lewis et al., 2024; Stacey et al., 2025).

In the 2024 update, we extracted data using the Guidance for Reporting Involvement of Patients and the Public 2 (GRIPP2) checklist (Staniszewska et al., 2011) on the extent to which patients or health consumers were included on the research team that developed the PtDA and on the research teams that conducted the randomized controlled trial (Stacey et al., 2024). Of the 149 PtDAs included in a network meta-analysis, 90 reported patient involvement in the PtDA development and 95 reported patient involvement in the field testing of the PtDA. However, only 10% of the newly added 104 studies reported patients were part of the research team. Our network meta-analysis revealed 7% higher knowledge for patients using PtDAs that had been developed with patients'/health consumers' involvement compared to only including clinicians on the development team.

Conclusion

PtDAs are a type of intervention for communicating evidence-based information in a format to facilitate patient engagement in decision making. These interventions are used by patients in preparation for discussion with their clinician or used in the consultation together with their clinician. Findings from 209 randomized controlled trials show high certainty of evidence that patients who use them have improved decision making process outcomes and moderate certainty of evidence that patients will achieve informed values-matched choices. Knowledge gaps remain, related to health-care system outcomes and challenges with implementing PtDAs following the trials. Findings highlight the importance of having patients/health consumers involved in PtDA research, whether in

Box 19.1 Patient perspective

Patient and caregiver perspective

Since my diagnosis with a rare, chronic disease in childhood and later as a caregiver for family members with health conditions, I've struggled with the complexity of decisions for myself or as a caregiver (e.g. decisions about surgery, prostate cancer treatment, joining a clinical trial, screening, genetic testing, osteoporosis).

When it comes to my own healthcare decisions, making use of PtDAs has enabled me to overcome feelings of helplessness that often accompany a lifelong medical journey. PtDAs equip me with the tools I need to understand the options, risks, and benefits and to reflect on the outcomes that are important to me. This enables me to be actively engaged in my care.

What stands out to me are how PtDAs address the sometimes-harsh realities of healthcare systems, where time to consult with physicians and other healthcare professionals is limited and rushed. Physicians are focused on presenting the options. There is often little, or no time left to discuss what patients value. What are the outcomes that are most important to them? How do the options align with their values and preferences? A PtDA offers an opportunity to think about all the facets of a healthcare decision in a holistic way.

In many cases, patients have to be proactive about seeking PtDAs as they are not a requirement for most healthcare decisions and not everyone—including healthcare professionals—is aware of their existence. I usually start with asking the physician for a recommendation; however, I'm not discouraged if that doesn't work out. Fortunately, PtDAs are easy to find with a simple Google search. Reviewing it in preparation for the appointment helps patients not to be overwhelmed by the amount of information presented at an appointment. It also leads to preparing good questions to make the most effective use of the appointment time.

I've often thought about what my decision making process was like before PtDAs. I've always had a process, but I was scattered and very dependent on what I heard from the physician, that is to say reactive rather than proactive. Aside from the knowledge, better understanding of risks and benefits, and the time to think about the outcomes that are most important to me and what I value in a treatment, what I have found to be beneficial are the conversations that PtDAs allow me to have with my family and close friends who accompany me in my healthcare journey. The best support often comes from a person who understands the challenges a patient must grapple with when making a healthcare decision. I like to complete the PtDA on my own to allow me time to reflect and then go through the PtDA with a family member or friend. Those conversations have been very important to me, and their impact goes well beyond the decision itself.

PtDAs have also been a valuable tool for me as a caregiver. They facilitate and guide discussions about all aspects of a healthcare decision and allow caregivers to learn what's important to the patient. I often discovered that what I assumed was important to my loved one was not what they valued most. And I felt good about gaining a better understanding of the complexity of the decision from their perspective and doing something concrete to help them make the best decision for their needs in this situation.

Another significant way that I've interacted with PtDAs is as a 'patient partner', collaborating with research teams in their development and in research about PtDAs. I have contributed to two Cochrane systematic reviews about PtDAs, research into how people made decisions during the early years of the COVID-19 pandemic, co-developing a PtDA, and a study to update the international standards for PtDAs. It is of utmost importance that patients and the public be involved in the development of patient decisions aids, their evaluation, and research into PtDAs. We know that patient engagement will result in better PtDAs and in research that addresses the issues that are most important to the users of PtDAs. Let's embrace that co-production and continue adding to the inventory of PtDAs and disseminating them widely.

their development and testing, or as partners on the research teams seeking to evaluate PtDAs or to conduct systematic reviews on their effectiveness.

See Box 19.1 for our patient perspective.

REFERENCES

Andrews, J. C., Schunemann, H. J., Oxman, A. D., et al. 2013. GRADE guidelines 15: going from evidence to recommendation—determinants of a recommendation's direction and strength. *J Clin Epidemiol,* **66**, 726–735.

Bowen, S., Graham, I. D. 2013. Integrated knowledge translation. In: Straus, S. E., Tetroe, J., Graham, I. D., Eds. *Knowledge Translation in Health Care: Moving from Evidence to Practice.* Wiley Blackwell.

Elwyn, G., Hutchings, H., Edwards, A., et al. 2005. The OPTION scale: measuring the extent that clinicians involve patients in decision-making tasks. *Health Expect,* **8**, 34–42.

Hamilton, C. B., Hoens, A. M., Mckinnon, A. M., et al. 2021. Shortening and validation of the Patient Engagement In Research Scale (PEIRS) for measuring meaningful patient and family caregiver engagement. *Health Expect,* **24**, 863–879.

Hoefel, L., O'Connor, A. M., Lewis, K. B., et al. 2020. 20th anniversary update of the Ottawa Decision Support Framework Part 1: a systematic review of the decisional needs of people making health or social decisions. *Med Decis Making,* **40**, 555–581.

Joseph-Williams, N., Abhyankar, P., Boland, L., et al. 2021. What works in implementing patient decision aids in routine clinical settings? A rapid realist review and update from the IPDAS Collaboration. *Med Decis Making,* **41**, 907–937.

Joseph-Williams, N., Elwyn, G., Edwards, A. 2014. Knowledge is not power for patients: a systematic review and thematic synthesis of patient-reported barriers and facilitators to shared decision making. *Patient Educ Couns,* **94**, 291–309.

Lewis, K. B., Smith, M., Stacey, D., Carley, M., Graham, I. D., for the Cochrane Review of Patient Decision Aids Research Team. 2024. Evaluation of an integrated knowledge translation approach used for updating the Cochrane Review of Patient Decision Aids: a pre-post mixed methods study. *Res Involv Engagem,* **10**(1), 21.

O'Connor, A. M., Rostom, A., Fiset, V., et al. 1999. Decision aids for patients facing health treatment or screening decisions: systematic review. *BMJ,* **319**, 731–734.

Stacey, D., Carley, M., Gunderson, J., et al. 2025. The effect of patient decision aid attributes on patient outcomes: a network meta-analysis of a systematic review. *Med Decis Making.* First published online February 19, 2025. https://doi.org/10.1177/0272989X251318640

Stacey, D., Légaré, F., Lewis, K. B. 2017. Patient decision aids to engage adults in treatment or screening decisions. *JAMA,* **318**, 657–658.

Stacey, D., Lewis, K. B., Smith, M., et al. 2024. Decision aids for people facing health treatment or screening decisions. *Cochrane Database Syst Rev,* **1**, CD001431.

Stacey, D., Suwalska, V., Boland, L., et al. 2019. Are patient decision aids used in clinical practice after rigorous evaluation? A survey of trial authors. *Med Decis Making,* **39**, 805–815.

Stacey, D., Volk, R. J. 2021. The International Patient Decision Aid Standards (IPDAS) Collaboration: Evidence Update 2.0. *Med Decis Making,* **41**, 729–733.

Staniszewska, S., Brett, J., Mockford, C., Barber, R. 2011. The GRIPP checklist: strengthening the quality of patient and public involvement reporting in research. *Int J Technol Assess Health Care,* **27**, 391–399.

20

Patient decision aids

Access and sustainability of up-to-date tools

Anja Fog Heen, Roger Bertozzi, and Thomas Agoritsas

Introduction

Healthcare providers and patients need some form of guidance to navigate the increasing complexity of modern medicine. A balance is needed between making the evidence accessible and actionable and not oversimplifying it into a single algorithmic pathway.

A one-size-fits-all guidance has a high risk of being perceived as too directive, as being viewed as a norm or standard, and therefore ignoring patients' individual characteristics, values, and context. Practitioners and patients need help to support their own decision making rather than feel compelled to follow guidelines (Montori et al., 2021). In other words, the key question is not 'How should I apply guidance?' but 'How is it useful in this individual context?', much like a compass that shows the direction, the captain and his crew determine the best route among different alternatives.

Various tools can guide decision making. Clinical practice guidelines, typically targeted at clinicians at the point of care, aim to provide trustworthy recommendations based on current best evidence. Patient decision aids aim to convey the same evidence to patients and clinicians in preparation for a clinical encounter or as support during a conversation between a patient and their clinician.

One of the fundamental challenges in maintaining the relevance and usefulness of guidance tools such as clinical practice guidelines and decision aids is the rapid evolution of medical knowledge and evidence. The production, dissemination, and uptake of these tools face similar challenges. They are often not based on the best available evidence, and often become outdated quickly as new research emerges. In addition, the update of guidelines and the use of patient decision aids is highly variable, and their production is very time-consuming. The work of updating a decision aid is similar to updating a systematic review and demands similar structured processes to ensure quality and trustworthiness. They also tend to be unwieldy and do not fit well into the constraints of real-life clinical practice—they are not easily accessible and actionable in the clinical workflow. All these factors limit their use (Agoritsas et al., 2015; Heen et al., 2021a, 2021b).

To meet some of these challenges, decision aids and guidelines have standards to ensure their quality and trustworthiness. For guidelines to be trustworthy, their development must be based on a rigorous methodology. This includes that guidelines should be based on a systematic review of the current best evidence and be developed transparently in terms of methods and potential conflicts of interest. Standards for guideline development and identification can be found in the comprehensive report *Clinical Practice Guidelines We Can Trust* published by the Institute of Medicine (now the Academy of Medicine) in 2011 (Institute of Medicine, 2011). These standards have gained acceptance from key guideline organizations such as the Guideline International Network, National Institute for Health and Clinical Excellence, and World Health Organization.

Additionally, incorporating perspectives from a diverse range of stakeholders, including healthcare professionals and patients, ensures that guidelines reflect varied clinical experiences and patient preferences, ultimately leading to more inclusive and patient-centred recommendations. Despite these standards and their endorsement from guideline organizations, most current guidelines imperfectly meet these standards, highlighting persistent challenges in guideline development and implementation (Kung et al., 2012; Armstrong and Bloom, 2017).

Similarly, the International Patient Decision Aid Standards (IPDAS) provide criteria for the development, evidence content, and implementation of decision aids. A central domain in IPDAS is the requirement that the information in the tools should be based on comprehensive, critically appraised, and up-to-date syntheses of scientific evidence (Witteman et al., 2021). However, a rigorous analysis of 471 excising decision aids reveals that most decision aids did not report an explicit update or expiration policy, as well as deficiencies in citing scientific references, and most did not report on evidence appraisal or the quality of evidence (Hoffmann et al., 2021). Similarly, an evaluation from 2018 showed that less than half of organizations developing decision aids had documented their approaches for evidence summarization. This underscores the need for enhanced adherence to IPDAS criteria to bolster the credibility and effectiveness of decision aids (Dannenberg et al., 2018).

The described challenges with guidance tools such as guidelines and decision aids have traditionally been addressed in silos. A multitude of actors are involved in the process from evidence being produced to its use at the point of care. Actors of evidence synthesis, guideline and decision aid developers, actors working to disseminate guidance, clinicians, patients, and those who evaluate and improve practice are all actors in the same system, where siloed communities and actors struggle within a poorly functioning evidence ecosystem.

Here information flow and utilization are inefficient and incomplete with evidence often being of limited reliability and relevance. Primary research too often represents waste for patients and society. The epidemic of flawed systematic reviews and guidelines often leave end users of evidence unable to make well-informed decisions. Implementation of evidence into practice may be delayed or not happen at all, with scattered attempts at measuring impact on healthcare performance and patient outcomes. The result is countries and healthcare systems struggling to maximize value in healthcare while continuing to waste resources under increasingly constrained budgets. And, how do we create and feed new more relevant, and reliable evidence into the loop, making this a true learning healthcare system?

Through developments and innovations of evidence ecosystems and learning health systems, we believe these challenges are better addressed by increasing value and reducing waste in healthcare and research by facilitating evidence flow, from its inception to documented improved care through links between currently siloed communities of people producing, synthesizing, disseminating, and implementing evidence into practice (Boutron et al., 2020; Vandvik and Brandt, 2020; Heen et al., 2021a).

As an example, clinical guidelines from prominent medical societies tended to be updated every 4 years on average. The COVID-19 pandemic made it obvious that decision makers—clinicians and patients alike—need more current guidance, and led to calls for living evidence synthesis and living guidance (Lamontagne et al., 2021; Vandvik et al., 2021). Similarly, shared decision making tools should adopt the same approach. Currently, many decision aids are not updated at all, partly because of limitations in funding after the development of the tool, often being developed as a part of a research project.

Publishing standards may act as an invitation to do better, for example, by having standards for updating, but is unlikely to result in the sustainable production, dissemination, and use of evidence-based guidelines and decision making tools, although the obvious potential harms of outdated tools can be if they are used at the point of care. Methods are needed within the evidence ecosystem to synthesize evidence in a rigorous and timely way. Pairwise comparisons of interventions (as occurs in randomized trials, and therefore in most systematic reviews) are increasingly replaced by large network meta-analyses comparing multiple interventions.

The body of evidence summarized by network analyses continues to increase in scale. For example, a recent review of drug treatment for type 2 diabetes included 816 randomized trials on 13 different drug classes (Shi et al., 2023). Such endeavours were exceptional a few years ago, yet they are likely to become the new standard for high-quality evidence synthesis, given that the number of relevant publications continues to rise almost exponentially, making it almost impossible to keep up using traditional standards for evidence synthesis, directly affecting the underlying evidence of both guidelines and tools for decision making.

Exploring avenues for the sustainability of decision aids involves navigating complex challenges, particularly in establishing partnerships with conventional vendors and stakeholders. Collaborative initiatives like Option Grids, originally developed by Professors Elwyn and Durand (Elwyn et al., 2013), later to engage with commercial vendors, provide access to resources for decision aid development and dissemination. However, while these partnerships can offer benefits, they also raise important questions regarding financial conflicts of interest, inherent in partnerships with commercial vendors.

Reliance on external partnerships for sustainability can be precarious. It may introduce vulnerabilities related to resource dependency and continuity. To mitigate these challenges, alternative avenues for decision aid sustainability have been explored. For instance, initiatives focused on public funding, philanthropic support, or government grants aim to reduce reliance on commercial partnerships but do not guarantee long-term viability of their development.

More than ever, to ensure sustainability, a closer collaboration between researchers, healthcare institutions, healthcare policymakers, patient partners, and advocacy groups are required. Such synergies are also needed to mutualize funding and human resources. Joint efforts between funding entities and stakeholders—commercial, non-commercial, and even governmental—could provide new opportunities to address these numerous challenges while increasing value and reducing waste (Chalmers and Glasziou, 2009). Independent funding or national-level grant competitions are unlikely to meet the data analysis demands of a new and more rigorous updated evidence landscape. Living collaboration across multiple stakeholders needs to replace projects that lack the resources to meet the challenges of accurately summarizing scientific evidence for a wide range of audiences.

Of course, creating such synergies brings new challenges as well, particularly in managing competing or even conflicting interests, whether financial or intellectual. Health disparities are increasing, both in terms of access to care and evidence-based resources. Evidence production and synthesis is heavily biased towards high-income countries and delivers tools that are much less adapted to low- and middle-income countries. Producing and adapting tools that serve everyone, including vulnerable, underserved, and diverse populations, is both an ethical requirement and a public health necessity. Paywalls (and delivery systems) continue to limit access to care and access to knowledge. Such challenges require innovations, vision, and high-level decisions from policymakers who wish to see a more equitable and healthier world emerging as inequity is inherently pathogenic.

Embracing open-access models and collaborative frameworks such as the evidence ecosystem can foster innovation and knowledge sharing while enhancing the sustainability of decision aids that serve everyone. Ultimately, achieving sustainability in decision aid development requires a multifaceted approach that balances collaboration with independence and transparency with innovation.

Technology can help in more than one way. Authoring and publication platforms offer opportunities to digitally structure data and structured assessment of evidence, guidance, and tools. These data can then be translated into various formats and tools that can be continually updated as new evidence emerges and accumulates, and the half-life of published evidence is diminishing (Vandvik et al., 2013, 2021; Agoritsas et al., 2015).

Integration of tools in electronic health records can make them more easily accessible at the point of care, possibly reducing some of the barriers to access and use, and thereby providing more opportunities for personalized approaches based on patient characteristics and context. But this degree of seamless integration requires user-centred approaches to overcome information overload for clinicians, alert fatigue, and ensure that decision support technologies are usefully embedded in workflows, and help users, clinicians, and patients alike.

The recent breakthrough in the usefulness of artificial intelligence (AI), particularly with the applicability of large language models, is likely to revolutionize many processes in the evidence-summarization ecosystem: evidence production, synthesis, living updates, and the creation of guidance are likely to change dramatically.

It may also deliver a more sustainable approach to the production of patient decision aids, infographics, and other innovating decision-support tools. AI might streamline repetitive processes and add value that we cannot yet imagine. However, technology-based optimism will not solve all access issues and may come with new costs, burdens, and ethical and political challenges. It may even further increase health disparities, notably among the poor in the most industrialized nations, and in the developing and least developed countries, despite the obvious benefits low-cost technology has brought so far to healthcare in unfavoured communities.

AI may lead to a new 'black box' phenomenon where we lack understanding of the processes involved, which may be susceptible to bias and to undue influence and interests. Principles of assessment of healthcare remain as applicable to new innovations as they have been to past innovations. Thus, we need to provide the same level of scientific, ethical, and sociopolitical scrutiny to AI as we did in the past for new medical treatments and interventions.

Additionally, digital disinformation and misinformation pose significant threats to the advancement of science, medicine, and decision making processes, as they have the capacity to influence individuals' cognitive and behavioural patterns regardless of their educational or socioeconomic backgrounds. The impact of social media on healthcare and patient–clinician communication is strong, with patients often bringing social media-derived concerns into clinical settings and discussing their experiences online (Luo et al., 2022; Kjaerulff et al., 2023).

The COVID-19 pandemic has highlighted the high prevalence of misinformation, as well as the importance of understanding and addressing the proliferation of health-related content on social media platforms. To effectively navigate these challenges, researchers, doctors, and healthcare professionals must recognize societal issues as integral components of their roles and acknowledge the significant influence wielded by social media in shaping healthcare perceptions and behaviours.

While patient decision aids have been primarily designed to support individual shared decision making, another potential strategy is to implement them more widely as educational resources and tools. In addition to a learning effect both for the patient and the clinician, a decision aid can help a doctor learn how to conduct a conversation and how to browse evidence from a patient and conversational perspective, instead of excessively relying on structured evidence recommendations or guideline-based algorithms. This approach shifts the focus towards cultivating conversational skills and adapting to individual patient needs. In addition, rather than focusing solely on implementing individual decision aids—an approach that has proven limited and unsustainable without extensive resources—there is a need to assess how a wide range of these tools can transform people's approach to shared decision making.

The future arrives quickly. The last decade has seen more progress than we can imagine in so many fields, from methods and standards to digitalization and the use of technology. However, we are no closer to ensuring equitable access to sustainable updated evidence and trustworthy knowledge and tools. Sustainability encompasses a broad spectrum of considerations beyond just methodological or technological aspects.

Achieving sustainability and accessibility in the evidence ecosystem requires a holistic approach. Key stakeholders, including professionals and patients, can call for regulations and clearer governance to address these challenges effectively, particularly with the emergence of AI. By focusing on regulatory frameworks and governance structures, we can work towards ensuring that the benefits of progress are equitably distributed and that the tools and knowledge necessary for decision making become accessible to all.

See Box 20.1 for our patient perspective.

Box 20.1 Patient perspective

Guidance is a natural human need

From looking at stars millennia ago to AI tools today, we have always been in search of directions to help navigate our existential journeys. Among them, safely and optimally managing our health from birth to death is fundamental because all other dimensions of our lives depend on our mental and physical well-being, while illnesses have enormous disruptive and destructive powers on the fate of individuals or societies. This applies also to states and to our international system, in the case of pandemics for example, or with environmental and civilizational pathologies such as obesity and allergies. Hence the paramount importance of guidance in the practice of medicine and in the governance of public health. It is therefore important to reflect on the meaning of guidelines and of decision aids from a patient's perspective, and this has a direct public health dimension, as societal acceptance of praxis is an integral part of the quality of medicine.

The work around the methodology of guidelines and their communication also determines in great part public perception and adherence, and here a note of caution must be sounded as doctors and patients may be inclined to perceive guidelines and decision aids in a normative way, rather than for what they are meant. In other words, the key question is not 'How should I follow?' but 'How are they useful?'

We need pedagogy after methodology, and in a sense, we must encourage the medical caregivers–patients ecosystem, or rather community, to reflect on the formulation and adoption of guidelines, and on how to best use guidelines and decision aids.

We can think of a metaphor to represent the function of guidelines: guidance is like a compass. The compass shows the direction, the captain (the healthcare community) determines the best route options, and the whole crew (all citizens) make the navigation safest for themselves, whatever the circumstances. That's how shared decision making tools, guidelines, and dialogue can work hand in hand to deliver the optimal cognitive and behavioural equation and the best possible healthcare at a point in time. This equation should optimally integrate, from the patient's perspective, an understanding of the limitations, adherence to the recommendations, and observance of the subsequent treatments.

Guidelines and decision aid tools constitute therefore a holistic and community-oriented, technologically and methodologically supported, partnership of minds in the day-to-day medical practice, respecting the 'art' of the practitioner and the intimate freedom of the patient. This works for the wider benefit of society, as the sum of successful treatments and healthier citizens positively impacts social cohesion, public finances, and economic productivity; in other words, it concurs with prosperity, well-being, and the pursuit of happiness.

The quality of the whole process, from elaborating guidelines to following them under the form of the patient's consent and adherence to their doctor's recommendation, constitutes a fundamental element of what is called 'the dignity of the patient': this inherent dignity is not served just by medical excellence, it is attained and supported when the patient's informed knowledge and understanding are embodied in their satisfaction, trust, adherence, and observance.

Guidelines-based medicine is in essence a holistic, community-oriented partnership of minds.

REFERENCES

Agoritsas, T., Heen, A. F., Brandt, L., et al. 2015. Decision aids that really promote shared decision making: the pace quickens. *BMJ*, **350**, g7624.

Armstrong, M. J., Bloom, J. A. 2017. Patient involvement in guidelines is poor five years after Institute of Medicine standards: review of guideline methodologies. *Res Involv Engagem*, **3**, 19.

Boutron, I., Crequit, P., Williams, H., Meerpohl, J., Craig, J. C., Ravaud, P. 2020. Future of evidence ecosystem series: 1. Introduction. Evidence synthesis ecosystem needs dramatic change. *J Clin Epidemiol*, **123**, 135–142.

Chalmers, I., Glasziou, P. 2009. Avoidable waste in the production and reporting of research evidence. *Lancet*, **374**, 86–89.

Dannenberg, M. D., Durand, M. A., Montori, V. M., Reilly, C., Elwyn, G. 2018. Existing evidence summarization methods cannot guarantee trustworthy patient decision aids. *J Clin Epidemiol*, **102**, 69–77.

Elwyn, G., Lloyd, A., Joseph-Williams, N., et al. 2013. Option grids: shared decision making made easier. *Patient Educ Couns*, **90**, 207–212.

Heen, A. F., Vandvik, P. O., Brandt, L., et al. 2021a. Decision aids linked to evidence summaries and clinical practice guidelines: results from user-testing in clinical encounters. *BMC Med Inform Decis Mak*, **21**, 202.

Heen, A. F., Vandvik, P. O., Brandt L, et al. 2021b. A framework for practical issues was developed to inform shared decision-making tools and clinical guidelines. *J Clin Epidemiol*, **129**, 104–113.

Hoffmann, T. C., Bakhit, M., Durand, M. A., Perestelo-Perez, L., Saunders, C., Brito, J. P. 2021. Basing information on comprehensive, critically appraised, and up-to-date syntheses of the scientific evidence: an update from the International Patient Decision Aid Standards. *Med Decis Making*, **41**, 755–767.

Institute of Medicine. 2011. *Clinical Practice Guidelines We Can Trust.* The National Academies Press.

Kjaerulff, E. M., Andersen, T. H., Kingod, N., Nexo, M. A. 2023. When people with chronic conditions turn to peers on social media to obtain and share information: systematic review of the implications for relationships with health care professionals. *J Med Internet Res*, **25**, e41156.

Kung, J., Miller, R. R., Mackowiak, P. A. 2012. Failure of clinical practice guidelines to meet institute of medicine standards: two more decades of little, if any, progress. *Arch Intern Med*, **172**, 1628–1633.

Lamontagne, F., Agoritsas, T., Siemieniuk, R., et al. 2021. A living WHO guideline on drugs to prevent covid-19. *BMJ*, **372**, n526.

Luo, A., Qin, L., Yuan, Y., et al. 2022. The effect of online health information seeking on physician-patient relationships: systematic review. *J Med Internet Res*, **24**, e23354.

Montori, V., Allwood, D., Heen, A. F. 2021. A moratorium on strong recommendations is needed. *BMJ*, **375**, n2887.

Shi, Q., Nong, K., Vandvik, P. O., et al. 2023. Benefits and harms of drug treatment for type 2 diabetes: systematic review and network meta-analysis of randomised controlled trials. *BMJ*, **381**, e074068.

Vandvik, P. O., Askie, L., Glen, F., Tendal, B., Agoritsas, T. 2021. COVID-19: living guidelines help fix cracks in evidence pipeline. *Nature*, **595**, 172.

Vandvik, P. O., Brandt, L., Alonso-Coello, P., et al. 2013. Creating clinical practice guidelines we can trust, use, and share: a new era is imminent. *Chest*, **144**, 381–389.

Vandvik, P. O., Brandt, L. 2020. Future of evidence ecosystem series: evidence ecosystems and learning health systems: why bother? *J Clin Epidemiol*, **123**, 166–170.

Witteman, H. O., Maki, K. G., Vaisson, G., et al. 2021. Systematic development of patient decision aids: an update from the IPDAS Collaboration. *Med Decis Making*, **41**, 736–754.

21

Large-scale implementation of shared decision making in Germany

Three case studies

Pola Hahlweg, Anja Lindig, Cordula Mühr, Kai-Uwe Parsons-Galka, Fülöp Scheibler

Current state and implementation needs of shared decision making in Germany

With the Law on Patient's Rights that passed in 2013, Germany has granted a legal claim to informed healthcare decisions based on a partnership between clinicians and patients and on comprehensive and comprehensible information (Bundesgesetzblatt, 2013). Numerous public organizations, reports, action plans, and funding initiatives have supported shared decision making (SDM) over the years (Hahlweg et al., 2022). In addition, SDM has been increasingly incorporated into medical students' and other healthcare providers' education curricula (Hahlweg et al., 2022). However, as in other countries, SDM implementation in routine healthcare is limited in Germany (Braun and Marstedt, 2014; German Federal Association of Statutory Health Insurance Physicians, 2016; Hahlweg et al., 2020). Several implementation efforts aim to close this gap. These range from initiatives to improve access to evidence-based information or developing patient decision aids and guidelines to SDM training studies and complex SDM implementation projects (e.g. see Hahlweg et al. (2022) for an overview of current developments). This chapter showcases three case studies of large-scale SDM implementation efforts in Germany: the PREPARED trial from Hamburg, the MAKING SDM A REALITY study in Kiel that developed the SHARE TO CARE programme, and efforts to make SDM a nationwide quality indicator. Two patient perspectives complement this chapter (Boxes 21.1 and 21.2).

Case study 1: PREPARED trial

From 2013 to 2020, a stepped wedge cluster randomized trial to develop and evaluate an empirically and theoretically based multicomponent SDM implementation programme in routine cancer

Box 21.1 Patient perspective

The patient perspective on SDM implementation in Germany—part 1

Kai-Uwe Parsons-Galka, cancer patient, chairperson of the bone marrow transplant patient support association in Hamburg (Germany)

Looking at SDM in Germany from the patient's perspective is a complex subject. I speak from my experience as an active member and chairperson of the bone marrow transplant patient association in Hamburg for more than 9 years as well as being a cancer patient myself. Over the years, I talked to numerous cancer patients and heard their stories and struggles. I try to summarize what I heard from them in the following.

Generally, human beings place a high level of trust in medical professionals, which is also due to their renown in society. In addition, many patients tend to have rather insufficient medical knowledge. Only a small minority seems to be interested in learning more about their own illness.

Patients need to have some knowledge about the existence of SDM. Furthermore, it's important to provide them with different easy-to-understand information and resources enabling them to make use of SDM if they wish to do so.

Good communication skills and an empathetic attitude in healthcare professionals are crucial for successful SDM. Patients need clear and understandable medical information about their health condition, treatment options, and potential outcomes. Training healthcare professionals in effective communication techniques and empathy, such as using plain language and ensuring patients understand the information provided, should be part of medical education, practical training, and examinations.

Another patient-relevant aspect to consider and clarify around SDM is liability. Who is responsible, if the patient and physician decided on a certain treatment together and the treatment turns out to harm the patient? Can the patient still claim for compensation? This is not to say that SDM should not be practised, but as a patient I ask for clarity regarding liability after SDM.

care (PREPARED trial) was conducted at the University Medical Center Hamburg-Eppendorf (UKE) and funded by the German Research Foundation (Scholl et al., 2018). This included a 1-year pilot study to develop the programme and a 3-year implementation trial to evaluate it, including outcome and process evaluation. Implementation research served as a theoretical underpinning for the pilot study and the subsequent trial, primarily the Consolidated Framework for Implementation Research (Damschroder et al., 2009). During the pilot study at the University Cancer Center Hamburg, a multi-method approach was used to assess the current state and needs regarding SDM. This included observation, focus groups, individual interviews, and document analysis (Hahlweg et al., 2015, 2017a, 2017b; Frerichs et al., 2016; Müller et al., 2016) and concluded with developing the SDM implementation programme. The programme comprised six strategies addressing three audiences (**Figure 21.1**): healthcare professionals, patients, and departments. We trained physicians and nurses in SDM. We distributed the German adaptation of the 'Ask 3 Questions' intervention (Lindig et al., 2020), an existing generic patient decision aid, and information materials. We revised quality management documents and reflected on the organization of tumour boards with relevant stakeholders.

The stepped wedge cluster randomized trial with three departments of the University Cancer Center Hamburg evaluated the programme's effects in routine cancer care, with SDM uptake from the patients' perspective, assessed by the nine-item Shared Decision Making Questionnaire (SDM-Q-9) (Kriston et al., 2010) as the primary outcome. No statistically significant differences between pre- and post-implementation were demonstrated for the primary outcome (Scholl et al., 2021). This was also true for most secondary outcomes (Scholl et al., 2021).

The process evaluation gave possible explanations for the limited effects and showed that although all implementation strategies had been rolled out at each department, there had been limited reach, variable doses, and several adaptations made during the trial (Scholl et al., 2021). In addition, a qualitative assessment of influencing factors on SDM implementation demonstrated the complexity of interconnected factors in all domains of the Consolidated Framework for Implementation Research (Hahlweg et al., 2023).

The results of this trial imply that other and more intensive approaches might be needed for a successful department-wide implementation of SDM in routine cancer care, as well as more comprehensive attention to the impact of influencing factors.

Case study 2: MAKING SDM A REALITY

The MAKING SDM A REALITY project aimed to implement SDM across an entire university medical centre in Kiel, Germany (Danner et al., 2020; Scheibler et al., 2024). It was funded from October 2017 to September 2021 by the German Innovation Fund of the Federal Joint Committee. The goal was to test the scalability of innovative forms of care that have been proven effective in smaller studies. If such testing succeeds, they can be recommended for standard medical care.

The four strategies of the SHARE TO CARE programme, the funded demonstration project, were to (1) provide SDM training for the physicians, (2) introduce patient activation interventions (e.g. Ask 3 Questions), (3) develop evidence-based, online patient decision aids in all departments, and (4) train specialized nurses in decision coaching (**Figure 21.2**).

The four strategies were implemented at the entire Kiel campus of the University Hospital Schleswig-Holstein, which treats around 220,000 patients annually. The Kiel campus has 25 departments, roughly 620 doctors, and 1100 nurses, making it one of the ten largest university medical centres in Germany.

Results demonstrated the feasibility and effectiveness of the large-scale implementation. The patient-reported measure called 'Perceived Involvement in Care' showed statistically significant and

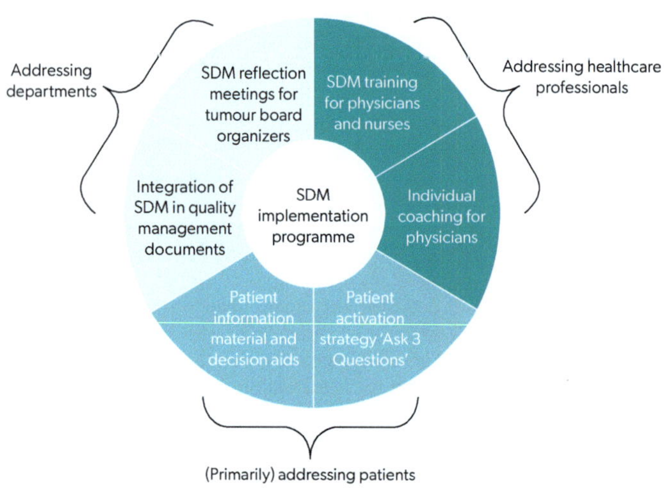

Figure 21.1 SDM implementation programme of the PREPARED trial.

Adapted from Hahlweg, P., Lindig, A., Frerichs, W., et al. 2023. Major influencing factors on routine implementation of shared decision-making in cancer care: qualitative process evaluation of a stepped-wedge cluster randomized trial. *BMC Health Serv Res*, 23, 840 under a Creative Commons Attribution 4.0 International License (https://creativecommons.org/licenses/by/4.0/deed.en).

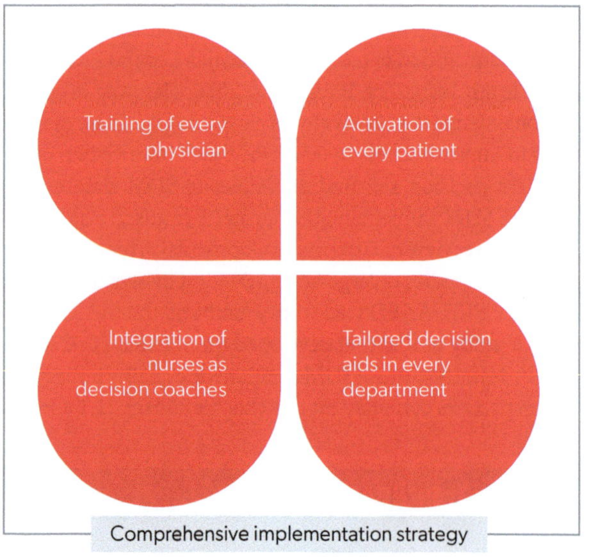

Figure 21.2 The SHARE TO CARE programme.

Reproduced with permission from Danner, M., Geiger, F., Wehkamp, K., et al. 2020. Making shared decision-making (SDM) a reality: protocol of a large-scale long-term SDM implementation programme at a Northern German University Hospital. *BMJ Open*, 10, e037575.

clinically meaningful increases in the score (Scheibler et al., 2024). Subsequently, the German Federal Joint Committee (2023) has recommended the project's strategies for standard care.

In Germany, the Federal Ministry of Health set up a commission to advise on modernizing healthcare in hospitals and basing it on current needs (German Federal Ministry of Health, 2023a). As a further consequence of the MAKING SDM A REALITY project, this commission incorporated the project's results into its activities. It recommended that successful SDM implementation become part of quality-related remuneration (German Federal Ministry of Health, 2023b). To this end, the effective introduction of SDM tools and methods must be demonstrated by evaluation, including patient assessments (German Federal Ministry of Health, 2023b). The instruments of the SHARE TO CARE programme were explicitly named by the commission as suitable for quality-oriented remuneration.

In the next years it will be apparent how many of the government commission's recommendations will be incorporated into German jurisdiction. This means there is a realistic chance that SDM will become a nationwide priority in Germany in the next few years.

Case study 3: SDM as a nationwide quality indicator

For this last case example, we stay at the policy level. In Germany, the government transfers tasks to the Federal Joint Committee (G-BA), the highest decision making body of the self-regulated organizations of health insurers and healthcare providers in Germany. On behalf of the G-BA, the independent scientific Institute for Quality Assurance and Transparency in Health Care (IQTIG) develops indicators to measure the quality of routine healthcare. So far, Germany almost exclusively uses clinical indicators or secondary data such as routine administration data. Patient-reported outcomes and experiences, especially SDM, as quality indicators are not used. This means that a central component of quality management has yet to be incorporated into the German healthcare system (Steinbeck et al., 2021).

In 2022, in the field of cardiac catheterization, a representative and mandatory patient survey with patient-reported outcome and experience measures (PROMs, PREMs) was introduced as a standard component of nationwide quality assessment for the first time in Germany (Blatt et al., 2023). The G-BA commissioned the development of a patient survey from the IQTIG based on the German Law on Patient's Rights (Bundesgesetzblatt, 2013). Central instruments within this survey are measures of patient information and SDM (Blatt et al., 2023). The G-BA has approved the development of further PREMs and PROMs as part of quality assessments in schizophrenia, schizotypal and delusional disorders, renal replacement therapy, outpatient psychotherapeutic care, and hospital discharge management (Blatt, 2022). Most of them include instruments to measure SDM. However, so far, none of these have been implemented in routine care by the G-BA.

The latest commission awarded to IQTIG in 2022 has been on the quality of the indication for hysterectomy in benign diseases (German Federal Joint Committee, 2022). Here, the focus of the patient-reported survey is, for the first time, on the process

Box 21.2 Patient perspective

The patient perspective on SDM implementation in Germany—part 2

Cordula Mühr, honorary patient representative on the G-BA in Berlin since 2004 on participation and co-determination on all levels

The current efforts to implement SDM have their precursors in long-standing participation movements in Germany. *'Nothing about us without us'* was the motto adopted by the disability movement, which formed in Germany in the 1960s to address the segregation and disenfranchisement of disabled people under National Socialism. Like the women's health movement in the 1970s and the so-called new social movements in the 1980s, it challenged hierarchical relationships in many areas of society, including the healthcare system, and advocated self-determination and participation. Although the Ottawa Charter of the World Health Organization (1986), for example, regarded empowerment and participation as integrated components of health promotion, citizen participation in the healthcare system was not a topic of legal discussion in Germany until 1999 (Badura and Schellschmidt, 1999).

In its 2002 report, the Expert Council for Concerted Action in Health Care (2002) called for improved participation of those affected through more information, consultation, and co-determination rights in decision making bodies of the healthcare system. Finally, on 1 January 2004, patient involvement on the policy level was legally manifested in Section 140f of the German Social Code V. This gave relevant patient organizations the right to co-consult and propose motions in healthcare decision making bodies that deal with healthcare issues, albeit without voting rights.

For 20 years now, the approximately 300 primarily honorary patient representatives in the G-BA have seen themselves as a counterweight to the other stakeholders by bringing the experiences of those affected into the deliberations. They also promote transparency about decision making processes and quality in medical care (Patient Representation in the G-BA, 2013).

Patient representatives in self-governing bodies must be systematically and sustainably strengthened so that they can adequately fulfil their legal mandate to help shape the healthcare system by giving voice to those who are underrepresented in the existing administration structures (Danner, 2023).

of decision making, explicitly including SDM. This highlights the potential of a close interlink between PREMs and PROMs in nationwide healthcare quality assessment and SDM implementation at a policy level.

Patient representatives play a pivotal role in the continuous improvements regarding mandatory and representative patient surveys, including SDM as standard components of healthcare quality indicators in Germany (Box 21.2). They have been campaigning for this since 2006 (Birkner, 2011). However, bringing this cultural change to the healthcare system and the minds of healthcare providers remains a challenge. To truly implement SDM, we need to understand how to bring evidence-based medicine and patients' informed preferences together in the treatment process (Sackett et al., 1996; McCormack and Elwyn, 2018).

Conclusion and outlook

By describing three large-scale SDM implementation efforts that have been undertaken in Germany and the views of two patient representatives, this chapter showcases the complexity of SDM implementation in routine care. The PREPARED trial demonstrates how implementation research can inform trials evaluating multi-component SDM programmes from preparation and development to implementation, evaluation, and interpretation of findings and stands as an example of a thoroughly planned and executed implementation trial with a distinct research focus. The MAKING SDM A REALITY project shows how hospital-wide implementation of SDM in a university medical centre with a strong focus on scalability can be undertaken and emphasizes the potential of such successful large-scale implementation projects to influence policy on the national level. The PREPARED trial and the MAKING SDM A REALITY project included SDM implementation strategies aimed at patients, healthcare providers, and whole departments. Furthermore, case study 3 and the patient perspective of Cordula Mühr (**Box 21.2**) showed how patient representatives can push for policy change regarding quality indicators and how SDM combined with other patient-centred tools such as PREMs and PROMs can improve quality in healthcare. Focusing on the person at the centre, the individual patient, Kai-Uwe Parsons-Galka (**Box 21.1**) highlighted the SDM-related challenges and needs of seriously ill people in healthcare in Germany. Taking everything together, it becomes apparent that successful SDM implementation is highly complex and needs changes on all levels: the individual, the dyadic, the organizational, and the system. Nonetheless, many promising activities are currently underway in Germany.

REFERENCES

Badura, B., Schellschmidt, H. 1999. Citizen participation—a challenge to different health care systems [in German]. German Federal Center for Health Education. Available at: https://shop.bzga.de/pdf/60610000.pdf

Birkner, N. 2011. Quality assurance in breast surgery: the aim is participatory decision-making [in German]. *Deutsches Aerzteblatt,* **108**, A96.

Blatt, K. 2022. Patient survey PCI: first year and outlook [in German]. Institute for Quality Assurance and Transparency in Health Care. Available at: https://www.g-ba.de/downloads/17-98-5402/PV1_1_Blatt_Patientenbefragungen-im-ersten-Jahr_2022-11-25.pdf

Blatt, K., Hassan, M., Volland, C., Messer, M. 2023. Patient-centred care with PREMs and PROMs: survey of patients with percutaneous cardiac intervention (PCI) and coronary angiography. *Z Evid Fortbild Qual Gesundhwes,* **178**, 8–14.

Braun, B., Marstedt, G. 2014. Shared decision-making at the doctor's: aspiration and reality [in German]. In: Böcken, J., Braun, B., Meierjürgen, R., Eds. *Gesundheitsmonitor 2014.* Verlag Bertelsmann Stiftung.

Bundesgesetzblatt 2013. *Law for Improving the Rights of Patients* [in German]. Bundesanzeiger Verlag.

Damschroder, L. J., Aron, D. C., Keith, R. E., Kirsh, S. R., Alexander, J. A., Lowery, J. C. 2009. Fostering implementation of health services research findings into practice: a consolidated framework for advancing implementation science. *Implement Sci,* **4**, 50.

Danner, M. 2023. Strengthening patient participation and representation in the Federal Joint Committee (G-BA) and other participation bodies in accordance with Section 140f SGB V for consideration in the Healthcare Reinforcement Act [in German]. Available at: https://www.bag-selbsthilfe.de/fileadmin/user_upload/News/2023/23-07-21_Forderungen_der_PatV_zum_GVSG__End.docx

Danner, M., Geiger, F., Wehkamp, K., et al. 2020. Making shared decision-making (SDM) a reality: protocol of a large-scale long-term SDM implementation programme at a Northern German University Hospital. *BMJ Open,* **10**, e037575.

Expert Council for Concerted Action in Health Care. 2002. Needs-based justice and economic efficiency [in German]. Available at: https://www.svr-gesundheit.de/fileadmin/Gutachten/Gutachten_2000_2001/Kurzfassung_Band1_2.pdf

Frerichs, W., Hahlweg, P., Müller, E., Adis, C., Scholl, I. 2016. Shared decision-making in oncology—a qualitative analysis of healthcare providers' views on current practice. *PLoS One,* **11**, e0149789.

German Federal Association of Statutory Health Insurance Physicians. 2016. Survey of insured persons by the German Federal Association of Statutory Health Insurance Physicians 2016 [in German]. Available at: https://www.kbv.de/media/sp/2016_Berichtband.pdf

German Federal Joint Committee. 2022. Decision of the Federal Joint Committee to commission the IQTIG to develop a patient survey on the process quality of the indication of hysterectomies for benign diseases from the patient's perspective [in German]. Available at: https://www.g-ba.de/downloads/39-261-5357/2022-03-18_IQTIG-Beauftragung_Patientenbefragung-Hysterektomien.pdf

German Federal Joint Committee. 2023. Decision of the Innovation Committee of the Federal Joint Committee in accordance with Section 92B (3) SGB V on the completed MAKING SDM A REALITY project (01Nvf17009) [in German]. Available at: https://innovationsfonds.g-ba.de/downloads/beschluss-dokumente/373/2023-02-23_MAKING-SDM-A-REALITY.pdf

German Federal Ministry of Health. 2023a. Government commission for modern and needs-based hospital care [in German]. Available at: https://www.bundesgesundheitsministerium.de/themen/krankenhaus/regierungskommission-krankenhausversorgung

German Federal Ministry of Health. 2023b. More quality and less bureaucracy in hospitals: government commission presents recommendations on minimum requirements [in German]. Available at: https://www.bundesgesundheitsministerium.de/presse/pressemitteilungen/mehr-qualitaet-und-weniger-buerokratie-im-krankenhaus-pm-20-10-23.html

Hahlweg, P., Bieber, C., Levke Brütt, A., et al. 2022. Moving towards patient-centered care and shared decision-making in Germany. *Z Evid Fortbild Qual Gesundhwes,* **171**, 49–57.

Hahlweg, P., Didi, S., Kriston, L., Härter, M., Nestoriuc, Y., Scholl, I. 2017a. Process quality of decision-making in multidisciplinary cancer team meetings: a structured observational study. *BMC Cancer,* **17**, 772.

Hahlweg, P., Härter, M., Nestoriuc, Y, Scholl, I. 2017b. How are decisions made in cancer care? A qualitative study using participant observation of current practice. *BMJ Open,* **7**, e016360.

Hahlweg, P., Hoffmann, J., Härter, M., Frosch, D. L., Elwyn, G., Scholl, I. 2015. In absentia: an exploratory study of how patients are considered in multidisciplinary cancer team meetings. *PLoS One,* **10**, e0139921.

Hahlweg, P., Kriston, L., Scholl, I., et al. 2020. Cancer patients' preferred and perceived level of involvement in treatment decision-making: an epidemiological study. *Acta Oncol,* **59**, 967–974.

Hahlweg, P., Lindig, A., Frerichs, W., et al. 2023. Major influencing factors on routine implementation of shared decision-making in cancer care: qualitative process evaluation of a stepped-wedge cluster randomized trial. *BMC Health Serv Res,* **23**, 840.

Kriston, L., Scholl, I., Hölzel, L., Simon, D., Loh, A., Härter, M. 2010. The 9-item Shared Decision Making Questionnaire (SDM-Q-9). Development and psychometric properties in a primary care sample. *Patient Educ Couns,* **80**, 94–99.

Lindig, A., Hahlweg, P., Frerichs, W., Topf, C., Reemts, M., Scholl, I. 2020. Adaptation and qualitative evaluation of Ask 3 Questions—a simple and generic intervention to foster patient empowerment. *Health Expect,* **23,** 1310–1325.

Mccormack, J., Elwyn, G. 2018. Shared decision is the only outcome that matters when it comes to evaluating evidence-based practice. *BMJ Evid Based Med,* **23,** 137–139.

Müller, E., Hahlweg, P., Scholl, I. 2016. What do stakeholders need to implement shared decision making in routine cancer care? A qualitative needs assessment. *Acta Oncol,* **55,** 1484–1491.

Patient Representation in the G-BA. 2013. Mission statement of patient representation in the G-BA [in German]. Available at: https://patientenvertretung.g-ba.de/was-wir-tun/leitbild-der-patientenvertretung/

Sackett, D. L., Rosenberg, W. M., Gray, J. A., Haynes, R. B., Richardson, W. S. 1996. Evidence based medicine: what it is and what it isn't. *BMJ,* **312,** 71–72.

Scheibler, F., Geiger, F., Wehkamp, K., et al. 2024. Patient-reported effects of hospital-wide implementation of shared decision-making at a university medical centre in Germany: a pre-post trial. BMJ *Evid Based Med,* **29,** 87–95.

Scholl, I., Hahlweg, P., Lindig, A., et al. 2018. Evaluation of a program for routine implementation of shared decision-making in cancer care: study protocol of a stepped wedge cluster randomized trial. *Implement Sci,* **13,** 1–10.

Scholl, I., Hahlweg, P., Lindig, A., et al. 2021. Evaluation of a program for routine implementation of shared decision-making in cancer care: results of a stepped wedge cluster randomized trial. *Implement Sci,* **16,** 1–17.

Steinbeck, V., Ernst, S.-C., Pross, C. 2021. *Patient-Reported Outcome Measures (PROMs): An International Comparison* [in German]. Bertelsmann Stiftung.

World Health Organization. 1986. *Ottawa Charter for Health Promotion*. World Health Organization.

22

Implementation of shared decision making in the USA

Two case studies

Dan D. Matlock, Chris Knoepke, Mayuko Ito Fukunaga, and Susan Strong

Introduction: contextual elements that influence implementation of shared decision making in the USA

In the USA, numerous professional societies and task forces have called for expanded utilization of shared decision making (SDM) in everyday clinical practice, with some also calling for SDM to be considered a quality indicator. More recently, the United States Preventive Services Task Force (USPSTF) expressed support for SDM broadly in relation to services 'across the spectrum of USPSTF recommendations' (Davidson et al., 2022). However, implementation of SDM needs to operate within the context of dominant reimbursement models. In the USA, fee-for-service remains the major practice-driving reimbursement paradigm, with a combination of public payers—chiefly Medicare and Medicaid—operated by the Centers for Medicare and Medicaid Services (CMS), private insurers, and vertically integrated organizations (e.g. the Department of Veterans Affairs, Kaiser Permanente) setting policies for the conditions under which clinicians are reimbursed for services provided to patients.

CMS' general movement towards 'value-based care' (see also Chapter 4) includes activities accurately characterized as either payment reform or promoting patient-centred care (including SDM), but these efforts have not had corresponding reimbursement polices outside of mandates for a small number of specific decisions. As a practical matter, SDM conversations (including review of patient-facing decision aids and other materials) represent either unreimbursed clinical time or can only be billable in a small number of specific circumstances. Aside from payment, Washington State enacted legislation increasing legal protections for physicians when patients sign consent acknowledging use of a decision aid (Pope and Hexum, 2013).

CMS' most affirmative effort towards leveraging reimbursement to support SDM has come in the form of mandated documentation of SDM in certain clinical circumstances, typically as a post hoc condition for withholding payment for the procedure of interest if an audit reveals that SDM had not occurred. In addition to lung cancer screening described in detail below, CMS has mandated SDM for two advanced cardiology procedures that carry such a mandate (Table 22.1).

Among the challenges inherent in increasing the use of SDM is understanding the manner in which it becomes routine. Multiple contextual factors influence whether an intervention will be implemented successfully or not. In addition to policy and reimbursement

Table 22.1 Examples of specified mandated SDM conversations for reimbursements

Lung cancer screening	Left atrial appendage occlusion	ICDs
The beneficiary must receive a counselling and SDM visit . . . including the use of one or more decision aids, to include benefits and harms of screening, follow-up diagnostic testing, over-diagnosis, false positive rate, and total radiation exposure	A formal SDM interaction with an independent non-interventional physician using an evidence-based decision tool on oral anticoagulation in patients with non-valvular atrial fibrillation before long-acting anticoagulation. The SDM interaction must be documented in the medical record	A formal SDM encounter must occur between the patient and a physician . . . or qualified non-physician practitioner (i.e. physician assistant, nurse practitioner, or clinical nurse specialist) . . . using an evidence-based decision tool on ICDs before initial ICD implantation. The SDM encounter may occur at a separate visit

Adapted with permission from Knoepke, C. E., Allen, L. A., Kramer, D. B., Matlock, D. D. 2019. Medicare mandates for shared decision making in cardiovascular device placement. *Circ Cardiovasc Qual Outcomes*, 12, e004899.

factors discussed above, implementation is also influenced by local hospital and clinic level cultural factors and available implementation and sustainability infrastructure. Additionally, work studying SDM in this context requires a focus not only on the effectiveness of SDM (in improving patient knowledge or reducing regret, for example), but its reach (i.e. the proportion of patients who actually experience SDM divided by the number who should), adoption (i.e. the rate at which professionals who could practise SDM choose to do so), and maintenance (whether and how professionals continue to use SDM once external support for it ends). Below are some examples of implementation in the USA.

Case studies

In this section, we present selected case studies that show how SDM has been attempted in different settings in US healthcare. These are lung cancer screening and heart failure decision making. The success (or otherwise) of each implementation case should be interpreted through a lens of the contextual elements discussed above. We also present a patient's perspective on how patient organizations are advocating for more SDM in decisions about heart failure management (Box 22.1).

Case study 1: lung cancer screening

The USPSTF recommends, and CMS mandates, SDM for lung cancer screening using at least one patient decision aid before proceeding with the initial lung cancer screening (Krist et al., 2021). Lung cancer screening is the only preventive service for which CMS mandates SDM. Originally, the CMS even specified the type of providers to conduct SDM and the contents of SDM. Although CMS reimburses SDM with a specific billing code (G0296), how to integrate SDM in lung screening workflow was left to each healthcare system and provider.

Since the USPSTF recommendation in 2013, many patient decision aids have been developed in various formats as tools to support SDM for lung cancer screening. Studies show that these decision aids improve patient knowledge and reduce patient decision conflict in the study settings (Fukunaga et al., 2020).

Due to the original CMS mandate in 2015 for the SDM visit to be with a physician or a qualified non-physician practitioner (physician assistant, nurse practitioner, or clinical nurse specialist), the initial implementation of SDM for lung cancer screening in the US clinical workflow happened in two ways: (1) in-person SDM counselling by ordering providers (e.g. primary care providers and pulmonologists) in routine clinic settings, and (2) in-person SDM counselling at lung cancer screening programmes.

Primary care is the frontline of patient-centred care. Primary care providers have played a significant role in cancer screening in the USA. Patients and primary care providers have a longitudinal therapeutic alliance, and many patients rely on their primary care provider's recommendations in cancer screening decisions. However, there are barriers unique to SDM for lung cancer screening in primary care settings. Since the eligibility for lung screening depends on a detailed smoking history, which is often missing or inaccurate in electronic health records, providers often need to begin by obtaining this detailed smoking history to determine their patients' eligibility before engaging in an SDM conversation. Lung cancer screening is still relatively new and patient awareness is still limited (Monu et al., 2020). Providers often need to explain the methods and process of screening before reviewing its benefits and risks with their patients. Providers themselves might not have enough lung cancer screening knowledge to weigh up the benefits and harms (Melzer et al., 2020).

To overcome the challenges in information exchange and value clarification, patient decision aids are integrated into the clinical workflow and electronic health records. In two studies, pre-visit delivery of decision aids increased patient knowledge, decision quality, and lung screening uptake in primary care settings. However, one study reported the occurrence of lung screening discussions, but not the extent of SDM, and the other study showed no difference in SDM in the two groups (Schapira et al., 2023; Walsh et al., 2023). Another study by Kukhareva and colleagues evaluated implementation of clinician-facing electronic health record prompts and electronic health record-integrated decision aids. The intervention increased lung screening uptake, although the decision aid itself was used by only 25% of the patients opting for lung screening (Kukhareva et al., 2023). Competing priorities, limited clinical time, and providers' SDM skills remain barriers to implementation of SDM for lung cancer screening in primary care settings.

Another model studied is an in-person SDM visit at the lung cancer screening programmes. Programme providers often receive SDM training, have more detailed lung cancer screening knowledge, and have time designated to focus on SDM counselling using decision aids. However, patients have often already decided to undergo lung cancer screening when they arrived at lung cancer screening programmes for 'SDM counselling'. In Mazzone and colleagues' study, 97% of the patients who received in-person SDM visits completed lung cancer screening, and it suggested that SDM counselling might have little influence on patients' decisions (Mazzone et al., 2017). Further, the requirement for an additional in-person SDM visit could become an additional barrier to patients receiving lung cancer screening. Since the COVID-19 pandemic, more lung cancer screening programmes and healthcare systems are using telehealth in their workflows. Tanner and co-workers showed no difference in lung screening decision and decisional conflict between in-person versus telephone SDM (Tanner et al., 2019). In its 2022 update, CMS removed the specification for the type of practitioner to conduct SDM and permanently adopted telehealth in SDM for lung cancer screening. These updates were welcomed to reduce barriers and increase access to lung cancer screening.

Community health workers and tobacco quitlines have established working relationships with vulnerable populations often at higher risk of developing lung cancer. Leveraging the trust between the patients and themselves, community health workers have a strong potential to reach vulnerable populations and provide culturally and linguistically tailored SDM counselling. Percac-Lima and colleagues conducted a randomized controlled trial comparing lay-patient navigation and usual care in community healthcare settings (Percac-Lima et al., 2018). In the intervention arm, lay navigators introduced SDM to 53% of patients during the patient navigation process. In state tobacco quitlines, Volk and co-workers showed a decision aid, compared to educational materials, improved the quitline clients' knowledge and reduced decisional conflict, but there was no difference in decision intention and lung screening completion (Volk et al., 2020). Additional work is needed to fully leverage the potential of community health workers and tobacco quitlines in SDM for lung screening.

In summary, there are some positive steps towards implementation of SDM for lung screening but it remains challenging in the USA despite CMS mandate and reimbursement.

Case study 2: heart failure decision making

Patients with heart failure face an array of complicated decisions. Early in the disease course, patients face decisions about medications to improve heart function and interventions such as implantable cardioverter–defibrillators (ICDs) to prevent sudden cardiac death. Later in the disease course, patients face decisions related to advanced therapies like the left ventricular assist device (LVAD) and heart transplant. In this case study, we will compare experiences with national SDM implementation efforts in two significant heart failure decisions, ICDs and LVADs.

The ICD is a surgically implanted resuscitation device that is about the size of a pacemaker. It sits under the skin of the chest with leads that connect to the heart muscle sensing the electrical rhythm of the heart and delivering a shock if it finds a potentially lethal arrhythmia. The ICD confers a significant reduction in mortality for a large subset of patients with heart failure with a reduced ejection fraction and is indicated as a preventive measure. It comes with both several surgical risks and the subsequent risks associated with getting shocked. If not properly deactivated, the ICD can cause significant harm at the end of life. More importantly, it involves a preference-sensitive trade-off between accepting a risk of dying suddenly and earlier versus living longer but with progressive heart failure. In an acknowledgement of the significant trade-offs associated with this device, CMS mandated SDM for ICDs (Table 22.1) (Knoepke et al., 2019). This mandate has stimulated a national implementation effort as sites aim to meet the mandate through implementing decision aids (Knoepke et al., 2022).

The LVAD in contrast does not have a mandate. It is a major surgical procedure designed to permanently implant an auxiliary pump next to the heart to provide additional cardiac output. This pump must be connected to a power source in the external environment. The survival benefits of the LVAD are impressive with absolute improvements in 1-year survival of over 60%. However, it is a major surgical procedure with a high perioperative mortality rate. Further, long-term risks include an annual stroke risk of 10% and a 50% risk of hospitalization for issues like bleeding or infection (Allen et al., 2017).

Both procedures have had national efforts for implementation of SDM. The ICD has seen a forced implementation of SDM largely spurred by the payment mandate. The LVAD has not had a CMS

Box 22.1 Patient perspective

From a patient lens, it is essential to emphasize that SDM is not a tool, a decision aid, or a mandate, but a human interaction—and often one with high stakes for individuals and their families. When mandating or implementing SDM interventions, government agencies, payers, clinicians, researchers, and decision scientists must find meaningful ways to integrate 'soft' concepts from qualitative research, the humanities, and the social sciences in particular principles of trauma-informed care, co-creation, and narrative medicine.

'What would it take for medicine and science to listen?' asks Dr Rita Charon, founder of the Narrative Medicine programme at Columbia University, New York. 'Most patients want us [doctors] to know not just what's the matter with them, but also what matters to them' (Charon, 2008) (see also https://nihrecord.nih.gov/2019/11/01/charon-espouses-power-narrative-medicine).

SDM is an inherently collaborative process, in which expertise is brought to the conversation not only by clinicians, but also by patients and family members who are themselves experts regarding the preferences, values, needs, and lived experience that contribute to an individual's treatment goals.

In its implementation, SDM ultimately requires a trusted relationship. SDM transcends the realm of mere clinical protocol; it underscores the significance of human interaction in healthcare delivery. Patients are not just passive recipients of medical advice—they are active participants in a collaborative dialogue with their healthcare practitioners. Trust, empathy, and mutual respect form the foundation of this relationship, fostering an environment where patients feel empowered to voice their concerns, preferences, and goals. Principles of trauma- informed care—psychological safety, trustworthiness and transparency, collaboration, empowerment, humility and responsiveness, and peer support—should be part of SDM as an intervention. Through high-quality SDM, patients are recognized as partners in their own care, contributing to more informed and personalized treatment decisions. Decision aids and other tools may be extremely helpful in standardizing information and making it easy to digest, but in and of themselves, they are only the starting point of SDM rather than an end point.

In the development of patient decision aids and best practice recommendations for SDM implementation, it is essential to incorporate meaningful patient involvement from the earliest planning stages by including a patient co-investigator and patient advisors to inform the project. This is where co-creation occurs, and knowledge is generated through the collaborative efforts of researchers working alongside additional stakeholders.

Academic institutions, government, industry, and non-profits all have incentive and responsibility to collaborate to provide relevant training, certifications, and/or degree programmes to equip patient partners to serve in roles as co-investigators and research advisors as empowered, equal team members. The establishment of the Patient-Centered Outcomes Research Institute (PCORI) in 2010 marked a significant shift in the involvement of patients in research, but the process of real change has been painfully slow. Patient involvement is viewed by most as important, but many gaps continue to be problematic in actual implementation. How do researchers identify and connect with patients who have lived experience, professional experience and skills, training, and networks that would enhance their project meaningfully? How do motivated patients with these assets connect with researchers who would benefit from the partnership? Perhaps PCORI or another agency could create a resource to match patients and researchers. How do patient advocates increase and develop their skills to contribute as professional team members, earning not only appropriate respect but also compensation? In many areas of patient advocacy and involvement, oncology leads the way.

Involving patients in research endeavours is paramount to advancing implementation. However, determining the most effective and efficient methods for engaging patients in research and understanding their perspectives can be complex. It requires a multifaceted approach that acknowledges the diversity of patient experiences, preferences, and needs. From co-designing research projects to participating in advisory panels, there are various avenues through which patients can actively contribute to shaping research agendas and methodologies. Embracing patient-centred research approaches not only enhances the relevance and applicability of study findings but also fosters a sense of ownership and empowerment. Through collaborative efforts between patients, researchers, and healthcare providers, the journey towards patient-centred care becomes a collective endeavour, guided by the principles of empathy, inclusivity, and mutual respect (Strong, 2020).

mandate but has instead followed the more traditional model of starting with a randomized trial of SDM demonstrating significant improvement in decision quality (Allen et al., 2017). Following this, funding by the Patient Centered Outcomes Research Institute supported a national implementation effort at the 175 accredited centres across the USA.

The differences in experiences of these two implementation efforts are informative. Despite the mandate, the ICD implementation has been met with challenges. First, the context of ICD decision making is often in the busy outpatient setting where staff are already stretched thin and time is at a premium (Knoepke et al., 2022). In contrast, the LVAD context has embedded LVAD coordinators who have already been tasked with patient education and patients are often 'captive' in the intensive care unit with much available time for conversations. Thus, implementing a decision aid for LVAD patients was much easier logistically as there were already dedicated people available to distribute the decision aid, making the logistics of supporting LVAD SDM much easier; over half of the 175 sites use the LVAD decision aid as a standard of care (Thompson et al., 2023).

Perhaps more importantly, qualitative work exploring these two implementation efforts showed differences of opinion among the clinicians in these areas. For the ICD, the mandate was seen as a box to check and the general feeling was that the importance of SDM was questioned, given that it is perceived as a low-risk procedure with life-saving benefits (Knoepke et al., 2022). In contrast, the LVAD is seen as a decision where the patient's perspective is paramount, despite the LVAD procedure conferring an almost ten times greater survival benefit than the LVAD. The procedural risks and burdens are perceived by clinicians to be great enough to warrant SDM (Thompson et al., 2023). These contrasting settings highlight two of the most important aspects predicting successful implementation—a belief among the providers that SDM is important and an infrastructure for delivering decision tools.

Conclusion

This chapter provides two examples of implementation in the context of the USA. There are, in fact, many examples we could have drawn from, many of which have been discussed in previous editions of this book. It is important always to remember that implementation is contextually bound, and even in the USA, where many of the economic pressures work against SDM, there are examples where SDM has been successful. Going forward, work will need to continue at multiple levels—at the policy level, efforts should continue to create incentives for the use of SDM. At the healthcare system and clinician level, it will remain important to continue to design workflows that make SDM as easy as possible including utilizing the potential of key staff and community workers. Finally, at the patient level, implementation will always be enhanced when patients are involved in the process so that the strategies that are designed meet their needs as well.

REFERENCES

Allen, L. A., McIlvennan, C. K., Thompson, J. S., et al. 2017. Effectiveness of an intervention supporting shared decision making for destination therapy left ventricular assist device: the DECIDE-LVAD randomized stepped-wedge trial. *JAMA Intern Med,* **178**, 520–529.

Charon, R. 2008. *Narrative Medicine: Honoring the Stories of Illness.* Oxford University Press.

Davidson, K. W., Mangione, C. M., Barry, M. J., et al. 2022. Collaboration and shared decision-making between patients and clinicians in preventive health care decisions and US Preventive Services Task Force Recommendations. *JAMA,* **327**, 1171–1176.

Fukunaga, M. I., Halligan, K., Kodela, J., et al. 2020. Tools to promote shared decision-making in lung cancer screening using low-dose CT scanning: a systematic review. *Chest,* **158**, 2646–2657.

Knoepke, C. E., Allen, L. A., Kramer, D. B., Matlock, D. D. 2019. Medicare mandates for shared decision making in cardiovascular device placement. *Circ Cardiovasc Qual Outcomes,* **12**, e004899.

Knoepke, C. E., Wallace, B. C., Allen, L. A., et al. 2022. Experiences implementing a suite of decision aids for implantable cardioverter defibrillators: qualitative insights from the DECIDE-ICD Trial. *Circ Cardiovasc Qual Outcomes,* **15**, e009352.

Krist, A. H., Davidson, K. W., Mangione, C. M., et al. 2021. Screening for lung cancer: US Preventive Services Task Force recommendation statement. *JAMA,* **325**, 962–970.

Kukhareva, P. V., Li, H., Caverly, T. J., et al. 2023. Implementation of lung cancer screening in primary care and pulmonary clinics: pragmatic clinical trial of electronic health record-integrated everyday shared decision-making tool and clinician-facing prompts. *Chest,* **164**, 1325–1338.

Mazzone, P. J., Tenenbaum, A., Seeley, M., et al. 2017. Impact of a lung cancer screening counseling and shared decision-making visit. *Chest,* **151**, 572–578.

Melzer, A. C., Golden, S. E., Ono, S. S., Datta, S., Crothers, K., Slatore, C. G. 2020. What exactly is shared decision-making? A qualitative study of shared decision-making in lung cancer screening. *J Gen Intern Med,* **35**, 546–553.

Monu, J., Triplette, M., Wood, D. E., et al. 2020. Evaluating knowledge, attitudes, and beliefs about lung cancer screening using crowdsourcing. *Chest,* **158**, 386–392.

Percac-Lima, S., Ashburner, J. M., Rigotti, N. A., et al. 2018. Patient navigation for lung cancer screening among current smokers in community health centers: a randomized controlled trial. *Cancer Med,* **7**, 894–902.

Pope, T. M., Hexum, M. 2013. Legal briefing: shared decision making and patient decision aids. *J Clin Ethics,* **24**, 70–80.

Schapira, M. M., Hubbard, R. A., Whittle, J., et al. 2023. Lung cancer screening decision aid designed for a primary care setting: a randomized clinical trial. *JAMA Netw Open,* **6**, e2330452.

Strong, S. R. 2020. *Decades After Diagnosis: The Unrecognized Trauma of Surviving.* American College of Cardiology Foundation.

Tanner, N. T., Banas, E., Yeager, D., Dai, L., Halbert, C. H., Silvestri, G. A. J. C. 2019. In-person and telephonic shared decision-making visits for people considering lung cancer screening: an assessment of decision quality. *Chest,* **155**, 236–238.

Thompson, J. S., Matlock, D., Mcilvennan, C., et al. 2023. Adopting a patient decision aid into routine practice for left ventricular assist device: diffusion of innovation characteristics. *J Cardiac Fail,* **29**, 636.

Volk, R. J., Lowenstein, L. M., Leal, V. B., et al. 2020. Effect of a patient decision aid on lung cancer screening decision-making by persons who smoke: a randomized clinical trial. *JAMA Netw Open,* **3**, e1920362-e1920362.

Walsh, J. M., Karliner, L., Smith, A., et al. 2023. LungCARE: encouraging shared decision-making in lung cancer screening—a randomized trial. *J Gen Intern Med,* **38**, 3115–3122.

23

Implementation of shared decision making in Denmark

A case study

Karina Olling, Marlene Würgler, Karina Dahl Steffensen, and Jan Faldt Bentsen

Introduction

The healthcare system in Denmark operates on universal principles, ensuring free and equal access to healthcare for all citizens. Funding is derived from general taxes. Denmark is geographically divided into five regions, see **Figure 23.1**. Each of the five regions organizes its own health services and assumes operational responsibility for hospitals, mental healthcare services, and agreements with the general practice sector. The Danish Ministry of Health, a governmental entity, is tasked with formulating overall healthcare policy, managing economic frameworks and legislation, and overseeing bodies such as the National Danish Health Authority and the Danish Patient Safety Authority.

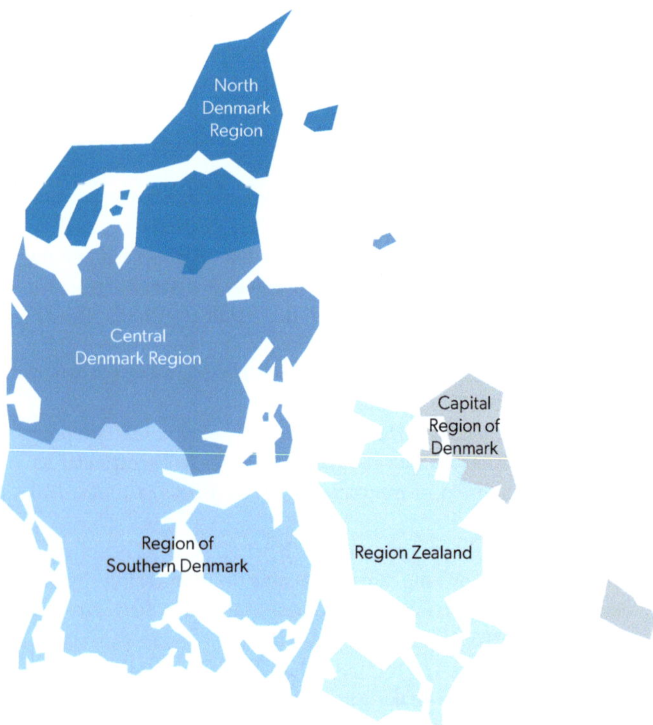

Figure 23.1 The five Danish Regions.

Danish patients are entitled to comprehensive information about their health conditions and treatment options, with explicit rights to informed consent, even for minors and adults without capacity, although rights to shared decision making (SDM) itself are not explicitly stated in current Danish healthcare legislation.

However, interest in SDM has gained momentum in Denmark over the past decade. Fifteen years ago, SDM was still in its infancy in Denmark. But the fundamental principles that patients should be involved in decisions, and that patients' personal preferences are crucial, have gained increasing attention. During the last 10 years, several regions and hospitals have established more systematic approaches to SDM implementation, reflecting the growing commitment to implementing these principles within the Danish healthcare system (Dahl Steffensen et al., 2022).

In 2019, the Region of Southern Denmark launched an ambitious effort to implement SDM in all hospitals in the region, establishing a systematic, generic approach based on SDM research, improvement methodology, and SDM experience (Steffensen et al., 2023). In the Region of Southern Denmark, representatives of patients and their relatives are actively engaged in the implementation of SDM at the highest organizational echelon. They participate in a regional steering committee that discusses important strategic matters concerning the implementation process in the region. Additionally, the five regional hospitals have councils comprising patients and/or their relatives, which partake in local initiatives. Moreover, patients or relatives are essential contributors to both strategic and operational initiatives within the Center for Shared Decision Making, which serves to support the implementation efforts throughout the region.

Since 2021, the Region of Southern Denmark and the Capital Region of Denmark have also worked closely together to develop a model for how SDM should be systematically implemented in the Capital Region (Copenhagen and surrounding area). There are now more than 80 departments, in different hospitals in the two regions, that have implemented SDM to a varied extent.

In the Central Denmark Region, the 'User-involving-hospital' programme has worked on the implementation of SDM through several projects and developed patient decision aids (PtDAs) for implementation in practice (Jorgensen et al., 2020). The other two Danish regions have a few departments as front-runners, which help build up experience for future more widespread implementation.

As yet there is no central organization to coordinate SDM initiatives and no central register of PtDAs or national portal to host them. The Region of Southern Denmark's Center for Shared Decision Making has created, tested and implemented a generic PtDA template (Olling et al., 2019)—Decision Helper™—following International Patient Decision Aid Standards criteria (Elwyn et al., 2006). The PtDAs are shared on the Center's website, which hosts a library of over 80 PtDAs. The PtDA template, shown in Figure 23.2, is now accessible nationwide, empowering healthcare professionals to develop high-quality PtDAs through www.cffb.dk. Patients and/or relatives play a crucial role in the development of all Decision Helpers, participating in collaborative workshops with clinicians during the development phase and engaging in testing phases of the Decision Helper™.

What worked for implementation of SDM in Denmark?

SDM is seen as a key driver in reshaping the mindset of individual clinicians and 'nudging' cultural change at a practice level to achieve a patient-centred culture in the Danish healthcare system. Clinical champions, who themselves have been involved in SDM implementation, share their positive experiences of practising SDM with other peers, leaders, and colleagues. They describe how starting to explore patients' preferences, life circumstances, and experiences with their disease(s) has a spillover effect on other practices and routines in the department, such as information materials for patients, ward rounds, and communication with patients and their caregivers. Over time, clinicians start to scrutinize these practices, reflecting on their effectiveness in preparing patients for involvement and ensuring active patient participation. This shifts the mindset of clinicians, making them aware of practices and routines that have been centred around the system's needs rather than being truly patient-centred (Cronholm et al., 2013).

Initiatives to promote SDM implementation typically encompass clinician training, the creation of PtDAs, and endeavours to activate patients (Joseph-Williams et al., 2021). These activities find resonance in the Danish context, where the predominant approach

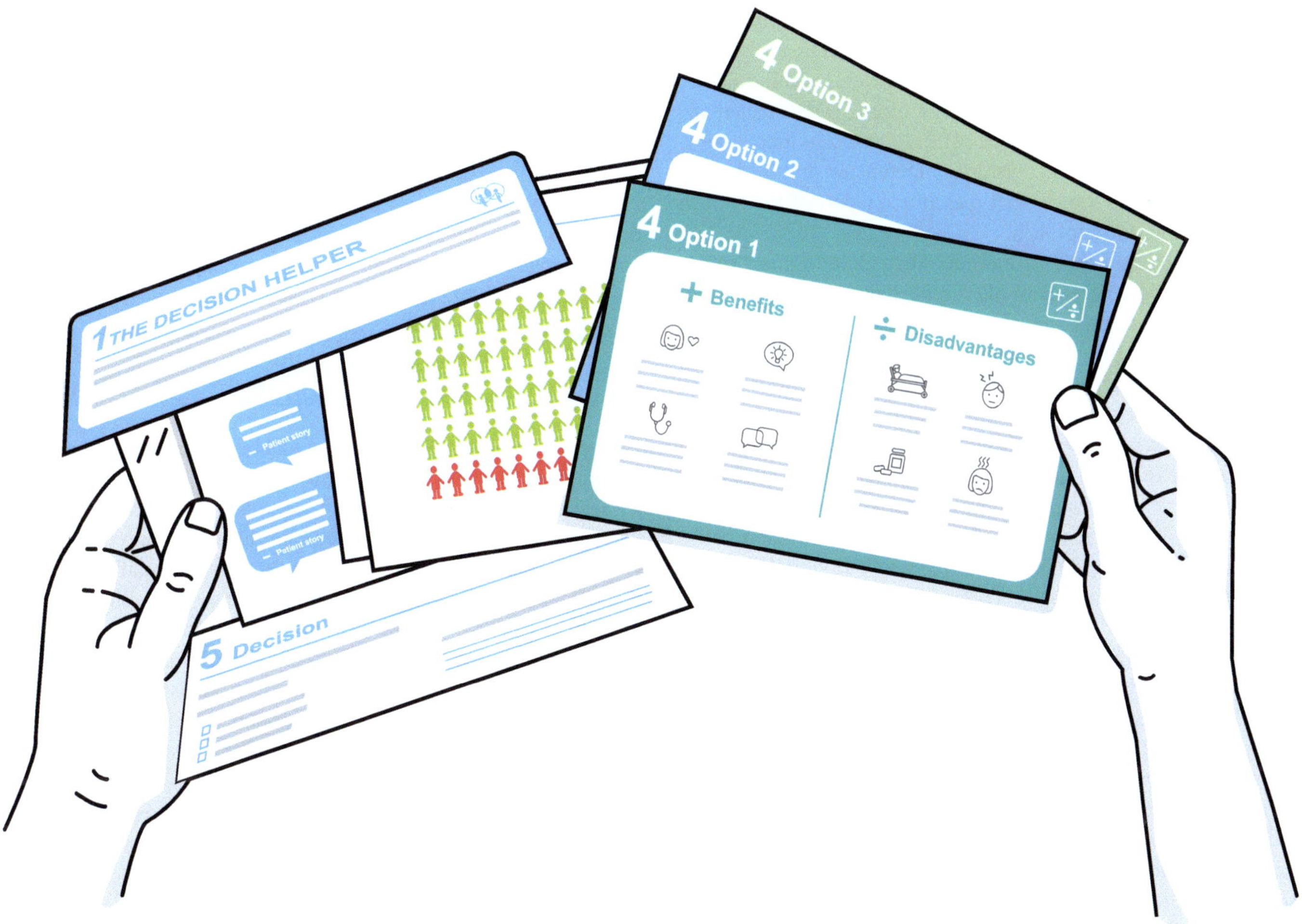

Figure 23.2 The Decision Helper template.

involves a 'train-the-trainers' model. Here, clinical champions learn to train their peers in SDM practices, and over the last few years, patients are more often invited to serve as co-teachers in the train-the-trainers courses. A range of PtDAs have also been developed and the Region of Southern Denmark in particular has embraced the challenge of providing opportunities for patients to be active in preparation and participation in SDM implementation activities.

The Danish approach develops these more usual initiatives by highlighting two further activities that are crucial to Denmark's implementation of SDM: (1) the imperative to involve leaders in implementation efforts and (2) the need to implement a systematic approach within hospital departments, supported by SDM experts, to create a robust system for SDM implementation that ensures long-term sustainability.

First, the belief that leadership is crucial for success with SDM implementation is based on the leadership role of understanding and articulating dilemmas closely connected to clinicians' everyday practice—this is a driver of cultural change itself. Dilemmas like: 'How do clinicians balance their knowledge about medical evidence with the patient's preferences and desires for how to live their life?' or 'How to create time for reflection and conversation with patients in a healthcare system where effectiveness and productivity is a strong guiding principle?' Leaders must articulate and acknowledge grassroots dilemmas like these if they want to succeed in implementing SDM. Leaders must also be able to handle clinicians' reactions and resistance to change, and enter into dialogue about clinicians' uneasiness with the new role (of SDM) or perceived disadvantages. They must be able to communicate, set goals, adjust workflows, and make sure the right competencies and skills are available to change the culture towards a more SDM-oriented approach (Holm-Petersen and Navne, 2015). All this calls for a systematic approach to increase leadership competencies, and leadership training programmes are for that reason a key part of the Danish SDM implementation approach.

Second, it is important to consider that, despite good intentions and positive outcomes of SDM reported in research studies, achieving sustained and comprehensive implementation has been a challenge. Tackling this, the Region of Southern Denmark has successfully integrated a systematic approach based on improvement methodology to promote implementation in clinical departments.

In this context, routine activities such as training sessions and the creation of PtDAs, when coupled with a meticulously planned process within clinical departments encompassing fixed elements like meetings, standardized agendas, and implementation activities, facilitate breaking the extensive implementation process down to manageable components. This process plan places an initial emphasis on implementation, gradually transitioning towards sustainability throughout the process (Steffensen et al., 2023). Various indicators are used to monitor the outcome of implementation efforts (e.g. a national survey of patient satisfaction by various parameters, process indicators such as number of clinicians trained and number of PtDAs developed, plus some indicators carefully chosen for the specific department). To support clinical departments in the complex intervention that is SDM implementation, a 'maturity matrix' (organizational development) tool has been developed and is used in both the Southern Denmark and Capital Regions. The tool helps in establishing goals, evaluating progress, and choosing next steps (Lund et al., 2024).

Box 23.1 Summary of what worked for the implementation of SDM in Denmark

- Patients and relatives actively engaged on the highest strategic level, in clinician training, in PtDA development, and in locally funded initiatives.
- Systematic process planning.
- Leadership training programmes.
- Clinical champions.
- Field observations of patient pathways.
- Pareto analysis of barriers and facilitators.
- Maturity matrix to establish goals and monitor progress.
- Carefully chosen indicators.
- Train-the-trainer model—clinical champions train clinician peers in SDM practices.
- Patient activation.

Last and also noteworthy, there are two distinct methodologies employed in preparing successful implementation efforts within clinical departments. Both approaches aim to provide departments with insights into specific challenges and strengths inherent in their cultural and workflow dynamics. The first method involves a Pareto analysis of barriers and facilitators, using a quantitative questionnaire distributed to all clinicians and departmental leaders. This analysis identifies critical areas where the greatest impact could be achieved by focusing on them during implementation. The second method involves conducting a series of field observations, shadowing patients and clinicians, to discern patterns and subsequently conveying insights derived from these observations back to the department. Both methods will contribute to building a system that is based on SDM implementation principles but adjusted to fit the specific department's needs.

All the above elements significantly contribute to the Danish initiative's comprehensive strategy for advancing SDM (for a summary of what worked see Box 23.1).

Challenges and milestones: advancing SDM in the Danish healthcare ecosystem

Progress with SDM implementation will be evident through systematic integration in various domains. Firstly, its inclusion in clinical guidelines will demonstrate a shift towards patient-centred care, reflecting the medical community's recognition of its value. Notably, the Danish Multidisciplinary Cancer Groups emphasize patient involvement in their recent strategy, aiming for 50% of their clinical guidelines to be linked to PtDAs. Secondly, integration into professional societies and educational curricula will signify the acceptance and endorsement of SDM among healthcare professionals and their leaders.

Furthermore, the inclusion of SDM into national and regional political agendas, along with the implementation of specific systematic initiatives at the local hospital level, would serve as a clear indication of policymakers' and administrators' commitment to promoting the integration of SDM in the future.

This emphasizes the importance of political and strategic support for SDM to become widely adopted in mainstream medical settings (Coulter, 2018). As SDM becomes systematically integrated into guidelines and clinician training, and is set as a goal in political agendas and strategies, it will signal a transformative change. This development will seek to empower patients and reinforce the importance of their active participation in healthcare decisions, setting a benchmark for comprehensive and patient-centred healthcare practices.

However, as with all cultural change there are several potential warning signs. One of the most widespread warning signs is the belief among clinicians and leaders that 'we are doing it [SDM] already'. Field observations and interviews with patients may suggest otherwise, showing that patients were not even aware of a decision to be made, let alone that they had a role to play in that decision. This is often compounded by the misconception of equating SDM with informed consent and the unidirectional communication this entails. This may indicate insufficient understanding of what SDM entails and a potential confusion about how it differs from the clinician's usual practice. Thus, (continued) training of clinicians should not be overlooked, and failing to prioritize this aspect serves as a warning signal. Such failure, if found, suggests a lack of acknowledgement by leaders that SDM entails a shift in the role and relationship between clinicians and patients, and the need to acquire and sustain new skills. If SDM training is inadequate or not given sufficient priority, there is a significant risk that successful and ongoing implementation of SDM will not be achieved.

Lack of leadership supporting and keeping a persistent focus on SDM implementation is another warning sign. Lack of leadership can lead to SDM being seen as optional for individual clinicians and not a systematic practice that is a part of the culture in the department.

Sometimes, in their enthusiasm, leaders have inadvertently provided clinicians and patients with a less comprehensive, 'light' model of SDM. This may, for example, overlook the need for actual skill development, solely focusing on checklists or simple tools to support the patient–clinician dialogue. These simplified models may not achieve the full extent of genuine SDM with patients, but can possibly contribute to incremental progress towards SDM and at least achieving the earlier stages of the maturity matrix.

Learning from past efforts is pivotal for future SDM implementation, such as continuing to focus on addressing misconceptions of SDM, ensuring clinician training, and developing leadership skills to drive and support the cultural change necessary to implement and sustain SDM. Envisaging the future, the aspiration is for tangible integration of SDM into clinical guidelines, professional societies, curricula, and political agendas, signifying progress towards patient-centred care. As Denmark progresses on its SDM journey, it is paramount to recognize that cultural shifts demand time, persistence, and comprehensive strategies. Viewing SDM as a catalyst for broader cultural change, leaders must continue to communicate its value, provide necessary training, and create an environment conducive to SDM. This commitment will not only solidify the foundation of SDM but also pave the way for a patient-centred healthcare landscape in Denmark.

See Box 23.2 for our patient perspective.

Box 23.2 Patient perspective

Perspectives on SDM implementation from a relative's or patient's point of view

Building a good rapport with me as a patient is very important. A good rapport means a close and harmonious relationship where the ones involved understand each other's feelings or ideas and communicate well. Therefore, the PtDA itself, the environment, the system, or the way it is used must never stand in the way. It is the purpose and process of SDM that is important from the first person I meet to the follow-up with my general practitioner. Some clinicians with many years of education and experience may think that they have mastered patients and relatives, but when the paradigm changes, everyone goes back to zero.

The roadmap to good implementation starts with the clinician's motivation for the idea itself and their desire to master it, and their leader's ability to inspire and help the clinician to use what has been learned, remove possible obstacles preventing SDM, and finally, also to keep the clinician on track through encouragement and follow-up.

In other words, the implementation strategy should start even before the clinician enters their training. The strategy should focus on changing the organizational culture and address activities that inspire clinicians throughout the organization and stimulate their desire to adopt SDM with patients before, during, and after treatment.

Successful SDM in healthcare is more than a single clinician's tool. It is a culture of team behaviour. Team members are guarantors, together securing the sustainability of a patient-agreed plan. If even one team member does not fulfil his or her task, it will influence a patient's treatment, showing that the chain is only as strong as its weakest link.

My motivation, trust, and stamina

The patient's comfort, motivation, and willingness are prerequisites for good rapport and are key to inviting the clinician into the patient's world, without bias. It's not easy to achieve an equal and neutral conversation with the least possible bias.

There will always be a bias—the clinician versus the patient. You cannot ignore it, nor should you hide it, but be honest and do your utmost to limit it.

I will as a patient or relative always listen to your expertise and if in doubt probably follow your advice, because of your expertise, provided I trust you.

My trust in you and a safe environment, embracing me and my situation, will set me free to make, probably the most difficult decision in my entire life—it's my future.

Trust is the core, and it is very delicate and can easily be crushed. When do I know that I can trust your advice? The health sector in Denmark is challenged with stories about shortages of resources, waiting lists, mistreatment, etc. So why should I believe in you and trust that you have the resources and competencies to successfully complete the treatment you suggest?

It is not only what you say, how you explain my options, the different treatments, the side effects and so on, but very much how I feel, how I perceive you as a person, our eye contact, your behaviour towards me, and at the same time your interaction with your colleagues, that tells me who you are as a person and perhaps makes me trust you.

Do I really feel that you are here for me, or are you just treating me like many other patients on the assembly line? At the end of the day, trust is a feeling.

As a patient, I will forget what you said and what you did, but I will never forget how you made me feel.

The trust you and I build in our relationship, does not live any longer than the congruence in the team treating and caring for me. You need to walk my path and talk with 'one voice' about my treatment, so that I don't experience different views between you and your colleagues about the diagnosis, doses of medicine, selections, treatment, and so on.

Congruence and alignment in the 'chain of clinicians' during my treatment keep my trust and motivation and help me through recovery.

REFERENCES

Coulter, A. 2018. *National Strategies for Implementing Shared Decision Making*. Bertelsmann Foundation.

Cronholm, P. F., Shea, J. A., Werner, R. M., et al. 2013. The patient centered medical home: mental models and practice culture driving the transformation process. *J Gen Intern Med,* **28**, 1195–201.

Dahl Steffensen, K., Mølri Knudsen, B., Finderup, J., Willemann Würgler, M., Olling, K 2022. Implementation of patient-centred care in Denmark: the way forward with shared decision-making. *Z Evid Fortbild Qual Gesundhwes,* **171**, 36–41.

Elwyn, G., O'Connor, A., Stacey, D., et al. 2006. Developing a quality criteria framework for patient decision aids: online international Delphi consensus process. *BMJ,* **333**, 417.

Holm-Petersen, C. N., Navne, L. E. 2015. What is leading patient involvement? An examination of goals and three individual models for patient involvement. *Tidsskrift for Forskning i Sygdom og Samfund,* **22**, 103–133.

Jorgensen, M. J., Pedersen, C. G., Martin, H. M., Lomborg, K. 2020. Implementation of patient involvement methods in the clinical setting: a qualitative study exploring the health professional perspective. *J Eval Clin Pract,* **26**, 765–776.

Joseph-Williams, N., Abhyankar, P., Boland, L., et al. 2021. What works in implementing patient decision aids in routine clinical settings? A rapid realist review and update from the International Patient Decision Aid Standards Collaboration. *Med Decis Making,* **41**, 907–937.

Lund, L., Hansen, D. G., Korsbek, L., et al. (2024). "Developing the tool SDM:KOMPASS. Supporting shared decision making implementation processes". *PLoS One,* **19**(11), e0312990. doi:10.1371/journal.pone.0312990

Olling, K., Bechmann, T., Madsen, P. H., et al. 2019. Development of a patient decision aid template for use in different clinical settings. *Eur J Pers Cent Healthc,* **7**, 1.

Steffensen, K. D., Hansen, D. G., Espersen, K., et al. 2023. 'SDM:HOSP'—a generic model for hospital-based implementation of shared decision making. *PLoS One,* **18**, e0280547.

24

Implementation of shared decision making in the Netherlands

A case study

Arwen H. Pieterse, Haske van Veenendaal, Dominique Sprengers, and Trudy van der Weijden

Introduction

Shared decision making (SDM) has taken off in the Netherlands in the past decade. Medical students, clinicians, and, increasingly, patients, have heard about SDM. Efforts to implement SDM could build upon evidence-based practice, which integrates three pillars in medical decision making: 'best research evidence', 'clinical expertise', and 'patient values' (Sackett et al., 1996). Evidence-based practice provides, in theory, fertile ground for embracing SDM. However, the transition from authority-based medicine to evidence-based practice has mostly focused on 'best research evidence' (Schoemaker and van der Weijden, 2016). Indeed, vast amounts of energy and time have been invested in compiling evidence (e.g. by conducting systematic reviews) and translating evidence into clinical practice guidelines, meanwhile neglecting the role of 'patient values'. SDM provides a method to address this pillar. In the following, we will describe the initiatives deployed in the Netherlands to implement SDM, describe success cases, and list major challenges encountered on the way.

Macro-level initiatives to implement SDM

SDM has been legally mandated in the Netherlands. Under the revised *Medical Treatment Contracts Act* (2020), clinicians have the legal duty to introduce the option of foregoing medical interventions and rather explore patients' preferences (Ubbink et al., 2021). In conjunction, the Dutch Ministry of Health has invested in research and implementation of value-based healthcare, with SDM as a central component of value-based healthcare. The Ministry has allocated €70 million in 2018–2022 to integrate patient-reported outcome measures (PROMs) and SDM in routine hospital care ('Outcome-based Care' programme, see https://www.uitkomstgerichtezorg.nl) (Damman et al., 2020).

Key stakeholders (e.g. Ministry of Health, Federation of Medical Specialists, Dutch Association of Hospitals, Federation of Nurses, and Netherlands Patients Federation) have concerted their efforts to implement value-based healthcare and SDM under the auspices of this Outcome-based Care programme. This has led to the development of decision support materials (e.g. infographics, patient decision aids), dashboards to present clinical outcomes and PROMs, training materials (e.g. e-learning), multiple pioneering examples of SDM implementation, and a 'roadmap' to help implement SDM. Products are freely accessible through an online learning and collaboration platform primarily aimed at clinicians (https://platformuitkomstgerichtezorg.nl/home/default.aspx). The website presents many practical examples and experiences with SDM, and explicitly invites clinicians to add success stories, learning opportunities, and resources. The decision tools developed add to the many available patient decision and conversation aids in Dutch, including some specifically targeting limited health-literate patients. Further, the Ministry launched a national SDM campaign in September 2021 ('Start a good conversation', see https://begineengoedgesprek.nl/) as a joint initiative with health insurers, professional bodies (general practitioners, medical specialists, paramedical professions, pharmacists), the Netherlands Patients Federation, and the Netherlands Federation of University Medical Centres. In September 2022, the Ministry, the Association of Dutch Municipalities, the Netherlands Federation of University Medical Centres, and representatives from the healthcare sector signed the Integral Care Agreement. A key topic in the agreement is delivering appropriate (high-value) care and de-implementing inappropriate (low-value) care through SDM and the deployment of PROMs.

Other national developments have occurred that should further support SDM implementation. First, national guidance on developing guidelines and standards of care ('AQUA-guide', 2021; see https://www.zorginzicht.nl/ontwikkeltools/ontwikkelen/aqua-leidraad (in Dutch only)) promotes SDM as a leading principle in

Box 24.1 Patient perspective

From SDM to *samen beslissen*

I agree with the general impression about the implementation of SDM in the Netherlands. We are proud to have changed the Dutch term for SDM. Clinicians and health services researchers quickly adopted the English term as a trendy concept. However, patients thought differently and we successfully turned it into the active verb 'decide together' ('*samen beslissen*'), nicely reflecting the work it takes to perform SDM. We are also proud that in many hospitals, the 'three good questions' ('What are my options?', 'What are the risks and benefits related to these options?', 'What does this mean for my situation?') have been implemented (Garvelink et al., 2019). Moreover, the Netherlands Patients Federation signed the Integral Care Agreement, even though it includes SDM as a rather abstract goal. The Federation's view is that 'Everyone can do SDM'.

preference-sensitive decisions. Relatedly, national guidance was developed on quality criteria for patient versions of guidelines and patient decision aids, the latter based on the International Patient Decision Aid Standards (http://ipdas.ohri.ca/) (van der Weijden et al., 2019). Second, the Dutch Healthcare Institute made grants available (yearly €5 million, 2021–2023) to improve SDM with target groups (frail elderly, children, lower health-literate people). Third, the Netherlands Organisation for Health Research and Development initiated research calls on SDM implementation, such as in primary, palliative, and elderly care. Finally, professional bodies, including the Federation of Medical Specialists, the Dutch College of General Practitioners, and the Federation of Nurses, have launched vision documents on SDM, pushed forward forerunners to promote SDM among colleagues, and identified SDM-specific competencies that have been integrated into qualifications for the medical educational curriculum (Federation of Medical Specialists, 2019; Baghus et al., 2021; V&VN, 2022). Indeed, SDM is frequently mentioned in the master plan for bachelor's and master's medicine programmes (Netherlands Federation of University Medical Centres, 2020). Our patient representative confirmed the overall movement towards SDM (Box 24.1).

Clinical examples of implementation strategies at local levels

Macro-level incentives to promote SDM implementation are tremendously helpful in supporting implementation efforts at regional and local levels. Having said this, we have not yet reached the desired level of application in local practice. Various observational studies show gaps between the ideal of SDM and actual performance (Roodbeen et al., 2021; van Veenendaal et al., 2021; Driever et al., 2022; Kuijpers et al., 2022; Baghus et al., 2024). A growing number of healthcare organizations are looking for a so-called *multilevel approach*, that is, defining region- or organization-wide ambitions to be achieved with actions deployed at multiple levels, each of which helps accelerate implementation (Scholl et al., 2018; van Veenendaal et al., 2022). This may involve leveraging macro-level factors described earlier, often as *extrinsic* motivators, and actions that can strengthen *intrinsic* motivation, which seem indispensable for a behavioural innovation such as SDM. The following are examples of such initiatives.

The Bernhoven case

Bernhoven Hospital is a medium-sized hospital (around 18,000 admissions/year, 2250 employees) that chose to explicitly adopt a hospital-wide, patient-centred '*Better care by less care*' approach in 2014, to reduce costs while preserving time for patients (Venhuizen, 2019). The hospital was reorganized to facilitate interdisciplinary collaboration, it was agreed with health insurers to move away from fee-for-service reimbursement, and SDM was adopted as an integral part of the strategy. Specifically, patients were encouraged to ask the 'three good questions' (Ask 3 Questions), were offered digital patient decision aids, and clinicians were trained. In co-creation between clinicians, other staff, general practitioners, and patients, it was determined when important choices are made in care pathways, what information is needed when, and how to best coordinate actions. Overall, the volume of medical interventions decreased by 16% in 3 years without patients turning to surrounding hospitals. Also, the hospital-specific mortality rate, as a measure of patient outcome, remained in line with the national average. Patients reported higher satisfaction, with 77% recommending Bernhoven in 2014 and 93% in 2018, and the hospital received the Dutch National Patient Hospitality Award in 2014, 2016, and 2017. Unfortunately, Bernhoven ran into financial problems. Reduced demand for care was no longer covered by long-term funding, and costs for housing and staff could not be reduced in the short term, probably due to long-term contracts and protective employment terms and conditions.

The breast cancer case

Breast cancer teams from more than 20 hospitals (25% of all Dutch hospitals) worked over an extended period (1–2 years) to increase SDM about surgery, systemic treatment, follow-up, and palliative care (Ankersmid et al., 2021; Perfors et al., 2021; Savelberg et al., 2021; van Veenendaal et al., 2021). The four-step model of SDM (Stiggelbout et al., 2015), widely adopted in the Netherlands, was introduced to clinicians, patient and clinician decision support tools (e.g. SDM pocket cards) were developed, and training and feedback were offered (e.g. communication skills training, feedback on consultations, and e-learning). In some cases, care pathways were redesigned, such as by adapting multidisciplinary team meetings, introducing patient reflection time ('time-out'), using PROMs, and/or redistributing tasks. Clinicians reported positive results for themselves (e.g. better structured, less hurried consultations), their patients (e.g. more sure about decisions), and their team (e.g. better task alignment) (van Veenendaal et al., 2022).

Implementation challenges at all levels

Promising initiatives such as those discussed have met resistance or failed for other reasons. The Dutch healthcare financing system is based on 'profit' through volume, and time allocated to talking with patients yields less than carrying out medical interventions. There have been well-intentioned attempts to secure funding to reward talking more. However, it is hard to claim (extra) time necessary for SDM, as time dedicated to SDM is often distributed over various consultations in the care pathway, with different clinicians and even care organizations involved, such as when clinicians from regional hospitals discuss patients with clinical experts from academic hospitals. If more SDM shifts the balance towards fewer medical interventions or the transfer of tasks to other care providers, financial problems may arise (as faced by Bernhoven Hospital), unless the changes coincide with increased healthcare demand (e.g. due to an ageing population). Solutions to this challenge, such as by offering 'population-based' financial incentives for health gains that can be achieved at regional level through collaboration between multiple healthcare parties, are still experimental (see https://www.zonmw.nl/nl/programma/uitkomstgericht-organiseren-en-betalen (in Dutch only)).

A second macro-level challenge relates to the AQUA-guide on developing clinical guidelines. It does not include explicit guidance on identifying and flagging preference-sensitive decisions, nor does it call for including evidence on variation in patient preferences regarding medical interventions. It therefore does not help create choice awareness in clinicians, a missed opportunity noted previously (Gärtner et al., 2019).

A third macro-level challenge relates to integrating SDM in efforts to keep high-quality healthcare affordable and accessible (e.g. Integral Care Agreement, Outcome-based Care programme). SDM may lose visibility and dedicated attention to its implementation. For example, grants aimed at improving SDM with target groups have already been cut. Finally, regarding education, SDM is addressed explicitly in just one-quarter of 78 undergraduate and postgraduate curricula for medical and nurse trainees and is hardly ever formally examined (Regioplan/Nivel, 2021).

Further, despite a large number of available decision support tools, many clinicians and patients remain unaware of their existence, nationwide implementation and maintenance strategies are lacking, and attempts at designing an open-access national library have failed so far. Decision support tools for primary and secondary care are offered through different platforms, and some are not open access. Moreover, only 2% of Dutch patient decision aids are appropriate for limited health-literate patients (Richter et al, 2025). Furthermore, the use of PROMs to foster SDM may, in fact, reinforce the focus on evidence relating to patient populations rather than on individual preferences and experiences.

Clinicians still have considerable scope to involve patients more in decisions (Roodbeen et al., 2021; Driever et al., 2022), including lower health-literate patients (Oosterveld et al., 2019). This is worrying. To date, the focus has mostly been on typical SDM decision situations, such as preference-sensitive decisions in oncology involving one clinician and one patient (and family). Increasingly, multidisciplinary teams are also involved, which makes incorporating patients' perspectives even more challenging. Moreover, many decisions in routine practice relate to elderly patients with multimorbidity, who often face complex decisions that require incorporating key issues from an individual's social domain. The latter necessitates extensive interprofessional teamwork distributed over time. These challenges require cultural changes, a point made by our patient representative (Box 24.2).

Box 24.2 Patient perspective

SDM requires a culture change

We recognize that performing SDM at a high level is not easily adopted. It is more than an add-on: it must be part of the medical culture. The challenge of sustaining healthcare resources may hinder the implementation of SDM, yet it could also create momentum and spark innovations that allow adding value for patients while saving costs. To illustrate, vulnerable elderly people with hip fractures are currently being offered the choice between surgery and conservative management in the Netherlands.

To improve implementation, perhaps there are win–win opportunities such as those in the Outcome-based Care programme. Data from PROMs, for example, may improve conversations by catalysing option talk (patient group-level evidence on the pros and cons of the options) and stimulate goal and preference talk. Embedding SDM in digital solutions might be promising but also risks leaving out patients with limited digital skills and/or lower health literacy.

There are also implementation challenges across various healthcare settings, such as when a patient moves from primary to hospital care. Holding a 'time-out consultation' with the general practitioner as part of the decision making process regarding oncological treatment is an interesting example in this respect (Wieldraaijer et al., 2019).

The intention of the 'time-out consultation' was to allocate time for patients to discuss the proposed treatment with their general practitioner, to check patients' understanding of all relevant information, and to consider if patients needed additional support. The Patients Federation also intends to take up the next challenge in implementing SDM by putting complex decision making (e.g. elderly people with multimorbidity) on the agenda.

To summarize, as patients we want to see attitudes changing. We need to keep working on normalizing *samen beslissen*. There is always some degree of choice to be considered for every clinician for every patient.

Conclusion and recommendations

There have been nationwide efforts to implement SDM in the Netherlands in recent years, including strong patient participation at the macro and meso levels. We expect that the uptake of SDM, SDM education and training, and SDM support tools will depend on ongoing promotion and facilitation at the macro level. Implementation strategies should be deployed at multiple levels, target clinician and patient behaviours, and aim to change care processes (van Veenendaal et al., 2022), and, importantly, involve all end-users in their design from the start. The uptake of SDM by individual clinicians and healthcare teams will depend on their choice awareness, good role modelling, and proficiency in involving patients. The recordings of routine consultations and team meetings for research and quality evaluations could increasingly be used as opportunities to learn in this regard, shifting attention to learning gains and away from 'doing SDM well or not'.

Despite fertile ground for SDM in the Netherlands, we face many hurdles ahead. In the coming years, healthcare sustainability will be increasingly challenging, and a key question is how to continue investing in SDM given the scarcity of resources. Moreover, SDM will remain limited if efforts to involve patients do not explicitly target those patients who are too often excluded: those who face barriers in accessing care and in becoming equal partners in healthcare decisions.

REFERENCES

Ankersmid, J. W., van Hoeve, J. C., Strobbe, L. J. A., et al. 2021. Follow-up after breast cancer: variations, best practices, and opportunities for improvement according to health care professionals. *Eur J Cancer Care,* **30**, e13505.

Baghus, A., Giroldi, E., Muris, J., et al. 2021. Identifying entrustable professional activities for shared decision making in postgraduate medical education: a national Delphi study. *Acad Med,* **96**, 126–133.

Baghus, A., Giroldi, E., van Geel, J., et al. 2024. Shared decision-making performance of general practice residents: an observational study combining observer, resident, and patient perspectives. *Fam Pract,* **41**, 50–59.

Damman, O. C., Jani, A., De Jong, B. A., et al. 2020. The use of PROMs and shared decision-making in medical encounters with patients: an opportunity to deliver value-based health care to patients. *J Eval Clin Pract,* **26**, 524–540.

Driever, E. M., Stiggelbout, A. M., Brand, P. L. P. 2022. Do consultants do what they say they do? Observational study of the extent to which clinicians involve their patients in the decision-making process. *BMJ Open,* **12**, e056471.

Federation of Medical Specialists. 2019. *Guide & Competence Set Training Medical Specialists: 'The Art of Shared Decision Making'* [in Dutch]. Federation of Medical Specialists.

Gärtner, F. R., Portielje, J. E., Langendam, M., et al. 2019. Role of patient preferences in clinical practice guidelines: a multiple methods study using guidelines from oncology as a case. *BMJ Open,* **9**, e032483.

Garvelink, M. M., Jillissen, M., Knops, A., et al. 2019. Implementation of the three good questions—a feasibility study in Dutch hospital departments. *Health Expect,* **22**, 1272–1284.

Kuijpers, M. M. T., van Veenendaal, H., Engelen, V., et al. 2022. Shared decision making in cancer treatment: a Dutch national survey on patients' preferences and perceptions. *Eur J Cancer Care,* **31**, e13534.

Netherlands Federation of University Medical Centres. 2020. *Medical Training Framework 2020* [in Dutch]. Netherlands Federation of University Medical Centres.

Oosterveld, M., Noordman, J., Rademakers, J. 2019. *Shared Decision Making in the Consulting Room: Experiences and Needs of People with Limited Health Literacy* [in Dutch]. Nivel.

Perfors, I. A. A., Noteboom, E. A., de Wit, N. J., et al. 2021. Effects of a time out consultation with the general practitioner on cancer treatment decision-making: a randomised controlled trial: time out with the general practitioner and cancer treatment decision. *Psychooncology,* **30**, 571–580.

Regioplan/Nivel 2021. [*Education and Training in Shared Decision Making: An Inventory*]. Nivel.

Richter, R., Jansen, J., van der Kraan, J., et al. 2025. How inclusive are patient decision aids for people with limited health literacy? An analysis of understandability criteria and the communication about options and probabilities. *Med Decis Making,* **45**, 143–155.

Roodbeen, R. T. J., Noordman, J., Boland, G., Van Dulmen, S. 2021. Shared decision making in practice and the perspectives of health care professionals on video-recorded consultations with patients with low health literacy in the palliative phase of their disease. *MDM Policy Pract,* **6**, 23814683211023472.

Sackett, D. L., Rosenberg, W. M., Gray, J. A., Haynes, R. B., Richardson, W. S. 1996. Evidence based medicine: what it is and what it isn't. *BMJ,* **312**, 71–72.

Savelberg, W., Boersma, L. J., Smidt, M., van der Weijden, T. 2021. Implementing a breast cancer patient decision aid: process evaluation using medical files and the patients' perspective. *Eur J Cancer Care,* **30**, e13387.

Schoemaker, C. G., van der Weijden, T. 2016. Patient preferences versus evidence-based medicine: did the pioneers of evidence-based medicine take the patient's preferences into account? [in Dutch]. *Ned Tijdschr Geneeskd,* **160**, D24.

Scholl, I., Larussa, A., Hahlweg, P., Kobrin, S., Elwyn, G. 2018. Organizational- and system-level characteristics that influence implementation of shared decision-making and strategies to address them—a scoping review. *Implement Sci,* **13**, 40.

Stiggelbout, A. M., Pieterse, A. H., De Haes, J. C. 2015. Shared decision making: concepts, evidence, and practice. *Patient Educ Couns,* **98**, 1172–1179.

Ubbink, D. T., Geerts, P. A. F., Gosens, T., Brand, P. L. P. 2021. Updated Dutch law demands shared decision-making [in Dutch]. *Ned Tijdschr Geneeskd,* **165**, D5775.

V&VN 2022. *Shared Decision Making in the Nursing Domain* [in Dutch]. Federation of Nurses.

Van der Weijden, T., Dreesens, D., Faber, M. J., et al. 2019. Developing quality criteria for patient-directed knowledge tools related to clinical practice guidelines. A development and consensus study. *Health Expect,* **22**, 201–208.

Van Veenendaal, H., Voogdt-Pruis, H., Ubbink, D. T., Hilders, C. G. J. M. 2021. Effect of a multilevel implementation programme on shared decision-making in breast cancer care. *BJS Open,* **5**, zraa002.

Van Veenendaal, H., Voogdt-Pruis, H. R., Ubbink, D. T., et al. 2022. Evaluation of a multilevel implementation program for timeout and shared decision making in breast cancer care: a mixed methods study among 11 hospital teams. *Patient Educ Couns,* **105**, 114–127.

Venhuizen, G. 2019. Can patient centred care plus shared decision making equal lower costs? *BMJ,* **367**, l5900.

Wieldraaijer, T., de Meij, M., Zwaard, S., Van Weert, H., Wind, J. 2019. Introducing a time out consultation with the general practitioner between diagnosis and start of colorectal cancer treatment: patient-reported outcomes. *Eur J Cancer Care,* **28**, e13141.

25

How to improve shared decision making in your practice

Using improvement methods to drive change

Alf Collins, Helen Bulbeck, and Paul Grundy

Introduction

This chapter describes how to implement shared decision making (SDM) in the *clinical microsystem* (Nelson et al., 2008), a setting where clinicians and health service managers work and where they can bring about change, for instance, a primary care clinic, a hospital ward, or an outpatient department.

SDM is a team activity. *For patients*, it is frustrating to encounter clinicians with varying degrees of skills in SDM across a care pathway. *For clinicians*, working in teams to bring about changes has advantages in terms of shared workload and team building.

Quality improvement

Quality improvement (QI) is the accepted approach to change in the clinical microsystem. It addresses three questions (Langley et al., 2009):

1. What are we trying to achieve?
2. How will we know that a change is an improvement?
3. What changes can we make that will result in an improvement?

QI encompasses a range of methods that 'give people closest to issues affecting care quality the time, permission, skills and resources they need to solve them' (The Health Foundation, 2021).

The methods draw on common principles:

1. Identify what you want to achieve.
2. Clarify the scope.
3. Understand opportunities and barriers.
4. Assemble a team.
5. Understand the evidence.
6. Construct a theory of change.
7. Methodically implement changes.
8. Develop high reliability.
9. Measure programme outcomes when all changes are embedded.

The rest of this chapter addresses these principles in turn.

Step 1. Identify the issue

The aims could be:

I want to get better at SDM in my own practice.
I want to get better at SDM in order to reduce post-surgical regret.
I want to ensure that all team members practise SDM to contribute to the safety agenda in our organization.

Learning point 1. Specify the primary objective and make it measurable. Consider whether achievement of that objective could lead to other downstream changes.

Learning point 2. Change programmes that contribute to an organizational priority are more likely to benefit from organizational support and to succeed (see also Chapter 23) (National Institute for Health and Care Excellence, 2021).

Step 2. Clarify the scope

Specify the patient population and the common decisions to be made. For a specialist this might be 'To ensure that everyone with osteoarthritic knee pain shares decisions in this clinic'. For a generalist, 'To ensure that everyone who sees me always shares decisions'.

It is tempting to want to share decisions with everyone. This is laudable, but QI tells us to break complex problems into achievable steps.

Learning point 3. Start small, in a focused population and with a single decision. Learn, embed the change into practice, then spread to other decisions in that patient population and/or to other patient populations. In QI, the phrase 'embed, sustain, spread' (Greenhalgh and Papoutsi, 2019) is often used.

Step 3. Understand opportunities and barriers

Prioritizing the patient population and the decision(s) to be made can be informed by a range of opportunities:

- Patient 'push'—demand for high-risk and/or low-value interventions (e.g. opioids for non-cancer pain) or patients demanding more involvement (e.g. many maternity services).
- SDM will contribute to an organizational priority.
- Safety concerns (e.g. high-risk surgery in people with frailty).
- High stakes decisions (e.g. decisions about length of life versus quality of life for people with advanced cancer).
- Decision making about low-evidence/low-value interventions (e.g. spinal injections for patients with back pain).
- Research relevant to your practice.
- Evidence of *unwarranted variation* (Atsma et al., 2020) where your team is an outlier.

Barriers to SDM (Joseph-Williams et al., 2017) include:

- The obverse of the above-listed opportunities
- Lack of support from colleagues or your organization.

Step 4. Assemble a team

A single clinician can implement SDM by developing skills via e-learning and using decision aids from a reliable source. However, high-quality healthcare delivery is a multidisciplinary activity so we recommend assembling a team comprising (National Institute for Health and Care Excellence, 2021):

- A clinical champion
- A patient leader
- A programme manager
- A senior leader who can help with managing obstacles.

Other team members could include experts in data, analytics, or digital systems.

A team approach is important in terms of spreading the workload, assembling a range of views, and sustainability. Change programmes that rely on the drive of a single team member may not be sustainable should they leave.

Learning point 4. Assemble a team bringing different perspectives and expertise. All patient-facing initiatives should be *co-designed* (National Institute for Health and Care Excellence, 2021), with patients engaged in all relevant aspects of programme design, as described in the patient perspective box (Box 25.1).

Step 5. Understand the evidence

The evidence supporting both SDM and QI when done well (Dixon-Woods and Martin, 2016) is strong. We therefore recommend a brief evidence synthesis *from implementation literature* to understand what others in your field/context have done. Otherwise, much of the evidence base about implementation of SDM using QI is signposted in this chapter.

Box 25.1 Patient perspective

Communication is central to human interaction, to everything we do. Without it, we cannot relate to those around us, make our needs and concerns known, or make sense of what is happening to us.

Any diagnosis of an illness is frightening and may impact someone's ability to communicate their needs clearly. A common theme at the point of diagnosis is the sense of isolation, a lack of voice, and the disempowerment that the patient feels; there is a feeling of loss of control. Nonetheless, a shift to being empowered can begin at the point of diagnosis, and a collaborative and interactive relationship between patients and their healthcare team can empower them to become involved in all decisions about management options.

SDM conversations should help to reframe problems, generate insights, shift dynamics, and change practice. Patients are concerned about vitality, role limitations, emotional well-being, mental health, and quality of life, and all of these elements of personhood are core to the decision making process. SDM done well means that patients can be people.

However, there remain major challenges to this for the patient, for example, from moving from the position of seeing the healthcare professional as an expert giving advice, to seeing them as an enabler who supports them to achieve their goals. There is also the challenge for the patient to move from seeing themselves as a passive recipient of care, to becoming activated and taking responsibility for their own contribution to improving health and well-being outcomes and being empowered to do so.

Patient advocacy can help establish SDM as a standard of care (National Institute for Health and Care Excellence, 2021). Involving patients in the design and delivery of SDM can be achieved through different advocacy roles, including:

- Navigation advocacy—being coached by an advocate before and after consultations
- Information advocacy—an advocate provides information between appointments
- Mediation/spokesperson advocacy—stating the patient's positions, needs, and interests on their behalf, if they cannot or do not wish to advocate for themselves
- Community advocacy—supporting co-design of SDM interventions.

Examples of where patients could be included in SDM co-design include:

- Development of driver diagrams and change ideas
- Development of decision aids
- Interventions to support patient preparation
- Feedback on improvement initiatives.

Most importantly perhaps, patient involvement at all levels of design and delivery can help to rebalance healthcare from an increasingly industrial process towards a shared endeavour, informed by one of humanity's most basic instincts—to care.

Learning point 5. To develop a further understanding of QI, resources such as that from The Health Foundation (2021) are invaluable.

Step 6. Develop a theory of change and an implementation method

QI is an umbrella term for a variety of approaches, and overlapping terms for these change methods are used, including *theory of change*, *logic models*, and *driver diagrams* (Institute for Healthcare Improvement, n.d.). The latter focus on changes specific to the microsystem and have been used in SDM implementation programmes such as The Health Foundation's 'MAGIC' programme in the UK (The Health Foundation, n.d.), so we will describe the use of driver diagrams here.

Driver diagrams: processes and outcomes

Driver diagrams rely on developing the following understanding of the relationship between processes and outcomes:

1. Specify a measurable *primary outcome*.
2. Develop a range of *secondary outcomes* (patient outcomes and system impact).
3. Identify groups of evidenced-based activities (processes) that *determine* the primary outcome. These are called *primary drivers* and ideally there should be three to five of them.
4. Identify groups of activities that feed into the primary drivers. These are called *secondary drivers* and ideally there should be three to five per primary driver.
5. *Discuss change ideas* that can feed into the secondary drivers.
6. *Clarify the enablers*—underpinning factors that help the programme succeed. Patient leadership and clinical leadership, a measurement system, and data management are enablers.

The driver diagram (Figure 25.1) demonstrates three primary drivers and two secondary drivers per primary driver. If these drivers are patient-facing, they are often called *care bundles*. The Institute for Healthcare Improvement describes bundles as 'structured ways of improving the processes of care and patient outcomes by deploying a small, straightforward set of evidence-based practices' (Institute for Healthcare Improvement, 2012).

Driver diagrams, the evidence base and context

QI programmes should be informed by method and evidence and take account of context (Coles et al., 2020). Context is usually team or organizational cultural factors that may sit outside the initial scope of the QI programme and that could enable or impede progress. Iterative programme design can help navigate the complexity that contextual factors often introduce.

Primary drivers should be evidence informed and have distinct face validity. Secondary drivers are often theoretically principled processes, and change ideas tend to gravitate towards contextual activities. We will explore drivers in more detail below.

Bringing together a range of stakeholders (as per step 4) to develop driver diagrams is an important approach to agree on the bundles of care that will be implemented (The Health Foundation, n.d.).

Primary drivers to improve SDM

The primary drivers are:

- Prepared patients
- Trained teams
- A supportive system.

We will consider these primary drivers in more detail below.

Enablers to improve SDM

As described above, enablers include:

- Assembling the right team
- Ensuring there is a data management and measurement system in place.

Learning point 6. The scope of the QI programme determines which activities are drivers and which are enablers. A sole practitioner may not require institutional support to become proficient at SDM, a small team might find such support beneficial (in which case it will become an enabler), while a larger programme might fail without such support (in which case it will be a secondary driver).

Secondary outcomes/system impacts

Improving the quality of SDM in a clinical microsystem will have predictable secondary outcomes. These outcomes could contribute to organizational priorities and could therefore gain significant senior support (see Chapter 23).

Learning point 7. Think about system priorities when considering the focal point of your QI programme. Understand the evidence base that links improved SDM to these outcomes (see also Chapters 17–24).

Secondary drivers to improve SDM

See Figure 25.2.

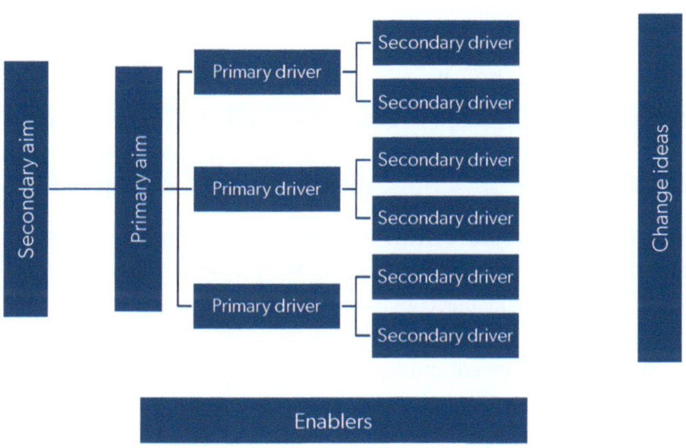

Figure 25.1 Driver diagram schema.

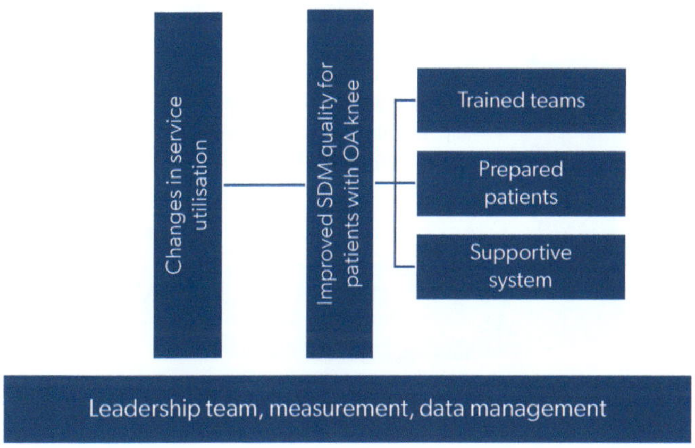

Figure 25.2 A worked example of an SDM driver diagram with three primary drivers.

Prepared patients

(See also Chapters 17–20.) Patients can be prepared to share decisions by ensuring that:

- They hold their own notes or have access to them
- Clinicians routinely write to patients, copying other clinicians
- Patients are provided with decision aids before their appointments (where appropriate)
- There is a systematic approach to 'nudge' patients to become involved in decision making, by using, for instance, BRAN (Academy of Medical Royal Colleges, 2023) or 'Ask 3 Questions' (A3Q) (Figure 25.3) (Shepherd et al., 2011).

Implementation of these approaches is highly context dependent. It is not feasible to give patients decision aids in a busy accident and emergency department or on a busy ward, but it is feasible to promote A3Q in these environments.

Trained teams

(See also Chapter 14.) Health professionals need to be trained to practise SDM to a high standard. There is a consensus that motivational interviewing and risk and uncertainty communication are core skills and e-learning in these approaches is widely available.

Organizations that are committed to *continuous learning* (Chapter 3) can provide teams with protected time to attend initial training and to develop their skills via communities of practice.

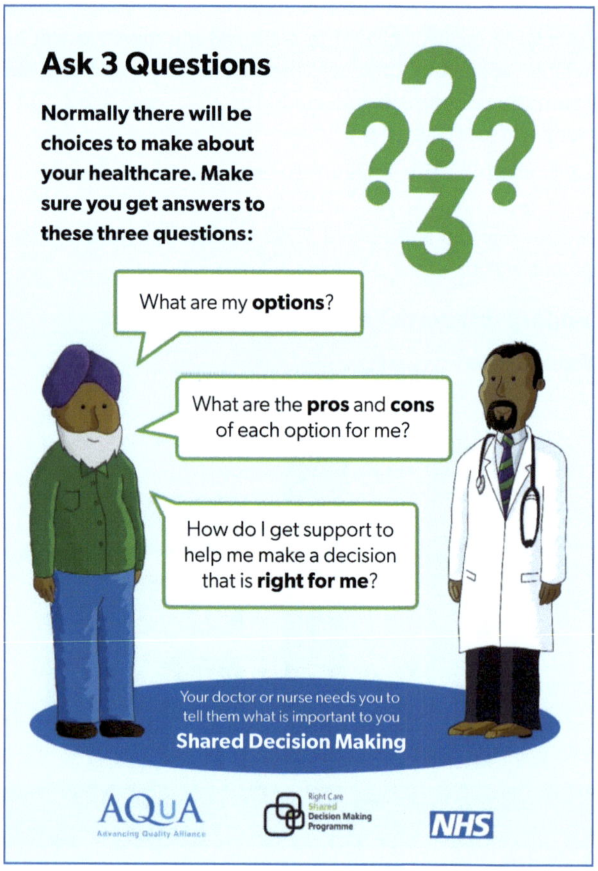
Ask 3 Questions
Normally there will be choices to make about your healthcare. Make sure you get answers to these three questions:
3
What are my **options**?
What are the **pros** and **cons** of each option for me?
How do I get support to help me make a decision that is **right for me**?
Your doctor or nurse needs you to tell them what is important to you
Shared Decision Making
AQUA
Advancing Quality Alliance
Right Care
Shared
Decision Making
Programme
NHS

Figure 25.3 Ask 3 Questions.
Reproduced from the Health Foundation MAGIC programme, AQUA, and NHS England 2012.

Supportive system

The healthcare system operates at three levels:

1. The clinical *microsystem*.
2. The *mesosystem*—a series of linked microsystems across a pathway of care *or* a local institution such as a primary care cluster or a hospital.
3. The *macrosystem*—a locality, region, or nation responsible for setting standards, training, regulation, and policy development.

Clinicians and operational managers can make many changes in their microsystem without institutional support, but will often need such support as outlined below.

Microsystem changes—little institutional support needed:

- Ensuring patients are prepared.
- Ensuring in-consultation decision aids are readily accessible in clinic.
- Ensuring there is a system to record that an SDM discussion has taken place, a decision reached, and actions agreed.

Mesosystem (institutional support) for SDM:

- Explicit board level engagement (often driven by organizational priorities to which SDM contributes).
- Clinical teams are given time and support to bring about the changes required.
- An explicit commitment to continuous improvement.

Step 7. Methodical implementation

- *Start small*. Displaying an A3Q poster in an outpatient clinic is easier than finding funding for a clinician training programme.
- *Celebrate early wins*. A survey demonstrating that 90% of patients became aware of A3Q after the above intervention helps build momentum.
- *Expect the programme to never actually 'end'*. Your programme will move forward over time, but there will be times of accelerated progress and of setbacks.
- *Adopt a strengths-based approach to learning*. Expect to learn about yourself, your colleagues, and change in a broad sense. Celebrate setbacks; this is where we learn the most.

Step 8. Establish high-quality, high-reliability processes

Secondary drivers are activities that often impact directly on patient experience (e.g. the processes within the prepared patient bundle), while some will take place 'behind the scenes' (e.g. many of the processes within the trained teams bundle).

There are two key components of these processes:

- Quality.
- Reliability—a high standard of care, delivered to as many patients as possible.

Establishing quality and reliability

Let us take implementation of A3Q as a worked example (Figure 25.3).

The desired outcome is that all patients ask questions in clinic. There are two primary drivers of this outcome:

1. Patients are prepared to A3Q.
2. Clinicians support patients to A3Q.

Driver 2 is covered by clinician training, so let's focus on driver 1—ensuring that patients are reliably prepared to A3Q.

Exploring change ideas with a range of stakeholders—*including, most importantly, patients*—can help to develop secondary drivers, for instance:

1. Appointment letters prepare patients.
2. Clinic receptionists prepare patients.
3. There are A3Q posters in the clinic.

Assume that all of these drivers are implemented at once. After perhaps a month it would be reasonable to understand whether patients are aware of, and feel equipped to, A3Q.

We can do this by using a survey. When doing so, it is important to remember a few design principles (Millstein and Agarwal, 2021):

1. *Framing the questions.* Tell patients why you are asking for their help and what you will do with their responses.
2. *Use plain, non-technical language.*
3. *Proximal, frugal, actionable survey items*:
   - If possible, survey patients as they exit the clinic.
   - Ask as few questions as possible (ideally three to five).
   - Consider actionable free text ('In order to ensure future patients are prepared to ask questions in clinic, what one change would you recommend we put in place?').
4. *Remember random sampling and variation*:
   - Driver 2 is a source of variability; perhaps not all receptionists are preparing patients. It is important to sample at times when different receptionists are in the clinic.

Most improvement surveys depend on randomly sampling just 20–30 patients (Etchells et al., 2015). Small samples like this can be highly informative; in this survey we might pick up that:

- The receptionist on Wednesdays wasn't preparing patients
- More than 50% of patients didn't recollect seeing A3Q in their appointment letter.

As a result, we could make changes to remedy these concerns and survey another 20 patients 2 months later.

Learning point 8. Patient-facing activities should be designed and improved using iterative patient feedback.

Plan-do-study-act

The example above is an illustration of continuous improvement. There are two *cycles of improvement* here:

- Cycle 1 = implementation of initial changes and a survey of reliability.
- Cycle 2 = implementation of further changes and another survey.

The second survey could uncover further potential for change, leading to a third cycle.

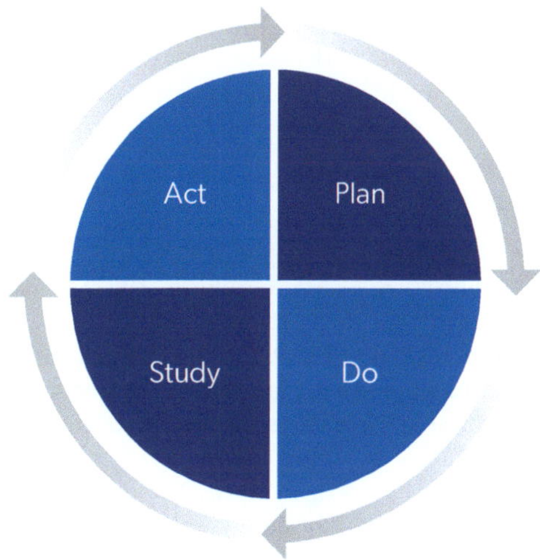

Figure 25.4 Plan-Do-Study-Act cycle.

These change cycles are referred to as 'Plan-Do-Study-Act' or 'PDSA' cycles (Figure 25.4) and are commonly used to help improve the reliability and quality of process changes (Reed et al., 2016).

Step 9. Measurement

The example demonstrates important aspects of measurement for improvement. Many such measures tend to help answer the question 'Have we reliably implemented processes to a high standard?' This is in contrast to measures that are used in clinical trials which usually ask questions like 'Does this intervention work?'

Another principle of QI is that outcomes are not optimized until all processes are reliably implemented to a high standard. Think of building processes into your microsystem as you would think of building a complex machine. The machine will only work optimally (the outcome) when all the components (the processes) are working smoothly and reliably together.

What this means is that you will spend much of your time deploying process measures. Some of the items in these measures can be taken from other questionnaires or surveys and some you will need to develop yourselves.

So measures of SDM that are in most common use (see Chapters 10 and 11) can be used in the context of QI to:

1. Assess the impact of a clinician training programme—but note that if the training programme has been put in place without preparing patients or ensuring that the system is supportive, the outcome will be suboptimal
2. Assess the impact of reliable implementation of all processes to a high standard.

Final remarks

QI encompasses a range of approaches, all with common principles. We have chosen to describe one particular (though almost universally recognized) approach in this chapter.

We hope that we have stimulated you to commit to co-production, to rigorous design of your work and to a way of working that motivates you and your team to become life-long learners.

REFERENCES

Academy of Medical Royal Colleges. 2023. BRAN patient leaflet. Available at: https://www.aomrc.org.uk/wp-content/uploads/2023/08/CWUK_patient_leaflet_100120.pdf

Atsma, F., Elwyn, G., Westert, G. 2020. Understanding unwarranted variation in clinical practice: a focus on network effects, reflective medicine and learning health systems. *Int J Qual Health Care,* **32,** 271–274.

Coles, E., Anderson, J., Maxwell, M., et al. 2020. The influence of contextual factors on healthcare quality improvement initiatives: a realist review. *Syst Rev,* **9,** 94.

Dixon-Woods, M., Martin, G.P. 2016. Does quality improvement improve quality? *Future Hosp J,* **3,** 191–194.

Etchells, E., Ho, M., Shojania, K.G. 2015. Value of small sample sizes in rapid-cycle quality improvement projects. *BMJ Qual Saf,* **25,** 202–206.

Greenhalgh, T., Papoutsi, C. 2019. Spreading and scaling up innovation and improvement. *BMJ,* **365,** l2068.

Institute for Healthcare Improvement. n.d. Driver diagram. Available at: https://www.ihi.org/resources/tools/driver-diagram

Institute for Healthcare Improvement. 2012. What is a bundle? Available at: https://www.ihi.org/insights/what-is-a-bundle

Joseph-Williams, N., Lloyd, A., Edwards, A., et al. 2017. Implementing shared decision making in the NHS: lessons from the MAGIC programme. *BMJ,* **357,** j1744.

Langley, G. J., Moen, R. D., Nolan, K. M., Nolan, T. W., Norman, C. L., Pronovost, L. P. 2009. *The Improvement Guide: A Practical Approach to Enhancing Organizational Performance,* 2nd edition. Jossey-Bass Publishers.

Millstein, J., Agarwal, A. 2021. Developing actionable survey questions to improve patient experience. *J Patient Exp,* **8,** 237437352199959.

National Institute for Health and Care Excellence. 2021. Shared decision making. NICE guideline [NG197]. Available at: https://www.nice.org.uk/guidance/ng197

Nelson, E. C., Godfrey, M. M., Batalden, P. B., et al. 2008. Clinical microsystems, part 1. The building blocks of health systems. *Jt Comm J Qual Patient Saf,* **34,** 367–378.

Reed, J. E., Davey, N., Woodcock, T. 2016. The foundations of quality improvement science. *Future Hosp J,* **3,** 199–202.

Shepherd, H. L., Barratt, A., Trevena, L. J., et al. 2011. Three questions that patients can ask to improve the quality of information physicians give about treatment options: a cross-over trial. *Patient Educ Couns,* **84,** 379–385.

The Health Foundation. 2021. Quality improvement made simple. Available at: https://www.health.org.uk/publications/quality-improvement-made-simple.

The Health Foundation. n.d. Implementing shared decision making. Available at: https://www.health.org.uk/publications/implementing-shared-decision-making

PART 6

The view from the clinical specialties

26

Shared decision making from the perspective of primary care

Leigh Sanyaolu, France Légaré, Adrian Edwards, and Susannah Fraser

Introduction

The strength of a country's healthcare system is dependent on the quality of its primary care services. In many countries, primary care is the first port of call for patients to access healthcare services; it acts as the 'gatekeeper' to more specialized care and provides both urgent and planned or ongoing care (Starfield et al., 2005). In 2021–2022 there were approximately one million encounters between the public and primary care in the UK's National Health Service per day (nearly three-fifths of all encounters) (The King's Fund, 2021). What goes on in primary care is vital for the overall healthcare system's effectiveness and efficiency (Starfield et al., 2005). It is also a major contributor to the overall experience of patients. Therefore, if we want patients to routinely experience shared decision making (SDM) throughout their care trajectory, it must be a routine part of primary healthcare service delivery.

Patients in primary care often present with undifferentiated or vague symptoms that can evolve with time; symptoms of both common and serious conditions also often overlap. As the population ages, the number of people with multiple and/or long-term conditions increases ('multimorbidity') (Chowdhury et al., 2023; Whitty, 2023). Although specialist services may also manage patients, these will generally focus on a specific condition or disease. There are numerous clinical guidelines to aid diagnosis and referral. Still, individual patients rarely fit these guidelines because they typically have more than one condition with competing 'best' management approaches.

It is often the role of general practitioners (GPs) and other primary care healthcare professionals (HCPs) to manage this complexity and coordinate long-term care. Primary care HCPs need to be skilled in this, integrating unique patient contexts, eliciting individual preferences and goals, and applying scientific and clinical experience to provide evidence-based care. The principles of SDM, a process for identifying and exploring options, patient preferences, values, and goals, and making decisions or plans with patients that reflect 'what is most important to them' (patients), are fundamental to value-based healthcare (National Institute for Health and Care Excellence (NICE), 2021a).

However, primary care is under extreme pressure due to the increasing demands on health and social care (e.g. over-medicalization, ageing, social inequities, etc.) coupled with the challenge of a declining workforce to meet these needs, which is a global problem that is likely to worsen due to increased workloads and burnout (Gunja et al., 2022). Nonetheless, primary care is resilient and has shown some ability to adapt to these challenges. For example, during the COVID-19 pandemic, primary care moved rapidly to provide remote consulting and played a pivotal role in the COVID-19 vaccination programmes. Primary care services need to continue to show this adaptability and play an important part in integrating SDM into routine care as recommended in key national guidelines such as from NICE in the UK (NICE, 2021a, 2021b).

SDM in primary care

NICE published its guidance on SDM in 2021 (NICE, 2021a). Before that guidance, there was limited practical advice on incorporating SDM into routine clinical practice. The collaborative process of SDM empowers individuals to make informed decisions about their care and make decisions that reflect 'what is most important for them' at that point in time. Decisions can include starting new treatment(s), or declining or discontinuing treatment. Other decisions can centre on tests, referrals to specialists, or access to non-medical services and support. We discuss how this could happen in practice through an example scenario concerning a woman examining preventive options for recurrent urinary tract infections (rUTIs), introduced first through the patient's perspective (Box 26.1).

The UK's NICE guidance describes several key components that HCPs should consider before, during, and after a SDM discussion. It provides specific advice on how this could look in clinical practice for each step. To illustrate this, we now map the guidance onto

Box 26.1 Patient perspective

'No decision about me, without me'

I am a patient who has suffered from rUTIs and interstitial cystitis/bladder pain syndrome for over 20 years now. I also work for the national charity Bladder Health UK offering advice and support to sufferers via an advice line.

Over the years of accessing services within the National Health Service, I feel that SDM rarely happens. I have found it difficult to have input into decisions about my care despite my firm belief that no decision should be made about my treatment without my view being taken into consideration—'no decision about me, without me'. It has also been difficult to obtain information about alternatives to a particular treatment being offered. I regularly find information on alternative treatments from Bladder Health UK rather than from my clinicians.

For example, as a sufferer of rUTIs, I was offered low-dose antibiotics, which I took for about a year. I was never entirely comfortable with this approach due to concerns about antibiotic resistance. No mention was ever made of an alternative antimicrobial product called methenamine hippurate. I only found out about this form of treatment by researching other options online. It has proved very successful for me, and I was prescribed it as soon as I asked.

I speak to many people on the advice line whose stories have led me to believe that the risks of surgery and interventions are not properly discussed, such as the risk to men of becoming incontinent after prostate surgery. People usually report that discussions focused mainly on the benefits of surgery.

Since the COVID-19 pandemic, access to primary care has become much more difficult. This is frustrating for patients and makes access to secondary care when it is needed even harder. GPs are very limited in the time they can spend with patients, making the routine integration of SDM even less frequent.

In my opinion, most sufferers would like to be an equal partner in deciding what would be best for them. It would be good if patients could be given as much information as possible - including the pros and the cons—about available alternative treatments and to be listened to when asking about new treatments or those that are available via other practices or providers. Some patients do extensive research on their condition as they want to know as much as possible about the causes and relief of symptoms and are very capable when contributing to their treatment plan. Others may not be so informed and would need more guidance. The outcome they are seeking from treatment may be quite different from the outcome the clinician is looking to achieve for them. We need to get the clinicians more focused on asking, 'What is important to you?' It would be a big help if the scenario described in this chapter were a commoner experience for patients.

a hypothetical scenario of a woman presenting in primary care with rUTIs (Box 26.2). The SDM decision considers long-term prevention, and for brevity, we have focused on long-term low-dose preventive antibiotics. We have chosen this scenario since there is evidence that women with rUTIs would like more discussion with their clinicians about the different preventive options (Sanyaolu et al., 2023).

Box 26.2 Hypothetical scenario to demonstrate how SDM might look in practice

Ms Davies is 58 years old and, since the menopause, has been having recurrent urine infections, with five in the last 12 months, all confirmed with a urine culture. She was referred to urology, and investigations, including an ultrasound scan and cystoscopy, were normal. Preventive antibiotics for 3–6 months were discussed at her last outpatient appointment. Ms Davies is unsure whether to start them and has made an appointment to discuss this with her GP.

Before the consultation

Before attending the consultation, individuals should be offered information in their preferred format about the decision they want to discuss with their HCP. This can help them consider, before the consultation: what are their priorities? What do they envisage as the outcome of the discussion and what questions would they like to ask during it? It is also important to consider whether the individual would require additional support (e.g. from a family member, carer, etc.) to help them understand any information provided before the consultation and support them to play an active role in the SDM discussion. In our scenario, this might involve sharing information or quality-assured patient decision aids (PtDAs) around rUTI prevention. A quality-assured PtDA is one that has been developed according to recognized standards, with contents that are both accurate and balanced (see Chapter 18). It is also important that the PtDA includes prompts to consider what is most important to the patient personally before the consultation.

During the consultation

At the start of the consultation, it is important to agree on the type or nature of the decision to be made, as this will inform the relevant options (Box 26.3). This is not trivial. For example, a decision

Box 26.3 Setting the agenda and encouraging patient participation.

GP: Good afternoon, Ms Davies; what can we do today?

Ms Davies: Good afternoon, Doctor. As you know, I have had several urine infections over the last year. I have seen the consultant and all my investigations were normal. They mentioned taking antibiotics daily for a few months. This isn't something I'd heard about before, but I am concerned about taking these and wanted to discuss these and other treatment options with you.

Setting the agenda

GP: Okay, thank you. If I understand correctly, you would like to discuss and explore whether to start taking antibiotics versus other treatments to prevent your urine infections? Were there any specific things you wanted to discuss?

Decision point: how to reduce the number of recurrent urine infections

Ms Davies: These urine infections are terrible and make me feel really unwell, so I wanted to know how good long-term antibiotics would be at stopping them. I have also read about antibiotics not working in the future if they are used a lot, and so I am worried about this. I also wanted to know what alternatives there are and how they compare.

GP: Okay, how about we talk about these antibiotics you could take every day for a few months, their benefits and risks, and any other potential options for you? I really want to know what you think about the possible outcomes of each option and what's most important to you in this situation. How does that sound?

Ms Davies: Thank you, that would be great.

Ensure individual knows they can ask questions and participate in the discussion

GP: As I go through each option, if anything is unclear or you have any questions, please interrupt me at any point.

Ms Davies: Thank you.

point such as 'What are my options to reduce recurring symptoms of rUTI?' is not the same as 'Should I take long-term antibiotics or not to prevent rUTI?' The patient and HCP can set an agenda and prioritize what is important to discuss. It is essential that patients know that they can participate in the decision as much as they prefer (Box 26.4). When discussing the different options, including 'watchful waiting' (i.e. not using antibiotics) and continuing the individual's current management, it is important to discuss the benefits and risks of each option and their consequences. This discussion should encourage patients to reflect and express their own personal priorities, needs, and preferences.

When discussing the benefits, risks, and potential consequences, the NICE guidelines advise on how this could be done (NICE, 2018). This information should be presented in the context of the individual's own preferences on the potential outcomes of each option and ideally be personalized. Where this personalized information is not available in a decision aid (or, in some decision situations, a risk calculator) then more general information should be presented, including how this relates to that individual. The guidelines also provide general advice about how risks and benefits should be discussed.

After the consultation

The guidelines advise that after the consultation or between consultations, individuals should be offered resources to help them understand what has been discussed and the decision made. This could include a PtDA matching the decision point (e.g. treatments to reduce rUTIs). Discussions should also include when the management option will be reviewed. Consider offering additional support for those who require it; this could include a follow-up appointment with an HCP or alternative if appropriate.

Box 26.4 Discussing management options and making a decision

Ms Davies: Thank you, Doctor. No, that all makes sense.

Give the patient time for questions and to make the decision

GP: You do not need to decide today if you don't want to. We can arrange a review in a few weeks if you want.
Ms Davies: No, I would like to start treatment today, please, and I would like to try the vaginal cream.

State the decision that has been made, document it and discuss what happens next, including when to review the decision and that the patient can change their mind or review it sooner

GP: That's not a problem at all. So, we're choosing the oestrogen cream, and I will write our discussion in your notes today, [GP gives directions on how to use the cream and advice regarding specific side effects and when to seek medical attention and agrees time for review]. If you have any questions, change your mind, or have concerns, you can always make an appointment at the surgery sooner. Here is the decision aid we used today, and there is a bit at the end where you can write down questions you have, so when we review your medication, you can talk this through with one of the GPs, nurses, or pharmacists at the surgery.
Ms Davies: Thank you, Doctor.

Challenges and evidence gaps

Changing care delivery

Implementing SDM in routine primary care has challenges, and successful implementation stories remain scarce. The structure of the primary care team is changing as has the mode of consultation, particularly during the COVID-19 pandemic. A significant proportion of consultations within primary care globally are now delivered via telephone or remotely (Neves et al., 2021). There are additional challenges and complexities of SDM with these consulting methods that need exploration including how traditional methods of SDM conducted in person can be translated to these different consulting formats. In addition, few studies of SDM implementation have evaluated the potential harms this could introduce (e.g. whether inequities are widened), and this is an important future research topic.

Changing primary care teams

Primary care teams have also changed over time, moving towards a multidisciplinary team model, with GPs complemented by allied HCPs such as mental health and advanced nurse practitioners, pharmacists, and physiotherapists, among others. This presents potential challenges for the implementation of SDM. Firstly, experience of SDM will likely differ between HCPs and training on implementing SDM may need to adapt for the various HCP groups. Currently, it is uncertain whether any interventions targeted only at HCPs are effective at increasing SDM (Légaré et al., 2018). Evidence does suggest that interventions are needed both at the HCP and patient levels, including both SDM and PtDA elements. Evidence on interventions with particular HCP disciplines is also lacking. Continuity between patients and HCPs also becomes challenging with the expanding clinical teams, more patients per practice, and reduced numbers of GP practices. How SDM will work across multiple consultations with various HCPs requires further research.

Increased demand and complexity

Other challenges to implementing SDM include increasing demand in primary care, increasing workload, and patient complexity. The number of patients per full-time equivalent GP has risen over time. The complexity of delivering primary healthcare continues to increase as the population ages and leads to the rising prevalence of long-term conditions and multimorbidity. This presents challenges for healthcare in general but also specifically for adopting and achieving SDM as 'routine' in primary care.

Where to start?

We have illustrated how SDM can be adopted, such as in the scenario around rUTIs. There is an almost infinite number of further scenarios reflecting the eclectic nature of primary care. With these challenges, how best to integrate SDM into this pressurized system is not clear but focusing on long-term conditions may be the best place to start, especially where SDM support tools already exist. Resolving this uncertainty is critical if we are to ensure that SDM becomes routine in primary care and a reality for patients across the healthcare spectrum.

REFERENCES

Chowdhury, S. R., Chandra Das, D., Sunna, T. C., Beyene, J., Hossain, A. 2023. Global and regional prevalence of multimorbidity in the adult population in community settings: a systematic review and meta-analysis. *EClinicalMedicine*, **57**, 101860.

Gunja, M., Gumas, E., Williams, R., II, Doty, M., Shah, A., Fields, K. 2022. Stressed out and burned out: the global primary care crisis — findings from the 2022 International Health Policy Survey of Primary Care Physicians. Commonwealth Fund. Available at: https://doi.org/10.26099/j2ag-mx88

Légaré, F., Adekpedjou, R., Stacey, D., et al. 2018. Interventions for increasing the use of shared decision making by healthcare professionals. *Cochrane Database Syst Rev*, **7**, CD006732.

National Institute for Health and Care Excellence. 2018. Decision aid for recurrent urinary tract infection (UTI) in postmenopausal women. Available at: https://www.nice.org.uk/guidance/ng112/resources/patient-decision-aid-on-reducing-the-chance-of-recurrent-urinary-tract-infection-uti-in-postmenopausal-women-pdf-6600984158

National Institute for Health and Care Excellence. 2021a. Shared decision making. NICE Guideline [NG197]. Available at: http://www.nice.org.uk/ng197

National Institute for Health and Care Excellence. 2021b. Standards framework for shared-decision-making support tools, including patient decision aids. Corporate document [ECD8]. Available at: http://www.nice.org.uk/corporate/ecd8

Neves, A. L., Li, E., Gupta, P. P., Fontana, G., Darzi, A. 2021. Virtual primary care in high-income countries during the COVID-19 pandemic: policy responses and lessons for the future. *Eur J Gen Pract*, **27**, 241–247.

Sanyaolu, L. N., Hayes, C. V., Lecky, D. M., et al. 2023. Patients' and healthcare professionals' experiences and views of recurrent urinary tract infections in women: qualitative evidence synthesis and meta-ethnography. *Antibiotics*, **12**, 434.

Starfield, B., Shi, L., Macinko, J. 2005. Contribution of primary care to health systems and health. *Milbank Q*, **83**, 457–502.

The King's Fund. 2021. The NHS in a nutshell: activity in the NHS. Available at: https://www.kingsfund.org.uk/projects/nhs-in-a-nutshell/NHS-activity

Whitty, C. J. M. 2023. Chief Medical Officer's annual report 2023: health in an ageing society. Available at: https://assets.publishing.service.gov.uk/media/65562ff2d03a8d000d07faa6/chief-medical-officers-annual-report-2023-web-accessible.pdf

27

Shared decision making in mental healthcare

Yumi Aoki, Lilisbeth Perestelo-Pérez, Hidetoshi Matsuura, and Yaara Zisman-Ilani

Introduction: shared decision making with people with severe mental illnesses

Integration of shared decision making in recovery-focused care

Since the beginning of this century, the treatment for severe mental illnesses (SMIs) such as schizophrenia, bipolar disorder, and depression has been increasingly recognized as user-centred, with a focus on recovery rather than alleviating symptoms. The concept of recovery involves adapting one's mindset, beliefs, emotions, aspirations, and abilities to lead a fulfilling life despite the challenges posed by illness. Recovery-oriented mental healthcare and shared decision making (SDM) are highly compatible, as both prioritize fostering collaborative interactions among individuals with SMIs, and their families, and healthcare providers. The movement valuing personal recovery, which originated from individuals with SMI, has become widely embraced at the national policy level in numerous Western countries and is now extending its influence to Asian and African nations as a global trend. This trend also underscores the growing interest in integrating SDM approaches into mental healthcare practices worldwide.

Concept of SDM in SMIs

Over the past 20 years, SDM with people with SMIs, and related research, has evolved rapidly, leading to various initiatives being implemented worldwide in practice. Aoki (2020) proposed a conceptual model based on a systematic review of 71 studies that focused on SDM with people with SMIs (Figure 27.1). This model comprises four key attributes: the user–healthcare provider relationship, communication between users and healthcare providers, user-friendly visualization of medical information, and involvement of various stakeholders. Antecedents such as complex illnesses and power imbalances act as barriers, yet SDM can overcome traditional power dynamics, promote changes, and improve relationships. Nevertheless, within the context of clinical practice, disparity in perceptions of SDM between healthcare providers and patients is frequent. It is essential to encourage engagement from both stakeholder groups to advance SDM.

Overviewing SDM interventions for people with SMIs

Global application of SDM with people with SMIs

Currently, SDM is globally practised and applied across various settings for individuals with SMIs (Aoki et al., 2022b). This encompasses choices regarding treatments and care across different stages, such as primary care, community mental health services, care facilities, nursing homes, outpatient psychiatric clinics, inpatient psychiatric hospitals, forensic psychiatry, care transitions, and discharge planning. Despite concerns about reduced capacity for decision making due to symptoms like hallucinations, delusions, manic states, or severe depression during the acute phase of SMI, SDM is considered feasible in psychiatry.

Strategies addressing concerns about decision making capacity involve contributions from various stakeholders involved in the SDM process. While the stakeholders involved may vary depending on the environment and the decision at hand, the understanding of SDM has been expanded beyond the dyad (individual user and service provider) recently in mental healthcare. For instance, interdisciplinary collaboration involving psychiatrists, psychologists, nurses, pharmacists, case managers, social workers, and occupational therapists is now usual, and SDM functions as a common concept that connects these professions with different expertise. Decision coaching, also as part of interdisciplinary care, aims to enhance participation in decision making for individuals by adopting a neutral stance towards each option, avoiding bias towards any specific choice, sharing the deliberative process with the user, and encouraging them to organize information, address enquiries, and clarify their values. Hamann et al. (2006) in Germany and Aoki et al. (2019) in Japan have implemented the practice of decision coaching by nurses, respectively, with inpatient schizophrenia patients and outpatient mood disorder patients (Aoki et al., 2022b).

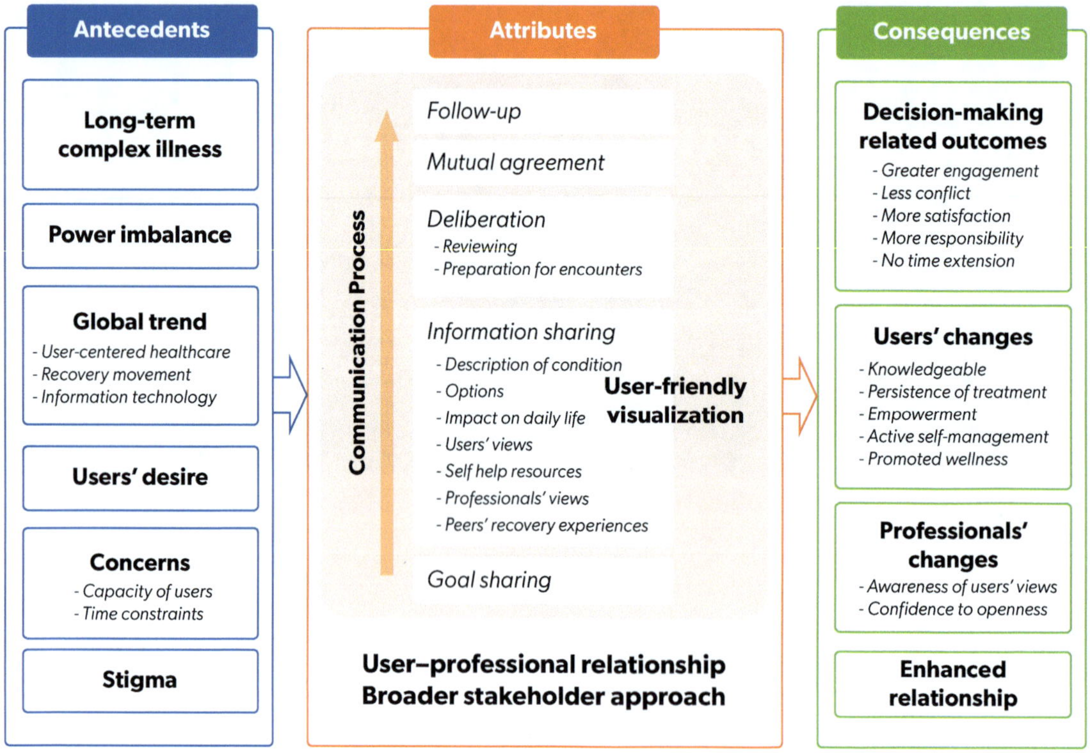

Figure 27.1 Concept model of SDM for adults with SMI.

Reproduced with permission from Aoki, Y. 2020. Shared decision making for adults with severe mental illness: a concept analysis. *Jpn J Nurs Sci*, 17, e12365.

Furthermore, the involvement of non-healthcare providers such as caregivers, family members, and peer supporters has been increasingly emphasized.

The involvement of these diverse stakeholders facilitates greater participation of the individual in discussions, which is desirable. Another strategy entails leveraging material resources, including decision support tools, alongside the contributions of human resources.

Effects of SDM for people with SMIs

Aoki et al. (2022b) conducted a systematic review and meta-analysis, focusing on randomized controlled trials of SDM interventions for individuals with mental health conditions. Examining 15 randomized controlled trials (n = 3141 participants), primarily involving adults from high-income countries in Europe, North America, and Asia with SMIs, the review found no significant differences in clinical outcomes. However, SDM interventions demonstrated potential in enhancing user participation in decision making immediately post-intervention (standardized mean difference 0.63, 95% confidence interval 0.26–1.01, three studies, 534 participants). The analysis also revealed that SDM interventions, even in acute psychiatric wards, did not result in adverse health effects or extended consultation times. This positive aspect could facilitate the clinical adoption of SDM. Nonetheless, despite these encouraging findings, the overall certainty of evidence remains low or very low. There are growing calls to employ research designs other than randomized controlled trials in SDM in mental health (Zisman-Ilani et al., 2021), and a further 'inclusive' (of other study designs) systematic review is imperative to strengthen the evidence base.

Overview of decision aids in mental healthcare

Role of decision aids in facilitating SDM in mental healthcare

Patient decision aids (PtDAs) are interactive tools that facilitate SDM (see Chapters 18–20). In the field of mental health, PtDAs are employed for various decision contexts, such as choosing between medication therapy and psychosocial interventions, selecting specific medications for pharmacological treatment, and deciding on services in community care. They play a crucial role in ensuring that service users have access to clear information to make informed choices about their mental healthcare.

Decision aids about treatment initiation for SMIs

Various PtDAs have been developed worldwide to assist in treatment choices for SMIs. The latest Cochrane review by Stacey et al. (2024) includes 71 different decisions, of which ten relate to mental health, and in seven of these the decisions focus on treatment choices for SMI. Among these, Hamann et al. (2006) developed a benchmark German PtDA for schizophrenia, integrating medication therapy and psychosocial interventions, including psychoeducation elements. For depression, starting with Loh et al. (2006) who developed a German PtDA, subsequent efforts by LeBlanc et al. (2015) led to the creation of an English PtDA for antidepressant therapy, incorporating visual cards comparing potential side effects. This was followed by Perestelo-Perez et al. (2017) developing an online version in Spanish, and Vigod et al. (2019) tailoring a DA for pregnant and planning women considering antidepressant treatment, showcasing diverse variations in development. For bipolar disorder, Aoki (2019)

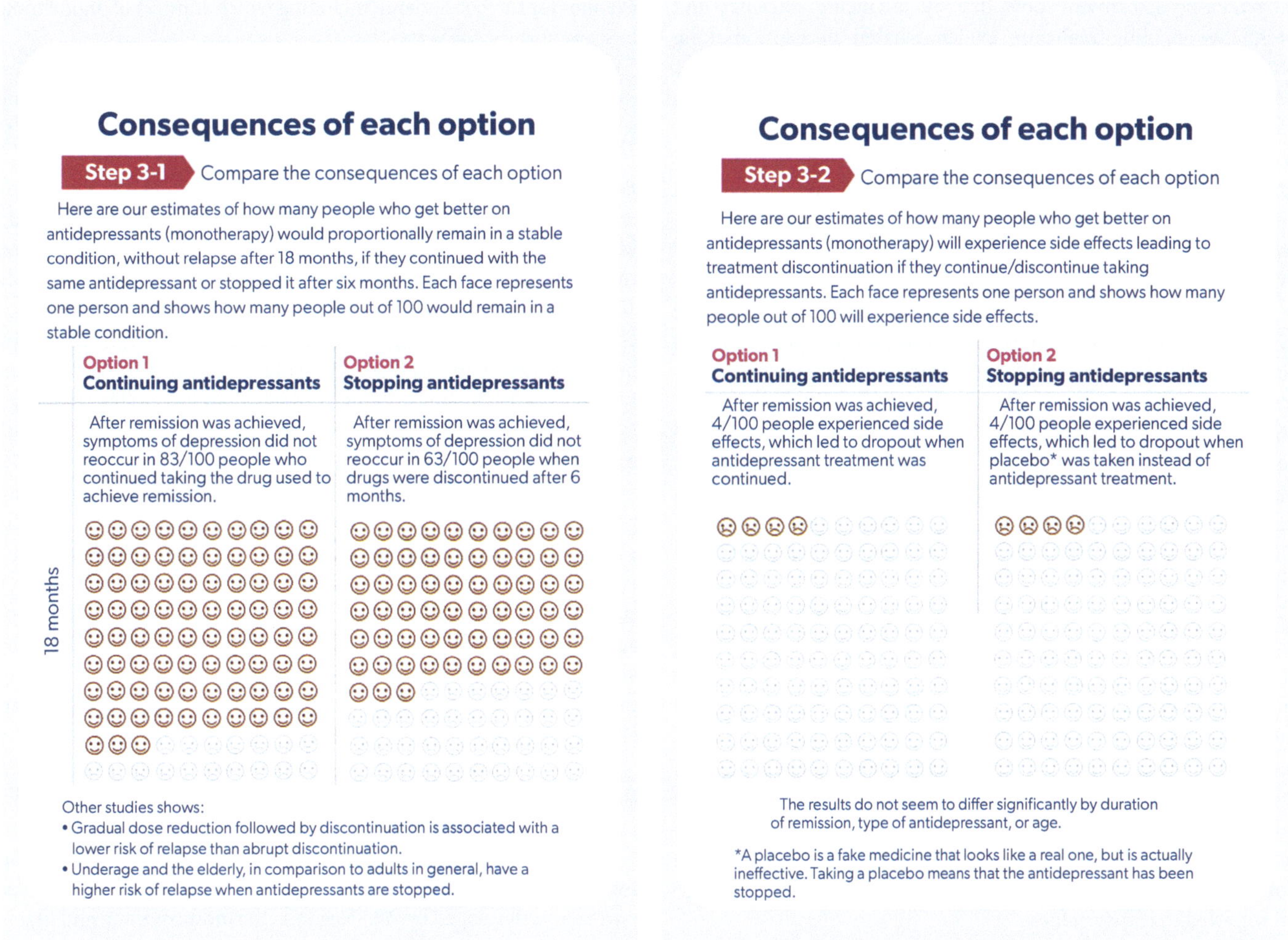

Figure 27.2 Comparison of pictorial diagrams illustrating outcomes for each option in a decision aid for major depressive disorder, considering discontinuation of antidepressant treatment after remission.

Reproduced with permission from Aoki, Y., Takaesu, Y., Baba, H., et al. 2022. Development and acceptability of a decision aid for major depressive disorder considering discontinuation of antidepressant treatment after remission. *Neuropsychopharmacol Rep*, 42, 306–314.

created PtDAs tailored for Japanese university students, addressing both depression and bipolar, and Fisher et al. (2020) from Australia also developed an online English PtDA specifically for bipolar disorder. This suggests an increasing interest in PtDAs for mental health disorders within the overall healthcare landscape. Alongside printed versions, online PtDAs have become more widespread, making them more accessible to wider user groups, although research shows that for individuals with SMI, the use of paper-based PtDAs is often preferred (Zisman-Ilani et al., 2017).

Decision aids for long-term management of mental health conditions

Mental health PtDAs support both initiating treatment and reassessing over time due to the long-term nature of many conditions. Aoki et al. (2022a, 2023a, 2023b) and Zisman-Ilani et al. (2024) developed various PtDAs to help individuals decide whether to continue or taper psychiatric medications. In Zisman-Ilani et al. (2024), a one-page table of the Antipsychotic Medication Decision Aid presents the three treatment options and information on risks and benefits based on literature, experts' opinion, and the feedback of individuals with lived experience of SMI. In each PtDA used by Aoki et al. (2022a, 2023a, 2023b), evidence from previous meta-analyses on the outcomes of each option, either continuation or tapering of medication, is compared using pictograms. Figure 27.2 illustrates an example of a PtDA for antidepressants. These aids are intended to serve as catalysts in addressing the tendency towards indiscriminate long-term use of psychotropic medications.

Digital innovation in SDM: challenges and prospects

In mental healthcare, conventional care methods are being supplemented by health technologies like PtDAs on smartphones, self-management systems accessible through the web, and online support groups. For example, the web platform PyDeSalud.com is a medical website developed in Spain to promote citizens' participation in healthcare decisions about highly prevalent diseases including depression (Perestelo-Perez et al., 2017). Using these innovations enables patients to access information and facilitate decision making more readily. There is potential also to link with existing electronic medical systems like electronic health records and screening assessment tools, thereby enhancing efficiency and potentially enabling real-time evidence-based decision making (Sedlakova et al., 2023).

A systematic review by Vitger et al. (2021) of digital interventions promoting SDM in mental healthcare, focused primarily on SMIs, found that digital SDM interventions in general can enhance patient activation, a sense of 'working alliance', and reduce decisional conflict. However, no effect has been observed on self-efficacy, empowerment, or the subjective level of patient involvement.

Given the considerable variations in how researchers are creating tools to facilitate SDM, there is a need for comprehensive guidance in both development and assessment of these tools. In this sense, the International Patient Decision Aid Standards criteria (http://ipdas.ohri.ca/), which ensure the quality of tools for SDM, would be beneficial. The criteria consist of items outlining the content to be included and the development process, such as whether PtDAs cover the pros and cons of each treatment option comprehensively and impartially, involve stakeholders in the development process, and cite the quality of evidence alongside its sources.

Future trials exploring the impact of digital SDM interventions should assess tool adherence/usage and seek participant evaluations. Reporting the observed impact of a tool alongside information on its usage will aid future trials and stakeholders in determining whether the effectiveness is contingent upon a specific level of adoption, and whether participants perceive the tool as meaningful. Evaluating the decision making process is crucial; by using the Ottawa Decision Support Framework, it is possible to assess whether appropriate information was provided, whether the provided information was deliberated upon, and whether a process was followed to clarify values.

Most studies have focused on web-based or computer software-based interventions, which limits exploration of different features or categories of systems. Future trials are warranted to develop and explore the impact of digital SDM interventions on SDM outcomes. There may be a growing demand for more interactive features in digital interventions. Telehealth platforms could facilitate direct communication with healthcare providers through video conferencing and chat functionalities. Users might also engage in posting feedback on medical information and psychological education content, receiving subsequent responses from healthcare providers. Additionally, artificial intelligence could potentially assist in managing these interactions. Online platforms where individuals can anonymously seek advice for uncertainties in the decision making process could also be valuable. Moreover, for people with SMIs, sleep deprivation can exacerbate symptoms, and individuals are more prone to metabolic syndrome due to the side effects of psychotropic medication. Therefore, managing daily sleep rhythms, blood pressure, and weight data with wearable devices and utilizing them as material during consultations is expected to be beneficial.

In conclusion, there is potential for digital interventions in mental healthcare, and further high-quality research is needed to understand their effectiveness and optimal features in supporting SDM (Vitger et al., 2021). Nevertheless, the intricacies of SDM, coupled with the potential offered by digital tools, open up numerous avenues for further research including which features of digital tools best support the SDM process.

Involvement of peer support workers

Peer support and SDM are important components in the provision of high-quality modern mental healthcare (Zisman-Ilani et al., 2022). Peer support workers are individuals who have navigated their own mental health challenges and are now in recovery. Peer support workers play a vital role in assisting others along their recovery journey and mitigating the risk of relapse. Both peer support and SDM have roots in addressing historical issues of coercion within psychiatric care, offering alternatives to limited treatment options, fostering self-determination, and expanding choices in treatment and services (Zisman-Ilani et al., 2022).

Peer support and SDM share conceptual parallels, emphasizing person-centred care, prioritizing outcomes defined by the individual, and striving for autonomy and recovery as primary objectives. Despite these commonalities and the potential for peer support to enhance SDM, interventions that effectively merge these approaches are scarce. There is a pressing need to integrate peer support into SDM frameworks within psychiatric services, using peer-facilitated decision support interventions to bridge this gap (Zisman-Ilani et al., 2022).

Currently, most of the peer support interventions conceptualize peer support workers in a preparatory capacity, primarily focused on supporting individuals with SMI in readiness for engaging in SDM with a psychiatrist or psychiatric nurse prescriber, particularly concerning medication management. CommonGround, a notable decision support centre, developed by Pat Deegan, is the most common and usable example for involving peers in preparing individuals with SMI to engage in SDM with a different provider (a psychiatrist or a psychiatric nurse prescriber (Deegan et al., 2024)). Prior to meeting with psychiatric care providers, peer support workers assist individuals in setting goals for medication treatment, discovering non-medical self-care strategies (personal medicine), and using CommonGround software to report progress and express concerns about medicine to the provider. This peer-led SDM system based on CommonGround software was adopted by Woltmann et al. (2011) in the USA and spread globally, including the implementation by Yamaguchi et al. (2017) in Japan, facilitating interactions among users of community mental health services, peer supporters, and multidisciplinary teams (Aoki et al., 2022b).

Other forms of peer support and SDM are open dialogue and social prescribing. Open dialogue is a person-centred approach to mental healthcare, fostering collaboration between a clinician, an individual undergoing a mental health crisis, and their social network, which includes family members, friends, and caregivers (Chmielowska et al., 2022). Within the open dialogue framework, peer support workers have the opportunity to assume more active and central roles in SDM, not just as supporting and preparing for SDM with other providers, but as both experts by experience and community navigators within their clinical teams (Chmielowska et al., 2022).

Social prescribing has paved the way for the most independent and active involvement of peer support workers, often referred to as 'peer-led SDM' (Zisman-Ilani et al., 2023). In a 'traditional' social prescribing model, typically facilitated by a physician, often a primary care provider, patients receive a 'prescription' in the form of a referral to a community link worker or navigator. Link workers assist patients in selecting non-medical support options within their community. Peer support workers are well positioned to deliver and facilitate social prescribing, as they are essentially link workers with lived experience. Leveraging their unique perspective, peer support workers can offer support, advice, and guidance regarding services and opportunities based on their lived experience and local knowledge of community resources. In social prescribing, peers lead the SDM, are in the driver's seat, and are truly engaged in the decision making, not in a preparatory or supportive role, but as decision makers (Zisman-Ilani et al., 2023).

See Box 27.1 for our patient perspective.

Box 27.1 Patient perspective

My primary psychiatrists and SDM

My journey with mental health began during my fourth year of university, when I was initially diagnosed with depression. Six years later, the diagnosis shifted to bipolar disorder, and since then I've undergone treatment with various psychiatrists. While not initially acquainted with the term 'SDM,' I've encountered a similar collaborative approach with certain psychiatrists who provided explanations, fostering a sense of trust.

Potential and expectations of SDM

The concept of personal recovery, extending beyond symptom improvement to finding one's authentic way of living, deeply resonates with me as a compelling aspect of SDM. The intersection of personal recovery and SDM is intriguing. It is fascinating to learn that SDM is applied across various mental health conditions, with distinct intervention methods and tools designed to facilitate dialogue. Ideally, the establishment of a specific SDM approach for bipolar disorder would be most welcome.

My personal recovery

My understanding of depression defined my twenties, and even after the diagnosis shifted to bipolar, effectively managing the illness remained a struggle. A turning point occurred at 28 when I engaged in 'social reintegration training,' designed for individuals with depression or bipolar disorder. Through this, I gained self-awareness of my illness and developed coping strategies. Joining the company operating the facility marked my successful return to society, allowing me to translate coping strategies into practical ones. Despite setbacks, I learned from failures, and now I can maintain stable work conditions even with mood fluctuations. Currently, I operate media (https://bipolar-work.com/) that provide insights into working with bipolar disorder, drawing directly from my personal experiences, allowing me to fully express myself and participate in society.

Information sharing with peers

In my current role, I interview individuals with lived experiences for media features, and I organize support groups for individuals with bipolar disorder, fostering nationwide as well as global online connections. Despite the abundance of information on bipolar disorder today, there is a significant gap between knowing the information and internalizing it to take meaningful action. Witnessing the exchange of coping strategies among peers fills this gap, creating a profound impact. The shared insights among individuals with similar experiences provide invaluable opportunities for personal growth and change.

Ultimately, this experience has enlightened me about the significance of SDM, a crucial approach that can lead to better treatment and support for us, the patients. I hope that SDM continues to spread and evolve, offering improved outcomes for individuals navigating the challenges of mental health.

Conclusion

The practice of SDM for individuals with SMI is advancing in line with the global trend emphasizing personal recovery. Various healthcare providers endorse SDM to facilitate active participation of individuals in decision making, aiming to achieve patient-centred healthcare while leveraging their respective expertise. The active involvement of peer workers is notable, emphasizing interaction among individuals with similar experiences. As evident from the perspectives of a service user in this chapter, this holds profound significance for facilitating personal recovery. The development and adoption of PtDAs tailored for SMI, considering various cultural backgrounds and target populations, have greatly progressed. These tools are increasingly used not only during treatment initiation but also when reconsidering treatment strategies, resulting in a wide range of variations. The need for digital PtDAs and digital interventions is expected to further expand and gain momentum in the future. Bottom-up research integrating users' viewpoints is anticipated to play a pivotal role.

REFERENCES

Aoki, Y. 2020. Shared decision making for adults with severe mental illness: a concept analysis. *Jpn J Nurs Sci*, **17**, e12365.

Aoki, Y., Takaesu, Y., Baba, H., et al. 2022a. Development and acceptability of a decision aid for major depressive disorder considering discontinuation of antidepressant treatment after remission. *Neuropsychopharmacol Rep*, **42**, 306–314.

Aoki, Y., Takaesu, Y., Inada, K., et al. 2023a. Development and acceptability of a decision aid for anxiety disorder considering discontinuation of benzodiazepine anxiolytic. *Front Psychiatry*, **14**, 1083568.

Aoki, Y., Takaesu, Y., Inoue, M., et al. 2019. Seven-day shared decision making for outpatients with first episode of mood disorders among university students: a randomized controlled trial. *Psychiatry Res*, **281**, 112531.

Aoki, Y., Takaesu, Y., Matsui, K., et al. 2023b. Development and acceptability testing of a decision aid for considering whether to reduce antipsychotics in individuals with stable schizophrenia. *Neuropsychopharmacol Rep*, **43**, 391–402.

Aoki, Y., Yaju, Y., Utsumi, T., et al. 2022b. Shared decision-making interventions for people with mental health conditions. *Cochrane Database Syst Rev*, **11**, CD007297.

Chmielowska, M., Mannocci, N., Tansel, A., Zisman-Ilani, Y. 2022. Peer support and shared decision making in open dialogue: opportunities and recommendations. *Front Psychol*, **13**, 1059412.

Deegan, P. E., Stiles, A., Rufo, M., & Zisman-Ilani, Y. 2024. Awakening on antipsychotic medication: A call to action. *Psychiatr Rehabil J*, **47**, 283–290.

Fisher, A., Keast, R., Costa, D., et al. 2020. Improving treatment decision-making in bipolar II disorder: a phase II randomised controlled trial of an online patient decision-aid. *BMC Psychiatry*, **20**, 447.

Hamann, J., Langer, B., Winkler, V., et al. 2006. Shared decision making for in-patients with schizophrenia. *Acta Psychiatr Scand*, **114**, 265–273.

LeBlanc, A., Herrin, J., Williams, M. D., et al. 2015. Shared decision making for antidepressants in primary care: a cluster randomized trial. *JAMA Intern Med*, **175**, 1761–1770.

Loh, A., Simon, D., Wills, C. E., Kriston, L., Niebling, W., Härter, M. 2007. The effects of a shared decision-making intervention in primary care of depression: a cluster-randomized controlled trial. *Patient Educ Couns,* **67**, 324–332.

Perestelo-Perez, L., Rivero-Santana, A., Sanchez-Afonso, J., et al. 2017. Effectiveness of a decision aid for patients with depression: a randomized controlled trial. *Health Expect,* **20**, 1096–1105.

Sedlakova, J., Westermair, A., Biller-Andorno, N., et al. 2023. Comparison of analog and digital patient decision aids for the treatment of depression: a scoping review. *Front Digit Health,* **5**, 1208889.

Stacey, D., Lewis, K. B., Smith, M., et al. 2024. Decision aids for people facing health treatment or screening decisions. *Cochrane Database Syst Rev,* **1**, CD001431.

Vigod, S. N., Hussain-Shamsy, N., Stewart, D. E., et al. 2019. A patient decision aid for antidepressant use in pregnancy: pilot randomized controlled trial. *J Affect Disord,* **251**, 91–99.

Vitger, T., Korsbek, L., Austin, S., Petersen, L., Nordentoft, M., Hjorthøj, C. 2021. Digital shared decision-making interventions in mental healthcare: a systematic review and meta-analysis. *Front Psychiatry,* **12**, 691251.

Woltmann, E. M., Wilkniss, S. M., Teachout, A., McHugo, G. J., Drake, R. E. 2011. Trial of an electronic decision support system to facilitate shared decision making in community mental health. *Psychiatr Serv,* **62**, 54–60.

Yamaguchi, S., Taneda, A., Matsunaga, A., et al. 2017. Efficacy of a peer-led, recovery-oriented shared decision-making system: a pilot randomized controlled trial. *Psychiatr Serv,* **68**, 1307–1311.

Zisman-Ilani, Y., Byrne, L. 2022. Shared decision making and peer support: new directions for research and practice. *Psychiatr Serv,* **74**, 427–428.

Zisman-Ilani, Y., Chmielowska, M., Dixon, L. B., Ramon, S. 2021. NICE shared decision-making guidelines and mental health: challenges for research, practice and implementation. *BJPsych Open,* **7**, e154.

Zisman-Ilani, Y., Gorbenko, K. O., Shern, D., Elwyn, G. 2017. Comparing digital vs paper decision aids about the use of antipsychotic medication: client, clinician, caregiver and administrator perspectives. *Int J Person Centered Med,* **7**, 21–30.

Zisman-Ilani, Y., Hayes, D., Fancourt, D. 2023. Promoting social prescribing in psychiatry-using shared decision-making and peer support. *JAMA Psychiatry,* **80**, 759–760.

Zisman-Ilani, Y., Parker, M., Thomas, E. C., et al. 2024. Usability and feasibility of the antipsychotic medication decision aid in a community program for first-episode psychosis. *Psychiatr Serv,* **75**, 807–811.

28

Shared decision making in paediatrics and child healthcare

Douglas J. Opel, Naomi Laventhal, Nancy Kuemin, and Seema K. Shah

Introduction

Implementation of shared decision making (SDM) presents unique challenges when the patient is a child. For instance, the intended beneficiary of SDM—the child patient—typically lacks the capacity to share in the decisions affecting their interests fully (Opel, 2017). Further, decisions made between surrogates (typically parents) and clinicians are subject to limits on surrogate decision making authority, constraining how 'shared' SDM can be in paediatrics (Opel, 2017). It is also likely that parents have never heard of SDM, yet they will value being deeply involved in decision making (Box 28.1).

Consequently, SDM in paediatrics must accommodate multiple goals, including protecting the child and respecting parental values and decision making authority, rather than singularly promoting patient autonomy, as SDM stresses for adults. These complexities require developing a nuanced conceptual understanding of SDM in paediatrics (Wyatt et al., 2015; Adams et al., 2017; Opel, 2017; Aronson et al., 2018) that addresses barriers to its adoption (Boland et al., 2019).

A process for implementing SDM in paediatrics

To help improve the implementation of SDM in paediatrics, a process was developed and validated for SDM with parents of young children that accounts for decisional and contextual features in the paediatric setting (Figure 28.1) (Opel, 2018). This process is intended for SDM involving non-adolescent children in which parents are the principal participants. Modifications of this process

Box 28.1 Patient perspective

Parents have never heard of SDM but even so . . .

It is unlikely that parents have heard of SDM, know what it means, or know what role doctors are expecting them to play in the process. What parents do know is their own history, their child's history, and their past experiences in healthcare settings. They know their child, even as a newborn baby; they know the child's place in the family, what they envision their life will be like, and how involved they want to be in making choices for their child's care.

One of the most effective ways to deliver excellent patient care is to develop trust with effective SDM. Parents of young children often recognize that healthcare teams are assessing their choices and behaviour regarding their child's care. At the same time, they are assessing whether they believe the providers have their child's best interests at heart.

Past healthcare experiences will shape how parents view their role in making decisions for their children. A parent may have experienced health literacy challenges or bias from care providers and resulting mistrust. They may feel out of place, be navigating the hierarchies existing among care team members, and they could be experiencing a wide range of emotions during their child's healthcare experience, whether it be an outpatient visit or a long hospital stay.

Parents need to know what is expected of them and their child, given his/her age, to be meaningful participants in SDM. They also need an opportunity to share their own expectations of the healthcare team. Patients and families have often reported that one thing they really need from providers is regular and clear communication—and that the team ensures their understanding of that communication. This includes sharing expectations and discussing how everyone can work together towards the child's best state of health.

Something important to recognize is that these conversations cannot be 'one and done'. They need to occur regularly, over time, whether hour to hour in the hospital, day to day, or at clinic visits over many years. Just as physicians report it is impractical to offer shared decision making for every decision in care, parents can feel overburdened by being consulted on every small thing. Parents and their children will have different capacities for, need for, or desire for SDM, so finding the right balance is crucial. Several factors could influence this participation, including overall health, emotions, maturity, experience with the healthcare system, and relationships with providers. Regular check-ins with parents and their children about roles and engagement in SDM are vital to its success.

Using the framework outlined in this chapter, with compassion and self-awareness of biases, is an important step in delivering the healthcare experiences patients and parents need. It is a skill requiring careful attention to parent and patient preferences, and practice can improve a provider's experience of meaningful connections with those they care for.

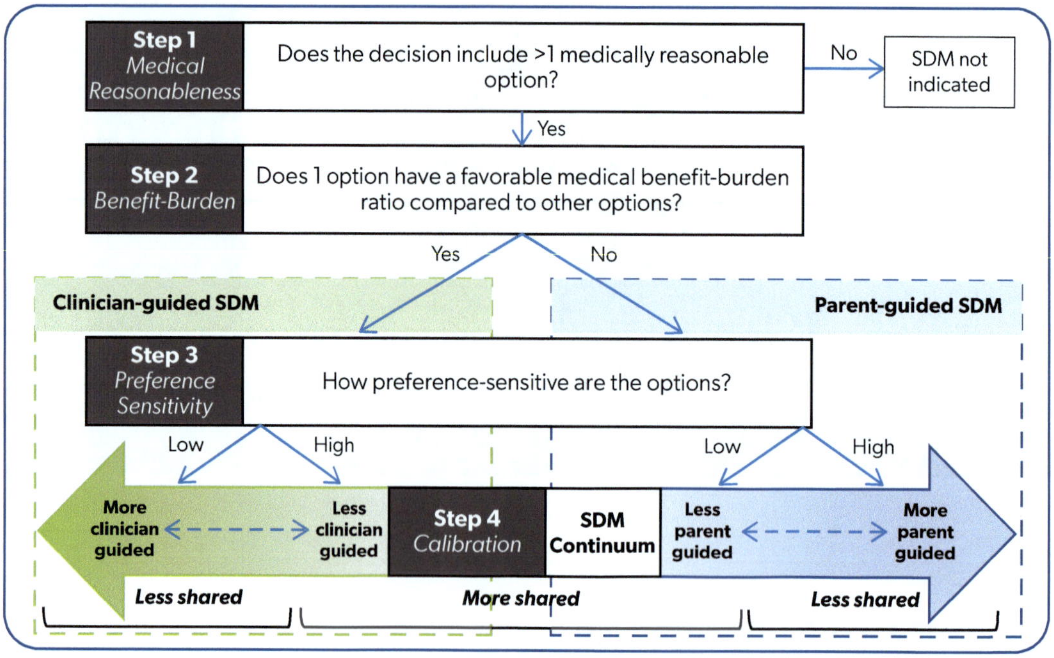

Figure 28.1 The process of SDM in paediatrics.

Reproduced with permission of the American Academy of Pediatrics from Opel, D. J. 2018. A 4-step framework for shared decision-making in pediatrics. *Pediatrics,* 142, Suppl 3, S149–S156.

may be needed for SDM involving adolescents, given the growing autonomy of adolescents, their legal authority to consent to specific treatments without parental permission, and power dynamics in the adolescent–parent dyad. This SDM process for parents of young children adapts prior conceptual work on SDM in the adult setting (Gwyn and Elwyn, 1999; Whitney, 2003; Murray et al., 2006; Whitney et al., 2008; Epstein and Peters, 2009; Kon, 2010; Muller-Engelmann et al., 2011) and integrates emerging consensus regarding the necessary components of SDM (Makoul and Clayman, 2006; Bomhof-Roordink et al., 2019; Eaton et al., 2022). It also accounts for the salient differences in decision making between paediatric and adult medicine. The overall goal of this process is to foster full implementation of SDM with parents of young children when appropriate (Makoul and Clayman, 2006; Bomhof-Roordink et al., 2019).

The process includes four steps, recognizing they may only sometimes happen sequentially. Step 1 ('Medical Reasonableness') determines whether there is more than one medically reasonable option; if there is only one option, there is no indication for SDM. In Step 2 ('Benefit–Burden'), paediatric clinicians must fulfil their obligations to ensure that surrogate decisions are aligned with the child's interests (Beauchamp and Childress, 2001). In this way, this Benefit–Burden step incorporates the best interest standard, a guiding principle underlying paediatric decision making (Streuli et al., 2021; Salter et al., 2023). Step 3 ('Preference Sensitivity') captures whether clinicians elicit parental values and preferences and integrate them into a discussion about the benefits and burdens of each option.

Finally, Step 4 ('Calibration') directs how much the clinician versus the parent should drive the decision. Here, SDM is visualized as a continuum, ranging from a clinician-guided SDM approach to a parent-guided one (Table 28.1). Certain decisional characteristics can help calibrate the version of SDM used in Step 4 (e.g. change the approach from more to less clinician-guided SDM), such as the urgency of the decision or whether the clinician or parent implements the care in question (Montori et al., 2006; Muller-Engelmann et al., 2011; Weiss et al., 2016).

Guidance on implementing each SDM step

Step 1 (Medical Reasonableness)

The key to implementing Step 1 (Medical Reasonableness) is determining that there is indeed a choice (i.e. more than one option). This can be challenging to determine, as there is no clear definition of what counts as a true choice. We propose that choice exists when there is more than one medically reasonable option, with medically reasonable defined as consistent with the standard of care (SOC). We have chosen this definition to help ensure what is reasonable at least reflects a consensus on a basic minimum. Indeed, the SOC requires physicians to provide 'minimally competent care' that other physicians would provide under the same circumstances and, as such, helps physicians uphold standards of professionalism and meet ethical obligations to provide competent medical care. Interventions ideally become the SOC because their safety and efficacy profiles are based upon quality scientific evidence, with professional guideline standards often helping promulgate evidence-based SOC (Guyatt et al., 2008). Since physicians who do not practise the SOC risk medical malpractice, negligence, and/or professional discipline, it seems appropriate that what is medically reasonable at least conforms to the SOC.

The Medical Reasonableness step is critical because when there is only one medically reasonable option, SDM is not the most applicable decision making model. Consider the treatment decision for a child who presents with a moderate acute asthma exacerbation.

Table 28.1 Details and example scenarios for each version of SDM in Step 4 (Calibration)

More clinician-guided	Less clinician-guided	Less parent-guided	More parent-guided
Explain each option and its risks and benefits to ensure the parent is fully informed			
Explain that all options are medically appropriate but convey which option is best based on reasoned estimation of the medical benefit–burden ratios		Explain that each option is medically appropriate and there is no consensus regarding which option is better	
Not preference-sensitive	**Highly preference-sensitive**	**Not preference-sensitive**	**Highly preference-sensitive**
Seek explicit parent agreement with the clinician-preferred option; if parent preferences change over the course of the discussion, try to persuade the parent to embrace the values and preferences that align with the preferred option	May try to persuade the parent to embrace the values and preferences that align with the clinician-preferred option, but remain more committed to working with the parent to reach a mutual decision aligned with the parent's values and preferences	May convey a preferred option based on clinician own expertise or experience, but mostly focused on working with the parent to reach a mutual decision aligned with the parent's values and emerging preferences	Commit to implementing the intervention that is most closely aligned with parent preferences
Example paediatric clinical scenarios potentially well suited for each version of SDM			
Surgical (vs medical) management in early uncomplicated appendicitis	Breastfeeding (vs formula feeding) a newborn	Local anaesthetic (vs oral anxiolytic) for simple laceration repair	Circumcision (vs no circumcision) of male newborn

Currently, the combination of short-acting beta-2 agonists and corticosteroids is the only medically reasonable option for initial treatment (Okpapi et al., 2012). As a result, a non-SDM, physician-led approach using a model of simple consent is appropriate (Whitney et al., 2003). This involves the physician explaining the intervention to the parent and, when appropriate, to the child, discussing the intervention's risks and benefits, and asking for the parent's consent. A physician might explain the lack of reasonable alternatives if the parent asks about other options.

There are several issues with the Medical Reasonableness step worth mentioning. First, there can be a lack of consensus on the SOC. However, this would suggest that more than one medically reasonable option exists, and moving to Step 2 is warranted. Second, whether there is >1 medically reasonable option––and therefore whether SDM is appropriate––does not necessarily depend on what parents think about the various options. For instance, some parents will refuse the one medically reasonable option, but whether this refusal is acceptable requires separate consideration (e.g. use of the harm principle to assess whether state intervention in parental decision making is justifiable (Diekema, 2004)). Consider two scenarios: treatment of moderate acute asthma exacerbation (as in the example above) and screening for congenital diseases in a neonate. In both scenarios, there is one medically reasonable option (to give short-acting beta-2 agonists and to screen), and therefore, a non-SDM, physician-led decision making approach is appropriate in both scenarios. Yet, whether parental refusal of the one medically reasonable option would be respected in these scenarios likely differs: parental refusal of short-acting beta-2 agonists would likely not be respected given the imminent risk of serious harm to the child, whereas parental refusal of newborn screening would not necessarily pose the same harm or require intervention (Committee on Bioethics et al., 2013).

Third, it is important to acknowledge that an element of subjectivity remains in determining what is medically reasonable. Clinicians need to be aware of how their own biases and values, for instance, may be influencing their determinations of reasonableness. Lastly, time can constrain the ability to implement SDM (Opel et al., 2023). For instance, even when there is more than one medically reasonable option for a clinical situation, the ability of a clinician to do SDM can be hindered by the fact that there are only 10 minutes allotted for the medical appointment. Time constraints may therefore require a disengagement from the four-step SDM process even though it may be clear via the Medical Reasonableness step that SDM is indicated. Though time pressure may occasionally justify deviating from SDM even though it is indicated, it requires vigilance on the part of the clinician so that this remains the exception rather than the rule.

Step 2 (Benefit–Burden)

Critical to this step is determining what constitutes a 'favourable' option. This involves a judgement based on evidence-based probabilities and magnitudes of the medical benefits and burdens of the options, along with assessing the uncertainty involved. What balance of probabilities and magnitudes is 'favourable' and which benefits and burdens to prioritize in this calculus will often vary among clinicians. Therefore, like the Medical Reasonableness step, this Benefit–Burden step is also susceptible to subjectivity and clinician bias. However, this step can help reduce such bias by making these judgements more explicit. For instance, when there is an absence of quality evidence favouring the medical benefit–burden ratio of one option over another, clinicians may still make assessments based on their experience or expert opinion; they should disclose they are doing so, however, and resist making *strong* recommendations.

Another factor to consider when determining the favourability calculus is the physician's dual duty to promote both the public's health and the health and welfare of the patient (American Medical Association, 2016). As such, this Benefit–Burden step should not only include benefit–burden assessments relative to the individual child's health but also include, where appropriate, benefit–burden assessments relative to the public's health. The weight that public health considerations deserve compared to those that affect the child's health, however, requires additional analysis.

Step 3 (Preference Sensitivity)

The intent of the Preference Sensitivity step is not to simply elicit what the parent would like to do. Rather, the clinician's role should be more expansive and include helping parents articulate their values and preferences (Epstein and Peters, 2009). Indeed, the ideal physician 'is a caring physician who integrates the information and relevant values to make a recommendation and, through discussion, attempts to persuade the patient to accept this recommendation as the intervention that best promotes his or her overall well-being' (Emanuel and Emanuel, 1992).

The justification for a more expansive clinician role in this step is threefold. First, a person's values and preferences are rarely clear or stable; rather, what one values and prefers is an ongoing process subject to one's capacity for change and reflection. Second, this process is relational (Sherwin, 1998). The development and revision of preferences are facilitated through our relationships and interactions with others—clinicians included. Third, this more expansive role aligns with the original intent for SDM to represent 'an appropriate balance' between patient autonomy and a clinician's obligation to promote the patient's health and well-being (President's Commission, 1982). Simply eliciting parent values and preferences falls short of this balance.

This is not to say that clinicians ought to coerce, manipulate, or be confrontational with parents and is not meant to infer that clinicians no longer have an obligation to acknowledge and communicate their own preferences. Rather, the Preference Sensitivity step is designed to empower clinicians to be involved in helping parents assess the worthiness of certain health-related values and prevent clinicians from presuming what parents prefer. Parents may not have a preference between available options despite evidence or experiences suggesting they should (and vice versa); the degree to which preferences matter in a decision may also vary (Madrigal et al., 2012). For example, a decision that is not typically preference-sensitive, such as which anticoagulant to use to treat a peripherally inserted central catheter-associated thrombus, might be highly preference-sensitive to some individuals who wish to avoid porcine-derived products such as heparin due to religious or cultural beliefs. The Preference Sensitivity step helps make explicit what parents prefer and how influential those preferences are to their decision making.

Step 4 (Calibration)

The Calibration step builds upon Kon's model for SDM (Kon, 2010) by incorporating additional variables beyond parent preferences to calibrate SDM (Montori et al., 2006). These variables include the urgency or clinical importance of the decision, the parent's desired level of involvement, whether the intervention is longitudinal (versus single event), and whether the intervention is implemented by clinicians or parents (Montori et al., 2006; Muller-Engelmann et al., 2011; Weiss et al., 2016). For instance, longitudinal interventions—such as those that occur in the context of chronic disease—may require calibrating the SDM approach to be more parent-guided. This is because of the increased opportunities for interaction between clinicians and parents, the potential for negotiation over time, and the need to maintain compliance. Contextual features of the decision may also change over time: patients might get sicker or have adverse effects from prior experiences with the intervention. As such, an SDM approach that was initially more clinician-guided may become less clinician-guided, or an SDM approach that was initially less parent-guided may become more so.

Who implements the intervention may also calibrate the version of SDM used. When parents are primarily responsible for implementation (e.g. nutrition management in a child who is overweight), SDM should be calibrated to align with this responsibility (i.e. a more parent-guided SDM approach). Likewise, when clinicians are primarily responsible for implementation, a more clinician-guided SDM approach is justifiable in order to accommodate the particular clinician's experience and comfort with the intervention as well as knowledge of unique system-level variables that may influence the success of implementing the intervention in the present clinical setting (e.g. the medically reasonable options to use ketamine or propofol sedation for fracture reduction in the emergency department).

Gaps in evidence

The four-step process for implementing SDM described above is intended for parents of young children. There remains a gap in how to implement SDM when the patient is an adolescent with emerging autonomy. In SDM with adolescents, unique factors must be considered, including power dynamics in the adolescent–parent dyad, the growing autonomy of adolescents, along with laws permitting independent adolescent decision making based on their status, condition, or maturity. Whether these factors can be accommodated by a modified four-step process or a novel process is needed requires further exploration.

Acknowledgements

Versions of this book chapter appear in *Pediatrics* (Opel, 2018) and *The Beautiful Complexity of Shared Decision-Making* (Lantos, 2021).

REFERENCES

Adams, R. C., Levy, S. E., Council on Children with Disabilities. 2017. Shared decision-making and children with disabilities: pathways to consensus. *Pediatrics*, **139**, e20170956.

Aronson, P. L., Shapiro, E. D., Niccolai, L. M., Fraenkel, L. 2018. Shared decision-making with parents of acutely ill children: a narrative review. *Acad Pediatr*, **18**, 3–7.

American Medical Association. 2016. *Code of Medical Ethics: Physicians and the Health of the Community*. American Medical Association.

Beauchamp, T., Childress, J. 2001. *Principles of Biomedical Ethics*. Oxford University Press.

Boland, L., Graham, I. D., Legare, F., et al. 2019. Barriers and facilitators of pediatric shared decision-making: a systematic review. *Implement Sci*, **14**, 7.

Bomhof-Roordink, H., Gartner, F. R., Stiggelbout, A. M., Pieterse, A. H. 2019. Key components of shared decision making models: a systematic review. *BMJ Open*, **9**, e031763.

Committee on Bioethics, Committee on Genetics, American College of Medical Genetics, Genomics Social, Ethical, and Legal Issues Committee. 2013. Ethical and policy issues in genetic testing and screening of children. *Pediatrics*, **131**, 620–622.

Diekema, D. S. 2004. Parental refusals of medical treatment: the harm principle as threshold for state intervention. *Theor Med Bioeth*, **25**, 243–264.

Eaton, S. M., Clark, J. D., Cummings, C. L., et al. 2022. Pediatric shared decision-making for simple and complex decisions: findings from a Delphi panel. *Pediatrics*, **150**, e2022057978.

Emanuel, E. J., Emanuel, L. L. 1992. Four models of the physician–patient relationship. *JAMA*, **267**, 2221–2226.

Epstein, R. M., Peters, E. 2009. Beyond information: exploring patients' preferences. *JAMA,* **302**, 195–197.

Guyatt, G. H., Oxman, A. D., Vist, G. E., et al. 2008. GRADE: an emerging consensus on rating quality of evidence and strength of recommendations. *BMJ,* **336**, 924–926.

Gwyn, R., Elwyn, G. 1999. When is a shared decision not (quite) a shared decision? Negotiating preferences in a general practice encounter. *Soc Sci Med,* **49**, 437–447.

Kon, A. A. 2010. The shared decision-making continuum. *JAMA,* **304**, 903–904.

Lantos, J. D. (Ed.) 2021. The Beautiful Complexity of Shared Decision-Making. Oxford University Press.

Madrigal, V. N., Carroll, K. W., Hexem, K. R., Faerber, J. A., Morrison, W. E., Feudtner, C. 2012. Parental decision-making preferences in the pediatric intensive care unit. *Crit Care Med,* **40**, 2876–2882.

Makoul, G., Clayman, M. L. 2006. An integrative model of shared decision making in medical encounters. *Patient Educ Couns,* **60**, 301–312.

Montori, V. M., Gafni, A., Charles, C. 2006. A shared treatment decision-making approach between patients with chronic conditions and their clinicians: the case of diabetes. *Health Expect,* **9**, 25–36.

Muller-Engelmann, M., Keller, H., Donner-Banzhoff, N., Krones, T. 2011. Shared decision making in medicine: the influence of situational treatment factors. *Patient Educ Couns,* **82**, 240–246.

Murray, E., Charles, C., Gafni, A. 2006. Shared decision-making in primary care: tailoring the Charles et al. model to fit the context of general practice. *Patient Educ Couns,* **62**, 205–211.

Okpapi, A., Friend, A. J., Turner, S. W. 2012. Asthma and other recurrent wheezing disorders in children (acute). *BMJ Clin Evid,* **2012**, 0300.

Opel, D. J. 2017. A push for progress with shared decision-making in pediatrics. *Pediatrics,* **139**, e20162526.

Opel, D. J. 2018. A 4-step framework for shared decision-making in pediatrics. *Pediatrics,* **142**, S149–S156.

Opel, D. J., Vo, H. H., Dundas, N., et al. 2023. Validation of a process for shared decision-making in pediatrics. *Acad Pediatr,* **23**, 1588–1597.

President's Commission for the Study of Ethical Problems in Medicine and Biomedical and Behavioral Research. 1982. *Making Health Care Decisions: A Report on the Ethical and Legal Implications of Informed Consent in the Patient–Practitioner Relationship*. The Commission.

Salter, E. K., Hester, D. M., Vinarcsik, L., et al. Pediatric decision making: consensus recommendations. *Pediatrics,* **152**, e2023061832.

Sherwin, S. 1998. *The Politics of Women's Health: Exploring Agency and Autonomy in Health Care*. Temple University Press.

Streuli, J. C., Anderson, J., Alef-Defoe, S., et al. 2021. Combining the best interest standard with shared decision-making in paediatrics—introducing the shared optimum approach based on a qualitative study. *Eur J Pediatr,* **180**, 759–766.

Weiss, E. M., Barg, F. K., Cook, N., Black, E., Joffe, S. 2016. Parental decision-making preferences in neonatal intensive care. *J Pediatr,* **179**, 36–41.e3.

Whitney, S. N. 2003. A new model of medical decisions: exploring the limits of shared decision making. *Med Decis Making,* **23**, 275–280.

Whitney, S. N., Holmes-Rovner, M., Brody, H., et al. 2008. Beyond shared decision making: an expanded typology of medical decisions. *Med Decis Making,* **28**, 699–705.

Whitney, S. N., McGuire, A. L., McCullough, L. B. 2003. A typology of shared decision making, informed consent, and simple consent. *Ann Intern Med,* **140**, 54–59.

Wyatt, K. D., List, B., Brinkman, W. B., et al. 2015. Shared decision making in pediatrics: a systematic review and meta-analysis. *Acad Pediatr,* **15**, 573–583.

29

Shared decision making in obstetrics and gynaecology

Johanna (Annemijn) W.M. Aarts, Laura Spinnewijn, Tina C. Foster, and Jolanda Wellen

Introduction

Obstetrics and gynaecology is a dynamic clinical specialty focused on treating women in distinctive phases of their lives. In recent decades, there has been a growing focus on comprehending how women's bodies, with their specific female organs, biological make-up, and functionality, differ from their male counterparts. This specialty is notably diverse, encompassing various subspecialties, all dealing with aspects of women's health and different types of typical 'female health problems'. These subspecialties include maternal–fetal medicine and obstetrics, reproductive endocrinology and infertility, urogynaecology, general (or benign) gynaecology, and gynaecological oncology.

Shared decision making (SDM) has significantly evolved within the field of obstetrics and gynaecology, with many national associations, such as the American College of Obstetricians and Gynecologists and the Royal College of Obstetrics and Gynaecology, incorporating it into their practice guidelines and viewpoints. A 2020 systematic review encompassing 35 studies, including 9790 women, evaluated patient decision aids in the field of obstetrics and gynaecology, reflecting the interest in this area (Poprzeczny et al., 2020). Gradually, SDM has found its way to clinical practice as well. However, it is essential to recognize that SDM has been embraced at least theoretically by some, but not all, women's health clinicians. Similarly, multiple challenges in improving clinicians' understanding of SDM remain, as well as in finding ways to provide support for executing SDM conversations.

In this chapter, we will reflect on the reasons why SDM has found its way into our clinical specialty, explore how the unique aspects of obstetrics and gynaecology impact its practical application, discuss the effects on both patients and clinicians of offering choices, and examine the persisting challenges in implementing SDM. We also include a testimony from our patient partner.

Women's voices

A key element of SDM is listening to patients, understanding who they are, their preferences, and what they find important when making health-related choices. High-quality conversations demand active listening. It facilitates and empowers patients to express their concerns and priorities. Perhaps because nearly every woman experiences events such as pregnancy and menopause, there is a relatively strong tradition of 'consumerism' in women's health. Carman and colleagues define consumerism as 'people proactively using trustworthy, relevant information and appropriate technology to make better-informed decisions about their health care options in the broadest sense, both within and outside the clinical setting' (Carman et al., 2019).

In the 1960s and 1970s, the women's health movement informed the development of organizations such as Lamaze International and the International Childbirth Educational Association. These initiatives opened the door for conversations about birth preferences, supported efforts to change practice, and ultimately succeeded in changing the childbirth experience for many women (Nichols, 1999). More recently, the Women's Global Network for Reproductive Rights, an international non-governmental organization advocating women's rights globally, has further amplified women's voices (Bracke, 2023). The resonance of women's voices has, therefore, progressively grown over time, influencing politics, ethics, and professional beliefs. Similarly, the 'medicalization' of menopause came to the fore in discussions about hormone replacement therapy in the wake of the Women's Health Initiative study as women engaged with their clinicians about indications for oestrogen replacement and discussions about the evidence (Women's Health Initiative, n.d.). As contraceptive choices have expanded, the need for informed discussions about choices and options has correspondingly increased.

Perhaps partly because of this tradition of questioning established medical practice, especially in the context of physiological events, the concept of SDM in women's health has gained familiarity. Decisions in obstetrics and gynaecology frequently involve discussions about deeply personal choices such as contraception, sexual health, and pregnancy termination. Inevitably, the decisions made by women in these sensitive situations will sometimes clash with the personal beliefs or ethics of healthcare providers. The intertwined narratives of women's emancipation and SDM have mutually supported each other, and SDM has important implications for mitigating health disparities (Durand et al., 2021). For instance, using a SDM tool for the possible routine induction of labour not only enhances pregnant women's knowledge and sense of empowerment but also improves clinicians' perceptions of counselling consistency and reduces the effect of implicit bias on specific alternatives discussed with patients (Peralta et al., 2023).

However, it is crucial to acknowledge that despite progress, women's voices often go unheard, and obtaining greater equity remains elusive in many settings. SDM demands that healthcare professionals have high-quality conversations using excellent communication skills, which are often difficult to achieve in times of urgency or unpredictable workload. There is a need to intensify efforts in educating clinicians to do better to support patients who have yet to be heard, ensuring that the principles of SDM become more widely accessible.

Choices that are unique to women and most women are confronted with

Throughout their lives, women are faced with an array of choices linked to their health, and then seek guidance from women's healthcare providers for screening, diagnostic, and treatment decisions. During obstetrical and gynaecological visits, clinicians and patients regularly discuss a range of sensitive topics, like prenatal and postpartum care, contraception options, family planning, and perimenopause and menopausal care. Some women also face treatment decisions related to gynaecological (pre)malignant conditions, impacting future fertility. Being infertile and undergoing these treatments imposes a significant psychosocial burden that directly affects quality of life (Verhaak et al., 2007). The emotional weight of possible infertility, coupled with the prospect of future childlessness, closely resembles reactions such as being diagnosed with a serious illness or mourning the loss of a loved one.

Most women encounter one or more of the above-mentioned issues throughout their lives. The individual significance of these issues is deeply personal, emphasizing the need to appreciate each patient's unique perspective on the quality of their life within the context of their personal priorities. This highlights the importance of understanding each individual patient's perspective on what matters in their own life. In some cases, a diagnosis may carry a deep level of stigma, or being confronted with a difficult treatment decision may present a significant ethical challenge. Decision making in such situations is not easy and requires sensitive counselling and guidance and is thus never straightforward. We advocate for tailored training in SDM for obstetrics and gynaecology professionals, recognizing the unique features inherent in decision making within women's healthcare settings. We believe that to achieve high-quality conversations, skills such as listening and eliciting preferences are pivotal, as our patient partner describes (Box 29.1).

Box 29.1 Patient perspective

The quality of the conversation is critical

The communication between doctor and patient holds immense importance for patients and doctors. This is especially important in the context of women's healthcare, where the conditions can sometimes pose life-threatening risks. As patients, we find ourselves navigating an unexpected situation, lacking knowledge, and feeling dependent on clinicians. We become uncertain about how our body works and afraid of an uncertain future. Also, the patient might feel dependent on the doctor based on a knowledge imbalance between the two. It is important for women to have a sense of control in uncertain times.

After reflection, I now recognize the significance of communication even more and the pivotal roles that both patients and doctors play in the SDM process. In addition to the obvious importance of explaining the diagnosis and possible treatments clearly, there are many other crucial aspects. One is having a strong relationship based on not making presumptions about the other's preferences. Careful listening, asking questions, and expressing your thoughts adequately as a patient is pivotal in that process. Another one is to reassess the situation and preferences regularly. While becoming more empowered and gaining more understanding about one's condition, these preferences could change.

It is crucial to have confidence in my doctors. Do they see me as an individual? Do they know my priorities and what is less significant to me? Suppose the doctor gains these insights into me as a person. In that case, my confidence will increase, opening up a space for joint exploration of possible solutions and collaborative decision making.

When I was faced with a tumour in both the ovary and the uterus, the primary source remained unknown. The decision whether or not to undergo chemotherapy (at the risk of over- or undertreatment) was left entirely in my hands. My work and my ability to do sports were key to me, so I wanted to know the impact of chemotherapy on these activities. My oncologist helped me think about these issues and restored in me a sense of 'control' that supported my choice of chemotherapy.

It was also important to reassess things often. There are different phases of illness, and preferences or needs may change. That is why it becomes necessary to reassess a patient's thoughts, feelings, and desires on a regular basis.

We wish to describe some unique features of managing situations in obstetrics and gynaecology. Many topics have ethical implications, such as considering elective abortion, which require appropriate counselling. Unintended pregnancies, often linked to the non-use or misuse of contraception, highlight the importance of thorough contraceptive counselling. For example, when choosing a contraceptive method, 50% of women feel professional pressure and many feel that their concerns about side effects are not well addressed during counselling (Dehlendorf et al., 2017). Respect for patient values and priorities should be at the forefront of these discussions, and this is the step of SDM that is often neglected or inadequately executed (Rake et al., 2022). More emphasis should be put on this part of SDM during the training of clinicians. This is particularly important in obstetrics and gynaecology, given that so many decisions are so personal and context dependent. In obstetrics and gynaecology, women often make treatment decisions that are not related to a medical problem; rather, they arise because of a normal physiological state, such as pregnancy or menopause, which occurs as part of life. There is a real risk, however, that clinicians can seem to view such physiological states as pathological, and as a disease rather than a situation where a medical intervention might not be required or desired. In these situations, SDM is especially important. For example, some women prefer minimal intervention in pregnancy and would not want labour to be induced unless strongly medically indicated. Others would be happy to end their pregnancy as soon as it is safe, and in light of newer evidence supporting the benefit of inducing labour at term, and would prefer that option.

Decision making for the realm of women's health is often time-sensitive. It may be extremely urgent, as in the case of whether or not to use special techniques such as a ventouse to help a mother in the final stage of giving birth, or highly time-sensitive, as with a new cancer diagnosis. The choices women make in such situations can significantly impact their well-being. This speaks to the need for clinicians to understand and practise SDM in various settings, typically without the assistance of patient decision aids. However. there can also be many tough choices when the timing is less urgent. For example, young patients with cancer face decisions about fertility preservation before undergoing cancer treatment. They may find the numerous treatment options overwhelming, especially when their decisions are time-sensitive, where they have to balance rapid decision making against the likelihood of regret at later stages.

Dealing with uncertainty

Women also deal with conditions where there are many reasonable options, such as the multitude of treatments for heavy menstrual bleeding. However, the lack of high-level evidence that helps compare these options introduces uncertainty and complexity. Less medical research is conducted on health conditions that affect women (Steinberg et al., 2021) and so clinicians often have to navigate a topic where the evidence is scarce.

In practice, we encounter several strategies that clinicians use to deal with uncertainty when discussing treatment options with patients. One strategy is that patients are encountered with a dump of information covering all treatment options. The choice is often left up to the patient without real deliberation of preferences or narrowing down of options after elicitation of the patient's personal situation. Another strategy is that clinicians lean highly towards protocolized pathways, despite a lack of solid medical evidence. The unpredictable outcomes of treatment decisions might fuel a tendency to shy away from SDM. Deviation from an established protocol could result in a negative outcome. Despite a patient's acceptance of those risks, a clinician may not feel comfortable honouring patients' wishes, especially in a potentially litigious field such as obstetrics. Also, in gynaecological cancers, which are, by definition, rare cancers with often limited evidence, treatment discussions are driven by protocols. This appears to constrain SDM (Spinnewijn et al., 2020). Clinicians put much weight on outcomes such as mortality and often seem to think that this is also most important to patients. Clinicians tend to adhere strictly to these protocols, leaving little room for patients to engage in the decision making process.

It becomes evident that when there is uncertainty or a lack of evidence, balancing imperfect evidence against partially informed patient preferences is necessary. A paradigm shift is needed: it is through SDM that both an evidence-based and patient-centred approach can be negotiated.

Summary

Obstetrics and gynaecology is a rewarding specialty with distinctive features that make SDM a core skill for clinicians who wish to be successful. This brings its own challenges in terms of communicating well and remaining up to date with developments in research. Patient decision aids are helpful but cannot be the be-all and end-all solutions. They can improve our efforts to achieve equity and can definitely be used as scaffolds for clinical conversations. Too often, however, there is no tool to address the unique situation that we face. We, therefore, advocate that clinicians become skilful professionals, and adept communicators, eliciting patient context and preferences, even when patient decision aids are absent.

REFERENCES

Bracke, M. 2023. Contesting 'global sisterhood': the global women's health movement, the United Nations and the different meanings of reproductive rights (1970s–80s). *Gend Hist*, **35**, 811–829.

Carman, K., Lawrence, W., Siegel, J. 2019. The 'new' health care consumerism. *Health Affairs Blog*, 5 March. Available at: https://www.healthaffairs.org/content/forefront/new-health-care-consumerism

Dehlendorf, C., Fitzpatrick, J., Steinauer, J., et al. 2017. Development and field testing of a decision support tool to facilitate shared decision making in contraceptive counseling. *Patient Educ Couns*, **100**, 1374–1381.

Durand, M. A., Yen, R. W., O'Malley, A. J., et al. 2021. What matters most: randomized controlled trial of breast cancer surgery conversation aids across socioeconomic strata. *Cancer*, **127**, 422–436.

Nichols, F. H. 1999. History of the women's health movement in the 20th century. *J Obstet Gynecol Neonatal Nurs*, **29**, 56–64.

Peralta, A., Drainoni, M. L., Declercq, E. R., et al. 2023. Development and testing of a decision aid to achieve shared decision-making for routine labor induction. *Birth*, **50**, 636–645.

Poprzeczny, A. J., Stocking, K., Showell, M., Duffy, J. M. N. 2020. Patient decision aids to facilitate shared decision making in obstetrics and gynecology: a systematic review and meta-analysis. *Obstet Gynecol*, **135**, 444–451.

Rake, E. A., Box, I. C. H., Dreesens, D., et al. 2022. Bringing personal perspective elicitation to the heart of shared decision-making: a scoping review. *Patient Educ Couns*, **105**, 2860–2870.

Spinnewijn, L., Aarts, J., Verschuur, S., Braat, D., Gerrits, T., Scheele, F. 2020. Knowing what the patient wants: a hospital ethnography studying physician culture in shared decision making in the Netherlands. *BMJ Open*, **10**, e032921.

Steinberg, J. R., Turner, B. E., Weeks, B. T., et al. 2021. Analysis of female enrollment and participant sex by burden of disease in US clinical trials between 2000 and 2020. *JAMA Netw Open*, **4**, e2113749.

Verhaak, C. M., Smeenk, J. M. J., Evers, A. W. M., Kremer, J. A. M., Kraaimaat, F. W., Braat, D. D. M. 2007. Women's emotional adjustment to IVF: a systematic review of 25 years of research, *Hum Reprod Update*, **13**, 27–36.

Women's Health Initiative. n.d. Changing the future of women's health: a landmark study since 1992. Available at: https://www.whi.org/

30

Shared decision making in cancer care

Karina Dahl Steffensen, Dawn Stacey, Liesbeth Boersma, and Mona Muusmann Petersen

Introduction

In the realm of oncology healthcare, the stakes are often high, decisions are frequently complex, and shared decision making (SDM) emerges as an indispensable paradigm. This chapter delves into the profound relevance of SDM in the field of oncology, where it has the power to transform the patient–provider relationship, enhance patient outcomes, and uphold the principles of patient-centred care (Kane et al., 2014).

> *Imagine a scenario*: John, a 67-year-old man, sits in the consultation room of his urologist, Dr Smith. Dr Smith informs John of the biopsy results indicating he has early-stage prostate cancer and introduces the need to make a treatment decision. The weight of the decision before him feels immense. Dr Smith presents John with four treatment options, each with similar benefits but different potential side effects and long-term complications (European Association of Urology, 2023). John grapples with a myriad of emotions, from fear and uncertainty to hope and determination. He yearns to comprehend his choices, the risks they entail, and how they align with his personal life circumstances.

This fictional narrative reflects the reality faced by countless oncology patients worldwide. The diagnosis of cancer is a life-altering moment, riddled with anxiety and confusion. Within this context, SDM holds profound significance, as it can empower patients to navigate diverse treatment options while clarifying their values for outcomes of options and align the available options with their overall preferences through a collaborative, evidence-based process. In the realm of oncology, where treatment options are often multifaceted and may carry significant side effects, SDM serves as a beacon of patient empowerment and autonomy.

The urgency of SDM in oncology is further underscored by the ever-evolving landscape of cancer care. The emergence of personalized medicine, with its array of targeted therapies and immunotherapies, has brought forth a dazzling array of new options. These options, while promising, can be overwhelming, leaving patients in a state of bewilderment without guidance. Moreover, cancer is not merely a physiological challenge; it is a deeply personal and emotional journey. Patients, like John, confront profound existential questions about their life, their goals, and their priorities. Their decisions extend far beyond medical considerations, encompassing quality of life, familial obligations, and personal aspirations. SDM acknowledges this holistic perspective and seeks to align treatment decisions with the patient's unique narrative.

As we embark on this exploration, it becomes evident that SDM is not just a framework; it is a lifeline for patients facing the daunting prospect of cancer. It represents a bridge between medical expertise and patient-centred values, offering hope, clarity, and dignity to those on a challenging path.

SDM implementation aspects in oncology healthcare services

In oncology, SDM is advocated at least for preference-sensitive decisions, that is, where there are two or more treatment options with similar overall and disease-free survival outcomes, but different toxicity profiles. For instance, John has four treatment options for prostate cancer including brachytherapy, external radiotherapy, surgery to remove the prostate ('prostatectomy'), or active surveillance. All options result in a very good overall survival but have different toxicities. Another example is early breast cancer, where breast-conserving therapy with radiotherapy or a mastectomy result in similar disease-free and overall survival rates, but obviously with completely different outcomes regarding body image. For these clear preference-sensitive decisions, several patient decision aids have been developed to support patients to participate in the SDM process. Although patient decision aids can be considered a good support for SDM, many more aspects should be considered to achieve SDM in clinical practice (Steffensen et al., 2023).

Several barriers have been mentioned when implementing SDM such as insufficient readiness for SDM by clinicians, patients, and the organization. A major hurdle is that many clinicians do not really know or understand what SDM comprises, and consequently feel that they already apply SDM. However, patient surveys indicate that they often do not feel involved in making decisions. When analysing the application of the four steps (choice talk, option talk, preference talk, and decision talk) of SDM described by Stiggelbout et al. (2015), it has been found that even clinicians who can be considered as early adopters of SDM, only properly apply the first two steps (i.e. making clear that a decision is to be made, and explaining the options), but often neglect the third step (i.e. eliciting patients' preferences and goals) before they come to the final step (decision) (Savelberg et al., 2020). This highlights the need for training clinicians.

Other hurdles frequently mentioned by clinicians are a lack of time during the consultation, stringent lead times in the care pathway (e.g. intervals from diagnosis to treatment, and used in some countries as quality indicators), and a perceived conflict between wishing to adhere to guidelines and applying SDM (Elwyn et al., 2013). In response to this perceived conflict, guidelines are beginning to define areas suitable for SDM situations where the balance between pros and cons of a specific treatment is unclear. In 2022, the 2017 Cochrane review of patient decision aids (Stacey et al., 2017) was referenced 110 times in clinical practice guidelines. In the Netherlands, chemotherapy is recommended for a survival benefit exceeding 5%, and it is a topic for discussion with the patient if the benefit is between 3% and 5%. These grey areas have boundaries as well, prompting arguments that SDM is always necessary, since the 'no treatment' or 'supportive care only' option should consistently be discussed with the patient. Another hurdle that may explain limited application of SDM by experienced clinicians is that they have developed their own methods of informing patients, and discussing treatment options with them, which may be difficult to change. Addressing this issue typically requires educational and behavioural change strategies tailored to different cultural backgrounds. Finally, some clinicians disagree with the application of SDM (Elwyn et al., 2013), which may reflect experiences that patients may become anxious and confused when multiple options are offered.

Patient readiness may represent another barrier for adequate implementation of SDM. While the patient co-author, Mona Muusmann Petersen, clearly is very ready for SDM, and has experience of being involved in many decisions taken during her patient journey, other patients may lack or have inadequate:

1. Understanding of and unfavourable attitude towards their role in SDM
2. Health literacy
3. Skills in communicating and in expressing oneself effectively
4. Confidence in raising their concerns and ask questions during consultation (fear of disrupting the clinician or lack of awareness that their opinion matters)
5. Self-awareness
6. Deliberation skills to anticipate consequences of the different options (Keij et al., 2021).

Characteristics that negatively influence elements of patient readiness are older age, emotional distress, some cultures, and lower education (Keij et al., 2021). Implementing SDM should address individual patient readiness, with efforts to enhance their preparedness for involvement.

Organizational readiness involves incorporating thinking time into care pathways, and fostering collaboration between clinical disciplines. In John's case, it is crucial for both the urologist and the radiation oncologist to offer well-balanced unbiased information on all treatments.

Decision aids available and their effectiveness

Patient decision aids are effective interventions to help prepare patients for SDM and may also be used to facilitate SDM in the consultation. At a minimum, patient decision aids make explicit the decision, identify the target audience, present well-balanced evidence-based information on options including their benefits and harms (e.g. side effects, long-term complications), and help patients clarify their values for features and outcomes of options (Stacey et al., 2017). Current formats for patient decision aids include printed materials and/or interactive online programmes.

A recent Cochrane systematic review of 209 randomized controlled trials evaluated patient decision aids compared to usual care (see Chapter 19) (Stacey et al., 2024). Within this review, there were 82 studies from 15 different countries, focusing on cancer decisions about screening (n = 45 studies on colorectal, prostate, breast, cervical, lung), treatments (n = 27 on breast surgery, prostate treatment, chemotherapy, skin cancer treatment, thyroid radiotherapy), prevention (n = 6 breast chemoprevention or prophylactic surgery), genetic testing (n = 5 breast), and supportive care (n = 2 for continence products for men, fertility preservation).

A sub-analysis of the 82 studies showed patient decision aids improve the quality of decisions and the decision making process. Quality decisions are defined as choices that match their informed values (risk ratio 2.63; 95% confidence intervals 1.73–3.98; ten studies with 5357 participants). People who used patient decision aids are more informed as indicated by 13% higher knowledge, 68% more realistic expectations, and 14% feeling less uninformed. Furthermore, 10% feel less unclear about their values. When prepared with patient decision aids, people take on a more active role, participating in decision making, with 43% less clinician-controlled decision making. This leads to 38% fewer patients being undecided. These 82 studies reported no harms from being given patient decision aids (e.g. no difference in decision regret or distress when compared to those receiving usual care). In a previous review of 105 studies of patient decision aids (46 focused on cancer decisions), there was no difference in outcomes when the decision aids were used in preparation for a consultation with their clinician or used with their clinician in the consultation (Stacey et al., 2017). In summary, patient decision aids can help prepare patients such as John for SDM.

Fictional scenario continued: John, who had early-stage prostate cancer, was faced with a difficult decision, given there were multiple options. When John received the biopsy results confirming prostate cancer, he was concerned about the risk of the cancer progressing. Given he was 67 years old and healthy, he immediately chose to have treatment rather than 'active surveillance'. His treatment options included surgery, external radiation therapy, or high-dose brachytherapy. To help him understand his options and determine what matters most to him, he was given a patient decision aid that described each of the options: the features (e.g. length of treatment, recovery), the benefits (e.g. reduced chance of cancer recurrence, removal of the cancer), and the harms (e.g. urinary incontinence, impotence, stool incontinence). When he completed the values clarification exercise, he valued having a shorter treatment duration and one that minimized the chance of impotence. He shared these values or what mattered most for him during his appointment with the prostate cancer specialist and together they agreed that he would have high-dose brachytherapy using radioactive seeds implanted into the prostate.

One of the challenges with patient decision aids is that they are not well implemented into the process of care. A Canadian study of three prostate cancer programmes in three different cities showed that 98% or 23% or 0% of men with early-stage prostate cancer received the patient decision aid (Stacey et al., 2020). Men who received the patient decision aid had positive experiences and over 80% felt informed, clearer about their values, and supported. Some urologists and radiation oncologists described consultations with men who had received the patient decision aid as easier with less need to provide education but others described continuing with their own method of discussing options. Using the patient decision aid was negatively influenced by the limited degree to which physicians were on board, low momentum since it was implemented, limited supply, English-only patient decision aids (one site also had men who required them in French), lack of an online version, and the limited extent to which the patient decision aid was normalized within the process of care. A recent review of evidence on implementation of patient decision aids recommended co-producing or co-adapting patient decision aids with patient partners, training of the entire healthcare team, preparing and prompting patients to participate, leadership support, and measuring outcomes for quality improvement (Joseph-Williams et al., 2021).

Gaps in evidence

Although SDM holds great promise in enhancing patient-centred care for individuals with cancer, there are several notable gaps in evidence.

A central query arises regarding the applicability of SDM within oncology healthcare systems informed by clinical guidelines. Clinical practice guidelines synthesize evidence and make cancer treatment recommendations. Although there is a shift with many clinical practice guidelines recommending use of patient decision aids, they often also lean towards recommending a single best treatment. This restricts the array of options presented by clinicians, potentially impeding the genuine essence of SDM. Thus, a gap develops between effective interventions (e.g. SDM, patient decision aids) and their fit within a clinical practice guideline-influenced environment.

Another gap is determining suitable clinical situations for SDM. Is it primarily suitable for preference-sensitive choices where there is equipoise among the options at hand, or should it be more universally applied, considering the omnipresent option of no treatment (or supportive care only)? This fundamental question challenges the boundaries of SDM. We need to explore the suitability and applicability of SDM across a broader range of healthcare decisions, and whether a deliberative process in which reasonable options are presented and thoughtfully considered can be promoted, even though there may not be genuine equipoise about the options.

There is a gap in measuring the effectiveness of SDM and interventions to facilitate SDM. What are the relevant outcomes for SDM? Traditional end points such as mortality and morbidity are not suitable when assessing the impact of SDM. SDM revolves around ethical considerations and how patients are engaged and involved in communication, irrespective of whether these efforts lead to extended lifespans. It is essential to recognize that SDM emphasizes that informed decision making should be considered a pivotal 'patient-relevant outcome' rather than merely focusing on system-centric end points. In doing so, one must be mindful of the potential gap between what truly matters to the patient and what can be quantified. This shift in perspective acknowledges the intrinsic value of SDM beyond conventional metrics. Moreover, we face the challenge that current patient-reported experience questionnaires often show significant ceiling effects, limiting their capacity to capture nuanced variations in decision making dynamics. Addressing these limitations is crucial for a more comprehensive and accurate assessment of the impact of SDM on patient experiences and outcomes, especially in oncology.

We need to investigate how to foster readiness for SDM among patients, doctors, and healthcare organizations. Readiness involves not only understanding the concept but also incorporating it into daily practices. This exploration requires a comprehensive understanding of the barriers and facilitators to SDM adoption at individual and systemic levels.

Conclusion

While SDM holds immense potential in cancer care, acknowledging and addressing the gaps in evidence is crucial for its successful integration. SDM and patient decision aids have positive outcomes for patients and the healthcare system. The challenge lies not only in expanding SDM beyond individual clinical trials testing interventions (including patient decision aids) and refining measurement tools but also in cultivating a culture of readiness that permeates throughout cancer healthcare systems. As we navigate these complexities, we can move closer to realizing the full benefits of SDM in the field of oncology.

See Box 30.1 for our patient perspective.

Box 30.1 Patient perspective

I have heard the words 'you have cancer' four times. The first time was in 1994 when I was 38 years old, and most recently in 2023. Throughout this journey, I have needed significant assistance in navigating this cancer journey and support with decisions along the way.

In the summer of 2023, I was diagnosed with a new aggressive form of breast cancer, leading to surgery to remove the affected breast that had cancer. Subsequently, a discussion about adjuvant post-surgical treatment followed. Unfortunately, the doctor was not entirely familiar with the concept of SDM. While I was aware of the concept, my focus at the time was solely on the anxiety surrounding my new cancer diagnosis.

I was unaware that there was a choice, and the conversation solely revolved around standard treatment, which I could not understand. I had believed that my personal situation and my previous cancer diagnoses would be taken into account. In fact, this was the fourth time I was diagnosed with cancer. This time, I did not actively participate in the conversation—I just felt emotionally upset. About 30 minutes into the consultation, an alternative option was presented by the oncologist. It was an option I could accept, and we agreed with this path forward. However, the experience left a deep impact on me, and I was upset for several days. It is incredibly important that the doctor is familiar with the

SDM concept, uses and follows the structure of SDM that may include a patient decision aid, and reads the patient's cues.

Over the last few years, the introduction of SDM into our cancer programme has made a significant difference for me. For most of my recent cancer diagnoses, I was able to make choices and this was entirely different from the original diagnosis 10 years ago.

Whenever I have received a cancer diagnosis, I have been in shock, and all initiative has disappeared. Making significant decisions without truly understanding the consequences has been challenging. While the doctor may have mentioned consequences during meetings, I did not comprehend them. I did not remember them. That is why, SDM is not just a method for me as a cancer patient—it is a crucial approach that restores a sense of empowerment and dignity in my efforts towards better health. It is an approach that values my role as an active participant in my own health and well-being.

To me, SDM means being heard, understood, and respected as an individual with unique needs and desires. It is an opportunity to share my concerns, preferences, and questions with my healthcare providers, and together find the solutions that feel right for me. This approach is vital because it allows me to take responsibility for my own health and make informed decisions about my treatment. It builds trust between me and my healthcare providers and fosters a sense of control in the midst of an often-overwhelming situation. When I actively participated in the decision making about my care, I gained a better understanding of my condition and treatment options. I felt more secure and less anxious, and my psychological and emotional well-being improved.

When I am not involved in the decision making about my care, there are serious consequences. I experienced this at the time when I was not included. I felt frustration, mistrust, and a sense of helplessness, and my quality of life deteriorated for an extended period. Not being involved can also lead to decisions that do not align with my preferences or values.

Based on my experiences and in discussions with others, I see that there is still a significant need for improvement to ensure that SDM does become an integral part of cancer care. This requires increased awareness and education among both healthcare providers and patients. It also involves creating an environment where I feel welcome to actively participate in the decision making process, and where healthcare providers are responsive to my needs and preferences.

Ultimately, SDM is a valuable approach that empowers cancer patients and enhances the quality of our care. It is the way forward to achieve more patient-centred and effective healthcare choices, and it should be a priority for all of us to promote this approach in cancer care.

REFERENCES

European Association of Urology. 2023. EAU-EANM-ESTRO-ESUR-ISUP-SIOG prostate cancer guidelines. Edition presented at the EAU Annual Congress, Milan 2023. EAU Guidelines Office. Available at: http://uroweb.org/guidelines/compilations-of-all-guidelines/

Elwyn, G., Scholl, I., Tietbohl, C., et al. 2013. 'Many miles to go …': a systematic review of the implementation of patient decision support interventions into routine clinical practice. *BMC Med Inform Decis Mak,* **13**, S14.

Joseph-Williams, N., Abhyankar, P., Boland, L., et al. 2021. What works in implementing patient decision aids in routine clinical settings? A rapid realist review and update from the International Patient Decision Aid Standards Collaboration. *Med Decis Making,* **41**, 907–937.

Kane, H. L., Halpern, M. T., Squiers, L. B., Treiman, K. A., McCormack, L. A. 2014. Implementing and evaluating shared decision making in oncology practice. *CA Cancer J Clin,* **64**, 377–388.

Keij, S. M., van Duijn-Bakker, N., Stiggelbout, A. M., Pieterse, A. H. 2021. What makes a patient ready for shared decision making? A qualitative study. *Patient Educ Couns,* **104**, 571–577.

Savelberg, W., Smidt, M., Boersma, L. J., van der Weijden, T. 2020. Elicitation of preferences in the second half of the shared decision making process needs attention; a qualitative study. *BMC Health Serv Res,* **20**, 635.

Stacey, D., Légaré, F., Lewis, K., et al. 2017. Decision aids for people facing health treatment or screening decisions. *Cochrane Database Syst Rev,* **4**, CD001431.

Stacey, D., Lewis, K. B., Smith, M., et al. 2024. Decision aids for people facing health treatment or screening decisions. *Cochrane Database Syst Rev,* **1**, CD001431.

Stacey, D., Taljaard, M., Breau, R. H., et al. 2020. A patient decision aid for men with localized prostate cancer: a comparative case study of natural implementation approaches. *Cancer Nurs,* **43**, E10–E21.

Steffensen, K. D., Hansen, D. G., Espersen, K., et al. 2023. 'SDM:HOSP'—a generic model for hospital-based implementation of shared decision making. *PLoS One,* **18**, e0280547.

Stiggelbout, A. M., Pieterse, A. H., De Haes, J. C. 2015. Shared decision making: concepts, evidence, and practice. *Patient Educ Couns,* **98**, 1172–1179.

31

Shared decision making in endocrinology

Naykky Singh Ospina, Victor M. Montori, Rene Rodriguez-Gutierrez, and Ruth Mccullars

The clinical need of shared decision making in endocrinology

Shared decision making (SDM) is a model of care where patients and clinicians work together to understand and address the patient's clinical situation (Hargraves et al., 2019; Montori et al., 2023b). While SDM is often viewed as the process of discussing evidence and considering patient values in decision making, this narrow definition is limited (Hargraves et al., 2019; Montori et al., 2023b). In reality, SDM offers a comprehensive method of care that allows patients and clinicians to navigate various clinical scenarios including:

- Weighing alternatives (e.g. which treatment alternative is best for me?)
- Negotiating conflicting desires (e.g. what do I want to do?)
- Solving problems (e.g. how do we manage and resolve the current situation?)
- Gaining existential insight (e.g. what really matters?).

SDM as a method of care can notably enhance the care of patients with endocrine conditions, particularly when we consider the various clinical scenarios in endocrinology where (1) multiple management or diagnostic options are reasonable, (2) patients' desires may not align with societal expectations, (3) complex situations necessitate consideration of practical issues, (4) there is low certainty in research evidence, and (5) serious health outcomes are possible (Rodriguez-Gutierrez et al., 2016).

Table 31.1 showcases endocrinology clinical situations where SDM can serve as a method of care. If patients and clinicians fail to engage in SDM to support clinical situations in endocrinology, the

Table 31.1 Clinical situations where SDM can support care in endocrinology

Clinical scenario	Key question	Goal of SDM
Patients with Graves' disease and their clinicians working together to understand if anti-thyroid drugs, radioactive iodine, or surgery is the best treatment option	Which alternative is best? (Weighing alternatives)	Identify the option for which the harms and benefits are more acceptable/beneficial for an individual patient
Patients with diabetes and their clinicians working together to understand which medication is the best treatment option		
In the care of patients with thyroid nodules, the decision to perform a thyroid nodule biopsy or to follow with surveillance ultrasound might require resolution of the conflict between general thinking that more is always better and the low risk of a clinically significant thyroid cancer	What do we want? (Negotiating conflicting desires)	Identify and resolve conflicts that might be influencing decision making
In the care of an older patient with diabetes who is experiencing frequent hypoglycaemia and there is a clinician recommendation to relax glucose targets but patient concern that hyperglycaemia even if transitory will be a sign of being a 'bad patient'		
Family members and clinicians caring for an older patient with type 1 diabetes who requires insulin injections but who has dementia and requires 24-hour care and support	How do we management and resolve the current situation? (Solving problematic situations)	Clarify the situation and consider different actions to improve/ resolve the situation
Family members and clinicians caring for a patient with severe hypercortisolism that is debilitating and requires active care and support and use of high-risk medication/ surgery for management		
Care of patients with anaplastic thyroid cancer or adrenal adenocarcinoma presenting in advanced non-treatable stages	What really matters? (Developing existential insight)	Identify what can give meaning and peace

quality of care and health outcomes for patients may be compromised. For example:

- There is a risk of not focusing on the best available evidence, potentially resulting in care that may not be safe or effective. For instance, prescribing suppressive levothyroxine therapy to prevent thyroid nodule enlargement—an effective strategy that is not recommended because of potential harms from hyperthyroidism.
- Inadequate consideration of patients' goals and priorities can lead to care that is generically correct, but may not make sense in the care of each patient. For example, recommending adrenal magnetic resonance image in a patient who prefers avoiding tight spaces, where a computed tomography scan is suitable.
- Decisions made without engaging in SDM may lack context awareness—offering recommendations that may be suitable for most patients, but which fail to address individual patient circumstances and comorbidities. For instance, intensifying treatment in a patient who is not improving because of overwhelming personal circumstances (e.g. adding insulin therapy in a patient who is forgetting to take oral glucose-lowering agents due to personal demands) in whom simplifying or adapting care could be more effective.
- Having patients complete diagnostic plans of care while feeling worried and confused about their value, meaning, or implications (Box 31.1).

Box 31.1 Patient perspective

From a patient perspective, methods of care that support involvement of patients in the decision making process and that support patient understanding of medical issues, next steps, and implications are extremely important and desired. When my primary physician found lumps in my thyroid, I was told what I needed to do, where to do it, and when to do it. It was hectic and terrifying. I underwent all the tests and procedures as I was instructed, without anyone actually clarifying what the outcome of all these tests could be. Because of the lack of communication, I imagined the worst, and my anxiety and depression worsened. Eventually, I was told the test results were 'inconclusive'. I felt like my whole life was in a state of upheaval.

When I sought a second opinion, I received care from a medical team that had a different approach to my care. They quickly reviewed my test results and within 3 days I was diagnosed with medullary thyroid cancer. I was informed of the typical treatment options and asked which options I preferred. Initially, I was hesitant to give much input since in the past (with my previous doctors) I had been told what steps I should take and was not included in any decisions regarding my treatment and considered this approach the norm for medical care. With this context, I eventually became more comfortable with being involved in the SDM process regarding my health. I began to feel more in control of what was happening to me, and I began to make strides towards improving my overall health and well-being. Now I feel like I have a good balance in my life as far as home life, work life, and taking care of myself. Patients are likely to adopt the approach of care that they receive even when it might lead to feeling out of control. Patients are also likely to need support to be able to participate in decision making if they have not previously received medical care with this approach.

Tools to support SDM in endocrine practice

SDM tools can help support SDM in practice. They include decision aids designed for use before the clinical visit, which help prepare patients for their consultation and improve their ability to collaborate with their clinicians. Alternatively, SDM 'encounter' tools could be used during the consultation to support collaborative conversations between patients and clinicians. Both patient decision aids and encounter tools typically provide descriptions of available options and summaries of the best available research evidence (Montori et al., 2017). A systematic review of 209 studies and 107,698 participants evaluated the effectiveness of SDM tools in practice. It found that use of these tools led to several improvements, including alignment between patients' values and care, patient knowledge, accuracy of risk perceptions, and decreased decisional conflict related to feeling uninformed (Stacey et al., 2024).

SDM appears to be rare in clinical practice, highlighting the need for tools that can support this method of care (Kunneman et al., 2018; Montori et al., 2023a). An analysis of 100 clinical visits recorded as part of trials involving SDM tools revealed that the initial step of SDM (creating choice awareness and considering different alternatives) was only evident in 22/50 (44%) of visits without a conversation aid. In a review of 100 video-recorded clinical consultations with patients with diabetes in primary care (31 without a conversation aid), some form of SDM took place in 86 of these visits; however, clinicians and patients took all the canonical steps of SDM in only 16 of these (Montori et al., 2023a).

Despite numerous opportunities for SDM and the established benefits, there are only a few SDM tools for use in endocrinology; even fewer that have been evaluated for effectiveness in randomized trials (Table 31.2), and most of these have focused on supporting patients with metabolic diseases and shared treatment decision making, particularly in weighing alternatives. Overall, benefits of these tools are consistent with the existing body of evidence (Stacey et al., 2024). A systematic review of 16 studies evaluating SDM and outcomes in patients with diabetes reported improved patient knowledge, risk perception, and decision quality but no association with glycaemic control, patient satisfaction, quality of life, medication adherence, or trust (Saheb Kashaf et al., 2017). Similarly, a systematic review of six studies of SDM tools in patients with osteoporosis found reduced decisional conflict, increased SDM, and increased accuracy of patients' perceived fracture risk with the use of tools compared with controls (Paskins et al., 2020; Nogues et al., 2022). Tools to support SDM for patients with thyroid nodules and low-risk thyroid cancer and treatment of Graves' disease have shown promising results in preliminary evaluations (Brito et al., 2015; Koot et al., 2023; van Deen et al., 2023).

Implementation of tools to support SDM in endocrine practice

Various barriers impede SDM implementation in the care of patients with endocrine conditions. These barriers encompass individual patient and clinician characteristics, contextual elements, and organizational- and systemic-level factors (Joseph-Williams et al., 2014,

Table 31.2 Selected randomized trials of tools to support SDM in endocrine care

Authors, year	Country	Clinical situation	Number of participants/setting	SDM tool	Primary outcomes
Metabolic care (diabetes, cholesterol, obesity)					
Moin et al., 2019	USA	Consideration of pre-diabetes prevention options	Multicentre, general practice; 351 patients receiving care with the web-based interactive tool by a clinical pharmacist, and 1028 patients selected from control clinics	During visit	Higher uptake of participation in the diabetes prevention programme, metformin, or both strategies at 4 months
Bailey et al., 2016	USA	Antihyperglycemic medication intensification	Multicentre, primary care and specialty clinic; 225 patients; 114 online tool and 111 usual care group	Pre-visit	Improvement in knowledge at 4–6 weeks
Denig et al., 2014	Netherlands	Prioritizing treatment goals and options in diabetes	Multicentre, general practice; 344 patients, 225 intervention and 119 usual care	Before and during visit	No differences in patient empowerment for setting and achieving goals
Arterburn et al., 2011	USA	Decision to have bariatric surgery	Single centre, specialty clinic; 152 patients; 75 video-based decision aid and 77 educational booklet	Pre-visit	Improvement in knowledge and value concordance at 3 months
Mann et al., 2010	USA	Treatment with statin	Multicentre, primary care; 160 patients; 80 encounter conversation aid and 70 control group (printed material)	During visit	Improvement of perceived risk of heart attacks. No difference in medication adherence at 3–6 months
Mullan et al., 2009	USA	Selection of antihyperglycemic agents	Multicentre, primary care; 85 patients; 48 decision aid group and 37 usual care (educational pamphlet)	During visit	Improved knowledge and involvement in making decisions At 6-month follow-up, there was better adherence in the usual care group, and no differences on haemoglobin A1c levels
Osteoporosis care					
LeBlanc et al., 2015	USA	Decision of treatment with bisphosphonates	Multicentre, primary care practices; 79 patients; 32 encounter decision aid, 33 Fracture Risk Assessment Tool (FRAX) score arm, and 14 usual care	During visit	Increase in patient knowledge in the decision aid arm about matters covered in the decision aid, and no difference in knowledge of matters not covered in the decision aid after the visit
Thyroid care					
Sawka et al., 2012	Canada	Patients with early-stage papillary thyroid cancer considering the choice of being treated with adjuvant iodine therapy	Single centre, specialist care; 74 patients; 37 computerized decision aid or 37 usual care	Pre-visit	Improved knowledge after the visit

2017; Scholl et al., 2018; Tang et al., 2022). Common barriers to SDM implementation include short clinical visits, clinicians' lack of self-efficacy and comfort in engaging in SDM, power imbalances between patients and clinicians during consultations, a healthcare delivery culture that does not prioritize or support SDM, and a lack of incentives or guidelines to support SDM (Joseph-Williams et al., 2014; Scholl et al., 2018; Tang et al., 2022). The historical context of endocrinology, which emphasizes evaluation of biochemical and mechanistic data with reliance on surrogate outcomes, may also play a role; but we are seeing a generational shift towards more patient-centred approaches in the care of patients with endocrine conditions (Dorsey-Treviño et al., 2019).

General strategies to address barriers include recommending SDM in clinical practice guidelines, providing postgraduate training in SDM, and establishing healthcare models that support high-quality, safe, effective, and patient-centred care (Joseph-Williams et al., 2014; Scholl et al., 2018; Barton et al., 2020; Tang et al., 2022).

One study explored implementation of an encounter conversation aid to help patients and clinicians decide on the need for statin therapy. During the study period, 7% of patients received care with the use of the tool and 48% of clinicians used the tool at least once. Both patients and clinicians factors were associated with the use of the tool in practice, underscoring the need for multilevel strategies to support implementation of SDM tools in practice (Martinez et al., 2024).

Summary and future steps for SDM in endocrinology

Incorporating SDM into the care of patients with endocrine conditions holds significant promise. Yet, there is a paucity of effective interventions and feasible implementation approaches. Healthcare systems that prioritize high-quality care—defined as care that is effective, safe, and patient-centred—should emphasize and facilitate clinical environments conducive to collaboration and co-creation of care plans between patients with endocrine conditions and clinicians. This includes ensuring access to care, providing adequate clinical visit time, training clinicians in evidence-based medicine and SDM, and making SDM resources available in practice. Furthermore, the development of methods to detect SDM in practice and to evaluate its impact on the extent to which resulting care plans 'fit' (meaning they respond well to the situation of each patient, reflect their goals and priorities, and are minimally disruptive of their lives), could further the adoption of SDM in endocrine practice (Kunneman et al., 2023).

Summary

This chapter describes SDM as a method of care that is integral to endocrinology, highlighting its role in helping patients and clinicians collaborate when navigating treatment choices and diagnostic and prognostic uncertainties. Through review of clinical scenarios in endocrinology, research evidence, and a patient narrative, it illustrates the potentially transformative impact of SDM, advocating for its widespread integration to ensure personalized and effective care in endocrinology.

REFERENCES

Arterburn, D. E., Westbrook, E. O., Bogart, T. A., Sepucha, K. R., Bock, S. N., Weppner, W. G. 2011. Randomized trial of a video-based patient decision aid for bariatric surgery. *Obesity,* **19**, 1669–1675.

Bailey, R. A., Pfeifer, M., Shillington, A. C., et al. 2016. Effect of a patient decision aid (PDA) for type 2 diabetes on knowledge, decisional self-efficacy, and decisional conflict. *BMC Health Serv Res,* **16**, 10.

Barton, J. L., Kunneman, M., Hargraves, I., et al. 2020. Envisioning shared decision making: a reflection for the next decade. *MDM Policy Pract,* **5**, 2381468320963781.

Brito, J. P., Castaneda-Guarderas, A., Gionfriddo, M. R., et al. 2015. Development and pilot testing of an encounter tool for shared decision making about the treatment of Graves' disease. *Thyroid,* **25**, 1191–1198.

Denig, P., Schuling, J., Haaijer-Ruskamp, F., Voorham, J. 2014. Effects of a patient oriented decision aid for prioritising treatment goals in diabetes: pragmatic randomised controlled trial. *BMJ,* **349**, g5651.

Dorsey-Treviño, E. G., Alvarez-Villalobos, N., González-González, J. G., et al. 2019. Outcomes that patients perceive and value are systematically unassessed in randomized clinical trials of endocrine-related illnesses: a systematic review. *J Clin Epidemiol,* **106**, 140–143.

Hargraves, I. G., Montori, V. M., Brito, J. P., et al. 2019. Purposeful SDM: a problem-based approach to caring for patients with shared decision making. *Patient Educ Couns,* **102**, 1786–1792.

Joseph-Williams, N., Elwyn, G., Edwards, A. 2014. Knowledge is not power for patients: a systematic review and thematic synthesis of patient-reported barriers and facilitators to shared decision making. *Patient Educ Couns,* **94**, 291–309.

Joseph-Williams, N., Lloyd, A., Edwards, A., et al. 2017. Implementing shared decision making in the NHS: lessons from the MAGIC programme. *BMJ,* **357**, j1744.

Koot, A., Hermens, R., Ottevanger, P., Netea-Maier, R., Stalmeier, P. 2023. Patient decision aids for patients with differentiated thyroid carcinoma: development process and alpha and beta testing. *Front Endocrinol (Lausanne),* **14**, 1162537.

Kunneman, M., Branda, M. E., Hargraves, I., Pieterse, A. H., Montori, V. M. 2018. Fostering choice awareness for shared decision making: a secondary analysis of video-recorded clinical encounters. *Mayo Clin Proc Innov Qual Outcomes,* **2**, 60–68.

Kunneman, M., Griffioen, I. P. M., Labrie, N. H. M., Kristiansen, M., Montori, V. M., van Beusekom, M. M. 2023. Making care fit manifesto. *BMJ Evid Based Med,* **28**, 5–6.

Leblanc, A., Wang, A. T., Wyatt, K., et al. 2015. Encounter decision aid vs. clinical decision support or usual care to support patient-centered treatment decisions in osteoporosis: the Osteoporosis Choice Randomized Trial II. *PLoS One,* **10**, e0128063.

Mann, D. M., Ponieman, D., Montori, V. M., Arciniega, J., McGinn, T. 2010. The Statin Choice decision aid in primary care: a randomized trial. *Patient Educ Couns,* **80**, 138–140.

Martinez, K. A., Montori, V. M., Rodriguez, F., et al. 2024. Clinician use of the Statin Choice shared decision-making encounter tool in a major health system. *J Gen Intern Med,* **39**, 1583–1589.

Moin, T., Duru, O. K., Turk, N., et al. 2019. Effectiveness of shared decision-making for diabetes prevention: 12-month results from the Prediabetes Informed Decision and Education (PRIDE) trial. *J Gen Intern Med,* **34**, 2652–2659.

Montori, V. M., Kunneman, M., Brito, J. P. 2017. Shared decision making and improving health care: the answer is not in. *JAMA,* **318**, 617–618.

Montori, V. M., Ruissen, M. M., Branda, M. E., Hargraves, I. G., Kunneman, M. 2023a. Problem-based shared decision making: the role of canonical SDM steps. *Health Expect,* **26**, 282–289.

Montori, V. M., Ruissen, M. M., Hargraves, I. G., Brito, J. P., Kunneman, M. 2023b. Shared decision-making as a method of care. *BMJ Evid Based Med,* **28**, 213–217.

Mullan, R. J., Montori, V. M., Shah, N. D., et al. 2009. The diabetes mellitus medication choice decision aid: a randomized trial. *Arch Intern Med,* **169**, 1560–1568.

Nogues, X., Carbonell, M. C., Canals, L., Lizan, L., Palacios, S. 2022. Current situation of shared decision making in osteoporosis: a comprehensive literature review of patient decision aids and decision drivers. *Health Sci Rep,* **5**, e849.

Paskins, Z., Torres Roldan, V. D., Hawarden, A. W., et al. 2020. Quality and effectiveness of osteoporosis treatment decision aids: a systematic review and environmental scan. *Osteoporos Int,* **31**, 1837–1851.

Rodriguez-Gutierrez, R., Gionfriddo, M. R., Ospina, N. S., et al. 2016. Shared decision making in endocrinology: present and future directions. *Lancet Diabetes Endocrinol,* **4**, 706–716.

Saheb Kashaf, M., McGill, E. T., Berger, Z. D. 2017. Shared decision-making and outcomes in type 2 diabetes: a systematic review and meta-analysis. *Patient Educ Couns,* **100**, 2159–2171.

Sawka, A. M., Straus, S., Rotstein, L., et al. 2012. Randomized controlled trial of a computerized decision aid on adjuvant radioactive iodine treatment for patients with early-stage papillary thyroid cancer. *J Clin Oncol,* **30**, 2906–2911.

Scholl, I., Larussa, A., Hahlweg, P., Kobrin, S., Elwyn, G. 2018. Organizational- and system-level characteristics that influence implementation of shared decision-making and strategies to address them—a scoping review. *Implement Sci,* **13**, 40.

Stacey, D., Lewis, K. B., Smith, M., et al. 2024. Decision aids for people facing health treatment or screening decisions. *Cochrane Database Syst Rev,* **1**, CD001431.

Tang, C., Wang, A., Yan, J. 2022. Exploring motivations and resistances for implementing shared decision-making in clinical practice: a systematic review based on a structure-process-outcome model. *Health Expect,* **25**, 1254–1268.

Van Deen, W. K., Spiegel, B. M. R., Ho, A. S. 2023. A narrative review of decision aids for low-risk thyroid cancer. *Ann Thyroid,* **8**, 3.

32

Shared decision making in thoracic surgery

Alessandro Brunelli and Janette Rawlinson

Introduction

The goal of this chapter is to demonstrate the relevance of shared decision making (SDM) in thoracic surgery. When does SDM make sense? The key is to consider situations where there is *clinical equipoise*, by which we mean that options exist where it is reasonable to compare them as potential ways to manage the issue at hand. This does not mean the options are perfectly balanced, only that they are alternatives where there are important trade-offs, and where the patient's views, priorities, and preferences can be considered as important inputs.

Examples of clinical scenarios in thoracic surgery

There are several examples of clinical equipoise situations in thoracic surgery.

Early-stage lung cancer where operative risk is high, and radiotherapy is a reasonable alternative

Stereotactic ablative radiotherapy (SABR; also known as stereotactic body radiation therapy) is a reasonable curative treatment for high-risk surgical candidates or for those patients refusing surgery (Wu et al., 2020; Pennathur et al., 2021). A multidisciplinary discussion is recommended, and, ideally, a referral to both the surgeon and radiation oncologist should be organized to discuss the relative risks and benefits of the two curative modalities in the context of patient preferences. Surgeons and radiation oncologists may have their own selection bias in presenting information about the risks and benefits of the two treatments. Ideally, a conjunct and coordinated meeting with the patient by both specialists in the same room at the same time would help to mitigate treating physicians' biases. This would require a coordinated approach and, ideally the use of information tools that could help both specialists to 'speak the same language' when presenting their unique impressions to the patient. Studies have shown racial disparities in the frequency of surgical versus radiation therapy (Cykert et al., 2010), and that the majority of patients with non-small cell lung cancer do not report being offered alternative treatment options (Hopmans et al., 2015). Patient preferences about how to manage early-stage lung cancer vary (Tong et al., 2016), and there are significant concerns by surgeons about the challenge of providing the correct amount of information with the most appropriate terminology to patients (Golden et al., 2017; Mokhles et al., 2017, 2018).

There is a widely acknowledged, long-standing debate about the comparative effectiveness of lung resection versus radiation for operable stage I non-small cell lung cancer (Samson et al., 2016). Trials that have attempted to study this question have not been able to recruit sufficient patients. For example, the SABRTooth trial paper stated as follows:

> We conclude that a phase III RCT [randomized controlled trial] randomising higher risk patients between SABR, and surgery is not feasible in the National Health Service. Patients have pre-existing treatment preferences, which was a barrier to recruitment. A significant proportion of patients randomised to the surgical group declined and chose SABR. (Franks et al., 2020)

This has led to questions as to whether randomized trials can provide a solution to this question (Subramanian and Meyers, 2018).

Lung cancer where different surgical approaches are possible (i.e. lobectomy vs sublobar resection)

Sublobar resection is a well-accepted procedure performed in high-risk patients or intentionally in peripheral small lung cancers. When performed as an alternative to lobectomy, patients should be informed of the increased risk of local recurrences and balance this risk with the reduced risk of morbidity and higher preservation of pulmonary function (Brunelli et al., 2021; Saji et al., 2022).

More locoregionally advanced lung cancer stages where a multimodal treatment is recommended.

The recent introduction of novel agents (i.e. immunotherapy and targeted systemic treatment to actionable mutations) with or without chemotherapy in the neoadjuvant, adjuvant, or perioperative treatment of locally advanced resectable lung cancer has multiplied the treatment options, often dependent on the molecular profile of the tumour, tumour stage, and the patient's fitness to undertake long multimodal management. In parallel, this has increased the complexity of the discussion with the patient to explain different possible treatment permutations. Several specialists usually participate in this discussion, including the respiratory physician, medical oncologist, radiation oncologist, surgeon, and lung cancer nurse. It is important that all these different individuals who often meet the patient at different times use consistent terminology and narrative to explain the treatment options in an understandable way. Patients often find this explanation overwhelming and difficult to retain. The use of an information aid tool and specific communication training targeted at healthcare professionals on how to convey this information appears to be necessary.

The definition of SDM stipulates that the best possible evidence is used as the basis for comparing options. This is not an easy task, especially as the information needs to be in a format accessible to people who do not typically consider scientific data. Patient decision support tools are becoming available for many decisions, and a highly cited systematic review shows that they increase patients' knowledge, lead to more accurate risk perceptions, and increase confidence in decisions (Stacey et al., 2024). Other beneficial outcomes are likely and are being evaluated (Elwyn et al., 2016). One advantage of such tools, if designed to be accessible to a wide spectrum of educational levels, and health literacy, is that they can help address health inequity (Durand et al., 2014).

In a recent study, Housten and colleagues described how to use available guidelines to create a decision support tool for patients with clinical stage I lung cancer deciding between radiation therapy and surgical resection (Housten et al., 2023). The work also highlights the challenges in implementing and evaluating the tool. This review may serve as guidance to implement similar tools in our specialty.

SDM is critical in those situations where the well-informed patient is undecided between treatments that are both reasonable to them (patient equipoise). The clinical team then assists the patient by providing subtle pros and cons of each treatment tailored to the patient's needs, values, and personal circumstances. SDM is equally relevant for the less informed patients who may be oblivious to recent changes in treatment and outcomes.

One of the keywords in the definition is 'support'. People are not accustomed to being asked to be involved in decisions and might even find the prospect a bit odd or uncomfortable. They expect clinicians to be experts, and rightly so. It is therefore important to explicitly say that you are describing options because the right decision relies on their input: there is no right answer because people's priorities, goals, and preferences vary. Ensure that the patient understands that you will support them to make the right decision, and never abandon them to make decisions where they feel anxious or confused (Quill and Cassel, 1995). In a recent systematic review exploring preferred decision making role using the control preference scale, 65% of respondents (pooled from five studies on SDM and early-stage lung cancer) preferred a collaborative role while only 28% preferred a more passive role (Dalmia et al., 2022). This is particularly important where patients might prefer their clinician to make recommendations and avoid the extra work and responsibility of decisions. People who are deeply anxious, have limited cognitive capacity, or feel unable to comprehend complex information may want more support than others. Nevertheless, they appreciate clinicians who understand their goals, preferences, and priorities as decisions are made: a modified and compassionate form of SDM.

It is also critical to consider the role of family members and care partners, or other surrogate decision makers. Sometimes other people have different perceptions of surgical risk and benefits, which may differ from the patient's and clinicians' views. Understanding these potential conflicting influences on decisions will be critical to achieving a successful collaborative process (Lee et al., 2023).

The human factor

Establishing a connection with patients during the appointment is essential to foster communication and create a safe environment for patients to express their values and preferences. An empathic approach to patients, utilizing appropriate verbal and non-verbal communication styles and practising active listening, signals respect and trust and that patients' concerns, fears, and values are considered (Brunelli, 2022). Too often, patients perceive doctors as being too busy to spend time with them. We are perceived as professional and competent but not very warm and approachable.

We traditionally struggle with these two dimensions: warmth and competence. We fear that if we behave too warmly or too empathetically with patients, we are perceived as less professional or competent.

This false concept has been disproven by studies showing that adopting an empathic non-verbal communication style increases not only patients' perception of physicians' warmth and empathy but also of physicians' competence (Kraft-Todd et al., 2017).

To connect with the patient during the first appointment, we first should accept the patient as a person, staying away from judgement and respecting their values and beliefs even if they differ from ours. When we meet a new patient for the first time and discuss what surgery will entail, risk estimation and communication represent the core of that discussion. Although patients may have variable perceptions of risk and weigh surgical risk subjectively, we still must present our opinion on the risks and benefits of that specific treatment.

To properly convey this information in an understandable and meaningful way to the patient, we first need to establish a safe connection with them. Empathy is about perspective-taking. Perspective-taking means adopting a holistic approach to patients to fully understand their situation and feelings. To achieve this important goal during the first encounter, we need to *attend* the meeting. Attending communicates that you respect and value the patient. In addition, being focused allows you to be sensitive to the patient's cues, the hidden hints of their main concerns. Rarely do patients shout out their main concern; most often, they whisper it. Therefore, we really need to remain attentive and listen carefully. Perspective-taking means exploring what matters most to patients. This is not necessarily morbidity, mortality, or survival. Increasingly patients value quality of life and independence more than the former traditional outcomes (Sullivan et al., 2019). One of the most frequent questions asked by patients during the first encounter is 'What will my life be like after surgery, will I be able to resume a good lifestyle?' This is what matters most to patients, and especially in frail, high-risk individuals, these aspects need to be carefully considered when discussing treatment choices.

Improving the doctor–patient relationship helps to relieve the psychological distress of lung cancer patients when they first meet the surgeon. Most patients describe the period preceding their first encounter with the surgeon as very stressful. Most, when they sit in front of us, are in a state of extreme anxiety and shock, often unable to fully grasp and retain all the complex information pertinent to their treatment. For most, when we first meet them, they are at

Box 32.1 Patient perspective

The shock of being told about lung cancer

I think that the incidental detection of serious illness, for example, at an emergency presentation, causes greater shock. Even ex-smokers are often stunned despite years of public health warnings. I found health-care terminology difficult to understand, especially when grappling with basic questions after a life-changing diagnosis. When patients ask, 'What does that mean?' it's not a cue for scientific information. Rather, they want to know about the impact on their everyday life. When I first met with the physician after my diagnosis of lung cancer, I wanted to know my life expectancy, if there was any treatment, whether I would lose my hair/weight, or if I could work or travel. I was more interested in information on my residual quality of life rather than complex statistics or medical terms. Many patients confess to hearing little besides the word 'cancer'. Visual aids, pictures, and diagrams help, especially if there is a language barrier. Offering information and videos/case studies to discuss with others can help.

My first appointment included mentally 'joining the dots' 7 weeks after accident and emergency department imaging revealed a 'lesion'. The surgeon showed the 'mass'/lobes on a drawing, explaining PET [positron emission tomography] scan and treatment. He then explained the likelihood of death and the complications of different treatments. I calmly asked, 'What won't I be able to do after surgery that I might do now?' and 'How could I get fit for surgery?' My reply to the question 'What do you usually do?' included distance swimming several times a week and full-time work. The surgeon's recommendation to keep active to recovery my previous level of fitness felt empowering.

It also seems important for patients to share their experiences with each other. Awaiting another appointment, an older lady sought my views. She seemed to be against having surgery. I explained my lobectomy years earlier and my full recovery. A man opposite explained he'd had his whole lung removed months earlier yet now walked his dog and played golf. Within 20 minutes she'd changed her views. Previously she thought: 'I've had my life so there's no point'. Now, she asked: 'How soon after surgery could I drive?'

their most vulnerable time. Our role is to find a way to facilitate connection and understanding through an empathic approach. Studies have shown that several cognitive biases may affect the outcome of SDM and most are linked to how the information is presented (Ozdemir and Finkelstein, 2018).

A patient representative describes in Box 32.1 the experience that she and others had with the diagnosis and management of lung cancer in the context of SDM.

In conclusion, thoracic surgery deals with serious life-threatening diagnoses, where there are trade-offs between different approaches and where people's views about the quality of their remaining time need careful discussion. Applying the principles of SDM in this context appears critical to empower patients to make decisions that best align with their priorities in life.

REFERENCES

Brunelli, A. 2022. European Society of Thoracic Surgeons Presidential Address 2022 Sawubona: bridging emotional and cognitive gaps through empathy and perspective taking. *Eur J Cardiothorac Surg,* **62**, ezac412.

Brunelli, A., Decaluwe, H., Gossot, D., Guerrera, F., Szanto, Z., Falcoz, P. E. 2021. Perioperative outcomes of segmentectomies versus lobectomies in high-risk patients: an ESTS database analysis. *Eur J Cardiothorac Surg,* **59**, 389–394.

Cykert, S., Dilworth-Anderson, P., Monroe, M. H., et al. 2010. Factors associated with decisions to undergo surgery among patients with newly diagnosed early-stage lung cancer. *JAMA,* **303**, 2368–2376.

Dalmia, S., Boele, F., Absolom, K., et al. 2022. Shared decision making in early-stage non-small cell lung cancer: a systematic review. *Ann Thorac Surg,* **114**, 581–590.

Durand, M. A., Carpenter, L., Dolan, H., et al. 2014. Do interventions designed to support shared decision-making reduce health inequalities? A systematic review and meta-analysis. *PLoS One,* **9**, e94670.

Elwyn, G., Durand, M. A., Song, J., et al. 2017. A three-talk model for shared decision making: multistage consultation process. *BMJ,* **359**, j4891.

Elwyn, G., Frosch, D. L., Kobrin, S. 2016. Implementing shared decision-making: consider all the consequences. *Implement Sci,* **11**, 114.

Elwyn, G., Frosch, D., Thomson, R., et al. 2012. Shared decision making: a model for clinical practice. *J Gen Intern Med,* **27**, 1361–1367.

Franks, K. N., McParland, L., Webster, J., et al. 2020. SABRTooth: a randomised controlled feasibility study of stereotactic ablative radiotherapy (SABR) with surgery in patients with peripheral stage I non small cell lung cancer considered at higher risk of complications from surgical resection. *Eur Respir J,* **56**, 2000118.

Golden, S. E., Thomas, C. R. Jr., Moghanaki, D., Slatore, C. G.; Early-Stage Lung Cancer Comparative Effectiveness Research Consortium. 2017. Dumping the information bucket: a qualitative study of clinicians caring for patients with early-stage non-small cell lung cancer. *Patient Educ Couns,* **100**, 861–870.

Hopmans, W., Damman, O. C., Senan, S., Hartemink, K. J., Smit, E. F., Timmermans, D. R. 2015. A patient perspective on shared decision making in stage I non-small cell lung cancer: a mixed methods study. *BMC Cancer,* **15**, 959.

Housten, A. J., Kozower, B. D., Engelhardt, K. E., et al. 2023. Developing an educational and decision support tool for stage I lung cancer using decision science. *Ann Thorac Surg,* **115**, 299–308.

Kraft-Todd, G. T., Reinero, D. A., Kelley, J. M., Heberlein, A. S., Baer, L., Riess, H. 2017. Empathic nonverbal behavior increases ratings of both warmth and competence in a medical context. *PLoS One,* **12**, e0177758.

Lee, A. C. H., Madariaga, M. L. L., Liao, C., Ferguson, M. K. 2023. Gender bias in judging frailty and fitness for lung surgery. *Ann Thorac Surg,* **115**, 356–361.

Mokhles, S., Maat, A. P. W. M., Aerts, J. G. J. V., Nuyttens, J. J. M. E., Bogers, A. J. J. C., Takkenberg, J. J. M. 2017. Opinions of lung cancer clinicians on shared decision making in early-stage non-small-cell lung cancer. *Interact Cardiovasc Thorac Surg,* **25**, 278–284.

Mokhles, S., Nuyttens, J. J. M. E., de Mol, M., et al. 2018. Treatment selection of early-stage non-small cell lung cancer: the role of the patient in clinical decision making. *BMC Cancer,* **18**, 79.

Nuyttens, J. J. M. E., de Mol, M., Aerts, J. G. J. V., et al. 2018. Treatment selection of early-stage non-small cell lung cancer: the role of the patient in clinical decision making. *BMC Cancer,* **18**, 79.

Ozdemir, S., Finkelstein, E. A. 2018. Cognitive bias: the downside of shared decision making. *JCO Clin Cancer Inform,* **2**, 1–10.

Pennathur, A., Brunelli, A., Criner, G. J., et al. 2021. Definition and assessment of high risk in patients considered for lobectomy for stage I non-small cell lung cancer: the American Association for Thoracic Surgery expert panel consensus document. *J Thorac Cardiovasc Surg,* **162**, 1605–1618.

Quill, T. E., Cassel, C. K. 1995. Nonabandonment: a central obligation for physicians. *Ann Intern Med,* **122**, 368–374.

Saji, H., Okada, M., Tsuboi, M., et al. 2022. Segmentectomy versus lobectomy in small-sized peripheral non-small-cell lung cancer (JCOG0802/WJOG4607L): a multicentre, open-label, phase 3, randomised, controlled, non-inferiority trial. *Lancet,* **399**, 1607–1617.

Samson, P., Waters, E. A., Meyers, B., Politi, M. C. 2016. Shared decision making and effective risk communication in the high-risk patient with operable stage I non-small cell lung cancer. *Ann Thorac Surg,* **101**, 2049–2052.

Stacey, D., Lewis, K. B., Smith, M., et al. 2024. Decision aids for people facing health treatment or screening decisions. *Cochrane Database Syst Rev,* **1**, CD001431.

Subramanian, M. P., Meyers, B. F. 2018. Surgical resection versus stereotactic body radiation therapy for stage I NSCLC: can randomized trials provide the solution? *Cancers (Basel),* **10**, 310.

Sullivan, D. R., Eden, K. B., Dieckmann, N. F., et al. 2019. Understanding patients' values and preferences regarding early-stage lung cancer treatment decision making. *Lung Cancer,* **131**, 47–57.

Taylor, L. J., Nabozny, M. J., Steffens, N. M., et al. 2017. A framework to improve surgeon communication in high-stakes surgical decisions: Best Case/Worst Case. *JAMA Surg,* **152**, 531–538.

Tong, B. C., Wallace, S., Hartwig, M. G., D'Amico, T. A., Huber, J. C. 2016. Patient preferences in treatment choices for early-stage lung cancer. *Ann Thorac Surg,* **102**, 1837–1844.

Wu, J., Bai, H. X., Chan, L., et al. 2020. Sublobar resection compared with stereotactic body radiation therapy and ablation for early-stage non-small cell lung cancer: a National Cancer Database study. *J Thorac Cardiovasc Surg,* **160**, 1350–1357.

33

Shared decision making in colon and rectal surgery

Srinivas Joga Ivatury, Helene Juul Würtz, Alexander T. Hawkins, and Craig Creelman

Introduction

Colorectal health and disease have a large effect on bowel function, thereby making choice of management vitally important. Regular bowel function contributes to overall well-being. Impacts on bowel function often change the daily life of the patient. Additionally, there are typically several options to manage disease ranging from doing nothing, dietary/lifestyle management, outpatient procedures, and formal operations. Our goal as surgeons is to assist patients in making the correct choice of management based on their preferences and values. Thus, high-quality shared decision making (SDM) is imperative in making these choices.

Patient preferences and features of daily life are essential knowledge for patients and surgeons to make informed, preference-sensitive decisions. Surgeons must also consider age, sex/gender, and comorbidities when making recommendations. Moreover, other aspects such as culture, family, and access to the nearest hospital are also important when discussing choice of management with patients with a colorectal disease. To make an informed and high-quality preference-sensitive decision, patients also need to know possible outcomes and risks of surgery and what to expect if surgery is not chosen. The trade-offs of risks and benefits of each option also need to be clear to the patient, before reaching a final decision on choice of management.

Across the spectrum of colorectal diseases, there are several management situations where patients must consider different options. Often the options presented have similar expected results or outcomes, but different 'costs' or risks. Clearly superior management recommendations are not always present in every case. One example concerns management of low rectal cancer where management options may include either surgery with a stoma or chemotherapy/radiation, especially for patients with comorbidities. An example in benign colorectal diseases concerns changes in lifestyle versus surgery for bleeding haemorrhoids. A particularly challenging example in benign inflammatory bowel diseases concerns deciding between surgery or medication for repeated Crohn's disease flare-ups.

Malignant colorectal polyps are a prime example of why SDM is an important skill for surgeons. The patient with a malignant colorectal polyp, with pathological evidence of cancer but uncertainty about its complete removal, retains a small risk of residual cancer. There are several management options: cancer surgery, surveillance, or no intervention. All options entail potential risks and benefits. However, which risks and benefits are most important when making this decision are subjective. Undergoing surgery entails removing part of the bowel to increase the possibility of removing residual cancer cells, but there are risks involved with the surgery. There is a high chance that the resected bowel specimen was cancer-free, resulting in the surgery having been unnecessary (also termed 'overtreatment'). Another option is to adhere to a surveillance strategy to heighten the chance of locating a possible recurrence without undergoing surgery. This entails frequent colonoscopy procedures, computed tomography scans, and magnetic resonance imaging. This strategy requires several visits to the hospital—several times a year—and undergoing multiple colonoscopy procedures including the need for multiple bowel preparations with laxatives. Moreover, there is the possibility that a future recurrence cannot be cured with surgery and, thus, a patient's fear of recurrence can be high. The final option is to choose neither of the above, avoid the need for going to the hospital, and hope that the cancer does not recur. However, a recurrence in this case could be fatal once ultimately detected and patient regrets might be very great.

This situation demonstrates the importance of listening to the patient's personal preferences and their ideas and goals in life. In this case, the trade-offs between preservation of bodily integrity and operative risks, long-term effects on bowel function and quality of life, and prevention of future recurrence must be considered and discussed. Only by asking questions, listening, and by explaining the benefits and risks of all the possible management options, can we enable patients to reaching the correct preference-sensitive decision on disease management.

Current status of SDM and its effectiveness

Overall, use of SDM remains nascent in the surgical treatment of colorectal disease. Despite several disease processes with multiple potential therapeutic interventions, formal SDM tools are lacking. There are several areas where facilitating SDM has been studied or actively promoted.

Diverticulitis

Diverticulitis is one of the most common gastrointestinal conditions with over 370,000 emergency department visits and 200,000 inpatient admissions in the USA each year (Peery et al., 2018). Less than 1% of these hospitalized patients require surgery for either free perforation or sepsis that does not improve with medical management. Most patients with diverticulitis are managed non-operatively (Hawkins et al., 2020). Of patients with uncomplicated disease, 20% will have recurrent diverticulitis, and 20% of those will have three or more lifetime episodes (Morris et al., 2014).

The only lasting treatment for recurrent diverticulitis is a sigmoid colectomy that surgically removes the section of the colon where diverticulitis develops. However, this involves the risk of complications from both anaesthesia and surgery. Without clear superiority between surgery and observation for recurrent diverticulitis, this decision is highly preference-sensitive and thus lends itself to SDM.

Current work in this area has included a qualitative study on surgeons' perceptions and a discreet choice study to understand the relative importance of many of the factors surgeons consider (Hawkins et al., 2022; De Roo et al., 2023). The qualitative study observed that surgeons mostly have discarded older dogma in recommending colectomy for recurrent diverticulitis based on the number and severity of episodes. Instead, decision making in recurrent diverticulitis is complex, involving multiple surgeon and patient factors and evolving over time. Surgeons struggle with this decision and education- or communication-based interventions that focus on SDM warrant development (Hawkins et al., 2022). In the discreet choice experiment, surgeons were less willing to offer an elective operation for scenarios with one lifetime episode of diverticulitis, if the most recent episode was managed with oral antibiotics only, if the patient had a strong preference to avoid surgery, or if the patient had no complaints about diverticulitis impacting their life. Patient preferences to avoid a stoma had little effect on surgeon decision making in this study (De Roo et al., 2023).

Future areas of study include understanding patients' perspectives of the decision making process and development of a decision aid.

Inflammatory bowel disease

Approximately 30% of patients with ulcerative colitis ultimately require surgery. Surgery for ulcerative colitis involves total proctocolectomy (large bowel removal) with permanent ileostomy or ileo-pouch anal anastomosis. These interventions have varied risks and benefits. Ileo-pouch anal anastomosis restores intestinal continuity, but can have lasting results on defecatory function. Permanent ileostomy usually requires fewer surgical procedures, but psychosocial adaptation to a permanent stoma is difficult. Patients with ulcerative colitis who are faced with the complex decision between ileo-pouch anal anastomosis and permanent ileostomy would benefit from SDM.

To address this problem, a decision aid was designed and tested (Cohan et al., 2016). Twenty-five patients were enrolled. After using the decision aid, patients' knowledge scores improved by 39% ($p < 0.006$), six patients changed their treatment preference, and eight reported increased certainty in treatment preference. Patient and surgeon satisfaction with the decision aid and the clinical encounter were high. Future directions include work on implementing the decision aid into clinical practice.

Colorectal cancer

Globally, colorectal cancer is the third most diagnosed cancer in males and the second in females, according to the World Health Organization GLOBOCAN database. Traditionally, cancer resection has not been considered a highly preference-sensitive decision—the cancer must be resected at all costs. However, in recent years, more personalized treatments have been developed for colorectal cancer. With all these new alternatives, clinicians need to understand and consider patients' opinions and values in selecting individualized therapies.

One area that has been a focus of formal SDM is in colorectal cancer screening. There are several different options for screening, each with their own trade-offs. This has sparked the development of decision support tools to engage patients and healthcare providers in making shared decisions about screening (Volk et al., 2018). Current research focuses on implementing these tools into health systems (PCORI, 2023). There is less work on SDM for colorectal cancer treatment (Goldwag et al., 2019).

Rectal cancer is a subset of colorectal cancer with greater treatment options including sequencing of adjuvant radiation and chemotherapy and alternative surgical procedures. While no formal SDM tools exist, there are several potential areas for study (see below). Despite acknowledgement of the need for better communication, SDM is infrequently mentioned in clinical practice guidelines and consensus statements from major societies and organizations (Maes-Carballo et al., 2023).

Gaps in evidence

Gaps in evidence for SDM in colorectal surgery exist due to complex preference-sensitive decisions and the availability of multiple surgical and non-surgical options. In addition, colorectal disease subtypes affect different age groups where preferences may differ. For example, fertility, returning to work, and childrearing may be more important to a younger person when making a preference-sensitive decision while physical strength, mental capacity, and independence may be more important to an older person. In general, these nuances have not been studied rigorously in colorectal surgery and are an identified gap in evidence. Below, we will review some examples of these gaps in colorectal surgery.

Choice between lifestyle modification and performing a procedure

Many colorectal diseases such as haemorrhoid disease and uncomplicated diverticulitis stem from dietary and toileting imbalances such as lack of fibre in the diet and excess time spent on the commode. These conditions are life-altering but not life-threatening. Patients seeking care are presented with a choice between lifestyle modification, increasing fibre and changing toileting behaviours, and surgical intervention, removal of the offending tissue (haemorrhoids). While surgery is the easiest option for people to understand, we know that dietary/lifestyle modification is the best option for overall health. We do not yet have a systematic way to present these options nor do we have robust comparative data for the dietary/lifestyle modification group compared with surgery, nor for best practices to ensure adherence to these modifications. Cynically, we can surmise that those who are compensated by doing more surgery would also have a bias towards surgery and, thus, no incentive to recommend or study dietary and lifestyle modification.

Choice between stoma and reconstruction after total mesorectal excision for rectal cancer

Major rectal cancer treatment is complex, and effects are life-changing due to short- and long-term treatment with chemotherapy, radiation therapy, and surgery. Colorectal surgeons generally lead the multidisciplinary team that treats rectal cancer and, therefore, are the ones who should be involved in SDM for rectal cancer. One major decision for rectal cancer treatment concerns choice of surgery, where many options exist including total mesorectal excision, local excision, and non-operative management. The risks, benefits, and postoperative/oncological outcomes are well known for these options. The lifestyle effects, often the most important to people, are not well studied either for each option or comparatively. Moreover, rectal cancer has substantial nuances which make assessment and decision making difficult, including different outcomes based on tumour location, pre-existing bowel dysfunction, and lifestyle factors. To address this, we must first have a systematic, large-volume collection of clinical, preference, and medical/lifestyle outcomes data in diverse populations. Deep machine learning may then be an avenue to help people make better choices for the treatment options that align with their preferences and values with modelling of potential outcomes and recommendations.

There are also two options regarding defecation after total mesorectal excision: re-anastomosis of the large intestine or permanent colostomy. There is equipoise for both options after an appropriate total mesorectal excision and both have substantial negative lifestyle effects; however, stigma against colostomy is significant among patients, the general population, and physicians (Eid et al., 2022). This stigma muddies the ability for people to make informed choices between the two options. There has been little work done on this. Future work must help tackle the stigma for patients and surgeons. We had embarked on a decision aid to facilitate this decision making but rectal cancer survivors noted that the entire journey from diagnosis to survivorship required more emphasis at the outset (Saunders et al., 2021). The survivors felt that a decision aid was important and that it should be easy to use and in multiple formats. Surgeons we interviewed also saw the benefit of a decision aid, but noted that it must not impede on their normal workflow (Goldwag et al., 2022).

Choice between medical management and surgery in inflammatory bowel disease

Inflammatory bowel disease is a lifelong inflammatory condition of the intestinal tract that manifests in various levels of severity and symptomatology. Inflammatory bowel disease is predominantly treated with medication to reduce the exaggerated immunological attack on the bowels. In some cases, initial or ongoing medical therapy fails to quell the inflammation fully and patients are faced with the choice of trying a new medication or considering surgery. This choice is most evident in Crohn's disease, where surgery is most often used to remove the damaged tissue with patients resuming medical therapy afterwards to prevent new damage. Current gaps in evidence include when the optimal time to consider surgery would be and what the patient-specific factors are that would predict success for a new medication over surgery or vice versa. Additionally, new and more targeted medications are being developed at a rapid rate so there is not enough experience to evaluate comparative effectiveness. Thus, surgeons and gastroenterologists tend to use 'gestalt' (or gut feeling) to suggest the right time for each treatment, knowing that patients will resume medication afterwards if surgery is chosen. Ulcerative colitis, which is the other inflammatory bowel disease, has a more straightforward decision making process in comparison as surgery is the final, irreversible step as the disease is limited to the colon and rectum. Once these are removed, ulcerative colitis is 'cured'. However, for ulcerative colitis, the complex decision making happens in the choice of surgery—whether to choose bowel reconstruction or a stoma—and with their different and significant impacts on daily life. As with rectal cancer surgery, ulcerative colitis surgery faces the same gaps in evidence to address pre-existing stigma for stomas (Taft et al., 2009).

See Box 33.1 for our patient perspective.

Box 33.1 Patient perspective

My rectal cancer experience by Craig Creelman

I was diagnosed with stage III rectal cancer in early 2021 after a few months of atypical bowel symptoms. I had just turned 49 years old.

In my first meeting with my treatment team, my new life was laid out for me. It was a very heavy meeting, and I did not know it, but I'd spend the next 6 months learning about my disease and trying to make a plan for the short term and how that plan would affect my life long term.

I couldn't believe that I, a lay person, was going to have to choose my treatment—something I thought the doctors would be doing. I guess I thought this disease was sort of 'boilerplate' and I'd just have a blueprint slapped on me, but there were treatment options now.

The first thing I did was call a close friend who was a retired doctor and laid the whole thing out for him. Little did I know that he would play an enormous role in helping me choose paths and make decisions. He then spent some time looking at the research on the options for treatment and laid out to me the data and pros and cons of both.

We decided on chemotherapy and radiation treatments prior to considering surgery. The treatment effects varied from negligible to severe nausea and extremity tingling. At its worst, the side effects affected my wife as well. It was tough for her. She was lonely—it's tough to foresee these things, even when they've been told to you, until you are in the middle of them.

After completion of treatment, we discussed a new approach to 'watch and wait' if the initial treatment effectively eliminated the cancer. I was very excited that I might be able to avoid surgery. I spent several months in scans and consultations to determine my eligibility and many statistics were thrown around.

The decision eventually became not about me but my loved ones. I decided that I would undergo the surgery with bowel reconnection albeit with a temporary bag (stoma). Surgery initially went smoothly, but there were complications that delayed my recovery. I had subsequent stoma reversal surgery after which my life changed. It became very clear to me right off that I had no control over my bowels. I knew it would take months if not years to get back to my normal but that I would figure it out.

I was trying to figure out what I could do to control my bowel habits but there was no one who could help—I was astonished. Most of the useful info I found was online—specifically British chat rooms. I felt like a ship without a rudder and like I was the first person ever to have this affliction. I didn't understand why there was no real formal support.

I tried several things to try to help. I changed my diet several times. I tried medication to regulate my bowels. I even tried a bowel irrigation system. Nothing seemed work. I was 15 months post bag and I needed something that I could rely on—even if it was a permanent bag. That was April 2023. I am now in the process of surgery to have a permanent colostomy surgery to remedy my bowel issues.

When I look back on my entire experience there was nothing that I would have done differently. It was important for me to shoot for the moon and try to get back to as close as normal as possible. What I mean is: once I have a permanent bag I will never look back and think I should have gotten a permanent bag from day 1—I needed to try everything regardless of result. I was in Miami this fall with my son all weekend and had a great weekend, but my system acted up Saturday afternoon and I had to bail on going to a college football game that night—I don't want to have to miss anything ever again and I'm down to one option which is a permanent bag. I am ready.

REFERENCES

Cohan, J. N., Ozanne, E. M., Sewell, J. L., et al. 2016. A novel decision aid for surgical patients with ulcerative colitis: results of a pilot study. *Dis Colon Rectum,* **59**, 520–528.

De Roo, A. C., Chen, Y., Du, X., et al. 2023. Polygenic risk prediction in diverticulitis. *Ann Surg,* **277**, e1262–e1268.

Eid, M. A., Goldwag, J. L., Gray, P. P., Shaw, R. D., Ivatury, S. J. 2022. Physicians perceive that ostomates have decreased quality of life but not overall health: an international survey of physicians. *Colorectal Dis,* **24**, 1602–1612.

Goldwag, J., Marsicovetere, P., Scalia, P., et al. 2019. The impact of decision aids in patients with colorectal cancer: a systematic review. *BMJ Open,* **9**, e028379.

Goldwag, J. L., Saunders, C. H., Read, J. T., Durand, M. A., Elwyn, G., Ivatury, S. J. 2022. A rectal cancer surgical decision aid is not enough: a qualitative study. *Dis Colon Rectum,* **65**, 1483–1493.

Hawkins, A. T., Rothman, R. L., Geiger, T. M., et al. 2022. Surgeons' perspective of decision making in recurrent diverticulitis: a qualitative analysis. *Ann Surg Open,* **3**, e157.

Hawkins, A. T., Wise, P. E., Chan, T., et al. 2020. Diverticulitis: an update from the age old paradigm. *Curr Probl Surg,* **57**, 100862.

Maes-Carballo, M., Gómez-Fandiño, Y., García-García, M., et al. 2023. Colorectal cancer treatment guidelines and shared decision making quality and reporting assessment: systematic review. *Patient Educ Couns,* **115**, 107856.

Morris, A. M., Regenbogen, S. E., Hardiman, K. M., Hendren, S. 2014. Sigmoid diverticulitis: a systematic review. *JAMA*, **311**, 287–297.

PCORI. Putting a decision aid into practice to support shared decision making for colorectal cancer screening. 2023. Available at: https://www.pcori.org/research-results/2023/putting-decision-aid-practice-support-shared-decision-making-colorectal-cancer-screening

Peery, A. F., Crockett, S. D., Murphy, C. C., et al. 2019. Burden and cost of gastrointestinal, liver, and pancreatic diseases in the United States: update 2018. *Gastroenterology,* **156**, 254–272.

Saunders, C. H., Goldwag, J. L., Read, J. T., Durand, M. A., Elwyn, G., Ivatury, S. J. 2021. 'Because everybody is so different': a qualitative analysis of the lived experiences and information needs of rectal cancer survivors. *BMJ Open,* **11**, e043245.

Taft, T. H., Keefer, L., Leonhard, C., Nealon-Woods, M. 2009. Impact of perceived stigma on inflammatory bowel disease patient outcomes. *Inflamm Bowel Dis,* **15**, 1224–1232.

Volk, R. J., Leal, V. B., Jacobs, L. E., et al. 2018. From guideline to practice: new shared decision-making tools for colorectal cancer screening from the American Cancer Society. *CA Cancer J Clin,* **68**, 246–249.

34

Shared decision making in care for older adults with multiple chronic conditions

Bianca Buurman, Ruth E. Pel-Littel, Gérard Hendriks, and Wim Roelofs

Introduction

Many older adults have multiple chronic conditions (MCC), defined as the coexistence of two or more chronic conditions. Older adults with MCC are frequent users of healthcare, use multiple medications, and are at risk of negative health outcomes. Healthcare decisions for patients with MCC are more difficult. First of all, because multiple conditions coexist, the traditional disease-oriented approach does not work. Guidelines often focus on single diseases and there is a lack of evidence around interactions between conditions and to what extent there are 'equal' treatment options (see also Chapter 53). This means that traditional models of shared decision making (SDM), such as with decision aids, are less applicable for older adults with MCC.

Moreover, older adults with MCC often value other outcomes, such as maintaining independence, reducing symptom burden, and quality of life, as more important than survival. So, in SDM, it is important first to identify the goals and health priorities that older adults have, so that the care and treatment options contribute to reaching a specific goal. As goals and priorities more often focus on remaining independent, maintaining social contacts, and a good quality of life, this also results in a broader approach to 'options' than just options from the medical perspective. Lifestyle adjustments, social interventions, and technological aids should also be examined as options to achieve one's goals.

Also, in older adults with MCC and frailty, there are more decision makers, such as a partner or children. Triadic decision making is often the standard with the older adult, as healthcare providers and family are partners in the SDM process. Although it is important to keep the perspective of the older adult central in the decision making process, the impact it has on the family is prominent too, such as the support that has to be provided at home.

Lastly, there are differences between older adults in the extent to which they want or can be involved in SDM. The ability to participate in SDM is dependent on the type of decision, cognitive abilities, and whether it is recognized that there is a decision to be made. Influencing factors are also anxiety, low self-efficacy, and low health literacy.

The American Geriatrics Society's Guiding Principles for the Care of Older Adults with Multimorbidity state that optimal care for older adults with MCCs should include eliciting and incorporating patient priorities into medical decision making (American Geriatrics Society, 2012).

This requires an approach to SDM in which, before discussing the benefits and harms of treatment options, personal goals are explored. In this chapter, we describe the steps of the 'dynamic model' of SDM with frail older adults. By following these steps, attention is paid to preparation, goals, choices, and decision making, so that older adults and their families feel supported to be involved in SDM. Perspectives from two patients and their sons, however, illustrate the difficulties of achieving SDM.

The 'dynamic model' for SDM with frail older adults

Van de Pol and colleagues created the dynamic model for SDM with frail older adults, by adding two steps on prioritizing preferences and life goals before discussing choices and options (van de Pol et al., 2016). Figure 34.1 schematically represents the SDM process elements. The arrows in the model highlight the dynamics, because reality is complex, and it may sometimes be necessary to go back to a previous step in the model.

To engage older adults in SDM, it is important that they are explicitly involved in each step. This means that the healthcare provider should involve the patient and their carers in the process, such as by explicitly describing what will be discussed. For example, at step 4 of the model (option talk), the caregiver might say, 'Now I am going to inform you about the pros and cons of this medication'. Or at step 5 (decision talk) 'Now it's time to discuss whether we can come to a decision'. We observed more than 200 video observations of conversations between older patients and geriatricians and found that very often the SDM process is very implicit and it is not clear to the patient that he or she is in an SDM process.

Let us take a look at the six steps of the model.

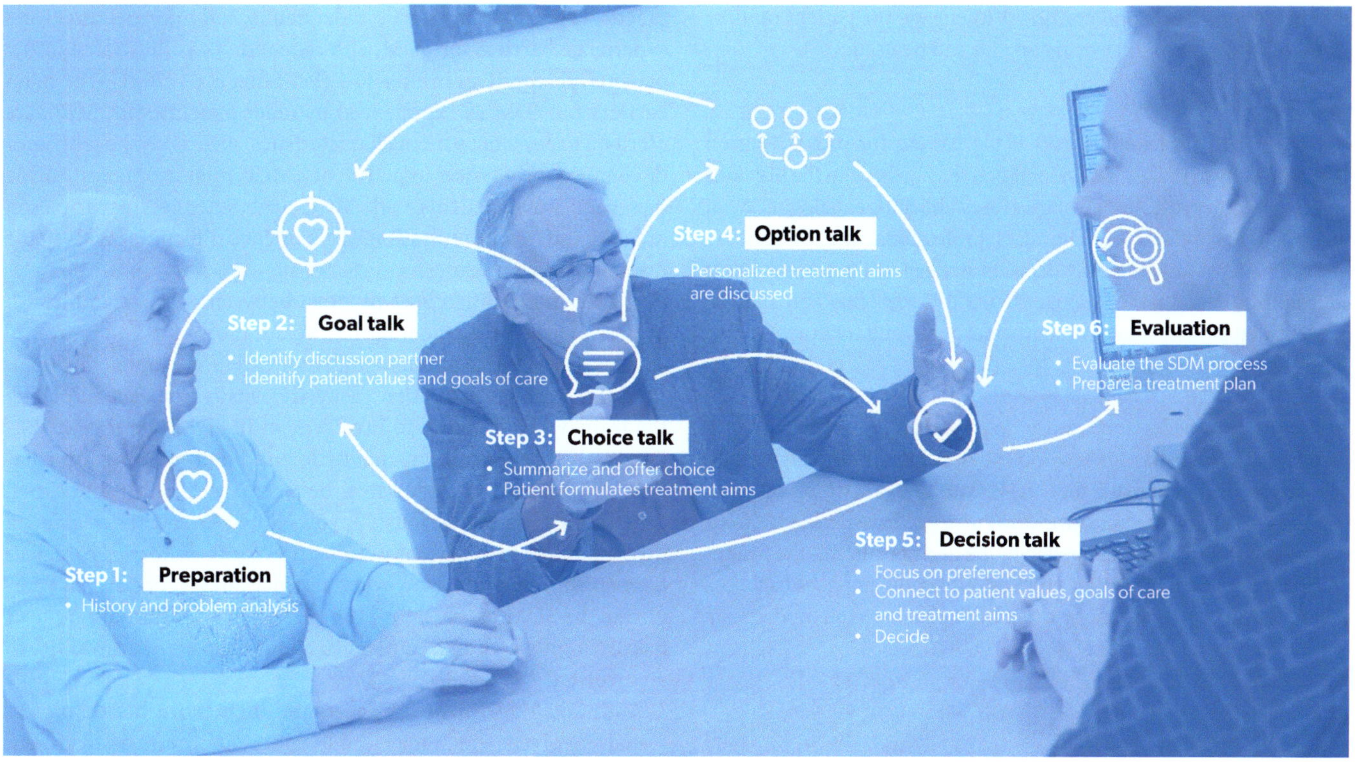

Figure 34.1 The dynamic model for SDM with frail older adults.

Step 1: preparation

The health professional starts the conversation by asking if the patient has previously discussed or documented anything about treatment in general or on specific issues (e.g. resuscitation, advance care planning). Has the patient thought about what he/she would like to discuss today?

Also, it is important to do a problem analysis, a functional assessment of all current problems. The extensiveness of the analysis depends on the situation and sometimes other caregivers can contribute. The comprehensive geriatric assessment is a useful tool. Clinicians should realize that not all problems are equally important to the patient; we prioritize the problems in consultation with the patient.

Patient preparation

Patients can be nervous before a conversation with a healthcare professional, so it can be very helpful if patients think about their personal goals and wishes before the conversation and preferably discuss this with their loved ones. Clinicians can facilitate this by sending a preparatory tool (Pel-Littel et al., 2020) or a 'Question Prompt List' (Brandes et al., 2015) to the patient beforehand. This helps in discussing goals in the next step.

Step 2: goal talk

In this step, the health professional explains that each patient is unique and has their own preferences and priorities. And that before choices can be made regarding the current problem, it is important to discuss what values are important in the patient's life. What makes a day a good day? What does the patient hope for, what do they fear? How does the patient rate their quality of life and what would need to change in their life to make these score 1 point higher? This helps to elicit fundamental goals (prolongation of life, functional autonomy, visit grandchildren, comfort, etc.).

During this discussion, the health professional also identifies whether the patient has sufficient decision making capacity (cognitive, emotional). If not, who is (by law) assigned to take the decisions?

Does the patient want to take decisions? If not, who does the patient designate (proxy decision maker)?

Step 3: choice talk

In this step, the health professional summarizes the preceding steps (the actual problem and the identified values and fundamental goals of care) and checks if the summary is correct. The health professional and patient formulate the treatment aims for functioning or symptom reduction. The health professional explains that there are several treatment possibilities, offers choice, and states that they will support the patient. They explain that while the health professional is the medical expert, only the patient can be the expert on treatment aims, priorities and preferences. The health professional checks if the patient (or proxy decision maker) has understood everything, summarizes again if necessary, and continues to engage the patient (and informal caregivers) in a dialogue.

Step 4: option talk

In this step the health professional lists personalized treatment options (according to the identified values, fundamental goals, and treatment aims) and invites the patient and informal caregiver explicitly to discuss options they think of (e.g. social interventions). Risks, benefits, and side effects of each treatment option must be discussed. The health professional checks which risks and side effects the patient is willing to take (opportunity/cost) and observes how the patient reacts and continues to engage the patient (and/or representative). If possible, decision aids can be used.

Step 5: decision talk

Now the health professional asks if the patient (or proxy decision maker) is ready to make a decision. If not, they go back to the previous steps. The health professional focuses on establishing a dialogue. What are the patient's preferences? The health professional makes a decision with the patient (and/or proxy decision maker). If the patient wants the health professional to decide, discuss this explicitly and align to the identified patient values, fundamental goals, and treatment aims.

Step 6: evaluation talk

The healthcare provider discusses the decision making process. To check whether the patient has understood the decision and the arguments, they can ask: 'I want to make sure I have explained everything clearly to you: can you tell me in your own words what we have decided?' (feedback method). Is everyone happy with the decision? If not, the healthcare professional enquires about the dissatisfaction and goes back to a previous step. If yes: they draw up a treatment plan based on the decision.

Barriers and facilitators to SDM with older patients with MCC

Barriers

Although both patients and health professionals identify the importance of SDM, implementation in daily practice is not yet common practice. Health professionals, older adults, and informal caregivers experience barriers for SDM with older adults as illustrated in the patients' perspectives in Box 34.1 (Pel-Littel et al., 2021). The main barriers for SDM as experienced by older patients with MCC are ascribed to personal patient characteristics, such as poor health and/or cognitive or physical impairments. MCC might complicate SDM in several ways: patients with MCC experience less participation in SDM and health professionals experience difficulties with single disease-based guidelines.

Furthermore, differences in views between patients and health professionals on treatment burden versus morbidity and mortality complicate SDM. Although informal carers are often the main caregiver for an older patient, they are usually not seen as 'part of the team' when it comes to involvement in SDM. Their contribution to the conversation is mainly focused on providing information and acting as a 'translator' between the health professional and the patient. But seriously involving the informal caregiver in discussing the implications of a decision for the informal caregiver happens infrequently. However, informal caregivers can also complicate the SDM process, for example, when an informal caregiver has different views on treatment or about the patient's capability to be involved.

Additionally, with MCC, there are often more health professionals involved, which may lead to conflicting views on treatment priorities, patient and caregiver involvement, and no one having an overview of a patient's case. Health professionals perceive poor interpersonal skills as a barrier to SDM and organizational barriers, such as time pressures and high turnover of patients. Financial

Box 34.1 Patient perspective

We share two stories of sons of older mothers with multiple conditions in hospital. The mothers are so vulnerable that support from their loved ones is needed in the decision making process. The general practitioner's (GP's) role in both cases was important: signalling, a listening ear, and 'thinking along'. In (family) discussions with healthcare providers, everyone's wishes were mostly well addressed. Yet there were also areas for improvement; in one case, for example, the transfer from hospital to a stay elsewhere and the lack of communication about the hospital's medication policy were lacking.

Gérard Hendriks

My mother, then 86, had many diagnoses: ovarian cancer, rheumatoid arthritis, transient ischaemic attack, psoriasis, chronic obstructive pulmonary disease, anaemia, lung cancer, but the most threatening one at the time was a stiffened heart valve. She often could not sleep from tightness and anxiety it caused. Things went from bad to worse and in the cardiology department it became clear that a TAVI (artificial heart valve) was among the possibilities, partly because this procedure could be done through the arm. However, the cardiologist explained that there could be major complications. For instance, there was a 20% chance of a brain haemorrhage, among a number of other unpleasant possibilities. My mother had plenty of life energy and wanted to get on with her life. But she could not and did not dare make a decision on whether or not to have the surgery. As a son, I felt I could not and should not make this decision for her, but I could support her in this decision. Help consisted of talking to my loved ones, but also by calling in her GP, who was so committed that she spoke to my mother in the hospital for an hour. Meanwhile, the cardiologist waited for my mother's decision. The GP also (obviously) could not decide for my mother, and after much back and forth and tears, my mother came up with a ruse. She said to me: 'Shall I do it then boy?' That was the maximum she could handle deciding. I nodded and said I would stand behind any decision she would make, including this one.

Wim Roelofs

My mother, 91, had increasing medical complaints, including heart problems. So bad that on her rounds in the neighbourhood, the GP regularly stopped by to enquire how she was doing. One Friday afternoon, the GP called me to say she would like to have my mother examined at the emergency room. By mutual agreement between the GP, my mother, and me, an ambulance was called. At the emergency room, all kinds of investigations were carried out. Sending her home was not an option. After admission to the geriatrics department, it soon became clear in the family interview that further treatment was not an option, given the various serious conditions.

In good consultation with the ward, the nursing approach was focused on keeping the patient 'as comfortable as possible' until transfer to another care facility. Some of this went well and some did not. For instance, my mother and I were happy with the arrangement that examinations and visits in the afternoon hours were limited to what was necessary. I did become increasingly worried about her apathetic behaviour; she was increasingly unresponsive. This was not how I knew my mother. After about 14 days, transfer was an issue. Finding a place in the region was difficult. I refused a place in a nursing home; not a good place for my mother. Then I managed to get cooperation from the hospital to get her into a hospice in her home town. This was very pleasant because expert and highly supportive palliative care was provided and immediate family members—some also at an advanced age—could say goodbye to her more easily here.

I was greatly surprised that the hospice followed a different medication policy. My mother became increasingly approachable and could even joke with her (great-)grandchildren again. However, it transpired that the hospital had, without her and my knowledge, greatly increased the sleep medication dosage. There are so many opportunities for more effective discussions and decision making with patients and family.

incentives, such as payments for productivity, are experienced as counterproductive to SDM, when 'doing nothing' is also an important option to discuss.

Facilitators

The commonest facilitator for SDM is an individualized approach in which healthcare professionals probe patient preferences. Older patients with MCC perceive that when they are explicitly encouraged to share information about personal values, priorities and preferences, and information about quality of life and functional status, this helps to formulate goals and find options that match patients' preferences. In addition, informal caregivers can be very helpful in facilitating SDM, for example, by helping the patient to formulate what is important to the patient.

Tools to facilitate SDM

There are several tools available to facilitate SDM and to monitor whether decisions made accord with the desired goals of the older patient with MCC. Those tools can be used for specific steps in SDM.

For step 1: preparation, there are two tools that can be used by patients to prepare for SDM.

Individualized patient reported outcome measures

This is a questionnaire that helps patients reflect on their health experiences and possible health problems. Questions are about daily functioning, pain, cognition, mental well-being, social activities, and quality of life. 'Individualized' stands for an individual prioritization by the patient about which items they want to discuss with the health professional. It is important to realize that an individualized patient reported outcome measure (iPROM) only reflects the patient's view. Perhaps a health professional identifies a health problem that the patient is unaware of or cannot identify due to memory problems. However, an iPROM indicates which problems are important to the patient. Although we focus here on using an iPROM as input for the SDM conversation, the iPROM can also be used to monitor the effect of the chosen interventions on patients' health. When iPROMs are used in a digital system, these data can easily be used not only to monitor one patient, but also to monitor groups of patients for quality improvement.

Patient preparatory tool

This tool can help the patient and informal caregivers prepare for the conversation. A patient preparatory tool could include an iPROM, but in addition it:

- Explains about SDM and explicitly encourages the patient to engage with SDM
- Asks about the patient's priorities: what do they want to discuss with the healthcare professional (agenda setting)?
- Asks what is important to the patient: what makes a day a good day? What does the patient hope for, what do they fear? How does the patient rate their quality of life and what would need to change in their life to score 1 point higher?
- Has a question for the informal carer: how do they feel; what are their worries; what do they hope for the patient?

For step 4: option talk, patient decision aids (PtDAs) can be used.

PtDAs

A PtDA provides information on different options for health problems and describes the pros and cons of each option (see Chapters 18 and 19). A PtDA also helps patients think about their preferences when choosing an option. Many countries have online PtDAs for many conditions. They can be very useful, but many do not take comorbidity into account. Comorbidities can influence the pros and cons of a treatment option. We think PtDAs should *not* be sent to older patients with MCC before the SDM process, because fundamental and treatment goal-setting are needed to focus on the specific health problem which is going to be addressed.

Training and competencies for SDM

Several competencies are needed for SDM. These competencies are applicable to doctors, nurses, and other allied health professionals. All make decisions with patients in various ways. First of all, it is important for all professionals to acknowledge that SDM leads to better quality of care because older adults are more likely to achieve outcomes that are important to them. It is important to understand the models of SDM and why PtDAs are more difficult to use for older adults. Professionals serve as coaches in this process of SDM and lead older adults and informal carers through the triadic process of SDM. This includes making sure that older adults and their carers can prepare at home by using preparatory tools. It requires communication skills in which older adults are equal partners in the SDM process and feel invited to participate in this process. Moreover, communicating goals and values of care are important in the network of care, so that all professionals work with the same goals.

The context for older adults and informal caregivers is very relevant information and should be assessed, so that decisions match with the context and preferences for care. In care for older adults, the comprehensive geriatric assessment can be used for a holistic assessment before exploring treatment options.

Gaps in evidence

The following gaps in evidence are evident, and which can inform new research:

- *How to address interprofessional SDM with older adults when multiple and various healthcare professionals are involved.* MCC often means that multiple healthcare professionals are involved. Often there is a lack of a coordinating specialist who is responsible for the care and treatment plan. There is little evidence around the organization and coordination of care for patients with MCC and the impact it has on health outcomes. Also, there is a need for better handovers of goals of care, so that patients do not have to start from scratch.

- *The long-term effects of SDM on personal health outcomes of older adults.* Most research on SDM focuses on immediate outcomes of the SDM process, such as whether patients are involved in SDM or whether the steps of SDM are followed. But SDM is a method to deliver better health outcomes by providing care that fits an older adult's needs. The middle- and long-term outcomes of SDM on personal health outcomes are not well known.
- *How to engage older adults with low health literacy in SDM.* SDM is traditionally seen as easier for older adults with high health literacy. They often have better access to information and a more comprehensive understanding of the complex language sometimes used. It is, however, of utmost importance that SDM is accessible and attuned to patients with low health literacy. By making informed decisions about health, adherence to care and treatment is higher. Thus, research on interventions to promote SDM among older adults with low health literacy is vital.
- *Interprofessional competencies for SDM.* We have outlined the competencies that are needed to perform SDM. Often it is assumed that SDM is mainly performed by doctors, but also nurses, psychologists, physiotherapists, and other allied health professionals make decisions with patients. Interprofessional competencies and collaboration for SDM should be studied.

REFERENCES

American Geriatrics Society. 2012. Guiding principles for the care of older adults with multimorbidity: an approach for clinicians: American Geriatrics Society Expert Panel on the Care of Older Adults with Multimorbidity. *J Am Geriatr Soc,* **60**, E1–E25.

Brandes, K., Linn, A., Butow, P., van Weert, J. 2015. The characteristics and effectiveness of Question Prompt List interventions in oncology: a systematic review of the literature, *Psychooncology,* **24**, 245–252.

Pel-Littel, R., Snaterse, M., Teppich, N., et al. 2021. Barriers and facilitators of shared decision-making in older patients with chronic conditions; a systematic review, *BMC Geriatr,* **21**, 112.

Pel-Littel, R., van Weert, J., Minkman, M., Scholte op Reimer, W., van de Pol, M., Buurman, B. 2020. The development of the evidence-based SDMMCC intervention to improve shared decision-making in geriatric outpatients: the DICO study. *BMC Med Inform Decis Mak,* **20**, 35.

van de Pol, M., Fluit, C., Lagro, J., Slaats, Y., Olde Rikkert, M., Lagro-Janssen, A. 2016. Expert and patient consensus on a dynamic model for shared decision-making in frail older patients. *Patient Educ Couns,* **99**, 1069–1077.

35

Shared decision making in cardiovascular care

Joshua B. Rager, Tod Papageorge, and Erica S. Spatz

Introduction

Cardiology is a diverse medical specialty encompassing general cardiovascular care and several subspecialties, including preventive cardiology, electrophysiology, interventional cardiology, structural heart disease, cardiomyopathy and heart failure, peripheral artery disease, and others. Within each specialty, there are growing diagnostic capabilities and options for treatment that include medications, procedures, and advanced therapies. Because of this, the role of shared decision making (SDM) is an essential part of modern cardiovascular care. Guidelines recommend SDM as best practice for several conditions and interventions (MacDonald and Turgeon, 2023).

SDM offers a more personalized approach to cardiovascular care; still, many challenges exist. Personalized risk calculation is a good example: numerical estimates can identify who will most likely derive benefit (or harm) from a given therapy. However, risk calculators add another wrinkle of complexity to SDM because communicating risk to individual patients can lead to several cognitive and heuristic biases. Eliciting patients' preferences, values, and goals is a complex skill, and many clinicians are not trained in these conversations. Moreover, matching a patient's goals with a specific care option requires knowledge about the care journey from the patient's perspective. A framework of SDM can support patient autonomy and health equity by giving information to patients about reasonable options and creating longitudinal, therapeutic alliances founded on mutual respect for each person's preferences and goals.

Several clinical areas in cardiology are obvious places for SDM and, as such, have seen particularly robust research into SDM models and the development of patient decision aids (PtDAs).

Atrial fibrillation management and care

Atrial fibrillation (AF) is an abnormal rhythm of the heart and can present with a variety of clinical manifestations. Multiple decisions often need to be made at diagnosis and in the ongoing care of a patient with AF, but key are (1) whether to manage AF with a rate or rhythm control method and (2) whether to prescribe anticoagulation for patients with high risk of stroke. Both decision points present opportunities to engage patients in a SDM process (Chung et al., 2021).

When AF is first diagnosed, a rhythm approach is often preferred. Evidence-based treatments to resume or maintain sinus rhythm include cardioversion, anti-arrhythmic medication, and ablation, but important trade-offs must be made. Cardioversion and ablation require time off work and sedation, include procedural risks, and are not 100% effective in maintaining sinus rhythm. Anti-arrhythmic medications come with the potential for toxicity but can be safe for the right patient with proper monitoring. The decision to *rate* control involves the use of lower-risk medications with less monitoring, but they may not be as effective in controlling symptoms or preventing recurrent episodes.

Another key decision in AF management surrounds treatment to reduce the risk of stroke from thromboembolism. Clinical eligibility for treatment with anticoagulation is guided by a risk score, abbreviated as CHA2DS2-VA and it still makes sense for the score to be 2 or greater has been endorsed as the threshold where a recommendation for anticoagulation should be given, but beyond this (and even below this) lies a vast gradation of risk for stroke, as well as bleeding. Luckily, several PtDAs and SDM strategies have been tested and validated. Four decision aids are highlighted in the 2023 American College of Cardiology/American Heart Association guidelines, wherein SDM and the use of a PtDA to guide AF treatments are recommended (Joglar et al., 2024). There is also an option to insert a left atrial appendage closure device as an alternative to anticoagulation in patients who have a history of bleeding; for this procedure to be reimbursed by Medicare, a physician other than the physician performing the procedure must engage the patient in SDM (Chung et al., 2021).

SDM models with PtDAs in AF have been shown to improve clinician satisfaction, increase patient knowledge, lower decisional conflict, enhance clinician–patient communication, and help patients make a decision (Man-Son-Hing et al., 2000; Kunneman et al., 2020). However, one of the challenges of AF is the dynamic nature of symptoms and clinical stability, which requires ongoing SDM. Trials showing the positive impacts of SDM interventions on decisional regret appear to lessen over time, suggesting that one-off, single SDM interventions may be insufficient (Wang et al., 2023). Furthermore, one-time use of a PtDA did not improve risk accuracy (Kunneman et al., 2020), and the impact of PtDAs and SDM on adherence to anticoagulation therapy is largely mixed (McAlister et al., 2005; Noseworthy et al., 2022).

Ischaemic heart disease: primary prevention, chest pain, acute coronary syndrome, and chronic ischaemic heart disease

Ischaemic heart disease is a main driver of premature death that afflicts millions of patients worldwide, and many more are at risk for atherosclerotic heart disease. Estimating one's 10-year risk of having a cardiovascular event is at the centre of risk assessment and SDM, enabling stratification into low, intermediate, or high risk (Arnett et al., 2019). If the risk is intermediate, or if there is uncertainty about one's risk, a coronary artery calcium score with a non-contrast computed tomography scan may be considered. Such estimates allow for a personalized approach to reducing the risk of cardiovascular disease and can enhance SDM (Mayo Clinic, 2015). One of the limitations is that several factors are not included in these risk calculators (e.g. family history of heart disease, pre-eclampsia, lipoprotein(a)), and risk may be over- or underestimated.

SDM tools to guide statin and blood pressure therapy for primary prevention of atherosclerotic heart disease have been shown to improve patient understanding of their risk, reduce decisional conflict, and possibly improve adherence to medications and reduce cardiovascular risk (Weymiller et al., 2007; Sheridan et al., 2014; Kask-Flight et al., 2021).

Regrettably, not all heart disease can be prevented, and chest pain is one of the most common reasons for emergency department visits. Of those presentations, there exists a wide range of patient severity and risk for acute coronary syndrome (i.e. heart attacks). The depth and appropriateness of SDM in these scenarios will fluctuate based on the acuity of the situation (Probst et al., 2017). In patients with low-risk chest pain, one large trial found that a PtDA improved patient knowledge, increased patient involvement, and patients were admitted less often (Hess et al., 2012). In higher-risk patients or those with acute coronary syndrome, patients describe reduced capacity to participate effectively and were relieved when the clinical care team made decisions for them, but once past this emergent phase, patients wanted to regain a more active role in their care (Wilson et al., 2017), highlighting further that as acuity changes, so too should the level of SDM and that one-time SDM is insufficient for most cardiovascular care.

Ongoing and iterative SDM is particularly meaningful for patients with chronic ischaemic heart disease (Coylewright, 2016). Research has shown that optimal medical therapy versus revascularization (e.g. stenting, coronary artery bypass graft surgery) are, on average, no different in preventing future heart attacks or death (Maron et al., 2020). However, some patients appear to benefit more from one approach than the other (Box 35.1) and patients with more chest pain at baseline are more likely to benefit from revascularization (Spertus et al., 2020); engaging patients in this decision is crucial.

Still, as with many other areas in medicine, clinician preference and practice can hinder patient-centred care, and an SDM intervention may not be enough to overcome entrenched physician practice. In this area, some clinicians report a lack of knowledge about SDM and are uncomfortable modifying their practices to include SDM (Coylewright et al., 2017). One PtDA trial showed that providing clinicians with the informed treatment preferences of their patients did not change what treatment that patient ultimately received (Doll et al., 2019). In addition to PtDAs and patient-level SDM interventions, interventions aimed at systems and clinician education and culture will be needed to improve patient-centred care.

Box 35.1 Patient perspective

'Shared decision is best' says a retired professor from Yale

As a retired Yale professor and an artist-photographer, I am used to being listened to and have learned to expect as much. So, the idea of SDM seems unremarkable to me: what physician or patient wouldn't want their working relationship based on honest communication? The difficulty, of course, is what to do about the physician's greater knowledge of the subject. Could it come down to everyone—especially the health professional—being willing to listen?

When I was first diagnosed with heart disease, prompted by problems with angina, my primary care doctor prescribed a 20 mg daily dose of rosuvastatin to help deal with the problem. I also received two stents, which, immediately and miraculously, I thought, relieved me of all discomfort. Having read various articles about statins, I was, like many people, 'philosophically' against taking them, but I went along with this prescription until pains in my legs convinced me that the dosage, if not the drug, had to change.

I was referred to the co-author of this chapter, Dr Erica S. Spatz, who, in response to my request (i.e. she listened), lowered the rosuvastatin dosage to 5 mg, which would be approximately 65% as efficacious as the amount I was taking.

So far, so good. Except that, with the passing years, I continued to have relatively high cholesterol levels. Given that I exercised regularly and followed an excellent diet, I wondered why. A review of my blood tests revealed the possible answer: I had been genetically 'gifted' with a high level of lipoprotein(a) in my blood, something which, at that time, was barely discussed in cardiological circles because there's little that can be done to lower that especially dangerous lipid. Although I had initially been sceptical about the hazard of cholesterol, this discovery led me to agree with Dr Spatz's suggestion to try the injectable drug Repatha to reduce my cholesterol level and, to a lesser degree, lipoprotein(a), something it did very effectively.

Eventually, though, I was forced last year to accept a third stent, even with my now extremely low cholesterol, primarily, if not entirely (I believe), due to my lipoprotein(a) levels. But at least I did all I could to deal with the problem.

This led me to conclude that I've been fortunate to have met doctors who have listened carefully to me and responded to my concerns. I'd say that I changed, too, by slowly accepting the principle that high cholesterol levels in the blood are unsafe. So yes, SDM and listening are good, if not the best, methods for developing a doctor–patient health plan.

Heart failure management and cardiac devices

As the population ages and as treatments for cardiovascular disease improve, there is a greater prevalence of congestive heart failure. Goal-directed medical therapy (GDMT) is the cornerstone of heart failure treatment showing improved quality of life, reduced hospitalizations, and lower mortality. Still, implementation is challenging, as GDMT requires frequent medication adjustments, which can result in greater pill burden, potential increase in out-of-pocket expenses, drug–drug interactions, and side effects. Whether or not cost should enter the SDM encounter is of considerable debate, but the addition of cost into an SDM model for GDMT is desired by patients (Dickert et al., 2020), and the degree of out-of-pocket costs impact patient willingness to accept treatment (Smith et al., 2019), although cost considerations are de-emphasized by clinicians (Venechuk et al., 2020).

Beyond GDMT, some patients with heart failure are at higher risk for sudden cardiac death, and implantable cardioverter–defibrillators (ICDs) have been shown to reduce this risk (Bardy et al., 2005). Implanting a resuscitative device is a value-laden decision. Discussions around the risk of sudden death, preferences for resuscitation, code status, and end-of-life care need to be included. Yet one study in Sweden found that 40% of patients with ICDs did not want to discuss this (Thompson et al., 2019), exhibiting the importance of assessing patient readiness for SDM. Although low, there are risks for complications of the procedure, infection, and a chance that an electrical shock is delivered when there is no life-threatening arrhythmia. Furthermore, two-thirds of patients will never receive a shock, highlighting the need to personalize risk and emphasize patient values (Merchant et al., 2020). SDM and PtDA use for ICDs is particularly consequential in the USA, as the largest public insurer (CMS) requires SDM and PtDAs for reimbursement. PtDAs for ICDs are now available and have been shown to be acceptable to patients (Wallace et al., 2021).

For patients with the most severe heart failure, transplantation is the gold standard, but a limited organ supply precludes transplantation for a vast majority of patients. Left ventricular assistant devices have been shown to extend life in such patients, but a left ventricular assistant device is a highly invasive procedure and requires considerable ongoing care and increased risk of serious harm or death. SDM with a PtDA has been shown to improve patient knowledge, reduce left ventricular assistant device use, and improve decision making, particularly in patients with low health literacy (Allen et al., 2018; Raymer et al., 2022). However, an SDM intervention has not been shown to improve concordance between patient preference and treatment received, highlighting potential other sources of influence (Allen et al., 2018). A website with decision aids to support complex cardiac device decisions is publicly available (https://patientdecisionaid.org/).

SDM gaps in cardiology

Despite the growing body of work on SDM and PtDA use in cardiology highlighted here, there are still several opportunities to advance patient-centred care in cardiology. Many barriers exist to implementing decision aids and realizing SDM in the everyday clinical environment, including system-level issues and the culture of medicine more broadly. Implementation research has begun to address these issues in both AF (Spencer-Bonilla et al., 2020) and cardiac devices (Matlock et al., 2020) and provide promising models for implementation (Matlock et al., 2020). But, to overcome these challenges, greater investment from healthcare systems, leaders, and government agencies will be needed if the promise of patient-centred care is to be realized. Such an integration will require a full view of the factors that go into the clinician–patient encounter and whether the current way in which healthcare systems are structured can be adapted to achieve this goal.

Importantly, as healthcare systems, society, and insurers target their focus on reducing healthcare disparities, especially in cardiovascular care, SDM may provide a mechanism for improving outcomes for patients of historically marginalized groups. While some PtDAs and SDM models in cardiovascular care have been explicitly designed with cultural, literacy, and numeracy tailoring (Sivly et al., 2022; Chiu et al., 2023; Thomas et al., 2023), some publicly available PtDAs may not apply to such populations (Bonner et al., 2019). At its core, SDM is about providing the best available evidence, being transparent about uncertainty, and supporting patient autonomy to achieve outcomes that are best aligned with individual values; time and training are necessary, and there needs to be intentional efforts to achieve health equity in decision making.

REFERENCES

Allen, L. A., McIlvennan, C. K., Thompson, J. S., et al. 2018. Effectiveness of an intervention supporting shared decision making for destination therapy left ventricular assist device: the DECIDE-LVAD randomized clinical trial. *JAMA Intern Med*, **178**, 520–529.

Arnett, D. K., Blumenthal, R. S., Albert, M. A., et al. 2019. 2019 ACC/AHA guideline on the primary prevention of cardiovascular disease: a report of the American College of Cardiology/American Heart Association Task Force on Clinical Practice Guidelines. *Circulation*, **140**, e596–e646.

Bardy, G. H., Lee, K. L., Mark, D. B., et al. 2005. Amiodarone or an implantable cardioverter–defibrillator for congestive heart failure. *N Engl J Med*, **352**, 225–237.

Bonner, C., Patel, P., Fajardo, M. A., Zhuang, R., Trevena, L. 2019. Online decision aids for primary cardiovascular disease prevention: systematic search, evaluation of quality and suitability for low health literacy patients. *BMJ Open*, **9**, e025173.

Chiu, H.-H., Chang, S. L., Cheng, H. M., et al. 2023. Shared decision making for anticoagulation reduces anxiety and improves adherence in patients with atrial fibrillation. *BMC Med Inform Decis Mak*, **23**, 163.

Chung, M. K., Fagerlin, A., Wang, P. J., et al. 2021. Shared decision making in cardiac electrophysiology procedures and arrhythmia management. *Circ Arrhythm Electrophysiol*, **14**, e007958.

Coylewright, M., Dick, S., Zmolek, B., et al. 2016. PCI Choice decision aid for stable coronary artery disease: a randomized trial. *Circ Cardiovasc Qual Outcomes*, **9**, 767–776.

Coylewright, M., O'Neill, E. S., Dick, S., Grande, S. W. 2017. PCI Choice: cardiovascular clinicians' perceptions of shared decision making in stable coronary artery disease. *Patient Educ Couns*, **100**, 1136–1143.

Dickert, N. W., Mitchell, A. R., Venechuk, G. E., et al. 2020. Show me the money: patients' perspectives on a decision aid for sacubitril/valsartan addressing out-of-pocket cost. *Circ Cardiovasc Qual Outcomes*, **13**, e007070.

Doll, J. A., Jones, W. S., Lokhnygina, Y., et al. 2019. PREPARED study: a study of shared decision-making for coronary artery disease. *Circ Cardiovasc Qual Outcomes*, **12**, e005244.

Hess, E. P., Knoedler, M. A., Shah, N. D., et al. 2012. The chest pain choice decision aid: a randomized trial. *Circ Cardiovasc Qual Outcomes*, **5**, 251–259.

Joglar, J.A., Chung, M. K., Armbruster, A. L., et al. 2024. 2023 ACC/AHA/ACCP/HRS guideline for the diagnosis and management of atrial fibrillation: a report of the American College of Cardiology/American Heart Association Joint Committee on Clinical Practice Guidelines. *Circulation*, **149**, e1–e156.

Kask-Flight, L., Durak, K., Suija, K., Rätsep, A., Kalda, R. 2021. Reduction of cardiovascular risk factors among young men with hypertension using an interactive decision aid: cluster-randomized control trial. *BMC Cardiovasc Disord*, **21**, 543.

Kunneman, M., Branda, M. E., Hargraves, I. G., et al. 2020. Assessment of shared decision-making for stroke prevention in patients with atrial fibrillation: a randomized clinical trial. *JAMA Intern Med*, **180**, 1215–1224.

MacDonald, B. J., Turgeon, R. D. 2023. Incorporation of shared decision-making in international cardiovascular guidelines, 2012–2022. *JAMA Netw Open*, **6**, e2332793.

Man-Son-Hing, M., Laupacis, A., O'Connor, A. M., et al. 2000. Development of a decision aid for atrial fibrillation who are considering antithrombotic therapy. *J Gen Intern Med*, **15**, 723–30.

Maron, D. J., Hochman, J. S., Reynolds, H. R., et al. 2020. Initial invasive or conservative strategy for stable coronary disease. *N Engl J Med*, **382**, 1395–1407.

Matlock, D. D., McIlvennan, C. K., Thompson, J. S., et al. 2020. Decision aid implementation among left ventricular assist device programs participating in the DECIDE-LVAD stepped-wedge trial. *Med Decis Making*, **40**, 289–301.

Matlock, D. D., Fukunaga, M. I., Tan, A., et al. 2020. Enhancing success of Medicare's shared decision making mandates using implementation science: examples applying the Pragmatic Robust Implementation and Sustainability Model (PRISM). *MDM Policy Pract*, **5**, 2381468320963070.

Mayo Clinic. 2015. Statin choice decision aid. Available at: https://statindecisionaid.mayoclinic.org/

McAlister, F. A., Man-Son-Hing, M., Straus, S. E., et al. 2005. Impact of a patient decision aid on care among patients with nonvalvular atrial fibrillation: a cluster randomized trial. *CMAJ*, **173**, 496–501.

Merchant, F. M., Levy, W. C., Kramer, D. B. 2020. Time to shock the system: moving beyond the current paradigm for primary prevention implantable cardioverter-defibrillator use. *J Am Heart Assoc*, **9**, e015139.

Noseworthy, P. A., Branda, M. E., Kunneman, M., et al. 2022. Effect of shared decision-making for stroke prevention on treatment adherence and safety outcomes in patients with atrial fibrillation: a randomized clinical trial. *J Am Heart Assoc*, **11**, e023048.

Probst, M. A., Kanzaria, H. K., Schoenfeld, E. M., et al. 2017. Shared decisionmaking in the emergency department: a guiding framework for clinicians. *Ann Emerg Med*, **70**, 688–695.

Raymer DS, Allen LA, Chaussee EL, et al. 2022. Health Literacy in Patients Considering a Left Ventricular Assist Device: Findings From the DECIDE-LVAD Trial. *Journal of Cardiac Failure*, **28**(8), 1318–1325.

Sheridan, S. L., Draeger, L. B., Pignone, M. P., et al. 2014. The effect of a decision aid intervention on decision making about coronary heart disease risk reduction: secondary analyses of a randomized trial. *BMC Med Inform Decis Mak*, **14**, 14.

Sivly, A., Gorr, H. S., Gravholt, D., et al. 2022. Enrolling people of color to evaluate a practice intervention: lessons from the shared decision-making for atrial fibrillation (SDM4AFib) trial. *BMC Health Serv Res*, **22**, 1032.

Smith, G. H., Shore, S., Allen, L. A., et al. 2019. Discussing out-of-pocket costs with patients: shared decision making for sacubitril-valsartan in heart failure. *J Am Heart Assoc*, **8**, e010635.

Spencer-Bonilla, G., Thota, A., Organick, P., et al. 2020. Normalization of a conversation tool to promote shared decision making about anticoagulation in patients with atrial fibrillation within a practical randomized trial of its effectiveness: a cross-sectional study. *Trials*, **21**, 395.

Spertus, J. A., Jones, P. G., Maron, D. J., et al. 2020. Health-status outcomes with invasive or conservative care in coronary disease. *N Engl J Med*, **382**, 1408–1419.

Thomas, K. L., Al-Khatib, S. M., Kosinski, A. S., et al. 2023. Facilitating shared decision making among black patients at risk for sudden cardiac arrest: a randomized clinical trial. *Ann Intern Med*, **176**, 615–623.

Thompson, J. H., Thylen, I., Moser, D. K. 2019. Shared decision-making about end-of-life care scenarios compared among implantable cardioverter defibrillator patients: a national cohort study. *Circ Heart Fail*, **12**, e005619.

Venechuk, G. E., Allen, L. A., Doermann Byrd, K., Dickert, N., Matlock, D. D. 2020. Conflicting perspectives on the value of neprilysin inhibition in heart failure revealed during development of a decision aid focusing on patient costs for sacubitril/valsartan. *Circ Cardiovasc Qual Outcomes*, **13**, e006255.

Wallace, B. C., Jones, J., Masoudi, F. A., et al. 2021. Development and piloting of four decision aids for implantable cardioverter-defibrillators in different media formats. *Pacing Clin Electrophysiol*, **44**, 1842–1852.

Wang, P. J., Lu, Y., Mahaffey, K. W., et al. 2023. Randomized clinical trial to evaluate an atrial fibrillation stroke prevention shared decision-making pathway. *J Am Heart Assoc*, **12**, e028562.

Weymiller, A. J., Montori, V. M., Jones, L. A., et al. 2007. Helping patients with type 2 diabetes mellitus make treatment decisions: statin choice randomized trial. *Arch Intern Med*, **167**, 1076–1082.

Wilson, T., Miller, J., Teare, S., et al. 2017. Patient perspectives on engagement in decision-making in early management of non-ST elevation acute coronary syndrome: a qualitative study. *BMC Med Inform Decis Mak*, **17**, 153.

36

Shared decision making in dermatology

Tessalyn Morrison, Rita Pipes, and Erin Foster

Introduction

Shared decision making (SDM) confers agency to patients by preparing them to anticipate choices between treatments, reviewing treatment options and making decisions that align with their values and preferences (Elwyn et al., 2012). Engaging patients as partners in decision making reduces paternalism common to the medical field when clinicians make decisions on behalf of patients. SDM is best used when multiple reasonable treatment options exist and in cases that depend on different aspects of the patient and disease. Dermatology is well suited to SDM because multiple treatment options are effective for many skin diseases. SDM helps incorporate important features of treatments, such as cost, route of administration, dosing frequency, and side effects, which are important factors in patient preferences and ability to adhere to medications as prescribed. As described, SDM helps patients become more collaborative (Box 36.1).

Patient preferences, symptoms, and quality of life are at the forefront of patient-reported outcomes research and education in dermatology. Patient support groups are active in research and advocacy, educating clinicians about life with skin disease. The current dermatology standard of care is transitioning from messy, uncomfortable topical medications applied all over the body to more liberal use of oral and injectable systemic medications. Many have direct-to-consumer advertising, and patients often prompt clinicians about these treatments. This is a challenge for clinicians, who must then provide information about treatment effectiveness, expected cost,

Box 36.1 Patient perspective

SDM as a way to become more collaborative

In 2022, at the age of 52, I was diagnosed with a chronic, 'rare' skin condition that I had never heard of. The provider gave me the diagnosis, provided little information, performed a biopsy that resulted in complications (some permanent), and prescribed medicine without clear instructions. I panicked and immediately began searching for information and a second opinion. I was fortunate that the provider I subsequently saw practised what I now know is SDM. She shared relevant details and treatment options for my condition and included me in treatment decisions. She solicited questions from me and addressed them. I realized that I had noticed symptoms for years, disregarded by previous providers. I also found support groups that helped deepen my understanding of my diagnosis and gave me a sense of community.

I began sharing my diagnosis with close friends and family, a diagnosis which is sensitive in nature and embarrassing to disclose. Several of them opened up about similar symptoms and their silent struggles. They sought care and were diagnosed with the same skin condition I have, which seems far more common to me now than 'rare' might indicate. I suggested to my provider that the public should be better informed and challenged her as to why a condition like this is not openly discussed, like cancer or heart disease. I have learned so much. My constant worry lessened. I am now better able to manage my condition, my treatment, and my overall well-being.

Reflecting on other serious health concerns I have had in my lifetime, I feel that if SDM had been practised, appropriate diagnosis and treatment would have happened sooner. I would have advocated for myself, sought second opinions, and followed treatment plans more readily.

I embrace SDM as a way to become more educated and collaborative. I felt empowered to be actively involved in SDM, though others may prefer a more passive role, which is also acceptable. I know several people who cannot decide for themselves for many reasons. Although we live in a time where data are available to anyone within seconds via a simple web search, not all people are inclined to gather the data. In some cases, they are discouraged by providers from doing any independent research. Some patients may end up more confused or overwhelmed than before diagnosis. In these cases, a patient may lean heavily on the support and expertise of their provider, who must try to determine what the patient understands and how to support decision making.

My provider could see that I was worried and needed more details on my condition and treatment. Although my care did not involve using a PtDA, I see how PtDAs and assessments provide a standardized way of documenting interest in SDM and how treatment decisions were made over time. Treatment plans can always be adjusted over time, as can a patient's involvement in the decision. Documentation of these changes and how decisions were made can help patients and clinicians track the care history.

We can all speak from experience that relationships benefit from open communication. SDM can enable open communication between patient and provider and lead to better outcomes, as it did for me. If the development of SDM tools is difficult, clinicians could put initial documents into use, and then commit to frequent reviews and improvements. Any tool as a starting point is better than no tool, and it will at least get these important conversations started.

and side effects and compare them with other treatment options. Therefore, conversations about such options are often avoided.

SDM is underutilized in dermatology. In a scoping review we performed in 2021, we identified only 29 studies on SDM practice in dermatology (Morrison et al., 2021), and there were only two studies of patient decision aids (PtDAs) appraised by the International Patient Decision Aid Standards (IPDAS) (Tan and Wolfe, 2012; McLellan et al., 2019). Since that publication, new data have emerged regarding patient preferences, detailing the needs related to SDM in patients with atopic dermatitis and psoriasis (van der Kraaij et al., 2020; Vermeulen et al., 2020; Foster et al., 2023; Yee et al., 2023). This research has shown that patients desire SDM in decisions around skin disease and express higher satisfaction with medical care when SDM is used (van der Kraaij et al., 2020; Vermeulen et al., 2020; Morrison et al., 2021; Foster et al., 2023; Yee et al., 2023). In 2022, the US Preventive Services Task Force issued a call for more collaboration and SDM between patients and clinicians in preventive health decisions, which include skin cancer prevention (US Preventive Services Task Force, 2022). This has been paired with the widespread adoption of SDM in the medical school curricula, meaning students are more familiar with the practice of SDM and will expect to use these skills (Durand et al., 2018).

Unique opportunities for SDM in dermatology

For most skin diseases, there are multiple treatment options, with varying effects on quality of life related to cost, route of administration, side effects, and dosing frequency. SDM is an important part of continuity care for dermatology patients as skin disease changes over time, and most patients have disease flares due to the natural history of their diseases and changing stressors in their lives. Patients are experts in their skin and can monitor whether a treatment works in real time. Given the continuity of care with ever-changing treatment options, the relationship between dermatologists and patients requires trust and shared decisions to ensure treatment success.

The principles of SDM are already relatively familiar to most dermatologists. Many clinicians already discuss patient preferences for topical formulations or timelines in which to expect symptomatic relief. Multidisciplinary care can be required for certain dermatological conditions, and clinicians use SDM among colleagues to arrive at a treatment decision. Allergists and dermatologists work together to treat atopic dermatitis and eczema, and wound care experts help people with ulcers, hidradenitis, or pyoderma granulosum. Skin cancer patients are cared for in collaboration with medical, surgical, and radiation oncologists. In complex medical dermatology, rheumatologists and dermatologists prescribe systemic treatments used in tandem or in sequence, often with significant side effects. In oral and genital diseases, dermatologists coordinate treatment with dentists, gynaecologists, and rheumatologists.

SDM is particularly important for dermatology patients who may experience adverse experiences with treatment, whether physical, emotional, or financial. Patients, especially those with systemic or rare diseases, often need to trial multiple medications to find one that may be effective and tolerable while dealing with visible disease. In surgical dermatology, significant scarring is left in areas of prior skin biopsies and cancer treatments. Many dermatological medications are expensive with variable insurance coverage, and very few cosmetic interventions are covered by insurance. Throughout this process, patients can experience stress, pain, and embarrassment with their skin disease and deal with financial hardship and regret. Understanding options, including the outlook for future options, can help patients navigate their care as preferences, priorities, and treatment options change over time.

Patient decision aids and other SDM tools

SDM tools, including PtDAs, are developed to provide evidence-based information to help clinicians and patients arrive at a decision that aligns with the patient's goals. These tools can come in various formats, including decision grids, narrative descriptions, videos, and other imagery. In a broad sense, all publicly available information supports patient decision making, highlighting the importance of SDM practices and PtDAs to organize and assess extensive amounts of information directed at patients. High-quality PtDAs can help standardize care practices, encourage clinicians to stay up to date with evidence-based care, and help clinical learners know what is important to discuss with patients.

In dermatology, some PtDAs have been evaluated in clinic settings available for acne (Cameron et al., 2018; McLellan et al., 2019; Hung et al., 2022), psoriasis (Renzi et al., 2006; Tan and Wolfe, 2012; Strohal et al., 2015; Cameron et al., 2018; van Huizen et al., 2023), basal cell carcinoma (Banks et al., 2022; van Delft et al., 2023), melanoma (Vaidya et al., 2021), hidradenitis suppurativa (McLean et al., 2020), and vitiligo (Shourick et al., 2021). There are also PtDAs available that have not been evaluated in the clinical setting for psoriasis (Smith et al., 2020; van der Kraaij et al., 2020, 2021; Vermeulen et al., 2020; Monks et al., 2021; Nahirney et al., 2021), atopic dermatitis (American College of Allergy, Asthma, and Immunology, n.d.), melanoma (Wilson et al., 2023), basal cell carcinoma (Junn et al., 2020; Wilson et al., 2023), eczema (Vermeulen et al., 2020), hidradenitis suppurative (McBride et al., 2020), and rosacea (InforMED, n.d.).

It is important to note that the end points in these studies vary and may not align with the goal of a clinician adopting the PtDA at their institution. Unfortunately, it is difficult to find copies of the PtDAs and determine which have been studied in clinical use. In reviewing PtDAs, clinicians and patients should be wary of conflicts of interest and commercial involvement.

The success of PtDAs depends heavily on the people using them: how they are presented and how they are received. Tools may need to be adapted based on the availability of medications, updated information about treatments, patient health literacy, visit lengths, access to electronic resources, and expectations around insurance coverage. These needs reflect reported barriers to using SDM. SDM, as a way of practising medicine, involves consistently adapting tools as new information arrives, meaning that clinicians should be involved in creating SDM tools for their practice.

Addressing challenges to implementing SDM in the clinic

Previously identified challenges to implementing SDM in dermatology include the need for more clinic time, formal training, and tools for discussing treatment options (Morrison et al., 2010). As

Table 36.1 Steps in creating a SDM practice in dermatology

Format	First steps	Next steps
Reflection	Review how you currently present options to your patients and what has made past encounters mutually satisfactory	Visualize what successful SDM looks like for you in your practice and create goals to meet this vision.
Education	Review evidence-based treatment information, including benefits, side effects, and monitoring practices Collect and review available patient resources and PtDAs related to diseases you treat	Request information about patient costs and coverage under common insurance plans Seek training opportunities for learning how to practise SDM
Experimentation	Create a PtDA prototype Tailor treatment discussions to health literacy, cultural practices, and accessibility needs	Create PtDAs and processes utilizing patient input Consider alternate formats of PtDAs, timelines for discussing treatment options, and accessibility to information
Measuring	Assess what patients understand about options presented at their visit Ask patients about their interest in SDM	Solicit feedback about patient satisfaction with the depth and clarity of options discussed
Sharing	Share SDM interest and practices with colleagues	Teach learners and practitioners about SDM Integrate SDM tools into the electronic health record

demonstrated in our scoping review, utilization of most SDM tools, including PtDAs, took less than 5 minutes (Morrison et al., 2010). In addition, the two validated PtDAs published online were designed to be used by the patient before or after clinic, not taking time away from discussion with the clinician (Tan and Wolfe, 2012; McLellan et al., 2019). The rapid pace of care in dermatology also presents an opportunity for using SDM. Most clinic visits are short, lasting at most 10–20 minutes, and there is rarely time to answer all questions about treatment. With clinicians spending more time charting and responding to patient messages, high-quality PtDAs can serve as time-saving tools to address the most frequently asked patient questions. As patients navigate extensive online information, PtDAs could also support clinicians in explaining treatment options. It can be optimal to have tools to help facilitate decision making both inside and outside the clinic visit and across multiple visits. Medicare reimbursement rules implemented in 2022 in the USA allow clinicians to bill specifically for time spent counselling the patient on treatment options. Dermatology has yet to follow other specialties in requiring the use of SDM for payment of services rendered, but this could also encourage more use of SDM in everyday practice.

In terms of training, medical schools have implemented curricula on SDM, and students are ready to practice SDM in dermatology (Durand et al., 2018). Online curricula exist and could easily be incorporated into dermatology residency didactics or grand rounds. Demonstration of SDM in the clinic by a dermatologist can sometimes remove the last remaining hesitation for a student or resident to use an approach that they have learned about in theory. There are not enough PtDAs or other SDM tools specific to dermatological conditions, but this is not the largest barrier to using SDM. In the authors' opinion, the largest barrier to implementing SDM in dermatology is an unwillingness to reimagine the patient–clinician dynamic towards patients knowing about treatment options sufficiently enough to advocate for treatment under the guidance of a clinician. When clinicians reorient their care practices to include patients in treatment decisions, they are likely to find or create the tools necessary to do so.

How to develop a SDM practice

SDM improves patient satisfaction and outcomes and has been outlined as the standard of care by the Centers for Medicaid and Medicare Services (Alston et al., 2014). No models or guidelines exist for incorporating SDM into dermatology practice specifically, though models for implementing SDM have been developed for general medical practice. The National Health Service has shared its SDM implementation model, which suggests involving SDM at all levels of care, providing SDM training for clinicians, tailoring SDM programmes to health literacy needs, and measuring the effects of using SDM (NHS England, n.d.). Implementing a complete practice of SDM requires professional and systemic change over time. We suggest a step-wise approach, starting with one's own clinical practice, including practice changes as possible and appropriate for the clinical setting (Table 36.1).

PtDAs can be adopted from those already published or newly created based on clinician needs and interests. The IPDAS Collaboration has provided minimal standards for what should be included in a PtDA (Joseph-Williams et al., 2014), which are more practical and achievable than prior standards for those wanting to design their own. Scales commonly used in dermatology measure interest in SDM (e.g. Control Preferences Scale), the success of SDM (collaborate), and disease activity (Dermatology Life Quality Index, SkinDex, Patient Global Assessment, and Visual Analog Scales) (Morrison et al., 2021). Clinicians may already be using some of these indices in the practice, for example, for prior authorization for biological treatments.

Conclusion

The need for SDM in dermatology is clear, yet the path forward for increasing the utilization of SDM in dermatology is not. While institutional policies and educational programmes are created, interested clinicians create and share SDM practices for their clinical environments. We suggest clinicians start with small incremental goals in improving their SDM practice, keeping aspirational goals for balanced decision making in mind. Future areas of focus should address systems to support SDM in dermatology through training for SDM in medical education, access to continued medical education, development of reimbursement mechanisms, integration of SDM tools into the electronic health record, advancing technology for SDM practices and evaluation, and sharing mechanisms for PtDAs and SDM practices among clinicians. As more therapies become available and standards of care change in dermatology, the mechanisms for disseminating evidence-based care must also improve so that clinicians can confidently present all treatment options. Finally, increasing transparency to patient costs and reducing unnecessary prior authorization processes would help clinicians provide information about cost which is vital for patients. While we address these systemic needs, we hope clinicians will recognize the need for SDM and its utility find ways to incorporate SDM into their practice.

REFERENCES

Alston, C., Berger, Z., Brownlee, S., et al. 2014. Shared decision-making strategies of care: patient decision aids. Institute of Medicine. Available at: https://nam.edu/perspectives/shared-decision-making-strategies-for-best-care-patient-decision-aids/

American College of Allergy, Asthma, and Immunology. n.d. Atopic dermatitis (eczema) shared decision making toolkit. Available at: https://college.acaai.org/practice-management/clinical-tools/

Banks, J., Odili, J., Zaidi, S., et al. 2022. The development and validation of a decision aid to facilitate patient choice of surgery versus radiotherapy for high-risk basal cell carcinoma. *Clin Exp Dermatol*, **47**, 1995–1997.

Cameron, M., Tan, J., McLellan, C., et al. 2018. Development of patient decision aids for plaque psoriasis and acne. *Dermatol Online J*, **24**, 13030/qt6z27q8bq.

Durand, M. A., DiMilia, P. R., Song, J., Yen, R. W., Barr, P. J. 2018. Shared decision making embedded in the undergraduate medical curriculum: a scoping review. *PLoS One*, **13**, e0207012.

Elwyn, G., Frosch, D., Thomson, R., et al. 2012. Shared decision making: a model for clinical practice. *J Gen Intern Med*, **27**, 1361–1367.

Foster, E., Loiselle, A. R., Thibau, I. J., Smith Begolka, W. 2023. Factors facilitating shared decision making in eczema: met and unmet needs from the patient perspective. *JAAD Int*, **11**, 95–102.

Hung, C. T., Chen, Y. H., Hung, T. L., Chiang, C. P., Chen, C. Y., Wang, W. M. 2022. Clinician-created educational video for shared decision-making in the outpatient management of acne. *PLoS One*, **17**, e0271100.

InforMED. n.d. Rosacea decision aid. Available at: https://www.informed-decisions.org/rosaceapda.php

Joseph-Williams, N., Newcombe, R., Politi, M., et al. 2014. Toward minimum standards for certifying patient decision aids: a modified Delphi consensus process. *Med Decis Making*, **34**, 699–710.

Junn, A., Shukla, N. R., Morrison, L., et al. 2020. Development of a patient decision aid for the management of superficial basal cell carcinoma (BCC) in adults with a limited life expectancy. *BMC Med Inform Decision Mak*, **20**, 81.

McBride, O., McLean, D., Samardzic, T., et al. 2020. Development of a hidradenitis suppurativa patient decision aid. *Dermatol Online J*, **26**, 13030/qt18p1n8tt.

McLean, D., McBride, O., Samardzic, T., Sisic, M., Dellavalle, R. P., Tan, J. 2020. Impact of a hidradenitis suppurativa patient decision aid on treatment decision making: a randomized controlled trial. *JAAD Int*, **1**, 190–199.

McLellan, C., O'Neil, A. I., Cameron, M., et al. 2019. Facilitating informed treatment decisions in acne: a pilot study of a patient decision aid. *J Cutan Med Surg*, **23**, 117–118.

Monks, G., Rivera-Oyola, R., Lebwohl, M. 2021. The psoriasis decision tree. *J Clin Aesthet Dermatol*, **14**, 14–22.

Morrison, T., Johnson, J., Baghoomian, W., et al. 2021. Shared decision-making in dermatology: a scoping review. *JAMA Dermatol*, **157**, 330–337.

Nahirney, M., Hum, M., Mathura, P., Dytoc, M. 2021. Psoriasis education tool for patient–physician decision-making about biologics: a pilot study. *Skin Therapy Lett*, **26**, 4–10.

NHS England. n.d. How to make shared decision making happen: shared decision implementation model. Available at: https://www.england.nhs.uk/personalisedcare/shared-decision-making/how-to-make-shared-decision-making-happen/

Renzi, C., Di Pietro, C., Gisondi, P., et al. 2006. Insufficient knowledge among psoriasis patients can represent a barrier to participation in decision-making. *Acta Derm Venereol*, **86**, 528–534.

Shourick, J., Ahmed, M., Seneschal, J., et al. 2021. Development of a shared decision-making tool in vitiligo: an international study. *Br J Dermatol*, **185**, 787–796.

Smith, C. H., Yiu, Z. Z. N., Bale, T., et al. 2020. British Association of Dermatologists guidelines for biologic therapy for psoriasis 2020: a rapid update. *Br J Dermatol*, **183**, 628–637.

Strohal, R., Prinz, J. C., Girolomoni, G., Nast, A. 2015. A patient-centred approach to biological treatment decision making for psoriasis: an expert consensus. *J Eur Acad Dermatol Venereol*, **29**, 2390–2398.

Tan, J., Wolfe, B. 2012. A patient decision aid for psoriasis based on current clinical practice guidelines. *Arch Dermatol*, **148**, 718–723.

US Preventive Services Task Force. 2022. Collaboration and shared decision-making between patients and clinicians in preventive health care decisions and US Preventive Services Task Force Recommendations. *JAMA*, **327**, 1171–1176.

Vaidya, T. S., Bander, T. S., Musthaq, S., et al. 2021. Validation of a patient decision aid for the treatment of lentigo maligna. *J Am Acad Dermatol*, **84**, 1751–1753.

Van Delft, L. C. J., Essers, B. A. B., Nelemans, P. J., et al. 2023. Effectiveness of a patient decision aid for patients with superficial basal cell carcinoma: a pre- and post-implementation study. *Patient Educ Couns*, **115**, 107907.

Van der Kraaij, G. E., van Huizen, A. M., Baerveldt, E. M., et al. 2021. Online decision aid for patients with psoriasis. *Br J Dermatol*, **184**, 981–983.

Van der Kraaij, G. E., Vermeulen, F. M., Smeets, P. M. G., Smets, E. M. A., Spuls, P. J. 2020. The current extent of and need for shared decision making in atopic dermatitis and psoriasis in the Netherlands: an online survey study amongst patients and physicians. *J Eur Acad Dermatol Venereol*, **34**, 2574–2583.

Van Huizen, A. M., Rietbergen, N. J., van der Kraaij, G. E., Ubbink, D. T., Spuls, P. I. 2023. Effectiveness and patient satisfaction of a Dutch patient decision aid for psoriasis—a pilot study. *J Dermatolog Treat*, **34**, 2186157.

Vermeulen, F. M., van der Kraaij, G. E., Tupker, R. A., et al. 2020. Towards more shared decision making in dermatology: development of evidence-based decision cards for psoriasis and atopic eczema treatments. *Acta Derm Venereol*, **100**, 5863.

Wilson, B. N., Shah, R., Musthaq, S., Vaidya, T.; American Society for Dermatologic Surgery/Advocacy (ASDS/A) initiative the Policy Priorities Work Group. 2023. Development of patient decision aids for the treatment of lentigo maligna and low-risk basal cell carcinoma. *J Am Acad Dermatol*, **88**, 440–442.

Yee, D., Kingston, P., Lee, K., Peterson, H., Korouri, E., Armstrong, A. 2023. Shared decision-making and satisfaction with care in patients with psoriasis: a population-based study in the United States. *J Am Acad Dermatol*, **83**, 920–926.

37

Shared decision making in vascular surgery

Elisabeth Smith, Daniel C. Norvell, Dirk T. Ubbink, Michael Mcloughlin, and David C. Bosanquet

Introduction

Vascular surgery is a surgical specialty that manages conditions affecting the circulatory system, including diseases of the arteries, veins, and lymphatic system. Vascular disease often develops over a period of years and is heavily influenced by the presence of risk factors such as smoking and diabetes. For this reason, many patients only require lifestyle modification advice and medications, such as antiplatelets and statins. Nevertheless, as many as 50% of vascular patients present urgently, sometimes requiring emergency surgical intervention (Royal College of Surgeons of England, n.d.). Surgical procedures range from endovascular angioplasties (the ballooning and stenting of narrowed or occluded vessels), to major surgery such as open abdominal aortic aneurysm (AAA) repair or major lower limb amputation. For those procedures where there is both time and opportunity to consider the risks and benefits of different surgical options, a shared decision making (SDM) approach is a viable and important paradigm. It should be considered an ethical and legal requirement of modern medicine.

Certain aspects of vascular surgery lend themselves to SDM, but it is challenging to adopt in other areas. Given the chronic and progressive nature of the underlying disease process, some patients can be identified early, to provide information and initiate non-invasive management. This information sharing, question asking and eliciting of values can take place over several months, or even years, giving patients the best chance of satisfactory SDM, should the need for intervention arise. Some vascular surgical interventions can be considered 'preventive', in that the patient is asymptomatic, yet is considering a potentially risky intervention to reduce the long-term risk of a catastrophic event (e.g. repair to prevent AAA rupture). In these circumstances, there is time for deliberation. Decisions regarding these types of procedures often delve into personal values and circumstances in the absence of a 'right' or 'wrong' choice (Xu and Prince, 2019). On the other hand, vascular disease frequently manifests as an urgent presentation mandating rapid intervention, such as aortic dissections or critical limb-threatening ischaemia. Life- or limb-threatening events can leave little time for careful consideration of risks and outcomes, and even less time for collaboration.

A significant amount of research has gone into the role of SDM in patient and clinical outcomes within vascular surgery, and how we can overcome barriers, and yet in practice it is very much still in its infancy. This is not due to doubts over its applicability to practice, ethical justification, or a lack of interest in its implementation, but rather due to deep-rooted organizational and cultural barriers. The modern-day healthcare system, with its targets and financial incentives, is designed for maximum patient turnover with minimal spend, and makes the deliberative, personalized approach that is SDM a challenge.

This chapter will explore patient and clinician experiences of SDM in the vascular surgery setting, and the data and risk stratification tools available for both physicians and patients to use in the SDM process.

SDM in vascular surgery

SDM in vascular surgery has the potential to improve both patient and surgeon well-being and satisfaction, reduce decisional conflict, and ultimately facilitate a more effective use of healthcare. A 2018 American study with over 63,000 respondents reported that 'poor SDM was associated with worse patient-reported health outcomes, worse established quality indicators, and higher healthcare utilization'(Hughes et al., 2018). Interestingly, the same report also found that those same consultations that rated SDM as poor resulted in lower rates of statin and aspirin use, two drugs recommended to most vascular patients to reduce their risks of secondary cardiovascular events as part of best medical therapy.

From the patients' perspective, several studies suggest they want and need more information about what to expect, both physically but also emotionally and psychologically. A large systematic review evaluating patient preferences in SDM found 71% of studies indicated that patients want to be active partners with their doctors in making healthcare decisions (Chewning et al., 2011).

SDM also has the potential to drastically change the way we manage common vascular conditions. The Dutch 2022 OVIDIUS study set out to improve SDM within vascular consultations with the use of decision support tools for patients, and training for

Table 37.1 Patient- and clinician-reported barriers to SDM and suggestions for better SDM in vascular surgery consultations

Barriers to SDM in vascular surgical consults		Suggestions for improving SDM in vascular surgical consults	
Perceived unequal patient/surgeon relationship	Santema et al., 2017	A good patient–clinician relationship based on trust	Santema et al., 2017
Poor clinician communication	Santema et al., 2017	Good communication	Santema et al., 2017; Leonard et al., 2023
Poor continuity of care (different clinicians)	Santema et al., 2017	Enough time for deliberation	Santema et al., 2017
Poor clinician preparation for consultation	Santema et al., 2017	Multidisciplinary team approach	Leonard et al., 2023
Patient characteristics (cognition, poor hearing/vision, acutely unwell)	Leonard et al., 2023	Sufficient and honest information sharing	Leonard et al., 2023
Patient overwhelmed by emotional/psychological distress from the idea of major amputation	Leonard et al., 2023	Feeling involved in the process of discussion, even if the final decision lay with the surgeon	Leonard et al., 2023
Emergency presentation necessitating urgent surgery	Leonard et al., 2023	Earlier provision and more detailed written information along with signposting to quality online information	Lecouturier et al., 2023
		Attendance of family at clinic appointments	Lecouturier et al., 2023
		Time to consider treatment options	Lecouturier et al., 2023

physicians. This improved SDM, as evidenced by a 9.1% increase in OPTION score (see Chapter 11), while also significantly improving patient knowledge, with AAA patients' knowledge increasing 40% after using a decision support tool. Notably, the intervention also resulted in patients choosing fewer surgical treatments; the number of patients with AAAs at treatment threshold who chose conservative treatment increased nearly fourfold, from 7.4% to 28.8%, while twice as many patients with intermittent claudication chose non-surgical treatment options (from 16% to 32%) (Stubenrouch et al., 2022). Consistent with SDM in other surgical fields, introducing SDM could result in fewer operations, enabling cost-saving and risk-eliminating benefits as a result.

Reassuringly, there is a growing body of evidence looking at SDM in vascular surgery, which shows a willingness and a want to enhance SDM in this field. Nevertheless, analyses of SDM behaviour in vascular surgery consultations by Santema and colleagues highlighted two interesting points (Santema et al., 2016). The first, that patients and surgeons consistently rated the level of SDM as significantly higher than what was observed (median SDM-Q-9 93% and median SDM-Q-Doc 84% versus median OPTION score of 31%[1]). One possible explanation is that there is a lack of understanding of SDM among patients and surgeons alike, and they have rated the overall satisfaction of the consultation, rather than the level of SDM. Second, the observed levels of SDM were below what may be considered 'baseline skill'. There is clearly a need for SDM education, not least to teach SDM, but to enhance clinicians' appreciation of its benefits and the opportunities for SDM in vascular surgery. Education and training in SDM for vascular surgeons can independently and significantly improve the level of SDM (Stubenrouch et al., 2022). A concept not well understood is hard to adopt, and even harder to implement.

Other barriers include the perception that SDM is time intensive, a concern that is not unfounded; studies have found that good SDM correlates with the duration of the clinical encounter (the longer the consultation, the better the observed SDM) (Peters et al., 2022). However, a 2023 systematic review and meta-analysis found that, once clinicians have been SDM trained, consultations do not necessarily take more time (van Veenendaal et al., 2023). Table 37.1 explores other perceived barriers to SDM in vascular surgery consultations and patients' suggestions for improvement.

Good surgeon communication (in terms of non-verbal skills and information provision) as a suggestion to help improve SDM may seem trivial, but it is a concept on which the success or failure of SDM is balanced. In a 2015 study into the decision making experienced by patients undergoing elective procedures for vascular problems, 90% of participants agreed with discussing all available treatment options. And yet in that same study, only 54% had been offered a choice between multiple treatment options and 48% had not been given alternate options (Corriere et al., 2015). Without tools to help facilitate SDM, its implementation is unlikely. Various decision support tools are available and should be considered for development to overcome these barriers and challenges to SDM implementation.

Bridging the gap—information provision, decision aids, and risk calculators

Evidence-based decision support tools and patient decision aids (PtDAs) (see Chapters 18–20), help mitigate some of the aforementioned barriers, by promoting more patient–physician conversations around treatment options. PtDAs are more than just educational materials (e.g. information leaflets). Effective PtDAs are developed and based on the International Patient Decision Aid Standards (see Chapter 18). In summary, these standards require that PtDAs have both an informational component that compares the risks and benefits of the potential options, and decision support elements that

1 SDM is measured by questionnaires: SDM-Q-9 is a patient-reported outcome measure, rating the perceived level of SDM experienced during the consultation. Similarly, the SDM-Q-Doc questionnaire is completed by the consulting doctor and rates their own perception of SDM behaviour. The OPTION (Observing Patient Involvement) instrument can be used to score SDM specific behaviour observed in a consultation.

guide the patient to choose an option that best matches their priorities and preferences. Indeed, it is this explicitness of identifying personal preferences, and 'what's important to me' (the patient), that seems to be often lacking in consultations. Traditionally, patients consistently report a lack of support when deliberating options (Peters et al., 2022), a perceived lack of respect of patients' opinions (Leonard et al., 2023), and a lack of opportunity to ask questions (Corriere et al., 2015). Conversely, several studies have shown the positive impact that PtDAs have on reducing decisional conflict and improving knowledge and decisional satisfaction (Coronado-Vázquez et al., 2020). A Cochrane review also highlights that PtDAs enabled more accurate risk perception by patients, and improved knowledge (see Chapter 19).

Three types of PtDAs (decision aids themselves, also consultation cards and decision cards) specifically for vascular conditions (AAA, carotid artery disease, intermittent claudication, and varicose veins) were designed and tested in 2021 with a good reception by both clinicians and patients (de Mik et al., 2021). Examples of other aids readily available for patients and physicians, include online modules for patients available at https://keuzehulp.medify.eu/KeuzehulpMedify/keuzehulp_medify.html (**Figure 37.1**) and the AMPDECIDE PtDAs (https://www.ampdecide.org/) (Norvell et al., 2021) (**Figure 37.2**).

Such aids that provide average patient risks are based on what is available in the literature; however, in the spirit of personalized care, risk calculators are an important adjunct to SDM. These provide patient-specific risks that are first interpreted by the surgeon, then carefully shared with the patient. The risks may include mortality and morbidity after various interventions, such as the likelihood of mobility after major lower limb amputation, and quality of life following AAA repair. A UK study of 13 such tools to predict outcomes following major lower limb amputation found, although largely reliable in predicting outcomes such as mortality or postoperative complications, there was a significant lack of tools that predict quality of life after such major surgery (Preece et al., 2021).

PtDAs and personalized risk prediction scores are important, not least because of the absence of reliable information elsewhere. Type 'what is vascular disease' into google, and within 0.36 seconds it retrieves an incomprehensible 467 million results (in 2024). A 2022 American study looked at the quality of online resources for patients with peripheral artery disease, and found that most are of variable quality, and are written at a level higher than the average US reading level, thus making them inaccessible. Furthermore, publications in leading surgical journals too often fall short in providing information relevant to SDM (Stubenrouch et al., 2020). Interestingly, websites from hospitals or healthcare organizations scored the lowest in terms of accountability, interactivity, structure, and content (Treffalls et al., 2022).

See **Box 37.1** for our patient perspective.

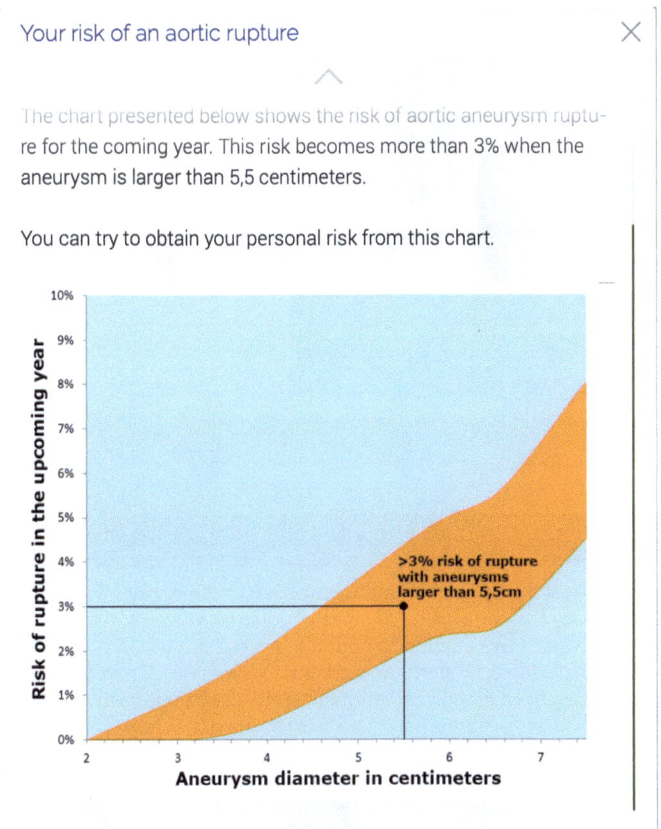

Figure 37.1 Risk representation for rupture of AAA.
Reproduced from Medify (https://medify.eu/).

Now what?

There is a need and a want to enhance SDM in vascular surgery, evident by the growing body of literature on the subject. SDM is significantly overreported in vascular surgery, with clinicians misinterpreting giving patients a choice with SDM; typically 'clinicians base(d) their own treatment decision predominantly on clinical factors rather than patient preference' (Lecouturier et al., 2023). We have also seen just how effective SDM can be, with better adherence to treatment, patients opting for non-surgical management, as well as improving important patient-reported outcomes such as satisfaction, well-being, and quality of life. Nevertheless, more development work is needed before SDM becomes integrated into the field, and there are certainly gaps in research that should be investigated. SDM has been well researched in AAA consultations, but more could be done to look at whether the findings are applicable to major lower limb amputation, carotid surgery, and diabetic foot complications, and what the state of SDM is in critical presentations requiring urgent surgery.

Despite these caveats, there is enough compelling evidence to develop both clinician SDM training and the implementation of PtDAs in consultations now, as there are several evidence-based PtDAs and risk calculators readily available for use. Lastly, the US Agency for Healthcare Research and Quality's SHARE programme has a comprehensive guide to training in SDM. The programme is an online platform that trains providers on the five steps of SDM, including identifying the risks and benefits of each option through conversation with patients about what matters most to them (Agency for Healthcare Research and Quality, 2024).

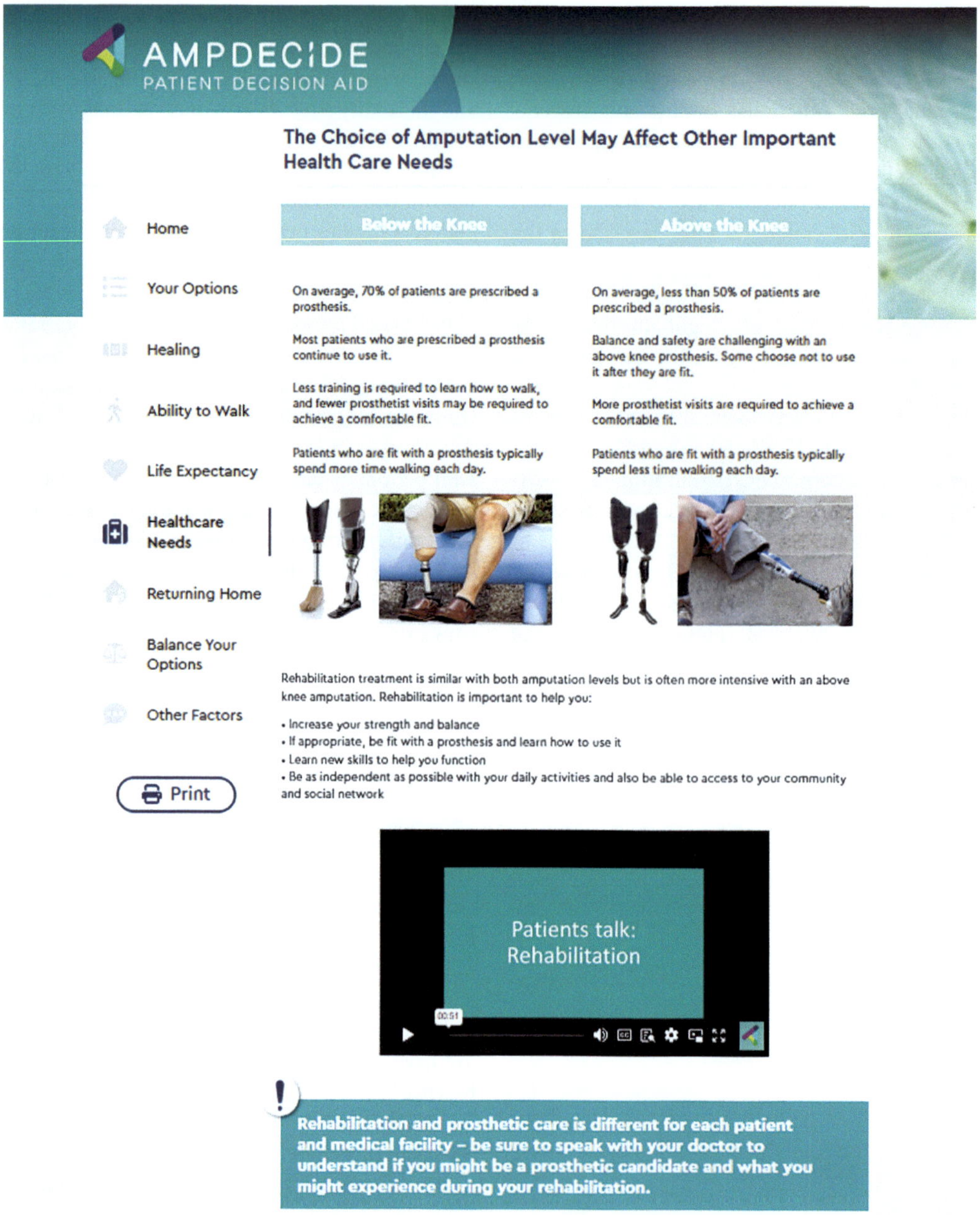

Figure 37.2 Example of the AMPDECIDE patient decision aids.

Box 37.1 Patient perspective

In January 2008, as my wife and I lay in bed, she suddenly said, 'I can feel a pulsation in your abdomen'. In response to her concern, I arranged a Doppler test, which revealed an AAA of 4.8 cm. I was also asked if I had stopped smoking. I realized it was serious, so I was keen to seek further information. My general practitioner referred me to a consultant surgeon who reassured me that imminent rupture was unlikely because of its size. A watching brief of regular scans would monitor the aortic diameter. The surgeon made himself available for follow-up questions and promptly responded. All treatments were thoroughly aired in plain language.

When the aneurysm reached 6.5 cm. I was offered a choice of an aortic stent or graft, with full explanations and associated risks. I was particularly alert to the risk to life that the graft option involved and having discussed the options with my family I decided on a stent. I was aware that this would involve regular follow-ups. The operation, in 2009, was a success.

For 3 years the computed tomography/X-rays came every 6 months, and annually thereafter. After 11 years of carefree freedom, a leak was found in 2020. I was advised to consider an endovascular extension to the stent, to which I promptly agreed. Success followed, apart from my experiencing a few months of discomfort in my left buttock when walking.

I began to feel progressively more bloated; my appetite was affected, and I lost a considerable amount of weight. In 2021, I developed a severe pain in my lower abdomen and following a 999 call I was admitted to hospital. Another leak was found and I was told this was more serious. I was initially placed in palliative care, because I was not in a good physical condition and an operation was ruled out. After several scans to determine the nature and location of the problem it was deemed possible to insert another extension. A team was assembled, and the outcome was again a success.

Annual ultrasound monitoring scan was carried out in July 2023. It showed that the aneurysm had increased from 7.3 cm to 8.5 cm over the previous 12 months. The surgeon advised me to stop driving. He organized a computed tomography scan so that he could determine the full nature of the problem.

It was then made clear to me that my situation was very serious, especially given my age (82 years) and the fact that other body systems were impaired. Because the graft operation was considered challenging, the advice of further surgical colleagues was requested. It was clearly stated, in the presence of my wife, that there was a 50/50 risk to life as well as possible problems with kidneys, bowels, and even some paralysis of nerves. I was repeatedly asked, in the light of these problems, whether I wished to proceed with the graft operation and my wife supported my complete and unreserved choice of proceeding. A team meeting was arranged where all the surgical team and supportive staff were to be gathered together to decide if the operation should go ahead. To my relief, the operation took place and was promptly considered a success.

I then spent several days in intensive care, during which time I developed a temporary psychosis, telling my family I needed rescuing from a clinic in France where I was being kept against my will! I am now fully recovered, regaining some of my lost weight and not missing my years without cigars!

In conclusion, I have enjoyed the frankness of discussions and the opportunity to discuss the pros and cons of all interventions with my family. Of interest, my three brothers have developed the same condition yet not one of them smoked. It is a testament to the skills of all involved that I was able to put the decorations on the family Christmas tree that year, which was my initial target before the surgery.

REFERENCES

Agency for Healthcare Research and Quality. 2024. The SHARE approach. Available at: https://www.ahrq.gov/health-literacy/professional-training/shared-decision/index.html

Chewning, B., Bylund, C., Shah, B., Arora, N., Gueguen, J. A., Makoul, G. 2011. Patient preferences for shared decisions: a systematic review. *Patient Educ Couns,* **86**, 9–18.

Coronado-Vázquez, V., Canet-Fajas, C., Delgado-Marroquín, M. T., Magallón-Botaya, R., Romero-Martín, M., Gómez-Salgado, J. 2020. Interventions to facilitate shared decision-making using decision aids with patients in primary health care: a systematic review. *Medicine (Baltimore),* **99**, e21389.

Corriere, M. A., Avise, J. A., Peterson, L. A., et al. 2015. Exploring patient involvement in decision making for vascular procedures. *J Vasc Surg,* **62**, 1032–1039.

de Mik, S. M. L., Stubenrouch, F. E., Balm, R. 2021. Development of three different decision support tools to support shared decision-making in vascular surgery. *Patient Educ Couns,* **104**, 282–289.

Hughes, T. M., Merath, K., Chen, Q., et al. 2018. Association of shared decision-making on patient-reported health outcomes and healthcare utilization. *Am J Surg,* **216**, 7–12.

Lecouturier, J., Stansby, G., Thomson, R. G. 2023. Information provision and decision-making in the treatment of abdominal aortic aneurysm: a qualitative study of patient experience. *PLoS One,* **18**, e0293354.

Leonard, C., Sayre, G., Williams, S., et al. 2023. Perceived shared decision-making among patients undergoing lower-limb amputation and their care teams: a qualitative study. *Prosthet Orthot Int,* **47**, 379–386.

Norvell, D. C., Suckow, B. D., Webster, J. B., et al. 2021. The development and usability of the AMPREDICT decision support tool: a mixed methods study. *Eur J Vasc Endovasc Surg,* **62**, 304–311.

Peters, L. J., Stubenrouch, F. E., Thijs, J. B., Klemm, P. L., Balm, R., Ubbink, D. T. 2022. Predictors of the level of shared decision making in vascular surgery: a cross sectional study. *Eur J Vasc Endovasc Surg,* **64**, 65–72.

Preece, R., Dilaver, N., Waldron, C.-A., Czerniecki, J. M., Twine, C. P., Bosanquet, D. C. 2021. A systematic review and narrative synthesis of risk prediction tools used to estimate mortality, morbidity, and other outcomes following major lower limb amputation. *Eur J Vasc Endovasc Surg,* **62**, 127–135.

Royal College of Surgeons of England. n.d. Vascular surgery. Available at: https://www.rcseng.ac.uk/news-and-events/media-centre/media-background-briefings-and-statistics/vascular-surgery/

Santema, K. T. B., Stoffer, A. E., Kunneman, M., Koelemay, M. J. W., Ubbink, D. T. 2017. What are the decision-making preferences of patients in vascular surgery? A mixed-methods study. *BMJ Open,* **7**, e013272.

Santema, T. P., Stubenrouch, F. E., Koelemay, M. J. W., et al. 2016. Shared decision making in vascular surgery: an exploratory study. *Eur J Vasc Endovasc Surg,* **51**, 587–593.

Stubenrouch, F. E., Cohen, E. S., Bossuyt, P. M. M., Koelemay, M. J. W., van der Vet, P. C. R., Ubbink, D. T. 2020. Systematic review of reporting benefits and harms of surgical interventions in randomized clinical trials. *Br J Surg Open,* **4**, 171–181.

Stubenrouch, F. E., Peters, L. J., de Mik, S. M. L., et al. 2022. Improving shared decision making in vascular surgery: a stepped wedge cluster randomised trial. *Eur J Vasc Endovasc Surg,* **64**, 73–81.

Treffalls, J. A., Treffalls, R. N., Zachary, H., et al. 2022. Quality analysis of online resources for patients with peripheral artery disease. *Ann Vasc Surg,* **83**, 1–9.

van Veenendaal, H., Chernova, G., Bouman, C. M. B., van Etten-Jamaludin, F. S., van Dieren, S., Ubbink, D. T. 2023. Shared decision-making and the duration of medical consultations: a systematic review and meta-analysis. *Patient Educ Couns,* **107**, 107561.

Xu, J., Prince, A. E. R. 2019. Shared decision-making in vascular surgery. *J Vasc Surg,* **70**, 1711–1715.

38

Shared decision making in breast cancer surgery

Adele Ketley, Sam Brunsden, Lynda Wyld, and Jenna Morgan

Introduction

Breast cancer treatment is increasingly complex with patients facing an array of difficult choices during their journey. In the early breast cancer setting, patients have a choice of surgeries, not just mastectomy versus breast conservation, but more nuanced options to optimize aesthetic outcomes and facilitate conservation. Axillary treatment, previously just a complete axillary clearance, may now include sentinel node biopsy, targeted axillary dissection, radiotherapy, or no axillary treatment. There are also increasingly complex options for adjuvant therapies. Radiotherapy to the breast may be whole breast, partial breast, intraoperative, or omitted entirely in some women. Systemic therapies have expanded; with new drugs such as immunotherapy, HER2-targeted therapies, PARP inhibitors, and cyclin-dependent kinase inhibitors alongside more established cytotoxic chemotherapy regimens. For all these options there are complex personal trade-offs to be made: balancing increased treatment toxicity and negative impacts on quality of life against survival benefits or better aesthetic outcomes.

In the advanced breast cancer setting, there have been huge advances with large numbers of new drugs proven to prolong life, albeit at the expense of varying toxicities. For a patient with terminal disease, deciding when to decline the next line of offered treatment can be a huge burden.

While many would say that survival is the most important outcome from cancer treatment, and indeed is the primary outcome for most cancer treatment trials, many women have different priorities. An excellent example is an older woman, nearing the natural end of her life, in whom the maintenance of independence and quality of life may be more important than prolonging life at any cost. Another example, eloquently described by our patient advocate co-author, relates to the perception that reconstruction is always desired after mastectomy and that a double mastectomy is not appropriate (Box 38.1). For many women, these are exactly the right options for them.

Box 38.1 Patient perspective

Shared decision making in breast cancer

In women with a breast cancer diagnosis, the difference between what patients want, and what clinicians think they want, can be either clearly or covertly apparent. In a very short and turbulent space of time, life-changing decisions are made requiring open discussion about patient values, beliefs, and lifestyle along with an evidence-based presentation of what treatments are clinically appropriate. When all the possible treatment pathways are not presented, or given an equal footing, then satisfaction with care and long-term outcomes can be detrimentally affected.

Having been diagnosed with multiple tumours, mastectomy was my best surgical treatment available. With a very busy and physically active lifestyle I did not want to prolong the recovery process with reconstruction alongside the necessary adjuvant therapies. While reconstruction was not something I wanted, asymmetry presented its own challenges which could be mitigated with a contralateral mastectomy, not just with reconstruction. The pressure that can be felt at this point when multiple members of the healthcare team question your decision without discussion about lifestyle and values can be both confusing and frustrating. A consultation process to facilitate and document an open discussion and a decision that considered both patient expectations and clinical expertise would have relieved much anxiety during this difficult decision making process.

With so much information available on the internet, the chance of misinterpretation of risk and appropriate treatments plus placing store in unreliable sources is great and potentially harmful. Patients who do not feel fully informed about all their options, or confident they have been listened to, often resort to 'Dr Google' which can erode satisfaction with long-term treatment outcomes and the healthcare team.

Alongside surgical options, the myriad of adjuvant therapies specific to various tumour types plus consideration of comorbidities and circumstances require very careful presentation by the clinicians involved. Patients facing a decision between breast-conserving surgery (BCS) and mastectomy or hormone therapy versus surgical resection need to understand the risk factors and implications to fully participate in a decision about treatment. The biggest challenge facing breast care units is time; without structure for a shared decision making (SDM) pathway, many patients find they are not afforded enough clinic time to feel confident in their choices and healthcare professionals feel frustrated in their efforts to provide the best care. In these circumstances, the role of the clinical nurse specialist is invaluable and improved access for patients to their support, outside specific clinic time, can greatly improve the patient experience.

Another significant trade-off for women with breast cancer is the effect on body image and sexual function that breast cancer treatment may cause. Most breast cancer treatments target elements that women may perceive as critical to their 'womanhood': loss of fertility, loss of the breast, loss of libido, hair loss, vaginal changes making intercourse painful, and induced menopause. For many women these are profoundly important to their sense of self and to their relationships. Many will therefore make significant sacrifices to preserve these sexual characteristics, even at the potential risk to survival, which may seem illogical to some healthcare professionals. The psychological issues interwoven with decision making are therefore hugely complex in breast cancer. It is for these reasons that breast surgery developed and promoted the role of the specialist nurse before any other cancer specialty, in recognition of the informational and psychological support that women need when making these choices.

Shared decision making (SDM) is a (UK) NHS priority which should improve equity of access to care, enhance patients' experiences of treatment, and ultimately improve long-term satisfaction and outcomes. Once again, our patient co-author's experience demonstrates that SDM is not always delivered, with some health professionals not prepared to listen to the patient's voice (Box 38.1). This shows a fundamental lack of respect to the patient. While healthcare professionals are the experts on the disease, the patient is the expert on themselves and their own needs and wishes. This is a key reason why formal decision support tools can be so useful, both to ensure optimal information is made available but also to explore the patient's priorities. This includes respecting the patient's wish to make the decision or delegate to the healthcare professional.

Many decision support tools have been developed to support women with early breast cancer treatment decisions (Table 38.1). Most focus heavily on survival or other disease-specific outcomes and some of the physical consequences of treatment with only limited attention to quality of life. This is perhaps understandable in that while clinicians are taught about a range of quality-of-life tools and domains and understand the concept, most patients have never been exposed to these concepts. Some academics have tried to develop metrics to display quality of life in a way that is accessible to a lay audience, but this has never been widely adopted clinically in the early cancer setting where cure is seen as the primary aim. In the advanced disease setting, where cure is no longer possible, there is much more recognition of the importance of quality of life and several tools have been developed to aid in decision making. These include Q-TWiST (Quality-adjusted Time Without Symptoms of disease or Toxicity) (Huang et al., 2019) which is a score that can be derived, usually in advanced cancer drug trials, to balance the negative and positive effects of treatment on both survival and quality of life. This is sometimes used to aid clinical decision making in the advanced disease setting.

An example of a SDM tool is MAGIC (MAking Good decisions In Collaboration) produced by The Health Foundation in the UK to aid patients and clinicians (The Health Foundation, n.d.). The project ran from 2010 to 2013 with the aim of embedding best practice in SDM across several clinical settings, including women with breast cancer who were choosing between mastectomy and breast-conserving surgery (BCS). The evaluation phase of the project found that the programme built awareness of SDM and successfully supported clinical teams in use of SDM and tools. Unfortunately, funding limits the availability and maintenance of these tools online and, even when resources are available, it does not lead to automatic implementation in a clinical setting. There are hindrances inclining clinical team attitudes, reorganization of care pathways, managerial support, and resource allocation.

The rest of this chapter will focus in more detail on two areas of breast cancer decision making where decision support tools have been designed to guide patients to support SDM.

Choosing between BCS and mastectomy

Surgery is the primary treatment for breast cancer, with the options of BCS or mastectomy, with or without reconstruction (Figure 38.1). There has been a rise in rates of BCS with only 41% of patients undergoing mastectomy in the UK in 2021 (MacNeill and Irvine, 2021). For patients opting for mastectomy, some may choose to stay flat while others go on to have reconstructive surgery. For those who do have reconstruction, this can be performed immediately at the time of mastectomy, or delayed until after adjuvant treatments. Some patients feel strongly that they do not want any period of being flat, so opt for immediate reconstruction. Others will have delayed reconstruction, due to prioritizing radiotherapy but which can negatively impact immediate reconstruction, or because of uncertainty about whether they wish for reconstruction. Patients also have a choice of reconstructive options, including implant-based and autologous techniques, such as latissimus dorsi or deep inferior epigastric perforator flaps. The Association of Breast Surgery and British Association of Plastic Reconstructive and Aesthetic Surgeons have acknowledged the importance of SDM in the context of breast reconstruction, recommending the use of decision aids, such as PEGASUS (Patients' Expectations & Goals: Assisting Shared Understanding of Surgery) (Gilmour et al., 2021).

Due to advances in oncoplastic breast conservation techniques (e.g. therapeutic mammoplasty and chest wall perforator flap surgery), and increasingly effective neoadjuvant chemotherapy, breast conservation of previously unresectable cancers is now possible, and more women now have the choice of BCS or mastectomy. Research has clearly demonstrated equivalent survival rates between the two techniques. Some more recent studies suggest BCS (with radiotherapy) has superior oncological outcomes compared to mastectomy, but these are limited by being observational studies (Xiang et al., 2022).

With comparable survival, several other considerations may affect treatment decision making. Patients prefer to be active participants in this decision making process (Caldon et al., 2008) and to enable effective SDM, patients need to be appropriately counselled about their surgical options and the associated issues.

There are practicalities involved in breast surgery choice relating to length of recovery and requirement for further treatment. Patients may prefer the low risk of adverse events associated with BCS or the decreased chance of requiring a second surgery mastectomy provides. BCS is viewed as generally providing cosmetically superior results then mastectomy although corrective surgery may sometimes be required. Mastectomy operations can be followed by either immediate or delayed reconstruction, although not all patients have these options due to comorbidities, smoking status, lack of donor sites, and so on. BCS and mastectomy have both been found to negatively impact quality of life, body image, and sexuality, with some studies suggesting mastectomy has a more negative impact (Gupta et al.,

Table 38.1 Table summarizing available SDM tools for breast cancer (not an exhaustive list)

Reference	Name of decision support tool	Decision supported by tool	Design	Evaluated in a clinical trial	URL
Setting: prevention or risk assessment					
Lee et al., 2019	CANRISK/BOADICEA	Genetic risk assessment to support risk management strategies	Online tool with data derived from UK cancer registry data and 156 case families to give predictions of an individual developing breast and ovarian cancer	Clinician acceptability evaluated in a multi-methods study showed the tool was acceptable to clinicians but there was apprehension about the impact of the tool on the consultation	https://canrisk.org/
Setting: early breast cancer					
Wyld et al., 2021	Age Gap	Older age specific decision about surgery versus primary endocrine therapy or adjuvant chemotherapy or not	Online tool with data derived from the UK cancer registry to give survival predictions tailored to patient age, fitness, frailty, and tumour characteristics. Supported by a downloadable booklet giving information about pros and cons of each option	Cluster randomized controlled trial evaluated performance showing enhanced patient knowledge and an impact on treatment allocation	https://agegap.shef.ac.uk/ (Figure 38.2)
Specht et al., 2005	Memorial Sloan Kettering (MSKCC): further axillary nodes after SLNB	Predicting further lymph node involvement after sentinel node biopsy	Online tool to assist decision about proceeding to completion axillary lymph node clearance. Based on regression model of 702 patients with lymph node metastases who underwent completion axillary node dissection in the USA	Outperforms clinicians' predictions but did not alter clinical management, based on 17 clinicians and 33 patients	https://nomograms.mskcc.org/Breast/BreastAdditionalNonSLNMetastasesPage.aspx
Raphael et al., 2021	BRASA	Adjuvant radiotherapy or not across a range of settings	Online decision aid containing information about how radiotherapy is performed and its side effects. Elicits patient preferences	Multi-centre pre- and post-intervention study showed no change in decision conflict but better informed decisions	https://beslissamen.nl/pda_launch.html?pda=tools/pda_borstradiotherapie_en/story.html
Candido Dos Reis et al., 2017	PREDICT	Adjuvant chemotherapy or not	Developed from a model based on UK cancer registry data and trial data. Allows survival outcome prediction based on patient age and tumour characteristics and allows personalization according to treatment selection (chemotherapy, endocrine therapy, trastuzumab, and bisphosphonates)	Prediction model validated across several international settings	https://breast.predict.nhs.uk/
Kalinsky et al., 2021	Genetic arrays, e.g. Mammprint, Oncotype DX	Adjuvant chemotherapy or not	Complex biological assays measuring an extended array of genes, the expression of which is converted via an algorithm into a risk score. This score is designed to predict the possible benefit of chemotherapy and so aid decision making	Mammprint validated in MINDACT and Ontcotype DX in the RxPONDER and TAILOR-X multi-centre randomized controlled trials	https://agendia.com/mammaprint/ 10

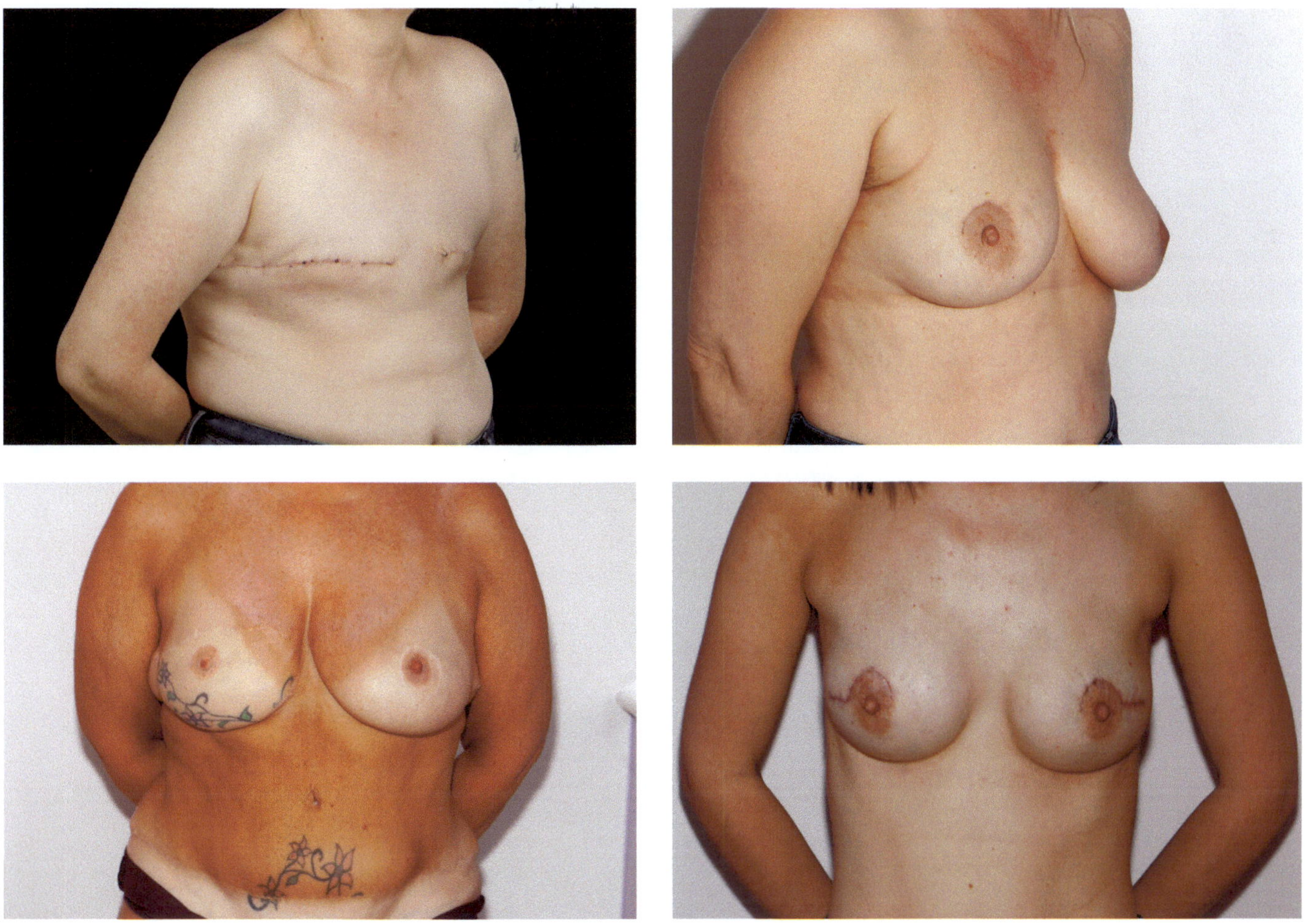

Figure 38.1 Example photographs of patients who have undergone different types of breast surgery, including (a) bilateral mastectomy; (b) BCS in the form of a wide local excision; and (c) right mastectomy with delayed autologous reconstruction (deep inferior epigastric perforator flap) and left symmetrizing breast reduction; (d) bilateral skin-sparing mastectomy and immediate implant-based reconstruction.

2022). Overall patient satisfaction with BCS is reported to be similar or higher than mastectomy satisfaction (Livingston-Rosanoff et al., 2020). In addition to the above reasoning, patients' personal feelings can affect their decisions. Women can choose mastectomy due to fear of recurrence, despite evidence against this, with patients feeling it is a more 'complete' operation, resulting in less anxiety. Some patients feel their breasts do not define them and choose to 'go flat'.

The most important element in SDM is patient choice after being appropriately counselled. Giving choice to patients contributes to more realistic expectations of outcomes and improvement in overall satisfaction. The choice between BCS and mastectomy is a personal and subjective topic which requires careful SDM between breast cancer patients and their clinicians.

Choosing between surgery and primary endocrine therapy for older women with operable breast cancer

Older women have inferior breast cancer survival outcomes compared to younger women due to presentation at a later stage and reduced treatment schedules. Decision making is complicated by the highly variable fitness levels of older women. Surgery is the primary treatment, but for older women with a reduced life expectancy and increased surgical risks, there are alternative treatments. These include primary endocrine therapy in women with oestrogen receptor-positive cancers, or primary radiotherapy in women with oestrogen receptor-negative cancers. In those who have surgery, adjuvant chemotherapy may also be offered, although the evidence for benefit in the over 70 age group is weak, especially in women with oestrogen receptor-positive cancers, and toxicity rates are higher. Consequently, patients over 70 years receive chemotherapy much less frequently than younger women.

For some older patients with significant comorbidities and with oestrogen receptor-positive cancer, primary endocrine therapy may be superior to surgery. Surgery and chemotherapy lead to more adverse events in patients over 70 years compared to other age groups, but these treatments can still offer cancer-specific and survival benefit for a select group of women. Many decision support tools exist for breast cancer patients but are not designed specifically for older patients. The Age Gap Decision Tool (Figure 38.2) fills this gap by providing patients aged over 70 years with an online algorithm, which takes into account survival data, comorbidities, and frailty (https://agegap.shef.ac.uk/). This tool helps women decide between

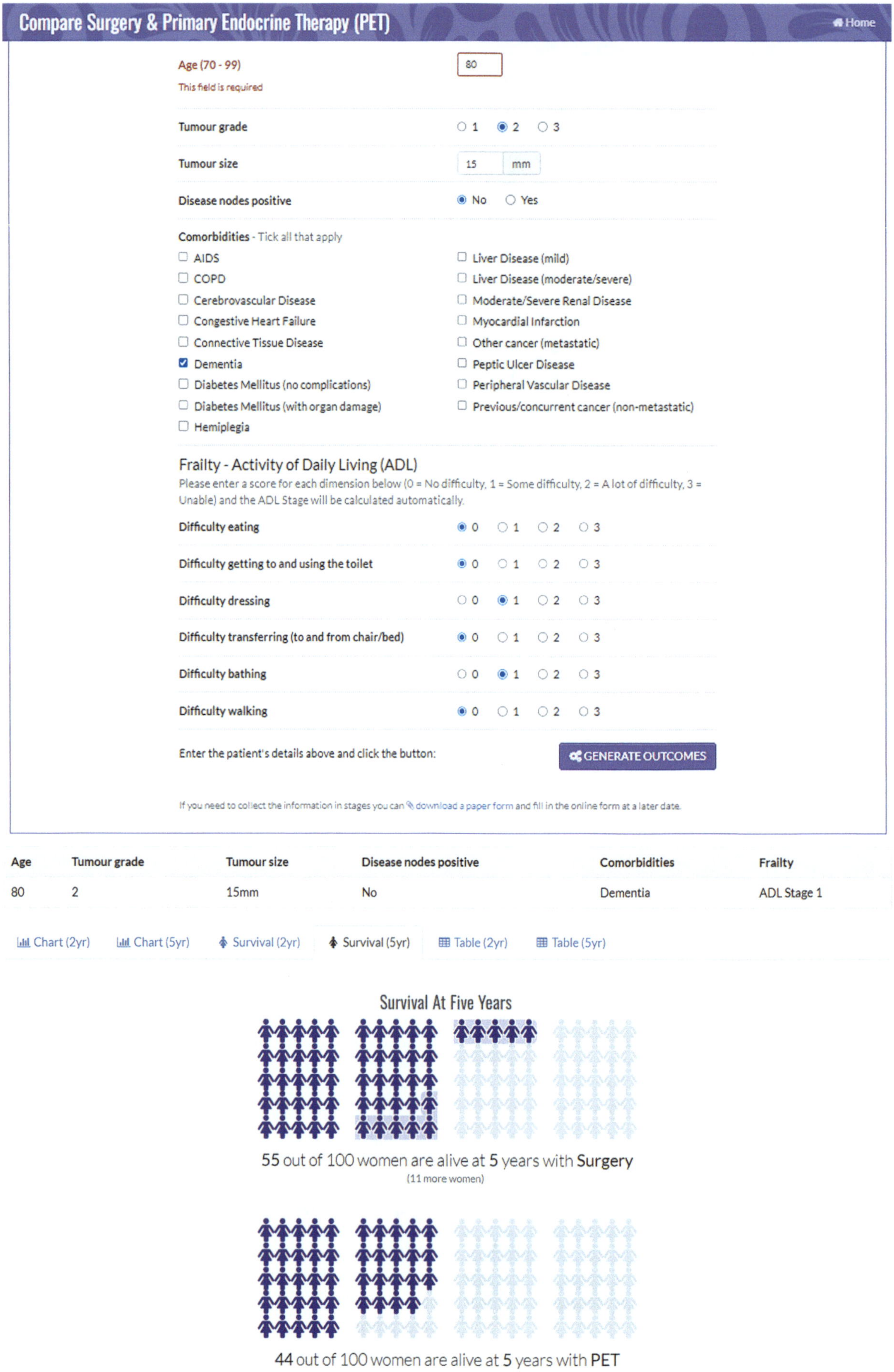

Figure 38.2 Screen shots of the Age Gap decision tool comparing primary endocrine therapy with surgery showing (a) the input screen and the results screens showing survival at 5 years in (b) pictogram style and (c) graphical style.

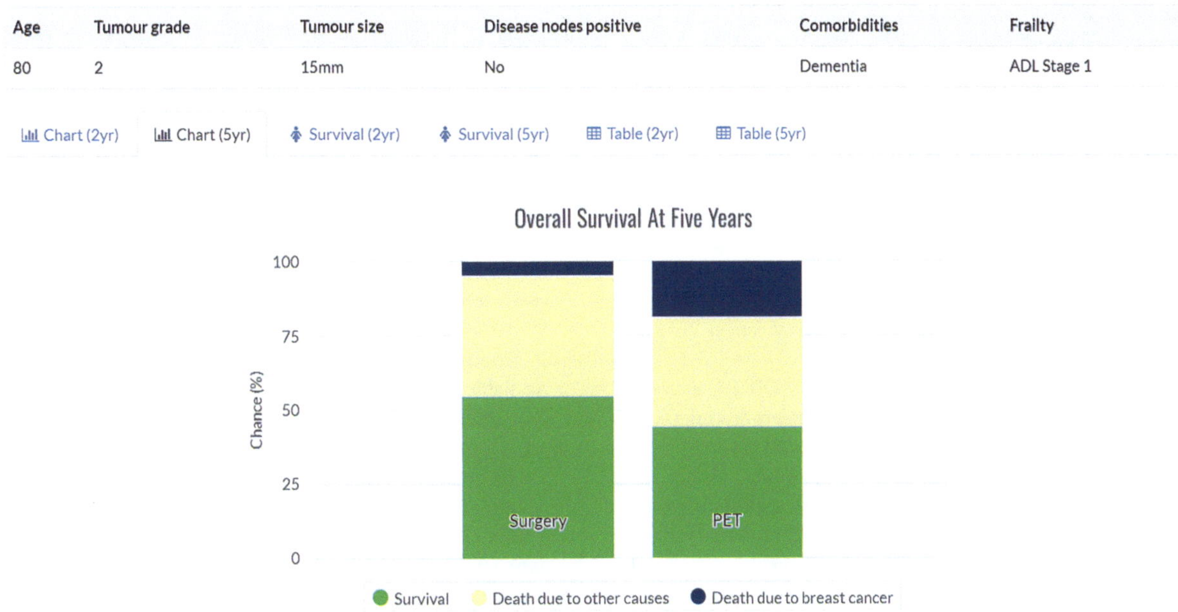

Figure 38.2 Continued

surgery plus/minus chemotherapy and primary endocrine therapy by producing a predicted survival outcome based on their specific characteristics.

The impact and benefit of surgery

Patients' decisions to have surgery are influenced by age, frailty, and comorbidities, including dementia (Burton et al. 2015). Breast cancer surgery is generally safe in those over 70 years, with surgery-related severe adverse events being rare (Morgan et al., 2020). However, a US study of very frail older patients in nursing homes found that those who had surgery for their breast cancer experienced high rates of morbidity, mortality, and functional decline (Tang et al., 2018). Surgery also negatively affects long-term quality of life and independence (Morgan et al., 2020). Older patients themselves value quality of life at least as strongly as length of life (Morgan et al., 2020) and, for some older women, surgery is not necessary as they have a very short estimated life expectancy due to frailty. For such women, primary endocrine therapy is a valuable alternative to offer. Identification of women for whom surgery is likely to confer little or no survival benefit is therefore key to this decision support tool.

The Age Gap tool was developed following International Patient Decision Aid Standards guidelines. It uses survival models developed from UK cancer registry data. Two models were developed: one for older women who were unfit, where outcomes from surgery and primary endocrine therapy could be compared; the second, for older women who had already had surgery and who were considering chemotherapy.

There was also an extensive process to determine the informational needs and preferences of older women considering these two choices. Ultimately, the data from patients and the models were incorporated into an online tool (https://agegap.shef.ac.uk/), piloted with patients and healthcare professionals, and evaluated in a cluster randomized trial with 1339 patients in 46 UK hospitals. Treatment allocation altered significantly as a result of using the tool. Despite the fact that most of the model outcomes favoured more, rather than less treatment, more women chose less aggressive treatment if the tool was used. Quality of life improved slightly when the tool was used. Patient levels of knowledge were enhanced. There was no detriment to survival. A detailed process evaluation was performed alongside the trial and feedback on the tool and its utility was very positive. The tool has since been made freely available and has been accessed over 100,000 times across 70 countries since it was launched.

See Box 38.1 for our patient perspective.

Summary

Breast cancer treatment is complex and decision making can be very challenging. A wide range of decision support tools are available and are effective to support SDM in breast cancer. Sadly, many women do not have access to these and still struggle to be heard when expressing their views. More training and education of healthcare professionals about the value of SDM and its implementation are needed.

REFERENCES

Burton, M., Collins, K. A., Lifford, K. J., et al. 2015. The information and decision support needs of older women (>75 yrs) facing treatment choices for breast cancer: a qualitative study. *Psychooncology*, **24**, 878–884.

Caldon, L. J. M., Walters, S. J., Reed, M. W. R. 2008. Changing trends in the decision-making preferences of women with early breast cancer. *Br J Surg*, **95**, 312–318.

Candido Dos Reis, F. J., Wishart, G. C., Dicks, E. M., et al. 2017. An updated PREDICT breast cancer prognostication and treatment benefit prediction model with independent validation. *Breast Cancer Res*, **19**, 58.

Gilmour, A., Cutress, R., Gandhi, A., et al. 2021. Oncoplastic breast surgery: a guide to good practice. *Eur J Surg Oncol*, **47**, 2272–2285.

Gupta, N., Pandey, A. K., Dimri, K., Jyani, G., Goyal, A., Prinja, S. 2022. Health-related quality of life among breast cancer patients in India. *Support Care Cancer*, **30**, 9983–9990.

Huang, M., Pietanza, M. C., Samkari, A., et al. 2019. Q-TWiST analysis to assess benefit–risk of pembrolizumab in patients with PD-L1-positive advanced or metastatic non-small cell lung cancer. *PharmacoEconomics*, **37**, 105–116.

Kalinsky, K., Barlow, W. E., Gralow, J. R., et al. 2021. 21-Gene assay to inform chemotherapy benefit in node-positive breast cancer. *N Engl J Med*, **385**, 2336–2347.

Lee, A., Mavaddat, N., Wilcox, A. N., et al. 2019. BOADICEA: a comprehensive breast cancer risk prediction model incorporating genetic and nongenetic risk factors. *Genet Med*, **21**, 1708–1718.

Livingston-Rosanoff, D., Trentham-Dietz, A., Hampton, J. M., et al. 2020. Evaluation of long-term satisfaction with breast surgery in patients treated for ductal carcinoma in situ: a population-based longitudinal cohort study. *Ann Surg Oncol*, **27**, 2628–2636.

MacNeill, F., Irvine, T. 2021. Breast surgery: GIRFT programme national specialty report. Available at: https://gettingitrightfirsttime.co.uk/wp-content/uploads/2021/09/BreastSurgeryReport-Jul21p.pdf

Morgan, J. L., George, J., Holmes, G., et al. 2020. Breast cancer surgery in older women: outcomes of the Bridging Age Gap in Breast Cancer study. Br J Surg, **107**, 1468–1479.

Raphael, D. B., Russell, N. S., Winkens, B., et al. 2021. A patient decision aid for breast cancer patients deciding on their radiation treatment, no change in decisional conflict but better informed choices. *Tech Innov Patient Support Radiat Oncol*, **20**, 1–9.

Specht, M. C., Kattan, M. W., Gonen, M., Fey, J., Van Zee, K. J. 2005. Predicting nonsentinel node status after positive sentinel lymph biopsy for breast cancer: clinicians versus nomogram. *Ann Surg Oncol*, **12**, 654–659.

Tang, V., Zhao, S., Boscardin, J., et al. 2018. Functional status and survival after breast cancer surgery in nursing home residents. *JAMA Surg*, **153**, 1090–1096.

The Health Foundation. n.d. MAGIC: shared decision making. Available at: https://www.health.org.uk/funding-and-partnerships/programme/magic-shared-decision-making

Wyld, L., Reed, M. W. R., Collins, K., et al. 2021. Bridging the age gap in breast cancer: cluster randomized trial of two decision support interventions for older women with operable breast cancer on quality of life, survival, decision quality, and treatment choices. *Br J Surg*, **108**, 499–510.

Xiang, W., Wu, C., Wu, H., Fang, S., Liu, N., Yu, H. 2022. Survival comparisons between breast conservation surgery and mastectomy followed by postoperative radiotherapy in stage I–III breast cancer patients: analysis of the Surveillance, Epidemiology, and End Results (Seer) program database. *Curr Oncol*, **29**, 5731–5747.

39

Shared decision making in urology

Giulia M. Ippolito, Roshan Paudel, Marty Chakoian, Jerry Thomas, and Danil V. Makarov

Introduction

Shared decision making (SDM) is well established as the standard of care for high-quality urological care. The American Urological Association first published a clinical consensus statement on the 'Implementation of Shared Decision Making into Urological Practice' in 2016 and subsequently updated the statement in 2022 (Makarov et al., 2016, 2022). The European Association of Urology guidelines are aimed 'to support shared decision making and ... the shift to individualised patient-centred care' (https://uroweb.org/guidelines). Several clinical practice guidelines within the American Urological Association and the European Association of Urology reference SDM within the context of urological disease.

However, the practice of SDM and decision aid use within urology are not as well understood. A survey of urologists' use of SDM and decision aids in differing clinical scenarios was distributed via the American Urological Association Annual Census in 2019 (Lane et al., 2020). This survey found that 77% of urologists self-reported that they regularly use four or more core steps in SDM in at least one clinical scenario (Lane et al., 2020). However, gaps in the SDM process were notable, and the proportion of urologists that self-reported regularly eliciting patient preferences varied between 54% and 66% based on the clinical scenario (Lane et al., 2020). Barriers to practising SDM in urology are consistent with non-urological studies, often driven by misperceptions surrounding time constraints and concerns about patient engagement (Lane et al., 2020).

Similarly to SDM use, decision aid use is also not well characterized and appears highly variable in current urological practice. In the same self-reported survey mentioned previously, urologists' use of decision aids varies between 40% and 58%, depending on the clinical scenario (Lane et al., 2020). This variation may be driven by the lack of availability of high-quality decision aids in several key clinical domains (Grüne et al., 2022).

Herein we will review the relevance of SDM and decision aids within urology with a clinical focus on prostate cancer, overactive bladder (OAB), and benign prostatic hyperplasia (BPH). We also provide insight into implementation of these tools in urological practice and gaps in evidence for future research.

Relevance of SDM to the care of patients with urological diseases

Advances in research have provided multiple options for treatment for urological conditions. These breakthroughs are often clinically equivalent, which makes many urological conditions preference sensitive. Some of the best studied preference-sensitive conditions in urology are prostate cancer, OAB, and BPH.

Prostate cancer

Prostate cancer is the fourth most common cancer worldwide. Intervention and treatment for prostate cancer vary widely based on the severity of disease. In some men, observation is a reasonable option whereas in others, intervention may be preferred. As the landscape of prostate cancer management has become more complex, the importance of SDM has gained prominence (Makarov et al., 2022). SDM may be employed in the screening, diagnosis, and treatment of prostate cancer with consequent effects on treatment decisions, patient satisfaction, and overall health outcomes. Prostate cancer management often presents complex choices with trade-offs between various healthcare states that are valued differently by different individuals and influenced by factors such as disease stage, patient age, and comorbidities.

SDM empowers patients by providing them with comprehensive information about the available treatment options, potential risks, and benefits. This collaborative approach ensures that decisions align with patients' values and goals, leading to increased satisfaction and adherence to the chosen treatment plan even when that plan is for no intervention (Elwyn et al., 2012). For example, patients exposed to a decision aid about prostate-specific antigen screening were less likely to choose prostate-specific antigen screening in pooled analyses (Stacey et al., 2017).

In the context of prostate cancer, SDM fosters informed decision making, allowing patients to actively participate in discussions about their diagnosis, prognosis, and treatment options. This process acknowledges the unique needs and values of individual patients, facilitating a personalized approach to care.

Studies have shown that involving patients in decision making leads to increased knowledge retention, reduced decisional conflict, and a greater sense of control over their health. Specifically within prostate cancer, patients who participate in SDM feel more informed or empowered, have higher satisfaction with their medical care, and report better quality of life and lower anxiety. They are less likely to have decisional regret and more likely to adhere to the medical plan. Such empowerment may be particularly important for long-term, anxiety-evoking decisions such as the decision to get prostate cancer surgery for early-stage prostate cancer, which can have long-term effects on sexual function.

Effective communication between healthcare professionals and patients is integral to the success of SDM. Open and honest discussions about treatment options, potential side effects, and expected outcomes build trust and strengthen the physician–patient relationship. Trust is crucial for patients to feel confident in their decision making process and fosters a sense of collaboration in navigating the complexities of prostate cancer care (Box 39.1). Research has demonstrated that patients who perceive their healthcare providers as trustworthy are more likely to actively engage in SDM.

Despite its benefits, several barriers hinder the implementation of SDM in prostate cancer care. Time constraints, limited resources, and varying levels of health literacy among patients are common challenges, although workarounds like videos and other technology-based approaches have been able to improve outcomes like patient knowledge without affecting clinic workflow. Additionally, physician attitudes and communication styles may influence the extent to which SDM is integrated into clinical practice. Physicians may be influenced by available resources; for example, a study within the Veterans Affairs hospital setting found that providers who had the robot available framed robotic prostatectomy more favourably than providers at institutions with no robot. Overcoming these barriers requires a multifaceted approach, including education and training for healthcare professionals, improved communication strategies, and the integration of decision aids to facilitate discussions.

There is consensus that SDM is a crucial component in the care of patients with prostate cancer. SDM enhances patient engagement, improves decisional outcomes, and fosters a collaborative approach to treatment planning. As healthcare continues to evolve towards patient-centred models, SDM will likely play an even greater role in prostate cancer care. Efforts to address barriers and promote effective communication will contribute to enhance patient experiences, improve treatment adherence, and, ultimately, enhance outcomes for individuals facing the challenges of prostate cancer.

Box 39.1 Patient perspective

Prostate cancer is exhausting. I know this as a 19-year survivor and from the many dozens of patients and caregivers I have worked with in my support group. So many decisions to make: should I get a prostate-specific antigen test? Do I need a biopsy? Should I go on active surveillance or opt for treatment? If so, which one? And if the cancer comes back, what then? How long can I put off androgen deprivation and other systemic therapies? Is there a clinical trial that might be appropriate for me?

Most diseases, and certainly most cancers, come with decisions for the patient. But because prostate cancer often lasts for years, with choice after choice and new therapies continually being developed, decision making can be overwhelming. Each step in the progression is new to us, and confusing. We need a trusted partner along the way, someone experienced with treatment options who can provide guidance and advice—our doctors.

But there is a power imbalance at play. We feel ignorant, frightened. Our urologists seem knowledgeable, experienced, and objective. We may be inclined to accept whatever recommendation they offer about what we should do, without considering other options. But it's our cancer, our body, our life to live in the aftermath of therapy. We have the right and the responsibility to select the treatment that is best for our individual situation, our values, and our vision of the future. Our job as patients is to work hard to understand our diagnosis, to fully comprehend the advantages and risks of each treatment option, to ask questions, and to communicate our values and our preferences. Our doctors are rightly concerned about helping us live longer, but we must advocate for the quality of life we want.

However, the other concern I hear often from the patients in my support group is not that their doctors are too dogmatic, but rather, that they may refuse to participate in decision making at all. This is particularly problematic for new patients who are struggling to come to terms with their cancer diagnosis. One man reported that his doctor carefully explained that he was a good candidate for either surgery or radiation, but when asked for a recommendation, held up his hand to signal *stop*. 'Oh, no, that's your decision, not mine,' the patient was told.

In contrast, after my salvage radiation for a recurrence, my radiation oncologist suggested that I stay on androgen deprivation therapy for 18 months. We talked and agreed that 6 months would probably be adequate and more consistent with my desire for an active life. That's how it should work. Doctors are equipped with an understanding of the nuances of treatment options and serve best when collaborating with patients to develop a treatment plan.

Any prostate cancer treatment can result in adverse side effects and lead to regret. But the patients in my support group most satisfied with their treatment are those who believe they made a reasonable and informed decision in partnership with their medical team.

OAB and incontinence

OAB syndrome is characterized by urinary urgency, frequency, nocturia, with or without urinary urge incontinence, in the absence of another obvious pathology. There is significant prevalence of OAB among the population, with some studies suggesting up to one-third of Americans suffer from OAB symptoms. OAB, though bothersome, is not life-threatening, and therefore the decision to seek and undergo treatment is preference sensitive. Traditional approaches to OAB treatment involve escalation of care from initial behavioural or conservative (non-pharmacological) therapies, pharmacological therapies, and ultimately to minimally invasive therapies such as neuromodulation or chemodenervation. However, this type of step therapy has been increasingly scrutinized within the context of OAB as a barrier to SDM and patient-centred care (Paudel and Lane, 2022).

Behavioural therapies (diet and fluid management, urge suppression, and bladder retraining) and non-pharmacological conservative therapies (pelvic floor physical therapy) all require significant patient engagement but offer very low risk profiles. Given that these are low-stakes preference-sensitive options with potential benefits, SDM to discuss trials of one or more of these options is generally recommended as an early intervention. Pharmacotherapy for OAB consists of anticholinergic or beta-3 adrenergic receptor agonists and can be paired with initial behavioural or non-pharmacological interventions; these medications are equally effective and differ mostly in their side effect profiles. While anticholinergic medications are the most accessible option to many, there are increasing concerns about safety of these medications on cognition and most patients cease anticholinergic therapy within 6 months due to inefficacy or adverse effects. Beta-3 agonist medications have few adverse

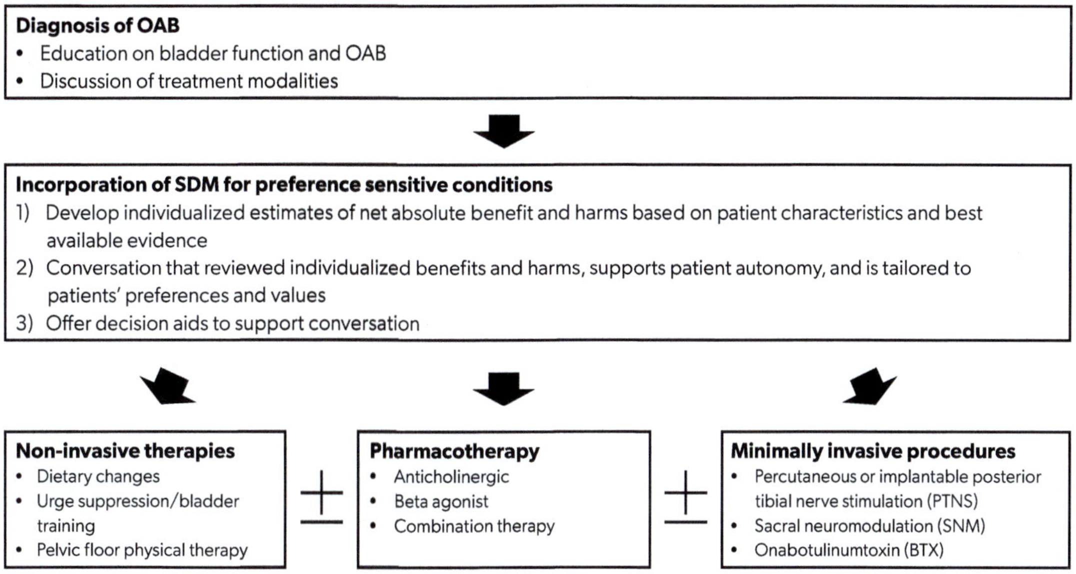

Figure 39.1 Potential strategy to increase incorporation of SDM into OAB practice.

effects but are currently often cost prohibitive due to lack of generic options.

Minimally invasive therapies consist of chemodenervation with onabotulinumtoxin, delivered by cystoscopic injection, or neuromodulation delivered in three modalities: sacral neuromodulation implant, a posterior tibial nerve implant, or percutaneous posterior tibial nerve stimulation with an acupuncture needle. Each of these interventions is equally effective, and again the main differences are in mode of delivery and side effect profile, making the decision to pursue any of these options also preference sensitive. Furthermore, there are data suggesting that therapies have similar clinical outcomes between categories. For example, data suggest pharmacotherapy may have similar outcomes to behavioural or non-pharmacological interventions and pharmacological therapy may have similar outcomes to chemodenervation.

Given the clinical equipoise, OAB ideally lends itself to SDM, but implementation of SDM in OAB is hindered by several barriers including physician- and policy-related barriers (such as insurance requirements necessitating pharmacotherapy before minimally invasive therapies). A potential model for SDM in OAB could follow the scheme represented in Figure 39.1.

BPH

BPH is defined by growth of the transitional zone of the prostate; it can lead to lower urinary tract symptoms associated with the storage and emptying of urine. Symptoms of BPH range from mild to severe, and in most cases the decision to seek and undergo treatment is patient-centred, but in severe cases, where life-threatening urinary obstruction can develop, the decision to undergo an intervention is no longer preference sensitive.

Treatment options for lower urinary tract symptoms caused by BPH include medication therapy (alpha blockers, 5-alpha reductase inhibitors, phosphodiesterase-5 inhibitor) and surgical therapy. There are 11 surgical interventions currently listed in the American Urological Association guidelines for the management of BPH (Foster et al., 2019). Complexity lies not only in the decision to undergo surgical intervention, but which intervention to pursue. Surgical guidelines recommend differing procedures based on prostate size, with some minimally invasive surgical therapies being indicated only for certain sizes of prostate. Further, medically complicated patients have more limited options based on evidence that particular surgeries are safer than others. These anatomical restrictions somewhat simplify the decision making, but men seeking surgical BPH treatment can be faced with between three and nine different surgical options that may all equally accomplish the patient's goals of care.

In men without medical complexity and with similarly sized prostate glands, the decision to pursue a particular therapy is highly preference sensitive. Often this decision rests on the patient's comfort with specific aspects of a procedure or its side effects and the availability of the particular surgical therapy. Some patients may favour an outpatient/office-based procedure to avoid the risk of anaesthesia, others may prefer a procedure that avoids the complication of retrograde ejaculation, while others prefer procedures that minimize the need for future treatments. Access to a favoured surgical option for BPH is variable as dissemination of all surgical techniques is not uniform and few surgeons offer all options. In this context, a major aspiration for SDM in BPH care is that urologists discuss all potential options for surgical therapy, even if that option is not one the urologist may perform, offering referrals if the patient chooses to pursue.

Decision aids in urology

Evidence-based patient decision aids (PtDAs) are essential tools created to support the SDM process for patients and providers. Decision aid use has been found to improve factors that affect SDM including short-term disease-specific knowledge, more accurate risk perceptions related to disease state, and clarification of patient values and preferences to tailor the SDM discussion (Makarov et al., 2022). Decision aids are not meant to supplant SDM, but to augment the urologist–patient SDM consultation. The availability of up-to-date and high-quality decision aids is highly variable, with most decision aids being focused on urological oncology and few available for functional, paediatric, or stone-related urological disease.

PtDAs are effective during the SDM discussion for prostate cancer screening. PtDAs for prostate cancer screening have been found to increase prostate cancer knowledge, intent to discuss screening, treatment satisfaction, and improve the patient–provider encounter, while reducing decisional conflict and anxiety among newly diagnosed men (Makarov et al., 2022). In spite of the benefits, a major limitation is the low use of decision aids among radiation oncologists and urologists for SDM about prostate cancer itself (Lane et al., 2020). The Ottawa Inventory currently includes eight decision aids related to prostate cancer screening or treatment (see also Chapter 18).

OAB treatment decisions are determined by patient preferences and values which is ideal for an SDM approach. However, PtDAs available to support patients with OAB are scarce with two only recently developed in 2021 (both for women only)—OABCare to elicit individual patient preferences and Streamlined, which is a mobile PtDA found to decrease decisional conflict (Chhatre et al., 2021; Khanijow et al., 2021). Further research is necessary to increase the availability of evidence-based PtDAs for preference-sensitive OAB treatments.

BPH treatment selection is ideal for a SDM approach considering the various options available for patients' medical or surgical therapy. It was one of the first clinical topics for which PtDAs were produced, and their use has led to lower rates of surgery among men previously treated with pharmacotherapy for BPH. There are two PtDAs for BPH available in the Ottawa Inventory as well as multiple web-based PtDAs available and currently being developed through research.

Leveraging implementation science to increase uptake of SDM in urology

Implementation science is an evolving field that offers a broad range of theories, models, and frameworks that can guide the implementation of SDM in routine practice. Practitioners in urology can consider these tools to contextualize the settings and help to assess barriers to implementation. Appropriate selection of these tools depends on the setting, the implementation goal, and the suitability of the model or framework to advance the goal. To support practitioners, implementation scientists have developed recommendations to help select the theories, models, and frameworks to advance the implementation goal (Moullin et al., 2020).

Effective design and implementation of SDM in routine urological practice remains a critical challenge. Numerous barriers to effective implementation have been documented (Makarov et al., 2022). Tools to assess barriers and identify potential solutions to overcome barriers have been developed, including a five-step process that guides the systematic intervention design for implementing evidence-based practices (Skolarus and Sales, 2015). Common barriers to SDM use and practical strategies for overcoming those barriers have also been proposed (Makarov et al., 2022). Once SDM is implemented, implementation science also offers tools to evaluate ongoing implementation, integration into routine practice, and to assess sustainability (see Chapter 25).

Implementation of SDM and PtDAs in clinical practice is not a one-time event. Once implemented, this practice requires sustained efforts, and long-term sustainability requires ongoing adaptation based on feedback from patients and practitioners. One example of this is how PtDA use for prostate cancer treatment was implemented successfully in the context of a statewide urological surgery collaborative in the USA as a quality metric (Lane et al., 2022). However the programme was ultimately not chosen as an ongoing quality metric after an initial pilot. Examples such as these underscore the importance of sustainability when designing interventions to implement SDM and PtDA use in urological practice.

Avenues for ongoing research

Scientific advances in medical care provide clinicians and patients with more treatment options for all aspects of urological care. However, with the increase of options, the implementation of effective SDM, and the availability of evidence-based decision aids, becomes increasingly important and the gaps in our current knowledge about SDM and PtDAs are readily apparent. Two of the most evident areas for research are in the dissemination and implementation of SDM in the urological workforce. While urology guidelines recommend SDM and PtDA use, there is no formal training on SDM within American urological training, though the Société Internationale d'Urologie offers online lectures on SDM in Urology for residents (http://tinyurl.com/sdmsiu). The lack of knowledge about SDM is evident in studies showing that urologists consistently skip key portions of SDM, such as patient preference elicitation (Lane et al., 2020). Clinician practice patterns have been directly linked to patient decisions even to use decision aids at all in their care (Makarov et al., 2022). How best to incorporate principles of SDM into the urological workforce remains an unanswered, but critical, question.

Another ongoing question is where the burden of creation and maintenance of high-quality decision aids should lie. A potential solution is to link decision aid creation with guideline creations, as has been proposed by the Making GRADE the Irresistible Choice (MAGICapp) organization (see Chapter 20). Linking SDM and PtDAs to clinical practice guidelines may be an opportunity for subspecialty societies to increase the dissemination and implementation of SDM in urology. However, this and other implementation strategies to increase uptake of SDM and PtDA use in urology have not yet been evaluated for acceptability, feasibility, or effectiveness and therefore are an open area for research.

REFERENCES

Chhatre, S., Newman, D. K., Wein, A. J., et al. 2021. Patient preference elicitation instrument, OABCare, to facilitate shared decision-making in the care of overactive bladder. *Neurourol Urodyn*, **40**, 791–801.

Elwyn, G., Frosch, D., Thomson, R., et al. 2012. Shared decision making: a model for clinical practice. *J Gen Intern Med*, **27**, 1361–1367.

Foster, H. E., Dahm, P., Kohler, T. S., et al. 2019. Surgical management of lower urinary tract symptoms attributed to benign prostatic hyperplasia: AUA guideline amendment 2019. *J Urol*, **202**, 592–598.

Grüne, B., Kriegmair, M. C., Lenhart, M., et al. 2022. Decision aids for shared decision-making in uro-oncology: a systematic review. *Eur Urol Focus*, **8**, 851–869.

Khanijow, K. D., Leri, D., Arya, L. A., et al. 2021. A mobile application patient decision aid for treatment of overactive bladder. *Female Pelvic Med Reconstr Surg*, **27**, 365–370.

Lane, G. I., Ellimoottil, C., Wallner, L., et al. 2020. Shared decision-making in urologic practice: results from the 2019 AUA census. *Urology*, **145**, 66–72.

Lane, G. I., Dupati, A., Qi, J., et al. 2022. Factors associated with decision aid use in localized prostate cancer. *Urol Pract*, **9**, 108–115.

Makarov, D. V., Chrouser, K., Gore, J. L., et al. 2016. AUA white paper on implementation of shared decision making into urological practice. *Urol Pract*, **3**, 355–363.

Makarov, D., Fagerlin, A., Finkelstein, J., et al. 2022. AUA white paper on implementation of shared decision making into urological practice. Available at: https://www.auanet.org/guidelines-and-quality/quality-and-measurement/quality-improvement/clinical-consensus-statement-and-quality-improvement-issue-brief-(ccs-and-qiib)/shared-decision-making

Moullin, J. C., Dickson, K. S., Stadnick, N. A., et al. 2020. Ten recommendations for using implementation frameworks in research and practice. *Implement Sci Commun*, **1**, 42.

Paudel, R., Lane, G. I. 2022. Delivering patient-centered care through shared decision making in overactive bladder. *Neurourol Urodyn*, **41**, 884–893.

Skolarus, T. A., Sales, A. E. 2015. Implementation issues: towards a systematic and stepwise approach. In: Richards, D. A., Hallberg, I. R. Eds. *Complex Interventions in Health: An Overview of Research Methods*, pp. 265–272. Routledge.

Stacey, D., Légaré, F., Lewis, K., et al. 2017. Decision aids for people facing health treatment or screening decisions. *Cochrane Database Syst Rev*, **4**, CD001431.

40

Shared decision making in orthopaedic surgery

Elizabeth A. Kroll, Adina Harri, Robert Schlegel, and Vincent D. Pellegrini Jr

Introduction

Shared decision making (SDM) is essential in orthopaedics due to the elective and highly discretionary nature of many orthopaedic procedures, as well as the subjective interpretation of their benefit to a diverse population of patients. The role of SDM in orthopaedics continues to develop with the potential to improve clinical encounters and outcomes (Slover et al., 2012, 2014; Klifto et al., 2017; Wilson and Probe, 2020; Riddle et al., 2021). In managing orthopaedic problems ranging from acute fractures to chronic conditions, there is often a ladder of treatment options escalating to surgical management. The progression through these options considers both the clinician's expertise with respect to the risks and benefits of the various interventions and the patient's treatment priorities and preferences. In the absence of a clear and definitive directive to the 'best' treatment, the management trajectory is often not clearly delineated by clinical guidelines and thus requires nuanced discussions where SDM plays a critical role, as highlighted in an interview conducted with a patient who underwent total hip arthroplasty (Box 40.1).

To accurately capture the nature of SDM in orthopaedics, an understanding of the contextual definitions of elective, subjective, discretionary, and patient preferences is required.

Elective may be defined as a medical intervention that is undertaken by choice and is medically *reasonable* but not medically *necessary* as a life-saving or essential disease-modifying intervention. One example might be a patient considering total hip replacement to relieve unrelenting osteoarthritic pain (Box 40.1). Such a procedure may be very desirable in the surgeon's opinion and hold the prospect of great benefit to the patient, but an elderly and sedentary individual may find the potential benefit to not sufficiently offset the apparent risk and elect not to proceed with surgery.

Subjective may be defined as the variation in any one person's (patient or physician) individual interpretation of a medical decision that is influenced, consciously or subconsciously, by their beliefs, emotions, and lived experience. For example, an individual with hip arthritis may have a relative who endured a debilitating infection following hip replacement that culminated in the removal of the prosthesis and an inability to walk independently. This person is much more likely to decline hip replacement than someone who has a cadre of friends who returned to active tennis play following their hip replacement surgery.

Discretionary may be defined as the quality by which a person's judgement influences their decision and implies that this judgement may be influenced by other unrelated, illogical, or even perverse incentives. A Dartmouth Atlas Project study (Fisher et al., 2010) illustrated this point by revealing that the rate of performance of hip and knee replacement varies widely depending on one's zip code in the USA, even when

Box 40.1 Patient perspective

SDM centres the conversation around the patient's experience:

> I want to see the patient be given permission to express what their life is like. I want to see clinicians willing to ask questions and listen to answers: 'How much is this getting in the way? What don't you do now that you used to do?'

The elective and subjective nature of orthopaedics makes SDM conversations particularly relevant:

> There does seem to be more of an element of decision making with orthopaedic surgery. As an example, I've had spine issues for years; the surgeon who saw my magnetic resonance imaging scan wanted me in surgery the next day. It's been 30 years since then, and I did not go along with it. SDM did not play a role in that encounter—there was not as much SDM 30 years ago. Unlike the symptoms of arthritis . . . which are incremental and go on for years, back pain comes and goes. I think SDM is even more relevant for the kind of pain that comes and goes. Risks become really relevant at that point.

Conversation aids prompt providers to listen to the patient's story:

> I think there's a significant benefit of using conversation aids if providers have the time for them. It's important for both parties to be involved, and the conversation aid allows for that to happen. I like the distinction between decision aid and conversation aid: conversation prompts should really be the way it goes versus relying on a cutoff score. The more you can get the provider to spend a little more time just listening, the better things will be.

all other patient characteristics are normalized to create similar populations within each geographic region. For example, someone in Colorado is five times as likely as someone in Louisiana to undergo hip replacement with similar types and severity of symptoms. This geographic variation in procedure utilization has been linked to the number of surgeons capable and ready to perform the desired procedure, revealing how non-medical market forces might influence a surgeon's judgement and thereby introduce a discretionary aspect to SDM conversations.

Finally, *patient preferences* may be defined as an individual's conscious rational interpretation, values, perceptions, life circumstances, and experiences that logically guide choices in a medical decision making process. For example, the same sedentary individual with advanced hip disease may judge the benefit of a hip replacement as relatively modest given that person's satisfaction with a sedentary lifestyle. This viewpoint might be radically different from the subjective assessment of the benefit of hip replacement by an octogenarian who still plays tennis but is now limited by hip pain and is not willing to accept that limitation in activities. In these two circumstances, differing patient lifestyle preferences guide an identical SDM conversation about undergoing the same hip replacement procedure, leading one to avoid surgery in the former and pursue it in the latter instance. The patient interview (Box 40.1) underscores the importance of asking questions about how a patient's symptoms impact activities of importance to them.

Together, these definitions elucidate the distinctive nature and critical importance of SDM in orthopaedics.

The place of SDM in orthopaedics

While SDM plays a role in many orthopaedic procedures, its utility is perhaps most clearly illustrated in the characteristically elective instances of joint replacement surgery. Total hip arthroplasty and total knee arthroplasty are regarded as nearly uniformly successful operations in improving pain and function in patients with arthritis. However, the decision to proceed and the timing of surgery remain quite subjective and highly discretionary (Riddle et al., 2014; Franklin et al., 2015; Nguyen et al., 2016). While the American Academy of Orthopaedic Surgeons has developed 'appropriate use criteria' (Porucznik, 2012) for the surgical management of osteoarthritis of the hip (American Academy of Orthopaedic Surgeons, 2017; Quinn et al., 2018a) and knee (Quinn et al., 2018b; American Academy of Orthopaedic Surgeons, 2022) to 'specify when it is appropriate to perform each procedure' (Porucznik, 2012), these complex guidelines assess patient medical comorbidities for the purpose of achieving medical optimization to reduce the risk of perioperative complications. While these criteria guide the surgeon in a risk–benefit analysis to avoid complications, they fall short of defining patient preferences and indications to perform the procedure.

Likewise, appropriate integration of SDM into clinical orthopaedic practice has some caveats. It is important to note that SDM does not necessarily factor into every clinical care decision—for example, it may not be expected for the surgeon to necessarily seek patient input regarding surgical approach, antibiotic selection, or postoperative restrictions. Nevertheless, some patients arrive with a clear idea of how they wish their operation would be performed, with which device, and with limited postoperative activity restrictions. As the definition of SDM suggests, some aspects of decision making are primarily within the surgeon's purview, subject to discussion perhaps but not typically where the patient's views are sought regarding the decision.

Total joint replacement: elective, subjective, and discretionary

Nevertheless, the importance of SDM in determining readiness for joint replacement, as well as most other orthopaedic procedures, is underscored by the subjective and individual nature of the interpretation of surgical outcomes. For example, while total knee arthroplasty is a generally very successful procedure, some studies suggest postoperative patient dissatisfaction rates ranging from 10% to 30% (Ayers et al., 2004; Franklin et al., 2008; Lavallee et al., 2016; Gunaratne et al., 2017; DeFrance and Scuderi, 2023). This is not surprising given that total hip arthroplasty and total knee arthroplasty address subjective quality-of-life issues in managing pain from chronic illness rather than seeking to cure life-threatening diseases. The outcome of total joint replacement, as reported by the patient, will be influenced by their preoperative goals and expectations, thus emphasizing the critical importance of a SDM discussion that incorporates patient preferences and their subjective experiences along with a careful assessment of where communication gaps can occur that can lead to unintended postoperative patient dissatisfaction.

Efforts at improving SDM in orthopaedic surgery have historically manifested in the form of decision aids. Tools such as informational pamphlets or online surveys aim to equip patients with knowledge to discuss their personal willingness and/or readiness for surgery. Numerous decision aids for orthopaedic procedures have been compiled by many organizations, such as the Ottawa Hospital Research Institute, including specific decision aids to assist in determining readiness for hip and knee arthroplasty (Healthwise, 2022a, 2022b). While some researchers suggest that these decision aids may contribute to lower rates of joint replacement utilization (Arterburn et al., 2012), others found that patients who underwent total hip and knee replacement after a decision making conversation that met accepted criteria for being 'informed' and 'incorporating patient preferences' correlated with improved patient-reported satisfaction and less regret (Sepucha et al., 2018, 2022).

Tools to facilitate implementation

Although comprehensive patient *decision aids* may be useful, briefer *conversation aids* may provide a distinct benefit to the SDM process. Decision aids are usually provided to the patient in preparation for a conversation regarding treatment options, whereas conversation aids are designed to be utilized during the SDM conversation to promote sharing of information, including surgeon views, patient priorities, subjective patient experience, and realistic expectations. Such aids (Box 40.1) can facilitate nuanced discussion and communication between the patient and clinician. While there are many decision aids developed for use in orthopaedics, there are fewer tools designed to facilitate the SDM conversation itself. Furthermore, while the benefits of decision aids in determining readiness for surgery are espoused, this has been argued to be relevant to the historic use of 'informed' decision making rather than actual 'shared' decision making (Riddle et al., 2021). Indeed, there is currently a paucity of research into the benefit of conversation aids in facilitating a SDM process, as well as a shortage of freely available conversation aids.

One such ‘conversation aid’ currently being studied is the Objective Performance Threshold Indicating Operative Need (OPTION) survey (Kroll et al., 2025). The OPTION survey seeks to identify criteria important to patients when considering the desirability of hip or knee replacement and was developed utilizing a modified Delphi method with collaboration between orthopaedic surgeons and patients who had recently undergone total hip arthroplasty or total knee arthroplasty. The resulting instrument was designed to facilitate a SDM discussion with the orthopaedic clinician regarding whether a patient is ready for total hip or knee replacement by interrogating pain, readiness for surgery, activity limitation, prior treatments, radiographic changes, and an understanding of patient treatment priorities. The survey is administered in two parts during the clinical encounter, with patient and surgeon each providing individual responses that jointly support a SDM conversation about whether to proceed with surgery based on consideration of patient expectations and the potential benefits of the procedure. The second part of the survey invites the patient to assess the quality of the SDM conversation. An important underlying assumption is that the patient is comfortable with their understanding of the risks, potential benefits, and anticipated postoperative course, such that their decision aligns with their own values, preferences, and experiences. While still under development, OPTION pilot surveys provide insight into the SDM conversation through a patient lens for determining readiness for joint replacement surgery (Kroll et al., 2025).

In the OPTION data, patient priorities in arthritis treatment varied with progression of the self-reported impact of their arthritis, including worsening pain, activity limitation, quality of life, and readiness for surgery. While patients consistently prioritized treating pain and removing activity limitations as important goals of surgery, they exhibited a particularly low tolerance for activity limitations and were accepting of long recovery times to eliminate even modest activity limitations. Conversely, neither the moderate importance attributed to avoiding complications nor the lack of concern over cost considerations fluctuated with worsening arthritis symptoms. These findings augment the literature delineating the variable characteristics of patients considering joint replacement (Ayers et al., 2004; Franklin et al., 2008; Nguyen et al., 2016). The imperfect relationship between symptom severity and radiographic disease was also revealed in the OPTION data; higher Kellgren–Lawrence grades (representing increasing arthritis severity) were associated with increasing patient-reported readiness for surgery, while patients reporting low pain levels had similar Kellgren–Lawrence grades to those reporting severe pain (Kroll et al., 2025). Orthopaedics relies heavily on imaging, which all too often invites surgeons to rely on imaging modalities over an in-depth patient history and physical exam. The OPTION data align with other studies demonstrating variable correlation between joint space changes and patient symptoms (Duncan et al., 2006; Bedson and Croft, 2008; Özden et al., 2020). These findings further warn against making assumptions regarding a patient's subjective pain levels based on imaging in the absence of both a physical examination and a purposeful conversation with the patient.

Furthermore, while patients and surgeons typically agree regarding symptom severity and readiness for surgery, the OPTION data revealed that when discordance occurred, surgeons most often underestimated the patient's self-reported symptoms, particularly pain (Kroll et al., 2025). These instances of disagreement were associated with lower patient-rated quality of SDM conversations (Kroll et al., 2025). This phenomenon has been previously explored, and healthcare providers have been shown to often underestimate patient pain (Berduszek et al., 2022), with the interpretation of pain severity differing depending on chronicity (Kappesser and de C. Williams, 2010). Collectively these findings highlight that surgeons may underestimate the degree to which patient-perceived pain is influenced by biopsychosocial factors. Furthermore, the OPTION data suggest poorly executed SDM conversations may be associated with discordant patient–surgeon perspectives regarding important clinical criteria (Kroll et al., 2025). In aggregate, OPTION survey pilot data amplify the literature by illustrating the complexity and diversity of patients who are considering total joint replacement and demonstrate myriad points in the determination of readiness for surgery that constitute pitfalls for miscommunication. Obvious benefits can accrue from deliberate and intentional discussions based on SDM and assist with the use of a ‘conversation aid’.

Practical application in orthopaedic practice

Notwithstanding that total hip replacement is one of the most successful procedures in the history of modern surgery (Learmonth et al., 2007) and joint replacement is also perhaps the most controlled demonstration of the importance of SDM in orthopaedics, the utilization of SDM extends into most elements of the field. The conversation with a professional athlete versus a sedentary individual differs dramatically when deciding how to manage a torn anterior cruciate ligament. When recommending how to manage an acute fracture, the surgeon should consider factors such as the patient's activity goals, job demands, and willingness to undergo surgical treatment in contrast with their likelihood of adherence to the often more stringent guidelines for non-surgical management. Indeed, in some cases, such as hip fractures, the risks of complications with non-operative care are so great that surgery can represent the ‘conservative’ treatment course. In such instances, the surgeon's expertise and experience may take precedence over a patient's hesitance to pursue surgery. Alternatively, when managing chronic low back pain, which is often best managed-non-operatively, the decision to pursue an operation relies heavily on the surgeon's discretion and obligation to emphasize medical management and outline realistic expectations and risks from surgical versus medical treatment despite a patient's eagerness to pursue surgery as a perceived solution for back pain. The differing role of SDM in hip osteoarthritis versus chronic back pain is highlighted in the patient interview (Box 40.1).

Successful outcomes in orthopaedics occur when patients achieve both an acceptable level of pain reduction and improvement in desired function, *as defined by the patient*. These outcomes are as complex as the preferences and backgrounds of the individuals being treated and are subject to the discretionary, subjective, and elective nature of orthopaedics. Accordingly, the nuances afforded by utilizing a SDM process in orthopaedics are a necessary and pivotal part of any patient–surgeon discussion that will afford patients the opportunity to achieve their greatest potential benefit from any treatment.

REFERENCES

American Academy of Orthopaedic Surgeons. 2017. Appropriate use criteria for the management of osteoarthritis of the hip. Available at: https://www.aaos.org/oahauc

American Academy of Orthopaedic Surgeons. 2022. Appropriate use criteria for the management of osteoarthritis of the knee. Available at: https://www.aaos.org/oakauc

Arterburn, D., Wellman, R., Westbrook, E. 2012. Introducing decision aids at group health was linked to sharply lower hip and knee surgery rates and costs. *Health Affairs,* **31**, 2094–2104.

Ayers, D. C., Franklin, P. D., Trief, P. M., Ploutz-Snyder, R., Freund, D. 2004. Psychological attributes of preoperative total joint replacement patients. *J Arthroplasty,* **19**, 125–130.

Bedson, J., Croft, P. R. 2008. The discordance between clinical and radiographic knee osteoarthritis: a systematic search and summary of the literature. *BMC Musculoskelet Disord,* **9**, 116.

Berduszek, R. J., Reinders-Messelink, H. A., Dijkstra, P. U., van der Sluis, C. K. 2022. Comparison between patient-reported and physician-estimated pain and disability in hand and wrist disorders. *Musculoskeletal Care,* **20**, 354–362.

DeFrance, M. J., Scuderi, G. R. 2023. Are 20% of patients actually dissatisfied following total knee arthroplasty? A systematic review of the literature. *J Arthroplasty,* **38**, 594–599.

Duncan, R., Peat, G., Thomas, E., Hay, E., McCall, I., Croft, P. 2006. Symptoms and radiographic osteoarthritis: not as discordant as they are made out to be? *Ann Rheum Dis,* **66**, 86–91.

Fisher, E. S., Bell, J. E., Tomek, I. M., et al. 2010. *Trends and Regional Variation in Hip, Knee, and Shoulder Replacement: A Dartmouth Atlas Surgery Report.* The Dartmouth Institute for Health Policy and Clinical Practice (The Dartmouth Atlas of Health Care). Available at: http://www.ncbi.nlm.nih.gov/books/NBK586141/

Franklin, P. D., Li, W., Ayers, D. C. 2008. The Chitranjan Ranawat Award: functional outcome after total knee replacement varies with patient attributes. *Clin Orthop Relat Res,* **466**, 2597–2604.

Franklin, P., Nguyen, U., Ayers, D., Weissman, N., FORCE-TJR Investigators. 2015. Improving the criteria for appropriateness of total joint replacement surgery: comment on the article by Riddle et al. *Arthritis Rheumatol,* **67**, 585–585.

Gunaratne, R., Pratt, D. N., Banda, J., Fick, D. P., Khan, R. J. K., Robertson, B. W. 2017. Patient dissatisfaction following total knee arthroplasty: a systematic review of the literature. *J Arthroplasty,* **32**, 3854–3860.

Healthwise. 2022a. Arthritis: should I have hip replacement surgery? The Ottawa Hospital Research Institute. Available at: https://decisionaid.ohri.ca/AZsumm.php?ID=1112

Healthwise. 2022b. Arthritis: should I have knee replacement surgery? The Ottawa Hospital Research Institute. Available at: https://decisionaid.ohri.ca/Azsumm.php?ID=1191

Kappesser, J., de C. Williams, A. C. 2010. Pain estimation: asking the right questions. *Pain,* **148**, 184–187.

Klifto, K., Klifto, C., Slover, J. 2017. Current concepts of shared decision making in orthopedic surgery. *Curr Rev Musculoskelet Med,* **10**, 253–257.

Kroll, E., Warren, C., Schlegel, R., et al. 2025. Shared decision-making in total hip and knee arthroplasty: understanding surgeon and patient perspectives regarding when it is time for operation. *J Bone Joint Surg Am,* **107**, 575–585.

Lavallee, D. C., Chenok, K. E., Love, R. M. et al. 2016. Incorporating patient-reported outcomes into health care to engage patients and enhance care. *Health Aff (Millwood),* **35**, 575–582.

Learmonth, I. D., Young, C., Rorabeck, C. 2007. The operation of the century: total hip replacement. *Lancet,* **370**, 1508–1519.

Nguyen, U.-S. D. T., Ayers, D. C., Li, W., Harrold, L. R., Franklin, P. D. 2016. Preoperative pain and function: profiles of patients selected for total knee arthroplasty. *J Arthroplasty,* **31**, 2402–2407.e2.

Özden, F., Nadiye Karaman, Ö., Tuğay, N., et al. 2020. The relationship of radiographic findings with pain, function, and quality of life in patients with knee osteoarthritis. *J Clin Orthop Trauma,* **11**, S512–S517.

Porucznik, M. A. 2012. What are appropriate use criteria? The next step on the road to quality. *AAOS Now,* July, 46. Gale OneFile: Health and Medicine. Available at: link.gale.com/apps/doc/A298615197/HRCA

Quinn, R. H., Murray, J., Pezold, R., Hall, Q. 2018a. Management of osteoarthritis of the hip. *J Am Acad Orthop Surg,* **26**, e434–e436.

Quinn, R. H., Murray, J. N., Pezold, R., Sevarino, K. S. 2018b. Surgical management of osteoarthritis of the knee. *J Am Acad Orthop Surg,* **26**, e191–e193.

Riddle, D. L., Jiranek, W. A., Hayes, C. W. 2014. Use of a validated algorithm to judge the appropriateness of total knee arthroplasty in the United States: a multicenter longitudinal cohort study. *Arthritis Rheumatol,* **66**, 2134–2143.

Riddle, D. L., Sando, T., Tarver, T., et al. 2021. Shared decision-making applied to knee arthroplasty: a systematic review of randomized trials. *Arthritis Care Res,* **73**, 1125–1133.

Sepucha, K. R., Atlas, S. J., Chang, Y., et al. 2018. Informed, patient-centered decisions associated with better health outcomes in orthopedics: prospective cohort study. *Med Decis Making,* **38**, 1018–1026.

Sepucha, K. R., Vo, H., Chang, Y., et al. 2022. Shared decision-making is associated with better outcomes in patients with knee but not hip osteoarthritis: the DECIDE-OA randomized study. *J Bone Joint Surg,* **104**, 62–69.

Slover, J., Alvarado, C., Nelson, C. 2014. Shared decision making in total joint replacement. *JBJS Rev,* **2**, e1.

Slover, J., Shue, J., Koenig, K. 2012. Shared decision-making in orthopaedic surgery. *Clin Orthop Related Res,* **470**, 1046–1053.

Wilson, C. D., Probe, R. A. 2020. Shared decision-making in orthopaedic surgery. *J Am Acad Orthop Surg,* **28**, e1032–e1041.

41

Shared decision making in public health

Balancing individual choice with the common good

Rachel C. Forcino, Robert M. Kaplan, Helen Leonard, and Christian von Plessen

The relevance of shared decision making to the decisions faced in public health

At first sight, shared decision making (SDM) and public health (PH) are not a good match. SDM promotes individual informed choice, while the goal of PH is to improve the common good. Individual choice and common good do not always align. Individual preferences might not be advantageous for the public, and common interest might require limiting individual choice. Quarantines and mandatory vaccination are classic examples of the latter and an individual decision for a costly treatment over a cheaper alternative might impact the common interest.

At second sight, however, individual-level SDM can very well serve the common good, and vice versa. For instance, it can improve uptake of and adherence to pandemic measures, including vaccines, screening programmes, and prevention measures (Politi et al., 2013; Scalia et al., 2022). Advancing the common good might also serve individual interests, as was the case of temporary pandemic lockdowns to protect individuals against infection. Even John Stewart Mill, a strong advocate for individual freedoms, recognized the right of public officials to restrict the activities of individuals when they are likely to harm others (Cerovac, 2022).

However, the individual advantage might not be visible at first sight. Hearing and convincing the persons concerned about their view of the arbitration between personal freedom and protection of the population might be required. This tension, fed by populists and amplified by social media, has resulted in intense ethical, political, and sometimes ideological debate. For decades, PH has viewed itself as more progressive than other medical disciplines. Members of the PH community typically embrace humanitarian causes and the dignity and autonomy of individuals. Yet, the roles of medicine and PH appear to have been reversed during the COVID-19 pandemic.

Patient involvement in coproduction has become widely accepted in the clinical practice of medicine and surgery and has increasingly become the default option for a wide range of conditions where no single intervention strategy is dominant. Central to the departure from more paternalistic approaches to SDM is the recognition that the patient and clinician share control of the decision process, where the patient has ownership of the ultimate decision and healthcare providers serve in a supportive and consulting role. In a relatively short period of time, SDM has gained significant footholds in medicine with papers describing SDM appearing in a wide range of medical specialty journals. Figure 41.1 shows the exponential increase in studies using 'shared decision making' as a keyword in medical journals but a slower increase in those using 'shared decision making' and 'public health' between 1993 and 2023. We also note a drop-off in studies using 'shared decision making' and 'public health' as keywords after the COVID-19 pandemic onset in 2020. This picture is reflected in practice, where SDM is less recognized in PH in comparison to clinical medicine.

In this chapter, we focus on the role and acceptance of SDM in PH in comparison to clinical medicine through five questions:

1. Is there a role for SDM in PH?
2. In which PH situations is SDM likely to be useful?
3. What adaptions need to be made to patient decision aids for the PH context?

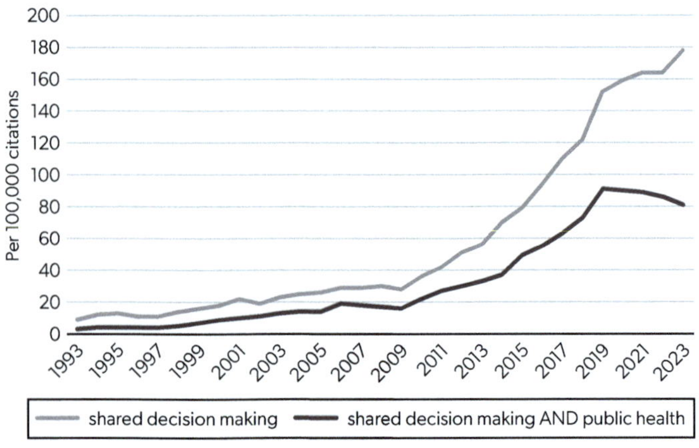

Figure 41.1 'Shared decision making' and 'public health' articles in PubMed: 1993–2023. To adjust for the substantial overall increase in publications, we show SDM publications per 100,000 citations on all topics.

4. Which conditions, including facilitators and barriers, should be considered in implementing SDM in the domains of PH?
5. Which controversies need to be addressed?

Current use of SDM in PH

Although community preferences are widely recognized as important and valuable, SDM has not been consistently used in PH decision making. Population screening programmes are aligned with PH priorities, such as limiting preventable disease and monitoring population health. Many screening tests offer substantial benefit to individuals and communities, including tests for common cancers with high morbidity and mortality burdens and effective treatments, such as colon and breast cancers. In these cases, widespread screening limits the individual burden of advanced disease by allowing for early diagnosis and potentially curative treatment, while also limiting the societal burden associated with costly treatment and disability resulting from advanced disease. As such, the PH focus is on promoting uptake. For other conditions, it is not clear that the benefits of screening outweigh the potential harms.

What is the potential role of SDM in PH?

Global panic accompanied the emergence of the COVID-19 pandemic in 2020, and many countries developed mandates for mask wearing. By December of 2020, vaccines were available, and campaigns were initiated to assure high uptake. Yet, as often is the case in healthcare, the evidence supporting these interventions was mixed. Studies both supported and refuted the benefits of masks (Jefferson et al., 2023), and while early clinical trial data suggested vaccines reduced the transmission of the SARS-CoV-2 virus, the benefit of initial doses and boosters did not appear to be as protective as expected. Evidence that vaccines prevented hospitalization and death came from observational studies, not from controlled trials (Fung et al., 2024). There were clear biases in these observational studies because healthy and wealthy people were more likely to accept the vaccine, while refusers tended to be from higher risk groups (Høeg et al., 2023).

Instead of directly confronting and communicating uncertainty, and presenting a more balanced view of findings, PH agencies emphasized the advice of leading authorities, politicians, sports heroes, and celebrities. Evidence evaluation and informed decision making was less prominent in the debate than the advice to trust known authorities, and those rejecting the vaccine were characterized as foolish and irresponsible (Hornsey, 2022). SDM, now well established in medical care, could have played a larger role in the pandemic PH decisions, providing people with transparent and comprehensive information about the potential harms and benefits of the vaccine and engaging them in the decision making process.

Overall, SDM has been largely neglected by PH officials, both during and prior to the pandemic. Applying SDM to vaccine acceptance and uptake requires a shift away from demanding adherence to PH authorities. Instead, the emphasis is on honest disclosure about what to expect. This requires a clear presentation of the risks and benefits of vaccination and an acknowledgement of the dependability or non-dependability of the available data.

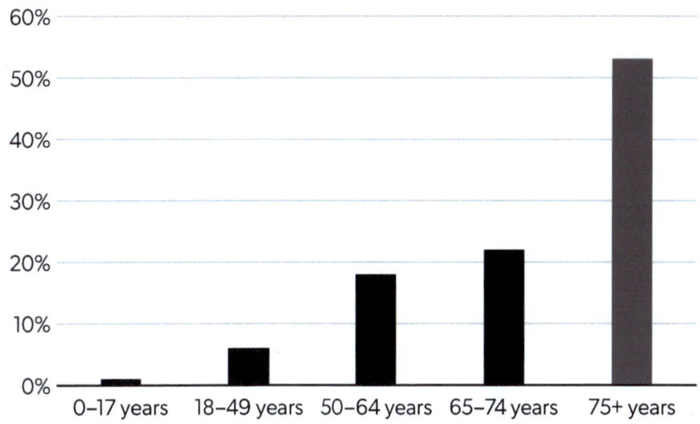

Figure 41.2 Share of COVID-19 deaths by age in the USA as of June 2023.

Source: data from Statista: https://www.statista.com/statistics/1191568/reported-deaths-from-covid-by-age-us/

However, communicating and understanding risks and benefits is not simple. COVID-19 communication campaigns imply that those accepting the vaccines have a 95% chance of avoiding infection while those injected with placebo have no protection; neither statement is factually correct. The Pfizer trial observed eight COVID-19 cases among 18,198 (0.04%) people who received the vaccine within 2 months of completing their second shot (Food and Drug Administration, 2022). In contrast, 162 of 18,325 volunteers who got the placebo (0.88%) got COVID-19. In other words, less than 1% of each group became infected, but among those who got sick, 95% were in the placebo group. We agree the vaccines were highly efficacious, but evidence accumulated over the last few years reveals that a substantial portion of vaccinated persons eventually got infected. In a campaign that vaccinates 200 million people we might expect about 80,000 COVID-19 cases. So, PH authorities must better prepare the public for the likelihood that some vaccinated people will still get sick (Wennberg, 2010).

Communication campaigns must recognize that one size does not fit all, and that SDM can play a role in COVID-19 vaccine decisions. The probability of serious consequences of COVID-19 infection increases with age (Figure 41.2). Clearly, those older than 65 years are at greater risk and should be more attracted to the potential benefits of vaccination. Teenagers and young adults have a much lower probability of becoming seriously ill or dying. Deciding not to take the vaccine is a riskier choice for an 80-year-old than for a 20-year-old. Decisions should ultimately be tailored to individual circumstances and preferences—this requires a SDM approach.

In which PH situations could SDM be useful?

PH spans numerous situations, touching many aspects of public life, and offers varied opportunities for SDM. Recommendations for the use of SDM by the US Preventive Services Task Force (USPSTF) offer several useful examples (USPSTF, 2018).

The USPSTF uses the best available evidence to make recommendations about preventive services, including screening, behavioural counselling, and medications that are used for prevention. Most of these recommendations concern services that are offered in primary care or that are referable by primary care physicians. Health problems in this domain do not usually have identifiable signs or symptoms. For each service, a systematic review of the literature is conducted, and the USPSTF makes a recommendation using categories defined in Table 41.1. The evaluation process is transparent, professional groups and the public have extensive opportunities to provide input, and the results are publicly available.

Services that receive an A or a B grade are recommended for use in practice. In the USA, the recommendations are important because any service receiving an A or a B grade is covered by both public and private insurers under the Affordable Care Act, without any financial cost to the person receiving the service. SDM is used to share information about the harms and benefits of these services and to identify personal preferences. Services that receive C grades are associated with a higher degree of uncertainty. These may involve gaps in evidence or equipoise between different possible courses of action. Services receiving C grades are considered ideal candidates for SDM discussions in which a health professional shares evidence-based information about the potential benefits and harms and supports the person to develop informed preferences. Services receiving a D grade are not recommended for use in practice and those receiving an I grade lack sufficient evidence to issue a recommendation. In the absence of sufficient evidence to recommend these services, the lived expertise of individual citizens and the professional experience of health professionals may determine whether individual autonomy should be prioritized through SDM despite the vacuum of evidence-based information.

Some screening programmes present opportunities for SDM. For example, colon cancers can be detected through both colonoscopy and fecal immunochemical testing. Despite equipoise in their clinical effectiveness for most people, these two tests have different requirements of the person being tested, including laxative preparation and sedation (colonoscopy) and independently collecting and submitting faecal samples (faecal immunochemical testing). They also have different requirements of health services, including high cost, time and expertise from gastroenterologists and anaesthesiologists, health system space, staffing, and other common resources for colonoscopy. Given the preference-sensitive nature of these trade-offs and differences in resources required, SDM can help to optimize this decision for the person screened.

What adaptions need to be made to patient decision aids for the PH context?

Patient decision aids presenting easy-to-understand evidence-based information are recommended to support SDM. These tools generally include information specific to individual-level benefits and harms of medical treatment, screening, or management alternatives. In contexts where individual health decisions interact with PH

Table 41.1 USPSTF grading of recommendations, suggestions for practice as well as, added by the authors, a potential place for SDM and occurrence in practice

Grade	Definition	Suggestions for practice	Example(s)	Need for SDM	Occurrence in practice
A	The USPSTF recommends the service. There is high certainty that the net benefit is substantial	Offer or provide this service	HIV prevention through pre-exposure prophylaxis Prenatal folic acid supplementation to prevent neural tube defects	No	Rare
B	The USPSTF recommends the service. There is high certainty that the net benefit is moderate or there is moderate certainty that the net benefit is moderate to substantial	Offer or provide this service	Screening for anxiety disorders in adults Screening for latent tuberculosis infection in adults and senior citizens	Yes	Common
C	The USPSTF recommends selectively offering or providing this service to individual patients based on professional judgement and patient preferences. There is at least moderate certainty that the net benefit is small	Offer or provide this service for selected patients depending on individual circumstances	Aspirin to prevent cardiovascular disease in adults Prostate cancer screening in adults ages 55–69	Yes	Rare
D	The USPSTF recommends against the service. There is moderate or high certainty that the service has no net benefit or that the harms outweigh the benefits	Discourage the use of this service	Screening for genital herpes Hormone replacement post-menopause	No	Rare
I	The USPSTF concludes that the current evidence is insufficient to assess the balance of benefits and harms of the service. Evidence is lacking, of poor quality, or conflicting, and the balance of benefits and harms cannot be determined	Read the clinical considerations section of USPSTF Recommendation Statement. If the service is offered, patients should understand the uncertainty about the balance of benefits and harms	Screening for skin cancer in adults Screening for obstructive sleep apnoea in adults and senior citizens	Yes/No?	Very common

Source: US Preventive Services Task Force (2018).

and the common good, information on societal harms and benefits should also be presented alongside individual-level information. For example, patient decision aids about COVID-19 prevention measures have also included information about societal benefits, such as a reduction in community transmission (Ottawa Hospital Research Institute, n.d.). By including societal-level evidence alongside individual evidence of harms and benefits, patient decision aids could better support people in making PH decisions that align with their personal values and preferences while also factoring in the common good.

What are the barriers and facilitators to implementing SDM in PH?

Despite the conceptual differences between PH and clinical medicine applications of SDM, the barriers and facilitators of SDM implementation are similar. Effective SDM implementation requires political backing—whether from a legislature (PH) or a health system leader (clinical medicine). As with health professionals in clinical medicine, PH officers and public administrators must learn to elicit and respect the perspectives of populations in policy decisions. Collaboration between PH and clinical medicine, particularly primary care, may be a promising avenue to both facilitate knowledge transfer about SDM and gather information from segments of the population that can better inform PH policy. SDM also requires substantial investments of time and resources (Joseph-Williams et al., 2019).

PH professionals may find that eliciting public preferences to guide decision making takes more time than autonomous action. Further, decision aids that simplify complex information are resource intensive to create and update following evolving evidence, as with the rapidly evolving evidence on COVID-19 vaccines. Finally, decisions are not mechanical, tool-dependent processes. Shared decisions in clinical care rely on trust and relationships between patients and clinicians, which differ from the trust and relationships at play between PH officials and populations. When considering the needs of populations, relying on interpersonal relationships that promote dialogue and build trust does not scale. Instead, mass communication campaigns and participatory governance approaches must build trust and rapport between PH officials and the public.

Which controversies need to be addressed?

Tension between individual autonomy and collective health and safety is the core controversy surrounding SDM in PH. This tension provokes questions about when SDM should be used in PH and when it may be inappropriate. For example, several health authorities worldwide mandate compulsory treatment for tuberculosis infection; this context, too, is subject to calls for SDM. Yet, when SDM is inappropriate, we must not offer the illusion of choice when there is none—that is, when an individual's choice would be unacceptable from a societal standpoint.

In cases where SDM is inappropriate from a societal perspective, SDM-aligned efforts may instead resemble participatory policymaking. While some sectors of government (e.g. land use permits), have substantial experience in gathering public input to inform policy decisions, PH has a more limited track record. A key question is therefore how to effectively and equitably apply SDM principles derived from clinical medicine to sharing policy decisions between PH authorities and representative segments of the populations that they serve. The impact of misinformation, spread quickly through social media in a global climate of political polarization, is an added hurdle to informed and shared PH decisions at the population level. This raises further questions about whether SDM is transferable from clinical care to PH—and whether its use in the PH context is appropriate, feasible, and desired by both PH officials and the populations they serve.

Next steps and future priorities

Incorporating SDM in PH practice appears to have great potential for empowering individuals and protecting communities. SDM in PH might help integrate and even reconcile individual interests and the common good. However, there are important gaps in evidence on the use of SDM in PH. Next steps must address gaps in expanding SDM models and approaches to address PH needs, improving SDM knowledge and skills among PH professionals, effectively and equitably applying SDM principles derived from clinical medicine to sharing policy decisions between PH authorities and representative segments of the populations that they serve, and developing and testing tools to support SDM in PH.

See Box 41.1 for our patient perspective.

Box 41.1 Patient perspective

As an individual and as a parent, I understand that PH advice is intended to improve health and protect people. The amount of information about keeping myself, my family, and my community healthy sometimes feels overwhelming, confusing, and changeable. Is it fat or carbs that are bad this week? What screening do I need?

In the past there was an expectation that people would follow expert advice unquestioningly, but society has moved away from the 'doctor knows best' approach and people want to understand why they are being told to do things. Yet, information directed to the public is often still in the form of straight advice ('Get your flu jab', 'Get screened') without explanation.

Although there are some areas where the evidence around PH advice seems very clear to experts in the medical community and it is a 'no brainer' that people should comply, it would still be helpful if the reasoning behind it could be shared with the people who are expected to follow the advice. It is even more important to do this where the evidence is not strong or where there are possible downsides to interventions. Screening for diseases offered by private companies, which on the face of it seems like a good idea to consumers, might serve as an example.

The ideal would be to have time to discuss information with staff. Given that this is not always practical for health practitioners or people who use their services, printed information such as patient decision aids are a useful supplement or alternative to discussions. They have been used in other areas, such as surgical operations, where complex information is presented in an understandable format for people to weigh up the evidence themselves and make decisions that are relevant and appropriate to them. Ideally this information should accompany invitations to screening or vaccination, giving time to consider the decision and ask any questions of health staff prior to attending.

This hunger for information will lead to people searching for information themselves—sometimes from sources that may not be reliable, as we saw in the COVID-19 pandemic. These sources include social media and trusted people in their communities who, although well intentioned, may not have the correct expertise. PH is historically not a common area for SDM and sharing evidence and information. A move towards seeing the public as partners in PH decisions, rather than passive recipients who follow instructions, may be a step forward in better preventative medicine, adherence to health promotion advice, and truly shared responsibility for PH.

Summary

Clinical medicine has made great progress in integrating the patient voice in the decision making process. PH should follow suit. From a practical perspective, empowering individuals as partners in the decision making process results in more acceptance of PH measures than top-down commands from experts. Shared medical decision making can help people use the best scientific evidence in support of choices that best fit their own personal circumstances.

REFERENCES

Cerovac I. 2022. *John Stuart Mill and Epistemic Democracy*. Rowman & Littlefield.

Food and Drug Administration. 2023. 2023–2024 COVID-19 vaccine formula: Pfizer/BioNTech clinical and preclinical supportive data. Vaccines and Related Biological Products Advisory Committee. Available at: https://www.fda.gov/media/169541/download

Fung, K., Jones, M., Doshi, P. 2024. Sources of bias in observational studies of covid-19 vaccine effectiveness. *J Eval Clin Pract*, **30**, 30–36.

Høeg, T. B., Duriseti, R., Prasad, V. 2023. Potential 'healthy vaccinee bias' in a study of BNT162b2 vaccine against covid-19. *N Engl J Med*, **389**, 284–285.

Hornsey, M. J. 2022. Reasons why people may refuse COVID-19 vaccination (and what can be done about it). *World Psychiatry*, **21**, 217–218.

Jefferson, T., Dooley, L., Ferroni, E., et al. 2023. Physical interventions to interrupt or reduce the spread of respiratory viruses. *Cochrane Database Syst Rev*, **1**, CD006207.

Joseph-Williams, N., Abhyankar, P., Boland, L., et al. 2021. What works in implementing patient decision aids in routine clinical settings? A rapid realist review and update from the International Patient Decision Aid Standards Collaboration. *Med Decis Making*, **41**, 907–937.

Ottawa Hospital Research Institute. n.d. A to Z inventory of patient decision aids. Available at: https://decisionaid.ohri.ca/AZinvent.php

Politi, M. C., Wolin, K. Y., Légaré, F. 2013. Implementing clinical practice guidelines about health promotion and disease prevention through shared decision making. *J Gen Intern Med*, **28**, 838–844.

Scalia, P., Durand, M. A., Elwyn, G. 2022. Shared decision-making interventions: an overview and a meta-analysis of their impact on vaccine uptake. *J Intern Med*, **291**, 408–425.

US Preventive Services Task Force. 2018. Grade definitions. Available at: https://www.uspreventiveservicestaskforce.org/uspstf/about-uspstf/methods-and-processes/grade-definitions

Wennberg, J. E. 2010. *Tracking Medicine: A Researcher's Quest to Understand Health Care*. Oxford University Press.

42

Shared decision making for screening

Jolyn Hersch, Rikke Nicoline Stokholm, Janice Tufte, and Carissa Bonner

Introduction

Screening for health conditions entails a complex array of potential consequences, including benefits (e.g. reducing morbidity and mortality) and harms (e.g. directly from invasive investigations, false positives, and overdiagnosis). Health conditions and screening modalities vary in their possible consequences, outcome probabilities, and benefit-to-harm ratios. These variations underpin different recommendations for whether and how to offer screening. Some forms of cancer screening are generally considered advantageous overall (e.g. bowel); some are viewed more negatively (e.g. prostate); while the benefit-to-harm balance is a closer call for others (e.g. breast) (Stefanek, 2011). Other fields have mixed evidence on the cost-effectiveness of organized screening (Oude Wolcherink et al., 2023) but are implemented opportunistically in clinical practice based on evidence for preventive treatment (e.g. cardiovascular risk assessment) (Australian Government Department of Health, 2023). Different study methods, population characteristics, and approaches to screening delivery can lead to contention around benefits and harms (Stefanek, 2011) complicating the task of policymaking about whether and how to screen. Despite these complexities, policymakers increasingly seek to enable informed decisions by giving balanced information to potential screening participants (Australian Government Department of Health, 2018).

The terms informed decision making and shared decision making (SDM) encompass a process where a person participates in making a healthcare decision after learning about a test or treatment and its potential consequences and considering their preferences. SDM, conceptualized in terms of a consultation, may be more relevant to primary care-based testing (e.g. cardiovascular risk), whereas for testing provided elsewhere (e.g. breast cancer), informed decision making may be a better term.

This chapter provides an overview of SDM about screening, highlighting relevant research and practice, using cancer and cardiovascular disease risk as contrasting examples of organized versus opportunistic screening approaches.

The need for informed (shared) decision making

Cancer

Public attitudes around cancer screening are highly positive, with people often supporting screening uncritically. A British survey documented widespread enthusiasm for cancer screening, with 89% of respondents considering it 'almost always a good idea' (Waller et al., 2015). Such attitudes may reflect unrealistic expectations: a systematic review of patient expectations of medical interventions, including 17 studies on screening, found people tend to overestimate benefit and underestimate harm (Hoffmann and Del Mar, 2015). This is unsurprising, given that messages about screening from public health organizations and advocacy groups have often emphasized benefits and minimized harms. This approach, persisting over decades, reflects the standpoint that persuasion is justified to maximize uptake. One frequently employed approach is to induce feelings of fear and vulnerability, then offer hope by framing screening as a simple means of protection (Stefanek, 2011; Woloshin et al., 2012). This has also engendered normative expectations that screening is the 'right' thing to do because of a social obligation to take responsibility for one's health (Willis and Baxter, 2003).

The messaging described above has been criticized as simplistic and overly positive. It is argued that, instead of promoting uptake, screening communication should primarily aim to tell people about harms and benefits to enable informed decisions (Stefanek, 2011; Woloshin et al., 2012). The ethical justification is that screening puts large numbers of healthy people at risk of harm by offering interventions they might not otherwise seek (Australian Government Department of Health, 2018). Advocates of this perspective note that screening can trigger a cascade of serious interventions, including invasive treatments with lasting consequences, and people who choose to screen (or not) must live with their decision and its repercussions. Moreover, although screening may be effective in reducing disease-specific mortality at a population level, the chance of any given individual avoiding a cancer death because of screening is small in absolute terms (see Figure 42.1 for an example

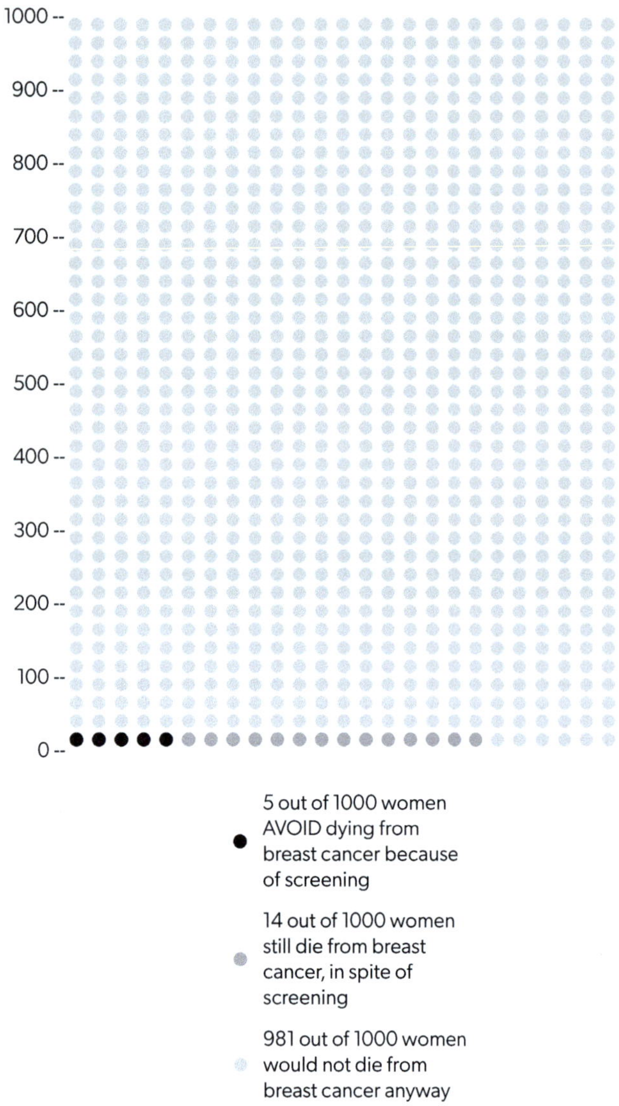

Figure 42.1 Breast cancer deaths avoided due to 25 years of biennial screening.

Source: icon array produced by https://iconarray.com/ using data from a published decision aid (http://hdl.handle.net/2123/16658).

from breast screening—noting, importantly, that the numbers will differ substantially among other cancers screened for, such as bowel or cervical cancer). Individuals may weigh attributes differently depending on their personal circumstances and psychological characteristics, and some might reasonably decline screening (Stefanek, 2011). Therefore, screening decisions are a good example of where helping people to be engaged and involved in informed/SDM may be particularly valuable.

Cardiovascular risk

In cardiovascular disease prevention, opportunistic risk screening is generally done in primary care. There is a lack of evidence to support whole population screening (Paige et al., 2023) so heart health checks are generally done by a general practitioner (GP) as part of another consultation. The health professional therefore plays a key role in communicating the benefits and harms of cardiovascular risk assessment and management. Clinical guidelines recommend using the 'absolute risk' approach to calculate a patient's overall risk of a heart attack or stroke in the next 5–10 years based on a combination of factors like age, sex, smoking, diabetes, blood pressure, and cholesterol (Australian Government Department of Health, 2023). Compared with separate assessments of blood pressure and cholesterol, absolute risk is a better way to identify which patients are at high cardiovascular risk and therefore more likely to benefit from medication, and may reduce overtreatment of patients at low risk. Some guidelines also recommend that GPs refer patients with certain risk factors to a cardiologist for additional tests, such as coronary artery calcium scoring (Australian Government Department of Health, 2023). However, there is mixed evidence for whether the incremental benefit outweighs the cost and harms such as radiation. This exemplifies how what appears to be 'simple' screening can lead to a succession of further investigations of uncertain value.

Recent guideline updates recommend SDM regarding medication for the prevention of cardiovascular disease. There is little benefit for low-risk patients to taking a statin or blood pressure-lowering medication, whereas the evidence strongly supports the efficacy of both medications for those at high risk (Australian Government Department of Health, 2023). However, thresholds for 'high risk' are somewhat arbitrary and differ between risk calculators and countries, meaning the same patient may be recommended to take one or more medications, or none, depending which guidelines are used in which country (Bonner et al., 2019a).

In addition, patients vary in their preferences around cardiovascular prevention (Bonner et al., 2019a). Some may prefer to change their lifestyle rather than consider medication, to avoid side effects. Importantly, while these medications are highly effective in reducing risk at a population level, the chance of an individual avoiding a heart attack or stroke due to taking medication is small in absolute terms (Figure 42.2). Using an absolute risk approach is essential to allow patients to weigh up benefits and harms of additional tests and medication for their risk level, but health professionals do not always communicate this information with patients (Bonner et al., 2019a).

Decision aids to support SDM in screening

Although screening providers and authorities have not always framed screening as an offer that citizens may reasonably take up or decline, there are now many evidence-based decision aids designed to support informed choice about cancer and prenatal screening (Stacey et al., 2024) (see also Chapter 19). Given the contrast with historical 'persuasive' messages, screening decision aids should make the decision explicit (e.g. to screen or not), describe why choice exists, acknowledge inherent uncertainties, and emphasize that there is 'no right or wrong answer' (Hersch et al., 2014). Decision aids should also identify shorter- and medium- or longer-term issues relating to decisions about screening participation, including the potential for regret if adverse events subsequently transpire, as described by the patient's perspective (Box 42.1). Extensive evidence shows that decision aids improve knowledge about cancer screening, thereby supporting informed decisions about participation (Stacey et al., 2024). However, the literature also highlights uncertainty about the validity of existing instruments to measure knowledge about breast, colorectal, and cervical cancer screening, demonstrating a need for further discussion to establish consensus around which elements of

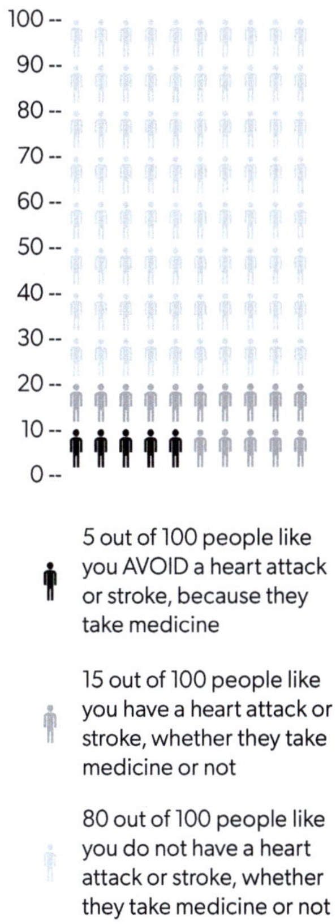

Figure 42.2 Heart attacks/strokes avoided due to 5 years of cholesterol-lowering medicine in patients at high cardiovascular risk.
Source: icon array produced by https://iconarray.com/ using data from https://checkyourheart.com.au/understand-risk/

knowledge are defined as critical to being sufficiently informed about cancer screening (Stokholm et al., 2024). A generalized measure of knowledge, applicable across multiple types of screening, may represent an important methodological advance that could benefit future research and practice, although whether this is possible remains uncertain (Larsen et al., 2022).

Ultimately, it is a health policy judgement whether individual deliberation and SDM are appropriate for a given intervention. Evidence on the preferences of well-informed members of the public can guide such judgements. Engaging a 'community jury', in which a representative sample of the target population deliberates together about benefits and harms, is a feasible way to elicit an informed, considered community view on questions of screening communication and policy. For example, an Australian community jury concluded that men should be able to make informed choices about prostate cancer screening, identified the need for better information, and recommended supporting GPs to better inform patients (Rychetnik et al., 2014).

Health literacy and inequalities

There are sometimes concerns that encouraging people to take a more active role in healthcare decisions might exacerbate inequalities. A systematic review investigating this question concluded that SDM interventions can be accessible to the wider community and indeed significantly improve outcomes for disadvantaged patient groups (Durand et al., 2014). Notably, though, interventions specifically designed to focus on the needs of disadvantaged patients

Box 42.1 Patient perspective

For screening discussions, SDM can be effective when benefit and harm information provided is relevant and aligns with the individual's health history, environment, and lifestyle. To reach a health screening decision, both clinician and patient should exchange information and convey appropriate knowledge in a manner where both come to a mutual understanding around the uncertainties, trade-offs, and benefits to screening while respecting patient preferences.

I better understand the benefit of screening after declining a recommended follow-up. Years ago, my primary care physician recommended screening and sent me home with a stool test. I completed the process and mailed the test card in. Within a week, an alert in my electronic messaging asked me to set up a phone appointment. During the call I found out I had 'failed the test' (in my words) as I had a positive occult blood test result. The clinician discussed a follow-up colonoscopy, noting that the procedure would not be billed as preventive due to the results of the stool test and, if polyps were removed, I would have to cover the full cost. Although the clinician provided current best evidence regarding why I should have a colonoscopy, at that time my priority was the cost associated with the procedure. What might have really helped me was a decision aid that clarified these trade-offs, in the short and long term, and helped me understand my own preferences, values, and what matters most to me.

I had no concerns for years afterwards, until I started having pain in my upper left abdomen and went to consult my primary care physician. A follow-up stool test showed nothing amiss. As the pain persisted, months later a scan was completed, then a colonoscopy (after changes to state laws on preventive health, this procedure was then covered by my insurance). The colonoscopy discovered a large colon tumour, leading to referral to a surgeon. I had a colectomy and spent 5 days in hospital. The moral to the story is: if I had followed-up the positive stool test years earlier, I would not have needed 12 inches of colon removed at great cost to everyone involved. I was fortunate that the large adenoma tumour was not cancerous. Recently I found out that advanced adenomas often do not show up positive on stool tests—reinforcing the fact that preventive screenings do save lives.

This experience enlightened me about the importance of screening and how I could have benefited, had I accepted the colonoscopy earlier. Many people today are cash strapped and if they have no symptoms after a positive screening test, too often will delay further testing. This can lead to devastating health outcomes. Because accuracy does vary between screening tests, another thing to discuss during SDM is what screening test might be the most reliable.

I know that there are more patients like me who face daily life challenges in multiple ways where preventive screenings are not at the top of their health priority list. Prioritizing SDM—supported by health systems—could result in better health outcomes and lower costs for everyone. It is important for clinicians to incorporate patient decision aids, enquire about 'What matters to you?' and discuss trade-offs in decision making visits. This makes sense to support the clinician–patient relationship where trust takes time to develop.

(such as those included in that review) probably differ from more generic decision aids that are commonly available in routine clinical settings. Developers of new resources must therefore pay attention to health literacy considerations in order to maximize utility for a broad population.

In cardiovascular disease prevention, decision aids exist for both testing and medication options, while cardiology procedures require hospital informed consent materials. However, reviews of these resources show they are rarely suitable for patients with lower health literacy (Bonner et al., 2019b). The language used in these documents is generally too complex for the average person to understand, meaning we cannot be confident they support informed SDM. Screening decision aids also vary in terms of their alignment with country-specific guidelines, so even high-quality tools developed in one country may not be applicable to another (Bonner et al., 2019b). This is a problem for implementation and scale-up of SDM resources. Nevertheless, evidence demonstrates that decision aids can improve knowledge about cardiovascular risk and management options.

Holistic decision making and the consequences of decisions

For decision aid developers, there are unique issues to consider in the cardiovascular disease context. One issue is that both lifestyle change and medication can effectively reduce cardiovascular risk, but most available tools focus only on the decision to take a single medication or not (Bonner et al., 2019b). Developers could take the approach of presenting all lifestyle and medication options equally to support a broad conceptualization of SDM. Or they could simply make a strong recommendation for lifestyle change and instead focus the SDM approach on the key decision where there is 'equipoise'—that is, about medication.

Furthermore, particularly for tests like coronary artery calcium scoring, patients do not receive information as part of an organized screening programme because current evidence does not support the cost-effectiveness of such a programme (Australian Government Department of Health, 2023). It is therefore important to engage with primary care providers and cardiologists to ensure decision support tools are acceptable to the stakeholders who can provide them to patients at the time of decision making. As higher costs can be involved with these specialist tests, patients also need information about financial implications, particularly for lower socio-economic population groups, and availability in rural areas which may add travel costs. Such costs may not be worthwhile for patients unless the test results will change their decision about taking preventive medication (Politi et al., 2023).

Challenges and future directions

One particularly contentious issue in some cancer screening contexts is overdiagnosis, which occurs when tumours are detected that would never otherwise cause harm. As there is no way to reliably distinguish cancers that would progress from those likely to remain indolent, overdiagnosis typically leads to overtreatment, even among screen-detected cases recognized as low risk (e.g. low-grade prostate cancer). A systematic review of cancer screening decision aids found that most tools did describe overdiagnosis and overtreatment using lay language. However, there was a lack of consensus regarding how to describe them and what terms to use (Housten et al., 2019). Overdiagnosis and overtreatment are complex and inherently uncertain concepts, challenging for both professionals and laypeople. Nonetheless, including this material, where applicable, is essential from an ethical standpoint to assist informed decision making. Co-designing resources in collaboration with persons with lived experience may be a valuable approach when developing materials involving such complex concepts.

Importantly, evidence-based scientific information presented in decision aids is just one of many factors shaping healthcare choices. Risk perceptions and screening decisions are likely influenced by personal experience, emotions and feelings of trust, as well as analytical risk assessments (Driedger et al., 2017). The long-standing use of emotive arguments to promote screening makes it difficult to communicate potential harms that experts now consider integral to properly informed decisions. A co-design process with patient involvement may yield useful insights regarding how to navigate these issues.

Clinicians are respected as credible sources of advice who can influence perceptions of screening and interpretation of risk information. In cardiovascular prevention, decision aids and visual risk communication tools have been integrated with clinical guidelines, GP risk calculators in medical software, and wider primary care systems that support quality improvement and education (Australian Government Department of Health, 2023). As the shift towards more informed, deliberative decision making is still relatively recent in certain cancer screening contexts, clinicians may not yet have sufficient training and capacity to engage skilfully in SDM. An important future goal, therefore, is to better support clinicians to communicate effectively about screening so they can help people understand the evidence about benefits and harms and guide them in clarifying their preferences. The importance of good communication and SDM will likely increase further with new complexities on the horizon, including risk stratification and genomic technology (Australian Government Department of Health, 2018).

Conclusion

When communicating about screening, whether through population-based programmes or in primary care, promoting uptake by emphasizing benefits and downplaying harms was once considered justified. However, with growing consensus that benefits and harms are sometimes delicately balanced, SDM is increasingly the recommended approach for choices about whether to undergo screening. To achieve this, people need high-quality information about screening outcomes based on the current best evidence. Furthermore, where appropriate, patients should have access to support from healthcare providers with the skills to support SDM. Despite challenges, it is possible to help people become better informed about screening (Stacey et al., 2024). Continuing efforts are vital to support people in all their diversity as they engage with their own informed preferences and participate in SDM about screening, if we want patients and citizens to be at the heart of the health system.

REFERENCES

Australian Government Department of Health. 2018. Population based screening framework. Available at: https://www.health.gov.au/resources/publications/population-based-screening-framework

Australian Government Department of Health. 2023. Australian guideline for assessing and managing cardiovascular disease risk. Available at: https://www.cvdcheck.org.au/overview

Bonner, C., Fajardo, M. A., Doust, J., et al. 2019a. Implementing cardiovascular disease prevention guidelines to translate evidence-based medicine and shared decision making into general practice: theory-based intervention development, qualitative piloting and quantitative feasibility. *Implement Sci,* **14**, 86.

Bonner, C., Patel, P., Fajardo, M. A., et al. 2019b. Online decision aids for primary cardiovascular disease prevention: systematic search, evaluation of quality and suitability for low health literacy patients. *BMJ Open,* **9**, e025173.

Driedger, S. M., Annable, G., Brouwers, M., et al. 2017. Can you un-ring the bell? A qualitative study of how affect influences cancer screening decisions. *BMC Cancer,* **17**, 647.

Durand, M. A., Carpenter, L., Dolan, H., et al. 2014. Do interventions designed to support shared decision-making reduce health inequalities? A systematic review and meta-analysis. *PLoS One,* **9**, e94670.

Hersch, J., Jansen, J., Barratt, A., et al. 2014. Overdetection in breast cancer screening: development and preliminary evaluation of a decision aid. *BMJ Open,* **4**, e006016.

Hoffmann, T., Del Mar, C. 2015. Patients' expectations of the benefits and harms of treatments, screening, and tests: a systematic review. *JAMA Intern Med,* **175**, 274–286.

Housten, A. J., Lowenstein, L. M., Hoffman, A., et al. 2019. A review of the presentation of overdiagnosis in cancer screening patient decision aids. *MDM Policy Pract,* **4**, 2381468319881447.

Larsen, M. B., Stokholm, R., Kirkegaard, P., et al. 2022. Making decisions on your own: self-administered decision aids about colorectal cancer screening—a systematic review and meta-analyses. *Patient Educ Couns,* **105**, 534–546.

Oude Wolcherink, M. J., Behr, C. M., Pouwels, X., et al. 2023. Health economic research assessing the value of early detection of cardiovascular disease: a systematic review. *Pharmacoeconomics,* **41**, 1183–1203.

Paige, E., Raffoul, N., Lonsdale, E., Banks, E. 2023. Cardiovascular disease risk screening in Australia: evidence and data gaps. *Med J Aust,* **218**, 103–105.

Politi, M. C., Housten, A. J., Forcino, R. C., et al. 2023. Discussing cost and value in patient decision aids and shared decision making: a call to action. *MDM Policy Pract,* **8**, 23814683221148651.

Rychetnik, L., Doust, J., Thomas, R., et al. 2014. A community jury on PSA screening: what do well-informed men want the government to do about prostate cancer screening—a qualitative analysis. *BMJ Open,* **4**, e004682.

Stacey, D., Lewis, K. B., Smith, M., et al. 2024. Decision aids for people facing health treatment or screening decisions. *Cochrane Database Syst Rev,* **1**, CD001431.

Stefanek, M. 2011. Uninformed compliance or informed choice? A needed shift in our approach to cancer screening. *J Natl Cancer Inst,* **103**, 1821–1826.

Stokholm, R. N., Stenholt, L., Lauridsen, H. H., et al. 2024. The validity of instruments to measure knowledge in population-based cancer screening targeting individuals at average risk—a systematic review. *Prevent Med,* **182**, 107940.

Waller, J., Osborne, K., Wardle, J. 2015. Enthusiasm for cancer screening in Great Britain: a general population survey. *Br J Cancer,* **112**, 562–566.

Willis, K., Baxter, J. 2003. Trusting technology: women aged 40–49 years participating in screening for breast cancer—an exploratory study. *Aust N Z J Public Health,* **27**, 282–286.

Woloshin, S., Schwartz, L. M., Black, W. C., Kramer, B. S. 2012. Cancer screening campaigns—getting past uninformative persuasion. *N Engl J Med,* **367**, 1677–1679.

43

Shared decision making in ophthalmology

Rashmi G. Mathew, Hannah M. Timlin, Olawale A. Akinrogunde, and Carrie J. MacEwen

Introduction

Ophthalmology is one of the busiest clinical specialities. In 2019/2020 there were over 9 million outpatient attendances in England (The Royal College of Ophthalmologists, 2021) and almost 10% of the entire National Health Service (NHS) waiting list is for ophthalmology (NHS England, 2023). Cataract surgery is one of the most common operations; over 450,000 cataract surgeries are performed each year in England, which is predicted to grow by 50% by 2035 (The Royal College of Ophthalmologists, 2022). There is unwarranted variation in referral practice (ranging from 40% to 92% of cataract referrals from primary care resulting in surgery), and there is eye health inequality between communities, such as ethnic minorities (The Royal College of Ophthalmologists, 2021) and low socioeconomic status (Armstrong et al., 2007; Denniston et al., 2019; Lawrenson et al., 2021).

While these facts present challenges for service delivery, they also make it one of the most ideal and vital specialties in which to implement good shared decision making (SDM) practice.

Good SDM could play a key role in addressing unwarranted variation and easing the pressures on ophthalmic health systems. If patients are knowledgeable about their condition and can express their values and beliefs, this would ensure that referrals are driven by patient preference; that patients are seen in the right setting; that patients understand the importance of adherence to treatment regimens, the implications of procedures, and the necessity of hospital attendance. SDM also has the potential to foster trusting relationships with patients, through open communication and building shared understanding. 'What matters to you?' needs to be the mantra that all healthcare professionals hold themselves accountable to, to do the best by their patients.

There are many examples of SDM and decision support tools being used in ophthalmology around the world, which we summarize in this chapter. Areas of focus include chronic ophthalmic conditions, such as glaucoma, age-related macular degeneration, diabetes, and cataract surgery. Our patient author also outlines his thoughts and experiences of decision making in clinical practice; this highlights the importance of understanding what matters to the patient and why a multidisciplinary team is pivotal in building patients' confidence in their healthcare team.

Driving the SDM agenda in ophthalmology

The UK White Paper 'Equity and Excellence: Liberating the NHS' (Department of Health and Social Care, 2010) set out the Government's vision of an NHS that puts patients and the public first, where 'no decision about me, without me' is the norm. It outlined the need for culture change within the NHS, to enable patient involvement to become routine practice, as well as accurate and accessible information to be made readily available to patients. A decade on, the General Medical Council released guidance stating that SDM and good consent practices are fundamental to good medical practice (General Medical Council, 2024).

The 2021 National Institute for Health and Care Excellence (NICE) guidance on SDM presents organizational and practice-level recommendations for SDM for adult patients making health and care decisions (NICE, 2021). The guidance outlines the importance of senior leadership accountability, which includes patient leaders, to ensure implementation of SDM across the organization. At a clinical practice level, it outlines how to support patients to be involved in SDM, including training, guidance on communicating risk, and using patient decision aids (PtDAs). NICE has also developed an online training package to enable clinicians to practically undertake SDM (NICE, n.d.).

Due to the high volume of cataract surgery, NICE developed guidelines for cataract surgery (NICE 2017), one aspect of which states that a decision for referral from primary care to the hospital eye service should be based on an understanding of 'how the cataract affects the person's vision and quality of life'—emphasizing the need to understand the patient's perspective through a SDM process. In 2023, the Academy of Medical Royal Colleges, in partnership with NHS England, set up an evidence based interventions programme for different specialties (Academy of Medical Royal Colleges, 2023). Taking the NICE guidance on cataract

Table 43.1 Examples of SDM in ophthalmology

Situations	Healthcare professionals involved	Setting
A patient with moderate glaucoma, who is insistent on having glaucoma surgery. With further exploration, their motivation is the desire to stop using eyedrops. SDM would ensure they understood the likelihood of still requiring drops after surgery and a consolidation of drops (if on multiple drops) or laser treatment might be better option for them	Glaucoma nurse specialist, specialist optometrist, ophthalmologist, pharmacist	Outpatient clinic
A patient with wet macular age-related degeneration, who requires repeated intravitreal injections every 6 weeks. The conversation may revolve around the patient's inability to attend frequent hospital appointments due to caring responsibilities	Ophthalmic nurse specialist, specialist optometrist, ophthalmologist, eye clinic liaison officer	Outpatient clinic
A patient who notices their vision is becoming increasingly blurred from cataract, but they are still able to undertake activities of daily living. On understanding the risks and benefits of surgery, they may choose to delay surgery and update their spectacles or even do nothing, over surgery	Optometrist, ophthalmic nurse specialist, ophthalmologist	Optometry setting in primary care/outpatient clinic

surgery one step further, one of its recommendations for ophthalmology is a formally documented SDM process between the referring primary care optician and patient, before they can be accepted into the hospital eye service. This is to ensure the right patients are seen in a timely way (Academy of Medical Royal Colleges, 2023) and that hospital eye service resources are used appropriately.

Ophthalmic workforce and decisions

Various healthcare professionals provide specialist ophthalmic care including ophthalmologists, ophthalmic nurses, optometrists, cancer nurse specialists, orthoptists, pharmacists, and eye clinic liaison officers. All these ophthalmic professionals independently discuss and make decisions with patients about their eye treatment and support (see Table 43.1 for examples), and thus need awareness of and training in SDM.

Training for healthcare professionals

The practice of medicine is traditionally paternalistic, and the shift to partnership may not come naturally to some. Our propensity to 'do', also affects the way we discuss options with patients. This can make us less neutral, thus finding ourselves being more persuasive in discussing options that we perceive as being in the patient's best interests, without fully exploring their needs and desires, or the option to do nothing. This is particularly relevant when there is a highly effective option for treatment, such as cataract surgery.

Other barriers to SDM exist, including the level of understanding of the evidence underpinning the options. It can be complex and the variations in levels of evidence and relevance of each to the needs and personal wishes of the individual without undue weighting need to be understood (Waddell et al., 2021).

To overcome paternalist attitudes/behaviours and these challenges and move towards a partnership approach, good-quality SDM training should be provided and is a key recommendation of the NICE SDM guidelines (NICE, 2021).

Having a framework for SDM is important because it enables healthcare professionals to understand and go through the necessary steps involved in supporting patients through a SDM process. The three-talk model of SDM, made up of 'team talk', 'option talk', and 'decision talk', is the most widely cited model (Elwyn et al., 2017). The mnemonic BRAN is also an excellent aide-mémoire for healthcare professionals to systematically go through the Benefits, Risks, Alternatives, and the option of doing Nothing (Choosing Wisely, n.d.).

Various training programmes are available to support the ophthalmological workforce. For example, NICE partnered with the University of Keele to develop a training package for SDM for healthcare professionals (NICE, 2021). Our group has also developed a free, online ophthalmology-specific SDM training module in 2020, in partnership with the Winton Centre for Risk and Evidence Communication, UK (SDM Ophthalmology, 2020). The module outlines the three-talk model (Elwyn et al., 2017) and uses common ophthalmic patient scenarios to walk the healthcare professional through the steps of SDM and outlines practical ways to optimize SDM. It also includes examples of PtDA tools, such as pictograms (see Figure 43.1 for a cataract decision aid), for communicating risk and options in simple visual ways that are easier to understand than words, statistics or numbers.

Tools to support ophthalmic SDM

Understanding what sort of partnership patients want and how they want information presented are key to SDM. In a qualitative study of existing information provision by 12 community optometry practices, participants defined high-quality information as concise with clear diagrams (Fylan and Grunfeld, 2002). Medical jargon and inappropriate layout of diagrams and too much text impeded their understanding. Participants also wanted the information to be pertinent to their own needs, rather than generic information.

A free online glaucoma patient education course has been developed in conjunction with patients, covering 'What is glaucoma?', 'What to expect when you attend a glaucoma clinic (including a virtual clinic)', 'Living with glaucoma', 'How to instil your eye drops', and 'Treatment options' (Hamid et al., 2023). After consultation with patients, the resource was developed in two formats, a long version and a short version, to suit patients' needs and their desire for different depths of understanding.

PtDAs are also key to improving patient involvement and supporting SDM. Studies have also shown that they improve knowledge and accuracy of risk perceptions and help patients to clarify values (Stacey et al., 2024). PtDAs show promising outcomes in ophthalmology (Shum et al., 2017; Ye et al., 2020). A study of a glaucoma PtDA developed in China found improvements in patient knowledge and adherence and reduced decisional conflict (Shum et al., 2017). Patient involvement in its development led to the inclusion of a chart where patients could compare 'common concerns' across the different options. Acceptance was fair, but the authors note that the short follow-up time was a limitation for conditions such as glaucoma. A randomized controlled trial of 773 patients in China found that 28% of participants in the PtDA intervention group were enabled to make an informed decision about their cataract surgery, compared to 6% of participants who received a standard information booklet (Ye et al., 2020). Participants who received the PtDA were also more satisfied with their knowledge, less likely to have decision conflict, and less likely to undergo surgery.

NHS England have created a range of PtDAs (guided by international guidelines, such as the International Patient Decision Aid Standards) on cataract, wet age-related macular degeneration, and primary open angle glaucoma. These are free to access for patients and healthcare professionals (NHS England, n.d.).

However, it has been suggested (Pieterse et al., 2019) that reading the PtDA in their own time can be laborious for some patients and some may not have time to do this, in the context of illness, caring responsibilities, and employment. Use of the PtDA after a consultation also inhibits focused discussions on what matters most to the patient (Pieterse et al., 2019); which could be identified if used prior to or during the consultation. As such, a personal briefing about the PtDA by a healthcare professional is an important factor in its usefulness, helping to ensure that patients know how to navigate the tool and use it effectively (Shum et al., 2017).

See Box 43.1 for our patient perspective.

Box 43.1 Patient perspective Reverend Olawale A. Akinrogunde

A few years ago, I had a particularly throbbing headache. I initially thought that it was because of my busy schedule. However, it continued unabated and when I couldn't cope any longer I saw my family doctor. They referred me the same day to Moorfields Eye Hospital A&E, London, where my intraocular pressures were high, in the early 40s (mmHg). The doctors stabilized the pressures, diagnosed ocular hypertension, and transferred me to the local glaucoma clinic. I then fell into the mistake that many of us make—I googled it (Ou, n.d.) and rapid fears and questions set in.

This is where I can share my positive experience of SDM (although I hadn't, yet heard this phrase). I would regularly speak with the doctors and nurses about the struggles that I had and they listened with rapt attention, wanting to help me. One particular nurse had such a calm voice. She was so professional, yet personable, and this attitude gave me the much-needed elixir for my 'white coat syndrome' and worry of losing eyesight.

The doctors prescribed an eye drop to bring the pressures down. However, I began to have nightmares and woke up with cold sweats. Eventually I couldn't sleep again for fear of the nightmares to come. At my next appointment, after explaining this, I was told that nightmares could be a side effect of the eyedrops. I also became very worried that I was going to lose my driving licence—as a local clergy, driving for pastoral visits is integral. There is a rumour that the Driver and Vehicle Licensing Agency is linked to the local glaucoma clinics in order to take licences off drivers—I was really scared! These nightmares continued until the medication was stopped and another eye drop was prescribed.

I am Nigerian by birth but have lived in the UK for over two decades. I return to Africa regularly to teach and spend time with extended family in Lagos. A few of my aunties raised concerns about my 'Western medication' advising that I seek alternative medication—meaning for me to seek 'Afro-Caribbean herbs' to help 'cure this glaucoma'! One in particular asked me to read up on glaucoma from an African perspective (Egbert, 2002). I don't have issues with African herbs because my late mother raised me on them, but I've become anglicized and would rather stick with medications from the UK. (I hope Africans reading this article wouldn't be upset with me!)

My consultant, then suggested that I undergo a laser treatment called selective laser trabeculoplasty (Moorfields Eye Hospital, 2020). She discussed this extensively with me and even asked for my contribution. She gave me ample time to think it through by recommending what to read to help me make an informed decision. At the next scheduled appointment, we both came to an agreed conclusion to proceed, which has been successful at lowering my eye pressure. I've told my extremely caring but concerned African sisters that 'I can see clearly now, the glaucoma is "gone"'.

What are current ophthalmic patients' experiences and outcomes of SDM?

From the literature, it is evident that treatment option discussions are inadequate; studies show them taking place in 5–50% of consultations (Smith et al., 2021; Sleath et al., 2023). Other studies report patients with age-related macular disease feeling hurried to make decisions and not being informed about the need for long-term treatment or the option of discontinuing treatment (Bian et al., 2019; Scheffer et al., 2022).

A study using the nine-item Shared Decision Making Questionnaire (SDM-Q-9) revealed patients with glaucoma felt the physician did not wish to understand how the patient wanted to be involved in decision making or ascertain which options the patient preferred (Sun, 2023). Another study using the SDM-Q-9 found that patients felt there were gaps in their involvement and eliciting their goals and expectations when undergoing strabismus surgery (Paduca et al., 2021).

A study exploring a glaucoma health coaching initiative found that 50% of patients had not previously been shown how to use their eyedrops (Taribagil et al., 2021). However, this could be an important factor in adherence; Sleath and colleagues found that eyedrop usage was positively associated with whether clinicians had explained how to administer the eyedrops to patients (Sleath et al., 2015). However, it should be noted that education and reading levels can also influence outcomes; those with higher education levels rated clinicians as more participatory (Sleath et al., 2023) and were also more likely to successfully administer their eyedrops (Kang et al., 2022).

The literature highlights aspects of current practice that require improvement, from explaining what the different options are, their implications, seeking patient input into decision making, and providing opportunities to ask questions. We all recognize these as challenges in our own practice, particularly when clinical pressures, such as appointment duration, overbooking of clinics, and staff shortages are not conducive to this.

Given the time and resource investment required for SDM, it is important that patient outcomes are evaluated. It is still unclear what the best measures are. The NICE guideline recommends research into the best outcome measures for gauging the effectiveness of SDM (NICE, 2021). Consensus is needed so that researchers and healthcare workers around the world can compare interventions more effectively, which will ultimately translate into effective clinical practice of SDM.

Future priorities

The ophthalmic workforce recognizes the need for SDM, yet face many obstacles to achieving it consistently and sustainably, including time, tools, and training. SDM must also be viewed through the lens of health inequalities. Many of the measures implemented may unintentionally exclude groups of people and widen inequalities, and lower education attainment is a recognized barrier to SDM with current methods (Kang et al., 2022).

As healthcare professionals who support increasingly diverse populations, how we build trust and cultural competence, overcome language barriers, and foster partnership become even more important. We also know that a significant proportion of our population don't have digital skills or access to technology; as we develop online patient resources, how do we ensure this doesn't disadvantage groups of people?

In ophthalmology, it is paramount that we also consider visual disability in SDM. Our patient author also highlights how differently patients view their care and what matters to them; he talks about family-based decision making and the importance of feeling cared for, in engendering trust. There are no easy solutions, but this requires time and partnership with our patient, and their significant others, to ensure no one is left behind and the benefits of SDM are for all.

Cataract Surgery Decision Aid

A cataract is a clouding of the lens inside the eye. When cataract develops, it prevents the light rays from passing through to the back of the eye, making it difficult to see.

Symptoms

Cataract is a normal ageing process and most people do not have any symptoms or problems. Patients may experience a gradual blurring of vision that is not corrected by their glasses. Some patients may also notice glare, particularly when driving at night and double vision when looking with one eye.

Treatment

Treatment Options	Benefits	Harms / Risks
No treatment	You avoid the risks of cataract surgery.	• Your cataracts do not need to be removed, particularly if they are not affecting your vision or lifestyle. • Your vision may gradually decline. • Your vision may fall below driving standards or worse. • You may not be able to do daily activities, particularly those that involve fine vision. • You may have an increased risk of falls. • You may have slightly higher risk of complications from cataract surgery if you wait until your cataract becomes very advanced.
Changing glasses	• Your vision will improve. • You avoid the risk of surgery.	• There may come a point when glasses are unable to improve your vision sufficiently. • Your glasses may need to be replaced more than once a year, so you will need to factor in the cost of new glasses.
Cataract Surgery	95% chance of Improving your vision	• 50 in 1000 risk of complications, the majority of which are minor, and may involve you taking drops more frequently or attending the clinic more often. • 10 in 1000 risk of needing further surgery if things do not go well for you during the first operation. • 1 in 1000 risk of loss of useful vision in the operated eye, which is usually due to infection or a severe bleed at the back of your eye. (see Figure 43.1)

What is Cataract Surgery?

Cataract surgery is an operation to remove the cloudy lens (cataract) inside the eye, It is usually performed under local anaesthetic, so you will be awake for the procedure, but your eye will be numbed. Once the cloudy lens is removed from the eye, it needs to be replaced with a clear lens implant, in order to be able to see properly.

What matters to me?

It is important to understand what matters most to your when considering the Treatment Options above. Please think about the statements below and place a cross along the horizontal line, to indicate how your cataract impacts you and what is important to your decision as to whether to undergo cataract surgery.

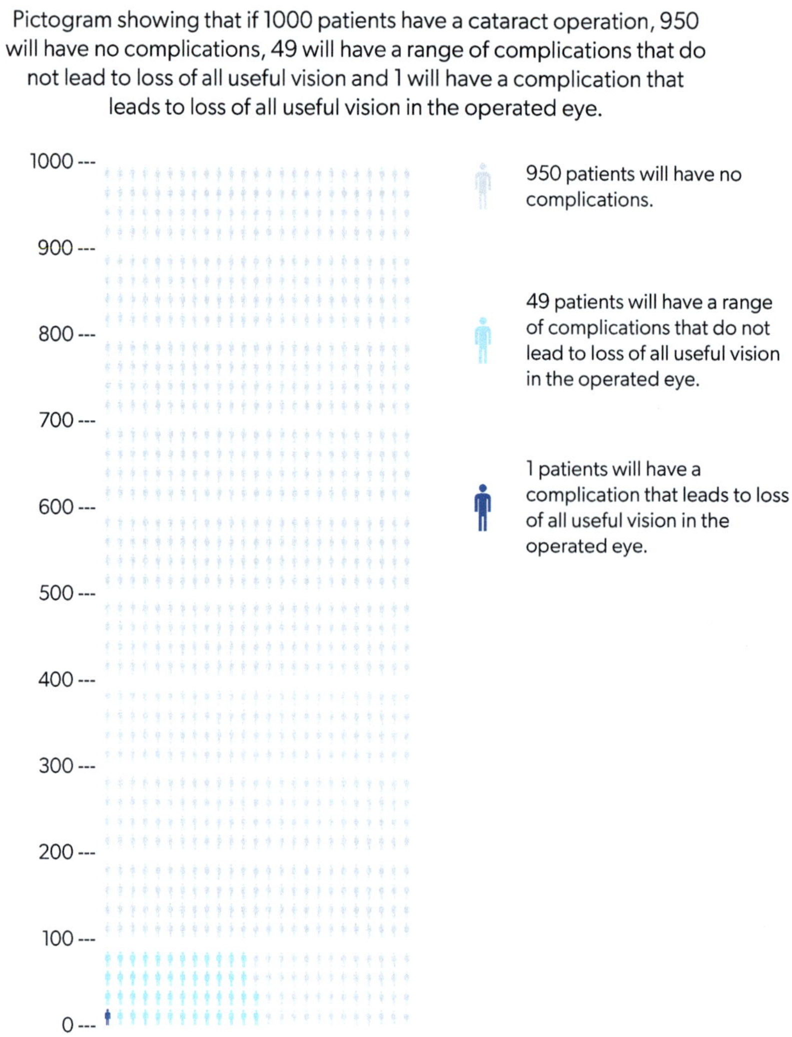

Figure 43.1 Pictogram within a cataract surgery decision aid.

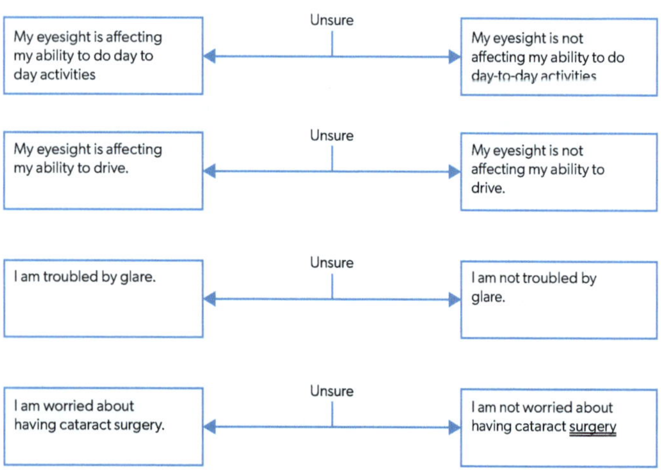

Please consider showing this decision aid to your family, friends, and health professionals, in order for them to best support you make your decision.

REFERENCES

Academy of Medical Royal Colleges. 2023. Evidence-based interventions. Available at: https://ebi.aomrc.org.uk/

Armstrong, K., Ravenell, K. L., McMurphy, S., Putt, M. 2007. Racial/ethnic differences in physician distrust in the United States. *Am J Public Health*, **97**, 1283–1289.

Bartalena, L., Baldeschi, L., Boboridis, K., et al. 2016. The 2016 European Thyroid Association/European Group on Graves' Orbitopathy guidelines for the management of Graves' orbitopathy. *Eur Thyroid J*, **5**, 9–26.

Bian, W., Wan, J., Tan, M., Wu, X., Su, J., Wang, L. 2019. Patient experience of treatment decision making for wet age-related macular degeneration disease: a qualitative study in China. *BMJ Open*, **9**, e031020.

Choosing Wisely. n.d. Choosing Wisely UK. Academy of Medical Royal Colleges. Available at: https://www.aomrc.org.uk/projects-and-programmes/choosing-wisely/

Denniston, A. K., Lee, A. Y., Lee, C. S., et al. 2019. United Kingdom Diabetic Retinopathy Electronic Medical Record (UK DR EMR) Users Group: report 4, real-world data on the impact of deprivation on the presentation of diabetic eye disease at hospital services. *Br J Ophthalmol,* **103**, 837–843.

Department of Health and Social Care. 2010. Liberating the NHS White Paper. Available at: https://www.gov.uk/government/publications/liberating-the-nhs-white-paper

Egbert, P. R. 2002. Glaucoma in West Africa: a neglected problem. *Br J Ophthalmol,* **86**, 131–132.

Elwyn, G., Durand, M. A., Song, J., et al. 2017. A three-talk model for shared decision making: multistage consultation process *BMJ,* **359**, j4891.

Fylan, F., Grunfeld, E. A. 2002. Information within optometric practice: comprehension, preferences and implications. *Ophthalmic Physiol Opt,* **22**, 333–340.

General Medical Council. 2024. Decision making and consent. Available at: https://www.gmc-uk.org/professional-standards/professional-standards-for-doctors/decision-making-and-consent

Hamid, S., Minakaran, N., Igwe, C., Baneke, A., Pedersen, M., Mathew, R. G. 2023. An online glaucoma educational course for patients to facilitate remote learning and patient empowerment. *BMJ Health Care Inform,* **30**, e100748.

Kang, J. M., Chatterjee, A., Rosdahl, J. A., et al. 2022. Health literacy and success with glaucoma drop administration. *Ophthalmol Glaucoma,* **5**, 26–31.

Killeen, O. J., Niziol, L. M., Cho, J., et al. 2023. Glaucoma medication adherence 1 year after the Support, Educate, Empower Personalized glaucoma coaching program. *Ophthalmol Glaucoma,* **6**, 23–28.

Lawrenson, J. G., Bourmpaki, E., Bunce, C., et al. 2021. Trends in diabetic retinopathy screening attendance and associations with vision impairment attributable to diabetes in a large nationwide cohort. *Diabet Med,* **38**, e14425.

Mapani, A. 2023. Distributed leadership: a new perspective on leadership in driving innovation and transformation in healthcare? *Hosp Admin Med Pract,* **2**, doi:10.54844/hamp.2022.0020.

Moorfields Eye Hospital. 2020. Selective laser trabeculoplasty (SLT). Available at: https://www.moorfields.nhs.uk/for-patients/information-hub/selective-laser-trabeculoplasty

NHS England. n.d. Decision support tools. Available at: https://www.england.nhs.uk/personalisedcare/shared-decision-making/decision-support-tools/

NHS England. 2023. New NHS measures to improve eye care and cut waiting times. Available at: https://www.england.nhs.uk/2023/05/new-nhs-measures-to-improve-eye-care-and-cut-waiting-times/

NICE. n.d. Shared decision making. Available at: https://www.nice.org.uk/about/what-we-do/our-programmes/nice-guidance/nice-guidelines/shared-decision-making

NICE. 2017. Cataracts in adults: management. NICE guideline [NG77]. Available at: https://www.nice.org.uk/guidance/ng77

NICE. 2021. Shared decision making. NICE guideline [NG197]. Available at: https://www.nice.org.uk/guidance/ng197

NICE. 2022. Macular degeneration—age-related: how common is it? Available at: https://cks.nice.org.uk/topics/macular-degeneration-age-related/background-information/prevalence/

Ou, Y. n.d. How long does it take to go blind from glaucoma? National Glaucoma Research. Available at: https://www.brightfocus.org/glaucoma/article/how-long-does-it-take-go-blind-glaucoma

Paduca, A., Arnaut, O., Beschieru, E., Lundmark, P. O., Bruenech, J. R. 2021. Shared decision making and patients satisfaction with strabismus care—a pilot study. *BMC Med Inform Decis Mak,* **21**, 109.

Pieterse, A. H., Stiggelbout, A. M., Montori, V. M. 2019. Shared decision making and the importance of time. *JAMA,* **322**, 25–26.

Scheffer, M., Menting, J., Roodbeen, R., et al. 2022. Patients' and health professionals' views on shared decision-making in age-related macular degeneration care: a qualitative study. *Ophthalmic Physiol Opt,* **42**, 1015–1022.

SDM Ophthalmology. 2020. Helping patients make informed decisions: communicating potential harms and benefits (ophthalmology). Available at: https://portal.e-lfh.org.uk/Component/Details/604821

Shum, J. W. H., Lam, W. W. T., Choy, B. N. K., Chan, J. C. H., Ho, W. L., Lai, J. S. M. 2017. Development and pilot-testing of patient decision aid for use among Chinese patients with primary open-angle glaucoma. *BMJ Open Ophthalmol,* **2**, e000100.

Sleath, B., Carpenter, D. M., Blalock, S. J., et al. 2015. Applying the resources and supports in self-management framework to examine ophthalmologist–patient communication and glaucoma medication adherence *Health Educ Res,* **30**, 693–705.

Sleath, B., Carpenter, D. M., Budenz, D. L., et al. 2023. Provider use of a participatory decision-making style with African American patients with glaucoma. *Patient Educ Couns,* **111**, 107679.

Smith, M., Bresolin, M., McCabe, R. 2021. Pilot study of clinician–patient collaboration in glaucoma. *Clin Ophthalmol,* **15**, 1715–1726.

Stacey, D., Lewis, K., Smith, M., et al. 2024. Decision aids for people facing health treatment or screening decisions. *Cochrane Database Syst Rev,* **1**, CD001431.

Taribagil, P., Thomas, S., Mathew, R. G. 2022. Glaucoma health coaching: a survey of eye drop instillation education. *J Glaucoma,* **31**, 351–355.

The Royal College of Ophthalmologists. 2021. Atlas of variation in risk factors and healthcare for vision in England. Available at: https://www.rcophth.ac.uk/news-views/vision-atlas-england/

The Royal College of Ophthalmologists. 2022. Changes in NHS cataract surgery in England 2016–2021: an analysis of national, regional and independent sector trends. Available at: https://www.rcophth.ac.uk/wp-content/uploads/2022/08/Cataract-Sector-Data-Report.pdf

Waddell, A., Lennox, A., Spassova, G., Bragge, P. 2021. Barriers and facilitators to shared decision-making in hospitals from policy to practice: a systematic review. *Implement Sci,* **16**, 74

Ye, G., Qu, B., Tham, Y. C., et al. 2021. A decision aid to facilitate informed choices among cataract patients: a randomized controlled trial. *Patient Educ Couns,* **104**, 1295–1303.

44

Shared decision making in otolaryngology

Elaine C. Thompson, Hannah Leavitt, Paul Hong, and Emily F. Boss

Overview of otolaryngology in the context of shared decision making

Shared decision making (SDM) is a patient-centred approach to medical care in which patients, families, and clinicians collaborate on a personalized treatment plan. Physicians and legislators alike have focused more attention on SDM as an approach to delivering patient-centred care and promoting health equity, and a provision of the US Affordable Care Act argues it is an ethical imperative (Drake and Deegan, 2009). The success of SDM extends to numerous medical fields, including oncology, neurology, critical care, psychiatry, cardiology, and general surgery (Stacey et al., 2024). This chapter specifically focuses on SDM in otolaryngology–head and neck surgery, a broad and diverse surgical specialty. Otolaryngology is uniquely poised to leverage SDM for patient care due to its mix of medical and surgical treatment options for both elective and essential conditions.

In otolaryngology, many conditions can be treated through various approaches and thus require consideration of complex treatment decisions. Substantial trade-offs in risks and benefits may make management decisions challenging for surgeons, patients, and families, resulting in widely variable outcomes and uncertainty about the best treatment course. Engaging the patient's perspectives, goals, and values in the process differentiates SDM from other healthcare models; Box 44.1 provides a patient's perspective on the significance of actively participating in decisions. The next section of this chapter explores clinical equipoise in otolaryngology subspecialties, focusing on how SDM can help patients and families navigate complex care decisions.

SDM in otolaryngology

Head and neck oncology

How patients with head and neck cancer navigate complex treatment decisions is one area of study in SDM research. Factors such as cancer type, location, and stage can change preferred management,

Box 44.1 Patient perspective

The significance of actively participating in decisions

In October 2022, I was diagnosed with postural orthostatic tachycardia syndrome (POTS) following a bout of COVID-19. Over the next 1.5 years, I grappled with persistent symptoms such as dizziness, nausea, balance issues, and migraines. Despite everyone attributing my symptoms to POTS (a circulation disorder with similar symptoms) it wasn't until I sought the expertise of an ear, nose, and throat (ENT) provider that a different path unfolded.

The initial ENT visit led to further testing, including an audiogram and an electronystagmography (ENG)/videonystagmography (VNG) test. Unfortunately, I had to discontinue the ENG/VNG test due to severe dizziness, leaving me disappointed and anxious about resolving my symptoms. With incomplete test results and no clear answers, I found myself managing my symptoms independently for the next 4 months.

Bedbound and desperate for relief, I decided to consult another ENT specialist. The prospect of yet another round of inconclusive results weighed heavily on me, as the constant uncertainty had taken a toll on my interactions with medical professionals. The anxiety leading up to each visit only exacerbated my symptoms.

However, this time was different. This ENT provider encouraged me to recount the beginning of my dizziness, starting in July 2022. Together, we meticulously reviewed the changes in my symptoms and the myriad of tests I had undergone. He acknowledged that I was the expert on my body, which encouraged me to be a part of finding a solution. The ENT professional took a thoughtful approach, asking probing questions and genuinely listening to my responses. This experience validated my symptoms and made me feel heard.

We discussed my goals and how my current state inhibited my ability to perform daily tasks. I didn't feel rushed to keep my responses brief and to minimize the impact on me of being disabled for the past 1.5 years. He then guided me through all of my options but highlighted the ones that aligned best with my capabilities at that point in time. I have followed up with that ENT professional multiple times, and each time we discuss my progress, the lingering symptoms, and the next steps forward—re-evaluating my preferences for treatment each time.

SDM to me involves a collaborative approach between healthcare providers and patients. It acknowledges the expertise of both parties and respects the patient's values, preferences, and goals. In my case, the ENT professional's willingness to engage in a dialogue, listen to my concerns, and involve me in the decision making process empowered me to take control of my health journey. It allowed me to make informed decisions that aligned with my needs and preferences, ultimately leading to a more effective management of my condition. This experience underscores the importance of fostering a healthcare environment where patients feel valued, respected, and actively involved in their care.

which may involve surgical resection, chemotherapy, and/or radiation. Treatment modalities range in their effect on oral intake, communication, and cosmesis, which can lead to dysfunction and disfigurement, resulting in isolation, anxiety, and depression (Dropkin, 1989). SDM emphasizes patient preferences and values, which helps patients navigate uncertainty, especially in vulnerable clinical scenarios (Forner et al., 2020).

Windon and colleagues investigated the experiences and needs of patients with oropharyngeal squamous cell carcinoma (OPSCC), deciding between surgery or radiation as their primary curative treatment. Through qualitative methods, authors found that decisions for surgery or radiation were motivated by the avoidance of toxic effects and the desire for physical tumour removal. Patients ultimately felt responsible for their decision despite multiple roles in decision making, and deference to their doctors' recommendations (Windon et al., 2021).

Patients with head and neck cancer are, however, at risk of decision regret. For laryngeal carcinoma, treatment decisions not only involve modality/approach but also consider post-treatment complications, which can lead to significant functional deficits. Shuman and colleagues investigated voice-related quality of life in patients with laryngeal cancer and found that patients with worse voice quality of life endorsed more decisional regret (Shuman et al., 2017). For patients with OPSCC, drivers of moderately strong regret include preoperative depression and frailty (Thomas et al., 2019), late symptom burden, and multimodality treatment (Goepfert et al., 2017). Of all factors, difficulty swallowing and feeling depressed carry the greatest risk of decisional regret (Goepfert et al., 2017).

While survivors of OPSCC have overall low rates of decision regret (Goepfert et al., 2017), transoral robotic surgery, a minimally invasive and de-intensified approach to surgical management of OPSCC, is associated with little to no decisional regret (Kwon et al., 2023). Kwon and colleagues examined decision regret in patients with early-stage OPSCC who were deciding between transoral robotic surgery or radiation therapy. Almost 85% who underwent transoral robotic surgery expressed no or mild decisional regret (Kwon et al., 2023).

Endocrine surgery

Management of indeterminant thyroid nodules typically involves thyroidectomy, yet in 75–80% of cases, pathology reveals a benign result (Taylor et al., 2016). Weighing the risks and benefits, as well as the uncertainty of the final diagnosis, can lead to decisional conflict. Taylor and colleagues performed a prospective study examining decisional conflict in patients with an indeterminant thyroid nodule and found one-third of patients had clinically significant conflict over the decision to pursue diagnostic thyroidectomy (Taylor et al., 2016).

Naunheim and colleagues conducted semistructured interviews to explore patient preferences, emotions, and attitudes towards diagnosing and managing thyroid nodules. Themes relevant for diagnosis included emotional response to the news, concern about cancer, reliance on expertise, and contextualization with past experience. For management, themes identified included bias to action, concern for metabolic concerns and medication side effects, fear of surgical complications, and convenience and financial considerations. The authors advocate for incorporating the patient perspective into the milieu of medical decision making (Naunheim et al., 2023).

Otology

Vestibular schwannoma

Management of internal auditory canal tumours may include observation, stereotactic radiation surgery, or surgical resection. Treatment decisions are significantly influenced by patient age, tumour size, growth, hearing status, and headache severity. Graham and colleagues examined decisional conflict in patients with newly diagnosed or growing vestibular schwannomas and found one-fifth of patients experienced significant decisional conflict. Most patients perceived a high degree of SDM, which was associated with reduced decisional conflict, suggesting that patient engagement in the decision process significantly reduced uncertainty (Graham et al., 2018).

Laryngology

Glottic insufficiency

Treatment of glottic insufficiency varies from watchful waiting, speech therapy, vocal fold injections, and thyroplasty. Vocal fold injection is a relatively low-risk procedure with minimal complications. A. Q. Liu and colleagues examined decisional regret after treatment with outpatient (in-office) vocal fold injections and found most patients had little to no decisional regret. Approximately 20% reported moderate-to-strong decisional regret, which was driven by the change in grade, roughness, and breathiness after injection. The authors conclude vocal fold injections are well tolerated and associated with relatively low decisional regret, reinforcing their role in glottic insufficiency management (A. Q. Liu et al., 2023).

Facial plastics and reconstructive surgery

Facial paralysis

Facial paralysis can cause a significant physical and psychological burden and impact quality of life. Smile restoration can be achieved through several surgical techniques, though differences in timing, smile spontaneity, and a number of procedures may elicit important patient preferences. Santosa and colleagues provide a framework for SDM in facial reanimation surgery, including a stepwise approach with example phrases for optimal communication (Santosa et al., 2019). The authors conclude the most appropriate choice depends on the patient's goals and circumstances, spotlighting the role of SDM.

Facial trauma

Y. Liu and colleagues examined SDM between patients seeking evaluation for facial trauma and reconstructive surgeons. The authors found patients with previous experiences of discrimination in healthcare and patients who experienced distress when choosing between treatment options felt that they participated less in the decision making process (Y. Liu et al., 2024).

Paediatrics

In paediatric otolaryngology, many conditions can be treated with various approaches, ranging from maximal intervention to watchful waiting. Navigating these decisions can prove challenging for parents, especially when considerable trade-offs in management strategies exist. Indeed, parents of children undergoing evaluation for elective otolaryngological procedure(s) report considerable decisional conflict (Boss et al., 2016). Decisional conflict is reduced in parents who perceive greater SDM with their clinician (Boss et al., 2016).

Parental perception of SDM in paediatric otolaryngology is mixed, with some studies reporting low levels of SDM (Evong et al., 2019), and others perceiving high levels (Hong et al., 2016). Interestingly, perception of SDM does not correlate with observed SDM behaviours. In other words, parents may leave an interaction feeling as though they were engaged in the decision making process despite few explicit SDM behaviours (Hong et al., 2016). These findings indicate that despite the growing popularity of SDM, there remains room for improvement in the implementation of SDM in practice.

Sleep-disordered breathing

Paediatric sleep-disordered breathing involves a spectrum of abnormal respiratory patterns, from snoring to obstructive sleep apnoea. The mainstay of treatment is adenotonsillectomy, which can significantly improve a child's quality of life (Baldassari et al., 2008). However, some evidence suggests watchful waiting may be equally effective (Marcus et al., 2013), suggesting a subset of children may improve over time without intervention.

Boss and colleagues conducted semi-structured interviews to explore parental factors influencing a decision to pursue adenotonsillectomy. Two major themes were identified: clinical factors and clinician interpersonal behaviours and communication. Specifically, parental decisions were influenced by fear of their child stopping breathing and behavioural and/or cognitive delays. Interpersonal and communication factors impacting a parent's decision include interpersonal characteristics (positive or negative) of the surgeon, clinician responsiveness, trust, and confidence (Boss et al., 2017).

Decision support tools in otolaryngology

Decision support tools are standardized, evidence-based education materials that facilitate SDM by providing information on the condition of interest and available treatment options. Importantly, decision support tools clarify patient values, which is a distinguishing feature from traditional educational materials.

Existing evidence illustrates many benefits of decision support tools and few, if any, disadvantages. Stacey and colleagues led a Cochrane review of over 200 randomized control trials in various clinical contexts, finding that patients given decision aids felt more equipped to make decisions and played a more active role in the process (Stacey et al., 2024). Decision support tools have also been shown to decrease decisional conflict, improve confidence in patients' chosen treatment, and reduce unnecessary variation in care and healthcare costs (Légaré et al., 2006).

Examples of decision support tools include Option Grids and decision aids. Option Grids compare facts about treatments in a simplified table with answers to a series of commonly asked questions (Elwyn et al., 2013). In otolaryngology, Option Grids exist for otitis media with effusion, sore throat, tonsillitis, and language options for deaf infants and children (EBSCO Health, n.d.).

Decision aids are multifaceted tools that come in various formats, such as booklets, brochures, and interactive online modules. Decision aids typically include (1) information on the condition; (2) incorporated evidence on treatment options, their risks, and benefits; and (3) elicitation of patient values.

In otolaryngology, relatively few validated decision aids exist, though this number is growing. The available decision aids are described below.

Chronic rhinosinusitis with nasal polyposis

A decision aid was created for patients navigating treatment options for chronic rhinosinusitis with nasal polyposis. This online interactive tool directs patients to read about management options, respond to statements about lifestyle and preferences, and print out their answers to facilitate a discussion at their next appointment (American College of Allergy, Asthma, & Immunology, n.d.).

Laryngeal cancer

Peterson and colleagues developed an online decision aid for patients with advanced laryngeal cancer deciding between radiotherapy, chemoradiotherapy, or total laryngectomy with adjuvant radiotherapy (Petersen et al., 2019). In addition to an overview of each treatment option, this aid details side effects and provides explanatory animations.

Oropharyngeal cancer

Bigelow and colleagues developed the first web-based decision aid for patients with OPSCC who are choosing between radiation therapy, chemotherapy, or transoral surgery (Bigelow et al., 2021). Heirman and co-workers created an interactive online decision aid for patients with early-stage oropharyngeal cancer in the Netherlands, comparing transoral robotic surgery and radiotherapy options and their short- and long-term side effects (Heirman et al., 2024).

Sleep-disordered breathing

Maguire and colleagues created a decision aid focusing on the treatment of sleep-disordered breathing in children. The tool is geared towards parents and compares watchful waiting and adenotonsillectomy and their associated risks (Maguire et al., 2016). Meier and co-workers further explored the feasibility of this prototype through a randomized control trial. Results revealed the decision aid was feasible among parents and surgeons, and that parents found the tool helpful. However, the use of the decision aids varied among surgeons, highlighting the need for improved SDM techniques for future investigations (Meier et al., 2019).

Obstructive sleep apnoea

Decision aids exist for paediatric (Williamson et al., 2022) and adult (Gulati et al., 2024) patients with obstructive sleep apnoea. Williamson and colleagues developed a brief questionnaire-based decision aid for parents of children who were candidates for tonsillectomy for obstructive sleep apnoea. The authors found that the use of the decision aid was associated with low decisional conflict and high decisional quality (Williamson et al., 2022). Gulati and co-workers created video-based decision aids for adults with obstructive sleep apnoea navigating positive airway pressure alternatives. They found that the high levels of decisional conflict pre-intervention improved after the use of the decision aid (Gulati et al., 2024).

Future applications and conclusion

There remains a dearth of investigations into SDM in otolaryngology, raising ample avenues for future study. Other opportunities for future research could examine conversational delivery and bias. How and when treatment options are presented by physicians can directly impact management decisions. Patients are more likely to choose surgery when outcomes are presented positively or when treatment decisions are made based on favourable framing (absolute vs relative risk) (Ozdemir and Finkelstein, 2018). Few, if any, investigations have explored these concepts with respect to SDM in otolaryngology.

In conclusion, SDM is a collaborative approach to medical care with particular applicability to situations of clinical equipoise. While accumulating evidence reveals the impact of SDM on the management of essential and elective otolaryngological conditions, ample opportunities remain for continued study.

REFERENCES

American College of Allergy, Asthma, & Immunology. n.d. Treating chronic rhinosinusitis with nasal polyps. Available at: https://acaai.org/resource/treating-chronic-rhinosinusitis-with-nasal-polyps/

Baldassari, C. M., Mitchell, R. B., Schubert, C., Rudnick, E. F. 2008. Pediatric obstructive sleep apnea and quality of life: a meta-analysis. *Otolaryngol Head Neck Surg,* **138**, 265–273.

Bigelow, E. O., Windon, M. J., Fakhry, C., Kiess, A. P., Seiwert, T., D'Souza, G. 2021. Development of a web-based, patient-centered decision aid for oropharyngeal cancer treatment. *Oral Oncol,* **123**, 105618.

Boss, E. F., Links, A. R., Saxton, R., Cheng, T. L., Beach, M. C. 2017. Parent experience of care and decision making for children who snore. *JAMA Otolaryngol Head Neck Surg,* **143**, 218.

Boss, E. F., Mehta, N., Nagarajan, N., et al. 2016. Shared decision making and choice for elective surgical care: a systematic review. *Otolaryngol Head Neck Surg,* **154**, 405–420.

Drake, R. E., Deegan, P. E. 2009. Shared decision making is an ethical imperative. *Psychiatr Serv,* **60**, 1007.

Dropkin, M. J. 1989. Coping with disfigurement and dysfunction after head and neck cancer surgery: a conceptual framework. *Semin Oncol Nurs,* **5**, 213–219.

EBSCO Health. n.d. My health decisions: current option grid patient decision aids. Available at: https://www.ebsco.com/health-care/products/my-health-decisions.

Elwyn, G., Lloyd, A., Joseph-Williams, N., et al. 2013. Option grids: shared decision making made easier. *Patient Educ Couns,* **90**, 207–212.

Evong, Y., Chorney, J., Ungar, G., Hong, P. 2019. Perceptions and observations of shared decision making during pediatric otolaryngology surgical consultations. *J Otolaryngol Head Neck Surg,* **48**, 28.

Forner, D., Noel, C. W., Shuman, A. G., et al. 2020. Shared decision-making in head and neck surgery: a review. *JAMA Otolaryngol Head Neck Surg,* **146**, 839–844.

Goepfert, R. P., Fuller, C. D., Gunn, G. B., et al. 2017. Symptom burden as a driver of decisional regret in long-term oropharyngeal carcinoma survivors. *Head Neck,* **39**, 2151–2158.

Graham, M. E., Westerberg, B. D., Lea, J., et al. 2018. Shared decision making and decisional conflict in the management of vestibular schwannoma: a prospective cohort study. *J Otolaryngol Head Neck Surg,* **47**, 52.

Gulati, A., Abdulbaki, H., Callander, J. K., Cai, Y., Chang, J. L. 2024. Video-based decision aids improve sleep surgery decision-making: a randomized controlled trial. *Laryngoscope,* **134**, 2958–2963.

Heirman, A. N., Dirven, R., van der Molen, L., et al. 2024. The development of a decision aid for patients with operable oropharyngeal carcinoma in the Netherlands—a mixed methods study. *Oral Oncol,* **149**, 106677.

Hong, P., Maguire, E., Gorodzinsky, A. Y., Curran, J. A., Ritchie, K., Chorney, J. 2016. Shared decision-making in pediatric otolaryngology: parent, physician and observational perspectives. *Int J Pediatr Otorhinolaryngol,* **87**, 39–43.

Kwon, J. J. Y., Liu, A. Q., Milner, T. D., Prisman, E. 2023. Decisional regret, symptom burden, and quality of life following transoral robotic surgery for oropharyngeal cancer. *Oral Oncol,* **146**, 106537.

Légaré, F., O'Connor, A. C., Graham, I., et al. 2006. Supporting patients facing difficult health care decisions: use of the Ottawa Decision Support Framework. *Can Fam Physician,* **52**, 476–467.

Liu, A. Q., Ji, Y., Hu, A. 2023. Do patients regret having in-office vocal fold injections for glottic insufficiency? *J Otolaryngol Head Neck Surg,* **52**, 33.

Liu, Y., Wamkpah, N. S., Ballamudi, A., et al. 2024. Shared decision-making in patients seeking surgery for facial trauma: the role of decisional conflict and perceived discrimination. *Facial Plast Surg Aesthet Med,* **26**, 333–338.

Maguire, E., Hong, P., Ritchie, K., Meier, J., Archibald, K., Chorney, J. 2016. Decision aid prototype development for parents considering adenotonsillectomy for their children with sleep disordered breathing. *J Otolaryngol Head Neck Surg,* **45**, 57.

Marcus, C. L., Moore, R. H., Rosen, C. L., et al. 2013. A randomized trial of adenotonsillectomy for childhood sleep apnea. *N Engl J Med,* **368**, 2366–2376.

Meier, J. D., Chorney, J. M., Fox, S. D., Hong, P. 2019. Decision aid prototype for treatment of pediatric sleep disordered breathing: a randomized pilot study. *Laryngoscope,* **129**, 229–234.

Naunheim, M. R., von Sneidern, M., Huston, M. N., et al. 2023. Patient experiences with thyroid nodules: a qualitative interview survey. *OTO Open,* **7**, e39.

Ozdemir, S., Finkelstein, E. A. 2018. Cognitive bias: the downside of shared decision making. *JCO Clin Cancer Inform,* **2**, 1–10.

Petersen, J. F., Berlanga, A., Stuiver, M. M., et al. 2019. Improving decision making in larynx cancer by developing a decision aid: a mixed methods approach. *Laryngoscope,* **129**, 2733–2739.

Santosa, K. B., Keane, A. M., Politi, M., Snyder-Warwick, A. K. 2019. Facial animation surgery for long-standing facial palsy: opportunities for shared decision making. *JAMA Facial Plast Surg,* **21**, 3–4.

Shuman, A. G., Larkin, K., Thomas, D., et al. 2017. Patient reflections on decision making for laryngeal cancer treatment. *Otolaryngol Head Neck Surg,* **156**, 299–304.

Stacey, D., Lewis, K., Smith, M., et al. 2017. Decision aids for people facing health treatment or screening decisions. *Cochrane Database Syst Rev,* **1**, CD001431.

Taylor, B. A., Hart, R. D., Rigby, M. H., Trites, J., Taylor, S. M., Hong, P. 2016. Decisional conflict in patients considering diagnostic thyroidectomy with indeterminate fine needle aspirate cytopathology. *J Otolaryngol Head Neck Surg,* **45**, 16.

Thomas, C. M., Sklar, M. C., Su, J., et al. 2019. Evaluation of older age and frailty as factors associated with depression and postoperative decision regret in patients undergoing major head and neck surgery. *JAMA Otolaryngol Head Neck Surg,* **145**, 1170–1178.

Williamson, A., Newby, M., Phillips, D., Carr, M. 2022. Development of a decision aid for parents who elect tonsillectomy for obstructive sleep apnea. *Ann Otol Rhinol Laryngol,* **131**, 617–621.

Windon, M. J., Le, D., D'Souza, G., et al. 2021. Treatment decision-making among patients with oropharyngeal squamous cell cancer: a qualitative study. *Oral Oncol,* **112**, 105044.

45

Shared decision making in gastroenterology and hepatology

Saam Dilmaghani, Johannah Ruddy, Ian Hargraves, and Jean Fox

Introduction

Gastrointestinal (GI) conditions are often chronic and incurable; treatment may only offer partial relief. They are frequently distressing, stigmatizing, and upend day-to-day life, including the freedom to travel, social activities, work, family, and diet. They may diminish patients' and their families' dignity and horizons of what is possible and meaningful in life. These very real problems hide euphemistically behind diagnoses such as inflammatory bowel disease (IBD). Still, they are the problematic situations that patients and clinicians grapple with in GI care and which should be served by SDM. Figure 45.1 summarizes the landscape of the challenges of GI illness, decision making, and SDM implementation.

Inflammatory bowel diseases

The major subtypes of IBD, ulcerative colitis and Crohn's disease, are increasingly prevalent chronic, life-limiting, relapsing/progressive, idiopathic, and inflammatory conditions. Therapeutic options for IBD have dramatically expanded over the last 20 years and range from topical medications to systemic immunosuppressants and biological therapies, all with varying degrees of benefit and risks.

Given the chronic nature of the condition, the multitude of treatment options and surveillance approaches, and the near certainty of relapsing symptoms, the need for SDM is clear. Many qualitative and survey studies have found that both paediatric and adult patients with IBD and their families desire an approach that is collaborative, informative, and caring (Lofland et al., 2017; Al Khoury et al., 2022). The need for SDM has also been acknowledged and advocated for by clinicians caring for these patients (Siegel et al., 2015).

A systematic review of IBD patient preferences found that their main concerns included using SDM in making treatment decisions (Al Khoury et al., 2022). Additionally, the investigators found that patients prioritized total symptom control rather than the time taken to achieve control, cared more about quality of life than endoscopic findings, and cared more about the risk of cancer compared to the priorities expressed by their providers. Interestingly, these

	Debility	Multi-morbid	Stigma	Stable sxs	Curable	Treatment burden	Number of options	Heterogeneity of options	Strength of evidence	Guideline/care consistency	SDM research or interventions	Clinician readiness
IBD	Severe	Likely	Common	Unlikely	No	***	***	**	**	***	***	*
IBS	Severe	Unlikely	Common	Unlikely	No	***	***	***	*	*	*	*
EoO	Moderate	Likely	Uncommon	Unlikely	No	***	**	***	**	**	*	*
GERD	Mild	Likely	Uncommon	Likely	No	**	**	**	*	***	*	*
BO	None	Likely	Uncommon	Likely	Yes	***	**	**	**	**	*	*
Obesity	Moderate	Likely	Common	Unlikely	No	***	***	***	**	*	**	*
CRC	-	-	Uncommon	-	-	**	**	***	***	**	**	*

Challenges of illness
Challenges to decision making
Challenges to SDM implementation

*** = Significant
** = Some
* = Minimal

Figure 45.1 Summary of disease, management, and shared-decision making considerations in gastroenterology. BO, Barrett's oesophagus; CRC, colorectal cancer; EOO, eosinophilic oesophagitis; GORD, gastro-oesophageal reflux disease; IBD, inflammatory bowel disease; IBS, irritable bowel syndrome; SDM, shared decision making; sxs, symptoms.

preferences conflict with current professional guidelines, which emphasize rapid disease control and endoscopic remission. This impedes using SDM to address the issues that matter to patients.

Numerous studies have attempted to explore the acceptability and effects of SDM in IBD (Lofland et al., 2017; Kim et al., 2021; Matula et al., 2022). For example, adult patients initiating biological therapies for a new diagnosis of IBD who engaged more in SDM were significantly more likely to report disease management self-efficacy (Lofland et al., 2017). Decision aids piloted in IBD care for medical and surgical decisions have been found to be acceptable and improve patient certainty and confidence (Kim et al., 2021; Matula et al., 2022).

Despite both theoretical and practical evidence for the need for SDM in IBD, there remain significant areas for improvement. IBD providers' awareness and knowledge of SDM are generally lacking, although one study estimated it could be as high as 75%. Even with education, barriers to implementing SDM among gastroenterologists have included concerns of time, reimbursement, and the limited availability of tools or aids (Siegel et al., 2015). There is no standardized recommendation or guidance for incorporating SDM in IBD care.

Irritable bowel syndrome

Disorders of the gut–brain interaction are a heterogeneous group of disorders characterized by GI symptoms without objectively quantifiable or observable findings. With an overall prevalence of 5–15%, the most common disorder of the gut–brain interaction is irritable bowel syndrome (IBS). Patients with IBS suffer from abdominal pain and varying stool frequency and/or consistency. These symptoms are intrusive, debilitating, and chronic and require individualized patient-centred care.

The pathophysiological mechanisms associated with IBS are diverse. Even with diagnostic testing, a large portion of patients are never provided with an explanation for their symptoms and are only unhelpfully and unilluminating told that testing was normal, and they have nothing wrong with them or they have 'idiopathic' IBS.

The absence of a definitive explanation for the patient's symptoms presents numerous challenges to care. For one, patients may experience frustration towards, dissatisfaction with, and mistrust of a healthcare system that lacks the tools and concrete understanding of their condition. Early on, the essential patient–physician relationship may struggle to establish its foundation if trust is questioned in physician uncertainty. Even if the relationship is built, it risks erosion over time as therapeutic trials likely continue to provide suboptimal results. This is commonly exacerbated by the discontinuity of care.

On the other hand, the lack of a specific aetiological mechanism could be a unique and yet unmet opportunity for SDM. This situation provides opportunities for collaboration that may otherwise be unavailable in other clinical specialties or GI diseases. For example, given minimal strong and definitive guidelines for management, physicians and patients are freer to experiment with treatments and maximize the patient's ability to find, sustain, and adapt the most situationally desirable approach for them.

While many therapeutic options exist, most have limited effectiveness and estimates of benefit due to limited high-quality studies and small sample sizes. As a result, guidelines provided by professional societies lack consensus recommendations for managing IBS. For example, the American College of Gastroenterology recommends *against* the use of an osmotic laxative (polyethylene glycol) and all antispasmodics for IBS. At the same time, the American Gastroenterological Association guidelines published the following year advocate using both of these options. This has led to uncertainty, confusion for patients and providers, and generally dissatisfactory symptom resolution. For example, a single-centre cross-sectional survey study of patients with IBS found that the average number of treatment attempts was estimated at 12 (ranging from 2 to 39) despite a non-response rate of around 75% (Dong et al., 2019).

Although society guidelines agree that SDM is integral to managing this incurable condition, direction on how to do this is slim and education for clinicians on how to incorporate SDM into their practice setting is lacking. Leaders have called for the explicit use of SDM, due not only to limited effective treatments available but also because a patient's situationally determined capacity to live with and manage IBS is determinative of outcomes. Unfortunately, the use of SDM in IBS may be less common than in other chronic conditions due to patient stigmatization and physician bias (Drossman et al., 2009; Fullwood et al., 2013). This issue must be addressed by professional societies and in medical education.

Colorectal cancer screening

Colorectal cancer (CRC) represents one of the most common and fatal malignancies in the world. In the USA, it is estimated that over 150,000 individuals will be diagnosed with the disease, and over 50,000 will die each year. Given that most CRCs develop slowly, survival from CRC depends on early diagnosis through early detection and removal of the precursors.

Many modalities exist for screening for CRC, which presents trade-offs between convenience, cost, and comprehensiveness, each with different recommendations for interval follow-up. However, there is a paucity of evidence comparing these modalities. Patient decision aids have been developed to help navigate these choices. An early systematic review of nearly 12,000 patients over 21 trials found that those who were provided with decision aids (including video and booklet formats) demonstrated greater knowledge of CRC and more interest in and a greater likelihood of completing screening compared to controls (Volk et al., 2016). Another systematic review suggested that SDM tools may benefit vulnerable populations most (e.g. lower health literacy and socioeconomic status), which could improve health equity (Herrera et al., 2023).

Yet, the uptake and implementation of SDM tools remain variable, and data to evaluate SDM practices in clinical care are sparse. Furthermore, professional guidelines for CRC screening and management recommend the use of clinical decision support tools to improve screening adherence but do not mention SDM aside from average-risk patients of advanced age, for whom the benefits of CRC screening are more ambiguous. An opportunity to increase the use of SDM would be to incorporate these recommendations in gastroenterology, family medicine, and internal medicine professional guidelines.

Oesophageal diseases

Eosinophilic oesophagitis is a chronic, incurable disease resulting in difficulty swallowing. Management options include elimination diets, antireflux medications, topical steroids, antibody infusions, and procedures. Despite substantial variability in the burden, potential benefits, and risks of these options, nearly half of patients with eosinophilic oesophagitis report not experiencing SDM (Chang et al., 2021), and nearly half of gastroenterologists report spending fewer than 10 minutes on patient education.

Gastro-oesophageal reflux disease (GORD) is a condition defined by symptoms due to reflux of gastric acid into the oesophagus. It is managed by lifestyle modification, antireflux medications, and surgery. Despite numerous options, for a variety of reasons, complete symptom resolution may not be achieved. In this context, experts recommend SDM strategies (Klenzak et al., 2018) so patients can choose their management options. However, no formal tools, aids, or educational materials have been developed or validated for GORD.

A small subset of patients with long-standing GORD may progress to Barrett's oesophagus, which is a precursor to oesophageal cancer. Professional guidelines have called for SDM with patients with only minor cellular abnormalities due to uncertainty regarding the rate of cancer progression (Krishnamoorthi, 2020). Early studies suggested that patients preferred more aggressive interventions to avoid oesophageal cancer (Yachimski et al., 2015). A tool to help navigate these decisions, Barrett's oesophagus Choice, has since been developed and pilot-tested (Krishnamoorthi et al., 2021) but has not yet been widely implemented, despite significantly improving knowledge, decisional comfort, and involvement compared to usual care.

Obesity

Obesity has reached epidemic proportions, with an estimated 42% of US adults affected in 2020, though the distribution of disease varies by demographics, such as socioeconomic status. Management options include lifestyle modification, pharmacotherapy, and surgical/endoscopic interventions. Although some have emphasized the need for SDM in obesity management, given the variable burden, benefits, and risks of each approach (Yanovski and Yanovski, 2024), there remains a paucity of data regarding the optimal way to incorporate SDM in clinical care. Given the increasing number of approved medications, early work has begun to characterize patient factors which may help to guide SDM (Donnan et al., 2022) and decision aids are being piloted (Moore et al., 2019).

Critically, obesity is associated with many diseases, including obstructive sleep apnoea, diabetes mellitus, heart disease, stroke, liver diseases, and GORD. To date, SDM strategies and tools are lacking to guide clinicians in communicating the risks of excess adiposity with patients. However, there is a potential danger in focusing too heavily on the risks of obesity as, for many patients, weight and the inability to sustain weight loss is a source of ongoing frustration and stigma. Commonly inadequately acknowledged in encounters is the evidence that the likelihood of sustained weight loss with most approaches is low. SDM has the potential to foster honest conversations of weight management and how to live with obesity.

Outstanding challenges and key priorities for SDM in gastroenterology and hepatology

Evidence limitations, including availability, quality, certainty, and applicability, pervade GI care, as do treatments with limited likely sustained benefit. In such situations, professional societies increasingly recommend the use of SDM. Some GI guidelines do, and this is likely to increase. This is to be encouraged.

However, when SDM is recommended, it is uncommon for guidelines to guide clinicians in using SDM in their practice. In so doing, they sustain the limited adoption of SDM. It is concerning that guidelines may promote SDM primarily to sidestep evidence and intervention limitations.

Historically, SDM research and interventions have stepped in to help patients and clinicians make preference-sensitive choices based on what is known about options, and there remain many opportunities to do this in gastroenterology. However, the lives of patients living with unpleasant, chronic, incurable, life-limiting GI illnesses are such that SDM focused on deciding between options may be inadequate. After many options have been tried and found unsatisfactory, as is common, repeatedly helping patients choose the next option becomes futile, uncaring, and off point. Instead, how to make the most of life with illness becomes the appropriate issue. Goal-centred SDM may be helpful in identifying points of focus, while problem-oriented models (Hargraves et al., 2019) focused more holistically on how to organize life and incorporate care practically also have promise.

See Box 45.1 for our patient perspective.

Box 45.1 Patient perspective

Living with a GI illness can markedly impact a patient's daily life. SDM serves as a crucial platform for patients to express their priorities and goals for treatment. For instance, a patient with IBS may prioritize minimizing medication use, even if it means only partial symptom relief. In contrast, another patient may prioritize complete symptom control and be open to different treatment options. The SDM approach ensures that the chosen treatment plan aligns with the patient's values and priorities.

The management of GI illnesses often necessitates ongoing adjustments and trying different approaches. The SDM approach fosters a collaborative relationship between the patient and the physician, wherein challenges can be openly discussed, and new treatment options can be explored. This approach is particularly helpful when initial treatments are not fully effective, underscoring the value of the patient's input.

When patients partake in treatment decisions alongside their clinician, they are likely to feel invested in the plan and have a better understanding of its rationale. This can lead to increased satisfaction with care and better adherence to treatment recommendations. Ultimately, the SDM approach enables patients to participate actively in their treatment, promoting patient-centred care in managing GI illnesses.

SDM in specific disease states

- IBD constitutes a complex spectrum of disorders that can be addressed through a diverse range of medications and therapies. SDM is a valuable approach to selecting the optimal course of treatment, considering factors such as symptom management and potential side effects.
- The management of IBS typically involves a combination of dietary modifications and medications. By utilizing SDM with your healthcare provider, you can explore and evaluate various treatment options to determine the most effective course of action.

- Oesophageal diseases, such as eosinophilic oesophagitis and GORD, may necessitate dietary modifications, medications, or procedures. SDM is an approach that can help evaluate the benefits and risks of each intervention, enabling you to make a well-informed decision and select the optimal management plan for your individual needs.
- A comprehensive management strategy for obesity comprises various interventions, including lifestyle modifications, pharmacotherapy, and surgical procedures. Incorporating SDM facilitates a collaborative discussion, enabling the patient and healthcare provider to evaluate the risks and benefits of each approach. This approach empowers patients to choose a weight management plan that aligns with their goals and preferences.

Current challenges in implementing SDM in GI care

Healthcare providers often lack adequate training or knowledge about SDM. This, combined with busy clinic schedules, makes it challenging for doctors to dedicate enough time to in-depth discussions. Moreover, the lack of standardized tools poses an additional challenge for clinicians in implementing SDM during consultations. Standardized resources are required to guide doctors in implementing SDM effectively.

Summary

In the field of gastroenterology, and especially in caring for patients with functional GI tract disorders, we often find ourselves without a best or gold standard of treatment, making these conditions ideal for SDM. SDM enriches the clinical interactions between healthcare provider and patient and may uncover misunderstandings or misconceptions on the part of both the clinician and the patient with regard to disease burden and treatment goals. Going forward, efforts must be made to expand the use of SDM in GI care. This could be achieved by developing decision aids for patients and providing interview guides for clinicians. But also, it will certainly require investing in awareness and educational campaigns, and possibly even reframing early-career training, to emphasize the usefulness and practical implementation of SDM in gastroenterology and hepatology. If implemented successfully, it will undoubtedly benefit both our care providers and patients burdened by these conditions.

REFERENCES

Al Khoury, A., Balram, B., Bessissow, T., et al. 2022. Patient perspectives and expectations in inflammatory bowel disease: a systematic review. *Dig Dis Sci,* **67**, 1956–1974.

Chang, J. W., Rubenstein, J. H., Mellinger, J. L., et al. 2021. Motivations, barriers, and outcomes of patient-reported shared decision making in eosinophilic esophagitis. *Dig Dis Sci,* **66**, 1808–1817.

Dong, Y., Baumeister, D., Berens, S., Eich, W., Tesarz, J. 2019. High rates of non-response across treatment attempts in chronic irritable bowel syndrome: results from a follow-up study in tertiary care. *Front Psychiatry,* **10**, 714.

Donnan, J., Huang, R., Twells, L. 2022. Patient preferences for attributes of Health Canada approved weight loss medications among adults living with obesity in Canada: a qualitative study. *Patient Prefer Adherence,* **16**, 911–923.

Drossman, D. A., Chang, L., Schneck, S., Blackman, C., Norton, W. F., Norton, N. J. 2009. A focus group assessment of patient perspectives on irritable bowel syndrome and illness severity. *Dig Dis Sci,* **54**, 1532–1541.

Fullwood, C., Kennedy, A., Rogers, A., et al. 2013. Patients' experiences of shared decision making in primary care practices in the United Kingdom. *Med Decis Making,* **33**, 26–36.

Hargraves, I. G., Montori, V. M., Brito, J. P., et al. 2019. Purposeful SDM: a problem-based approach to caring for patients with shared decision making. *Patient Educ Couns,* **102**, 1786–1792.

Herrera, D. J., van de Veerdonk, W., Berhe, N. M., et al. 2023. Mixed-method systematic review and meta-analysis of shared decision-making tools for cancer screening. *Cancers (Basel),* **15**, 3867.

Kim, A. H., Girgis, A., De Cruz, P., et al. 2021. Development and feasibility of a web-based decision aid for patients with ulcerative colitis: qualitative pilot study. *J Med Internet Res,* **23**, e15946.

Klenzak, S., Danelisen, I., Brannan, G. D., Holland, M. A., van Tilburg, M. A. 2018. Management of gastroesophageal reflux disease: patient and physician communication challenges and shared decision making. *World J Clin Cases,* **6**, 892–900.

Krishnamoorthi, R. 2020. Endoscopic therapy or surveillance for Barrett's esophagus with low-grade dysplasia: time to involve patients in shared decision making. *Gastrointest Endosc,* **92**, 575–577.

Krishnamoorthi, R., Hargraves, I., Gopalakrishnan, N., et al. 2021. Development and pilot testing of decision aid for shared decision making in Barrett's esophagus with low-grade dysplasia. *J Clin Gastroenterol,* **55**, 36–42.

Lofland, J. H., Johnson, P. T., Ingham, M. P., Rosemas, S. C., White, J. C., Ellis, L. 2017. Shared decision-making for biologic treatment of autoimmune disease: influence on adherence, persistence, satisfaction, and health care costs. *Patient Prefer Adherence,* **11**, 947–958.

Matula, K. A., Minar, P., Daraiseh, N. M., Lin, L., Recker, M., Lipstein, E. A. 2022. Pilot trial of iBDecide: evaluating an online tool to facilitate shared decision making for adolescents and young adults with ulcerative colitis. *Health Expect,* **25**, 3105–3113.

Moore, J., Haemer, M., Mirza, N., et al. 2019. Pilot testing of a patient decision aid for adolescents with severe obesity in US pediatric weight management programs within the COMPASS Network. *Int J Environ Res Public Health,* **16**, 1776.

Siegel, C. A., Lofland, J. H., Naim, A., et al. 2015. Gastroenterologists' views of shared decision making for patients with inflammatory bowel disease. *Dig Dis Sci,* **60**, 2636–2645.

Volk, R. J., Linder, S. K., Lopez-Olivo, M. A., et al. 2016. Patient decision aids for colorectal cancer screening: a systematic review and meta-analysis. *Am J Prev Med,* **51**, 779–791.

Yachimski, P., Wani, S., Givens, T., et al. 2015. Preference of endoscopic ablation over medical prevention of esophageal adenocarcinoma by patients with Barrett's esophagus. *Clin Gastroenterol Hepatol,* **13**, 84–90.

Yanovski, S. Z., Yanovski, J. A. 2024. Approach to obesity treatment in primary care: a review. *JAMA Intern Med,* **184**, 818–829.

46

Shared decision making in neurology

Constanze Stolz-Klingenberg, Michaela Prigge, Walter Maetzler, and Christoph Heesen

The many reasons why shared decision making is essential in neurology

Neurology as a medical specialty encompasses all diseases of the central and peripheral nervous system and muscles, ranging from persistent headaches to chronic and progressive conditions such as multiple sclerosis (MS), epilepsy, or Parkinson's disease. Neurology and its mostly chronic diseases have a natural affinity for the application of shared decision making (SDM) for numerous reasons. Once such a disease has been diagnosed, the patient and physician enter into a long-term collaboration in which the treatment works particularly well if the patient and the physician work together as a team over the long term. As a disease progresses, it often affects patients' physical, cognitive, and psychosocial health, which can vary in severity and symptoms from person to person. The difficulty in predicting the course of many neurological diseases and the limited efficacy of drug treatments make it imperative that patients play an active role in their treatment decisions. This is particularly true as some chronic progressive diseases, such as MS, are often diagnosed in young adulthood. It is at this stage of life that far-reaching personal decisions are usually made, such as career choices or family planning. SDM allows the patient's circumstances and personal life plans to be analysed in relation to the different aspects of the disease and its treatment options.

Furthermore, recent developments in medical research have led to a broad range of treatment options for many neurological diseases, which differ in terms of side effects, efficacy, and type of application. In such cases, effective patient–physician communication is crucial for optimal and individualized decision making. However, this process can be challenging since patients and doctors often have different treatment goals. Although the doctor's primary goal is to slow down disease progression through medical therapeutics, patients' perspectives are different (Col et al., 2018; Heesen et al., 2018). This difference in priorities highlights the importance of active participation from both the patient and their loved ones in these decisions. In the context of progressive diseases, cognitive impairments may arise, making relatives increasingly important for these treatment decisions. However, many relatives do not feel adequately informed or involved to support treatment decisions or make decisions on behalf of the patient (Schubart et al., 2008). SDM allows family members to learn about the preferences of a patient who is still able to make decisions early on, so that they can become active advocates for the patient's wishes later on.

See Box 46.1 for our patient perspective.

Box 46.1 Patient perspective

SDM in neurology

'Idiopathic Parkinson's disease.' I received this diagnosis on 30 March 2015 as a 50-year-old woman. Briefly and concisely formulated by the neurologist. After an examination that took no more than 5 minutes. Prior to the diagnosis, I spent approximately 2 years attempting to understand my symptoms and seeking diagnoses through physiotherapy, occupational therapy, and visits to doctors from various specialisms. I visited the Centre of Excellence for Parkinson's Medicine at the UKSH in Kiel, Germany, but they were unable to diagnose my condition despite numerous examinations. They suggested prescribing Lyrica (pregabalin) and antidepressants, but I declined. I was sure that something was wrong with my body and refused the treatment. I still remember the day I received my diagnosis very clearly. I have not forgotten the despair, the confusion, and the reluctance to accept my diagnosis. I immediately registered with the German Parkinson's Association, but I was devastated by the news. Although I finally had a diagnosis, it was not the one I had hoped for. For 4 weeks, I struggled with my emotions. My husband, three grown-up children, and I cried and talked a lot.

I decided not to give up. Although I have Parkinson's disease, I believe I can still achieve a lot in my life. My motto since being diagnosed with Parkinson's disease almost 9 years ago has been: 'I have Parkinson's—Parkinson's does NOT have me!'

Since my diagnosis, I have been collaborating with my doctor on an equal footing to develop a personalized therapy. Parkinson's disease is constantly changing, so I must be vigilant of any changes. While the doctor can only observe my body from the outside, I have a unique understanding of my body from the inside. As an intensive care nurse, I can offer my expertise objectively. I have a realistic self-perception. It would have been helpful to have more information about the symptoms of my illness as it progressed. This would have prevented me from being unsettled, for example, by visual disturbances and allowed me to categorize them correctly. I had to acquire a lot of knowledge from lectures and specialist journals. My doctor recognizes the expertise I bring to the consultation and decision making process.

The symptoms of the disease have increased over the years, and I now work 60% while receiving a reduced earning capacity pension since November 2020. As an intensive care nurse, I retired early from bedside care and have been teaching nursing since 2016. I find it fulfilling to work with young people in my dream job. However, due to the long-term strain, I have decided to say goodbye to work life. I have recently applied to the pension insurance fund for a 100% reduction in earning capacity. Although I am sad, I am mostly content because I am doing quite well. I have several health issues, including agraphia, anosmia, spasms in my right leg, subtle tremor, dyskinesia, visual disturbances, impaired fine motor skills, sleep disorders, and incontinence. Despite these challenges, I maintain a positive outlook and manage my daily life with motivation. While I no longer drive, I can still navigate on foot. I enjoy staying active and spending time with loved ones.

Spotlight on two groups of neurological diseases: preference-sensitive decisions in MS treatment and in the treatment of neurodegenerative diseases

MS and SDM

Persons with MS (pwMS) are mostly highly competent young adults who in most cases experience no long-lasting major disabilities in the early years of their disease (Jakimovski et al., 2024). MS is a poorly understood, highly heterogeneous disease with only partially effective treatments. While survey data from 20 years ago indicate a preferred SDM approach among pwMS (Heesen et al., 2004) recent studies indicate an even higher level of desired autonomy (Giordano et al., 2018).

MS is the neurological disease about which most research on strategies to stimulate SDM has been undertaken. PwMS suspect a potential MS diagnosis before undergoing diagnostic procedures (Heesen et al., 2009). A prerequisite of SDM is evidence-based patient information to support informed choices. However, there are very few controlled studies of patient information in MS (Köpke et al., 2018). Patient handbooks on all available immunotherapies have been developed in Germany and were made available via the German Self-Help Society and the German Clinical Competence Network for MS. For the first time these handbooks made risk information on benefits and risks of MS immunotherapies available for pwMS based on absolute risk reduction and absolute risk increases (Schneider et al., 2022). Early trial work in the German setting has shown that evidence-based patient information in a group education format leads to a change in relapse management behaviour, with fewer treated relapses and if treated, more oral treatments (Köpke et al., 2009).

Another trial of a single group education session combined with a booklet showed more informed choices in initiating immunotherapy in MS among recently diagnosed pwMS (Köpke et al., 2014). Moreover, treatment adherence was enhanced in the intervention group. While group education programmes cannot adapt to individuals' timely needs, a nurse-led decision coaching education programme has been developed. A two-centre pilot trial showed more informed choices in the intervention group (Rahn et al., 2018). However, a multicentre randomized trial was prematurely terminated because of difficulties of recruiting patients, itself largely due to the lack of time among MS nurses. This underlines the structural health system barriers for new approaches in clinical decision making. Magnetic resonance imaging (MRI) is a crucial biomarker tool for MS diagnosis with limited prognostic value but valuable relevance in monitoring immunotherapies in MS. While there is substantial risk of overestimating MRI findings in relation to prognosis, a web-based MRI education programme has been accepted enthusiastically by pwMS (Freund et al., 2022). A recently finished trial showed increased risk knowledge about MRI among pwMS who received the educational programme compared to controls. Finally, work from Italy reports a high level of autonomy in the palliative care setting (Borreani et al., 2014).

Quantitative risk information is a key element of patient information. However, patients also search for personal testimonials and individual narratives. Based on work from medical sociologists in Oxford, the Dipex foundation (https://dipexinternational.org) has developed a framework to collect individual patient experience data on several diseases based on audios and videos (https://healthtalk.org). Following this concept, a German website with short videoclips of all immunotherapies has been built up, with high acceptance among pwMS (Sippel et al., 2021). However, the impact on patient decision making is not yet clear.

Taken together, while a number of facets of SDM have been studied in MS, most of the work is based on a limited number of centres. Multicentre or even international intervention studies are largely missing. Based on the experience of work in the field for 20 years, the time is now to make these happen, perhaps notably supported by digital health applications.

Neurodegenerative diseases and SDM

Neurodegeneration typically starts in specific brain regions and spreads as the disease advances. The loss of nerve cells can cause a range of symptoms that vary from person to person, including memory, speech, and motor disorders, as well as loss of orientation, mood swings, and changes in personality. The more common neurodegenerative diseases include Alzheimer's and other dementias, Parkinson's disease, and Huntington's disease. Given the potential severity of symptoms and associated cognitive impairments, it is worth investigating whether SDM is feasible and desirable for patients with neurodegenerative diseases, and how it can be integrated into routine care.

As in other areas of neurology, most patients receiving treatment for neurodegenerative diseases desire an active and responsible role in treatment decisions. A survey of 120 people with Parkinson's disease in the Netherlands found that 93% of patients wanted to participate in SDM (Nijhuis et al., 2019). In cases of disagreement with their doctor, the patients prefer to either make the final decision themselves or seek a second opinion, rather than leaving the choice of treatment solely with the doctor (Zizzo et al., 2017).

Regarding dementia, nearly 250 surveyed patients in the UK also expressed their desires to have a say in all of their medical decisions or to make the decisions themselves (Miller et al., 2016). Summarizing, the answer to whether SDM is desirable in patients with neurodegenerative diseases is a clear yes. However, there have been few structured initiatives for practical SDM implementation in this field.

Good information for patients is fundamental to enable active participation. This can be supported by providing evidence-based decision aids in addition to medical consultations. The above-mentioned Dutch study involving 120 Parkinson's disease patients showed that the amount of information provided during a consultation can be overwhelming for patients (Nijhuis et al., 2019). Despite effective communication during the consultation, patients were unable to process all the information, suggesting a need for more time and opportunities for reflection. While 77% of patients with Parkinson's disease reported feeling well informed, only 41% of those patients could recall all three available treatment options after the consultation. Such a hidden knowledge gap can hinder participation in decision making. The study showed that active patients require effective information tools to manage the responsibility of decision making.

Dutch neurologists treating Parkinson's disease are creating an Option Grid patient decision aid, a website with additional information, and a value clarification tool for patients and professionals facing the decision of advanced treatment options: continuous subcutaneous apomorphine infusion, deep brain stimulation or levodopa–carbidopa intestinal gel (Nijhuis et al. 2018). The benefits and acceptability of the (decision aid) intervention have yet to be assessed. During consultations with people with Alzheimer's disease, a single-page memory and organization aid improved their understanding and perceived ability to make decisions (Rubright et al., 2010).

Embedded in an SDM intervention at an entire university hospital in Kiel, Germany, 12 decision aids are provided to patients as part of the SHARE TO CARE project in the neuromedical centre. With regard to neurodegenerative diseases, the decision aids about the treatment of advanced Parkinson's disease (medication pump or deep brain stimulation) and for the treatment of severe tremor (medication, ultrasound, or deep brain stimulation) are particularly relevant. The decision aids include text, images, and video, as well as interactive areas. The medical and nursing teams are trained to discuss options with patients in the context of their preferences. Patients are specifically encouraged to be actively involved. The intervention was not evaluated specifically concerning patients with neurodegeneration. However, for the neuromedical centre as a whole, after implementation of the intervention, 142 patients reported feeling significantly better prepared for and more involved in their treatment decisions (Stolz-Klingenberg et al., 2022) compared to another cohort of 109 patients investigated before implementation of the intervention.

In conclusion, SDM initiatives are slowly emerging in the field of neurodegenerative diseases, underlining that there is considerable potential to meet the wishes of patients to be involved in decision making.

Barriers and potentials for practising SDM in neurological care

Effective SDM necessitates a comprehensive understanding of the roles of both the doctor and the patient. Patients should be cognizant of their responsibility for their own body and contribute their expertise regarding their unique circumstances. The doctor should be receptive to discussing the advantages and disadvantages of treatment options with consideration of the patient's concerns and preferences. Ascertaining decision making capacity in cognitively impaired patients can be challenging, especially when it depends on the patient's daily norm. Early involvement of relatives can help make the process transitional towards being more supported in decision making.

A survey of 13 neurologists from five Dutch hospitals identified lack of time, continuity of care, and lack of evidence about all available treatment options as the greatest barriers for patient engagement in Parkinson's disease (Nijhuis et al., 2019). At various levels, there is potential for improvement. Patients require greater empowerment and access to better information. This can be achieved through activation campaigns in hospitals, social media, and by involving patient representatives and self-help groups. In the context of medical care, a lasting change in values is needed. Patients should be encouraged to take responsibility for their own health and to be aware of the consequences of their treatment decisions.

The production of decision aids can support the provision of information and can provide the knowledge needed to support an active decision maker. Researching the necessary evidence for a decision aid is time-consuming, so sharing and updating the existing decision aids in national and international networks is necessary. During such an exchange, a shared learning process should take place to identify success factors and barriers in production and implementation of decision aids. Those learnings can assist working groups in developing decision aids tailored to their specific decision making situations and allows for the pooling of resources to develop a support tool for a wider range of decision making situations. Furthermore, it is important to critically examine the format and structure of decision aids to determine which type—analogue, digital, or a combination of both—would be most beneficial for patients with the respective condition.

Conclusion

In summary, neurology involves many preference-sensitive decisions, and most patients wish to be well informed and actively involved. While initiatives to promote SDM in neurological care are scarce, the few available show that SDM can be successfully implemented in clinical care. There are also initial indications that patients with cognitive impairments and mild-to-moderate dementia can also participate actively in decision making. However, the findings are limited, and further research is urgently needed. Additionally, the early involvement of relatives in the SDM process for chronic progressive diseases has received little attention.

To intensify SDM activities in neurology, it is crucial to strengthen international networking among SDM players. This will help to pool resources and gain insights into the efficient creation of decision aids or successful SDM coaching. Active contributions from the relevant patient organizations can also be highly effective and are essential to sustaining a SDM culture in neurology.

REFERENCES

Borreani, C., Bianchi, E., Pietrolongo, E., et al. 2014. Unmet needs of people with severe multiple sclerosis and their carers: qualitative findings for a home-based intervention. *PLoS One*, **9**, e109679.

Col, N. F., Solomon, A. J., Springmann, V., et al. 2018. Whose preferences matter? A patient-centered approach for eliciting treatment goals. *Med Decis Making*, **38**, 44–55.

Freund, M., Schiffmann, I., Rahn, A. C., et al. 2022. Understanding Magnetic Resonance Imaging in Multiple Sclerosis (UMIMS): development and piloting of an online education program about magnetic resonance imaging for people with multiple sclerosis. *Front Neurol,* **13,** 856240.

Giordano, A., Liethmann, K., Köpke, S., et al. 2018. Risk knowledge of people with relapsing-remitting multiple sclerosis—results of an international survey. *PLoS One,* **13,** e0208004.

Heesen, C., Haase, R., Melzig, S., et al. 2018. Perceptions on the value of bodily functions in multiple sclerosis. *Acta Neurol Scand,* **137,** 356–362.

Heesen, C., Schäffler, N., Kasper, J., Mühlhauser, I., Köpke, S. 2009. Suspected multiple sclerosis—what to do? Evaluation of a patient information leaflet. *Mult Scler,* **15,** 1103–1112.

Heesen, C., Kasper, J., Segal, J., Köpke, S., Mühlhauser, I. 2004. Decisional role preferences, risk knowledge and information interests in patients with multiple sclerosis. *Mult Scler,* **10,** 643–650.

Jakimovski, D., Bittner, S., Zivadinov, R., et al. 2024. Multiple sclerosis. *Lancet,* **403,** 183–202.

Köpke, S., Kasper, J., Mühlhauser, I., Nübling, M., Heesen, C. 2009. Patient education program to enhance decision autonomy in multiple sclerosis relapse management: a randomized-controlled trial. *Mult Scler,* **15,** 96–104.

Köpke, S., Kern, S., Ziemssen, T., et al. 2014. Evidence-based patient information programme in early multiple sclerosis: a randomised controlled trial. *J Neurol Neurosurg Psychiatry,* **85,** 411–418.

Köpke, S., Solari, A., Rahn, A., Khan, F., Heesen, C., Giordano, A. 2018. Information provision for people with multiple sclerosis. *Cochrane Database Syst Rev,* **10,** CD008757.

Miller, L. M., Whitlatch, C. J., Lyons, K. S. 2016. Shared decision-making in dementia: a review of patient and family carer involvement. *Dementia,* **15,** 1141–1157.

Nijhuis, F. A. P., Elwyn, G., Bloem, B. R., Post, B., Faber, M. J. 2018. Improving shared decision-making in advanced Parkinson's disease: protocol of a mixed methods feasibility study. *Pilot Feasibil Stud,* **4,** 94.

Nijhuis, F. A. P., van den Heuvel, L., Bloem, B. R., Post, B., Meinders, M. J. 2019. The patient's perspective on shared decision-making in advanced Parkinson's disease: a cross-sectional survey study. *Front Neurol,* **10,** 896.

Rahn, A. C., Köpke, S., Backhus, I., et al. 2018. Nurse-led immunotreatment DEcision Coaching In people with Multiple Sclerosis (DECIMS)—feasibility testing, pilot randomised controlled trial and mixed methods process evaluation. *Int J Nurs Stud,* **78,** 26–36.

Rubright, J., Sankar, P., Casarett, D. J., Gur, R., Xie, S. X., Karlawish, J. 2010. A memory and organizational aid improves Alzheimer disease research consent capacity: results of a randomized, controlled trial. *Am J Geriatr Psychiatry,* **18,** 1124–1132.

Schneider, A., Fasshauer, E., Scheiderbauer, J., et al. 2022. Development and evaluation of evidence-based patient information handbooks about multiple sclerosis immunotherapies. *Mult Scler Relat Disord,* **60,** 103728.

Schubart, J. R., Kinzie, M. B., Farace, E. 2008. Caring for the brain tumor patient: family caregiver burden and unmet needs. *Neurooncology,* **10,** 61–72.

Sippel, A., Riemann-Lorenz, K., Scheiderbauer, J., et al. 2021. Patients experiences with multiple sclerosis disease-modifying therapies in daily life—a qualitative interview study. *BMC Health Serv Res,* **21,** 1141.

Stolz-Klingenberg, C., Bünzen, C., Coors, M., et al. 2022. Sustainability of large-scale implementation of shared decision making with the SHARE TO CARE program. *Front Neurol,* **13,** 1037447.

Zizzo, N., Bell, E., Lafontaine, A.-L., Racine, E. 2017. Examining chronic care patient preferences for involvement in health-care decision making: the case of Parkinson's disease patients in a patient-centred clinic. *Health Expect,* **20,** 655–664.

47

Shared decision making in emergency medicine

Fernanda Bellolio, Kasey Boehmer, and Erik Hess

What, when, and why

The emergency department (ED) is the gateway to care for patients with various illnesses and injuries and provides a safety net for patients otherwise unable to access care. In the high-stakes, fast-paced environment of emergency medicine (EM), shared decision making (SDM) can play a crucial role (Hess et al., 2015). SDM is especially relevant when there is more than one reasonable option, or when the benefits and harms of different options are uncertain or depend on the patient's values and preferences. SDM in EM has the potential to improve quality, safety, and outcomes; lead to increased patient satisfaction; better patient understanding; reduce decisional conflict; and promote patient autonomy (Grudzen et al., 2016).

SDM is appropriate in the ED when there are two or more reasonable management options, the patient or their care partner are willing and able to engage in decision making, and there is time to make the decision. A cross-sectional survey of emergency physicians assessed perceptions of SDM's appropriateness for different scenarios. SDM was reported to be most frequently appropriate for deciding on invasive procedures (71.5%), computed tomography (CT) scanning (56.7%), and post-ED disposition (56.3%). Among the specific clinical scenarios, the use of thrombolytics for acute ischaemic stroke was felt to be most frequently appropriate for SDM (83.4%), followed by lumbar puncture to rule out subarachnoid haemorrhage (73.8%) and cranial CT for paediatric minor head injury (69.9%) (Probst et al., 2016). Surveyed ED patients reported involvement in SDM 49% of the time. The most common decisions were admission versus discharge (19%), medication options (17%), and follow-up care (15%) (Schoenfeld et al., 2019). Evidence suggests that the time SDM adds to decisions is minimal (Hess et al., 2016). SDM can sometimes save time if the patient prefers a less intensive option than the ED team might have otherwise pursued.

In 2016, the Society for Academic Emergency Medicine organized a consensus conference, 'Shared Decision Making: Development of a Policy-Relevant Patient-Centered Research Agenda'. During this 1-day conference, clinicians, researchers, policy-makers, patients, care partners, funding agency representatives, and content experts interacted to define high-priority areas for research in several domains: (1) diagnostic testing; (2) policy; (3) dissemination, implementation, and education; (4) development and testing of SDM approaches and tools in practice; (5) palliative care and geriatrics; and (6) vulnerable populations and limited health literacy. A series of articles were published describing the state of SDM in the ED context and provided research priorities for SDM to increase quality of care and patient-centred outcomes. Examples included discussing the need for more research on diagnostic testing in the ED and how SDM can be incorporated into diagnostic testing (Barrett et al., 2016); the need for funding to evaluate the implementation of SDM in the ED and its impact on patient outcomes (Dodd et al., 2016); and approaches that facilitate SDM involving older adults (Hogan et al., 2016), as well as dissemination and implementation of SDM in clinical practice (Kanzaria et al., 2016). The conference generated a consensus definition of SDM in EM, identified key domains and topics for SDM research in EM, developed a conceptual model and framework for SDM interventions, and proposed best practices and methods for SDM education and training in EM (Grudzen et al., 2016). This conference was the accelerator for further investigations of the role of SDM in EM, and several studies have been conducted in EM since the conference.

Special considerations

Special consideration is needed when studying vulnerable populations, those with limited health literacy, those at the end of life or with life-limiting chronic illness, and persons living with dementia.

Vulnerable populations

SDM may be particularly important for vulnerable populations, such as older adults, those with housing insecurity, persons with homelessness, immigrants, refugees, and people with substance use disorder or mental health conditions who often face health disparities and are exposed to higher rates of social determinants of health that affect health outcomes and care preferences. Vulnerable populations disproportionately suffer from increased chronic disease burden. EDs have a unique position within the healthcare system and serve as a safety net for patients, regardless of race, ethnicity, religion, country of origin, sexual orientation, socioeconomic status, or medical diagnosis (Castaneda-Guarderas et al., 2016).

Vulnerable populations are less likely to trust the healthcare system, leading to social and economic consequences. SDM interventions increased knowledge, informed choice, participation in decision making, decision self-efficacy, preference for collaborative decision making, and reduced decisional conflict. Furthermore, SDM interventions appeared more beneficial to disadvantaged groups than higher literacy/socioeconomic status patients (Durand et al., 2014). An example in the ED is the Head CT Choice decision aid which resulted in less decisional conflict in non-white parents and greater physician trust in socioeconomically disadvantaged parents (Skains et al., 2020) (**Table 41.1**).

Limited health literacy

The prevalence of limited health literacy and numeracy among patients who attend the ED is as high as 88% (McNaughton et al., 2011). SDM in the ED may be especially challenging for patients with limited health literacy who may have difficulty understanding medical information, communicating their needs and preferences, and participating in decision making. For example, a patient with low health literacy may not understand the risks and benefits of antibiotics for acute bronchitis or may defer to the clinician's recommendation without expressing their concerns or questions. The clinician can use plain language, teach-back methods, visual aids, and open-ended questions to enhance the patient's comprehension, involvement, and empowerment in the decision making process.

The Chest Pain Choice trial (Table 47.1) demonstrated that the decision aid benefited all sociodemographic groups similarly, with greater knowledge transfer in patients with higher numeracy and greater physician trust in patients with low health literacy (Rising et al., 2018).

Specific recommendations for printed material in the ED have been suggested, including focusing on one or two main messages; using analogies that are familiar and culturally appropriate; using short sentences and conversational style; limiting medical jargon; presenting numerical information in tables or pictographs; using natural frequencies rather than relative risks, and using words like 'half' and 'one-third' (Griffey et al., 2016).

Life-limiting illness and palliative medicine

SDM in the ED is crucial for patients with life-limiting illnesses, those with complex medical and psychosocial needs, and those enrolled in palliative care or hospice (George et al., 2016). For example, a patient with advanced cancer and dyspnoea may have a preference for symptom relief, comfort measures, or hospice care, or they may prefer aggressive treatment, intubation, or intensive care unit admission.

There is growing interest in SDM among patients living with dementia. Patients with cognitive impairment and dementia and their care partners want to be involved in decision making regarding their health in the ED (Carpenter et al., 2016, Seidenfeld et al., 2023).

Examples of SDM in the ED

Decisions that are commonly encountered in the ED include diagnosis, treatment, and disposition decisions (Table 47.1).

- *Diagnosis decisions*: involve determining the most likely cause of the patient's symptoms and deciding whether to perform further tests or interventions to confirm or rule out the diagnosis.
- *Treatment decisions*: SDM is used to discuss the benefits and harms of interventions like thrombolysis for ischaemic stroke or antibiotics for conditions such as acute otitis media, sinusitis, or bronchitis. For example, a patient may prefer to avoid antibiotics if they are concerned about side effects or resistance, or they may prefer antibiotics if they are worried about complications.
- *Disposition decisions*: disposition is a common situation in which SDM is practised in the ED setting. Hospitalization versus continuing care at home is a complex decision that needs to be tailored to individual patient needs.

Gaps in evidence

Despite being accepted and preferred by patients and clinicians, SDM is frequently not incorporated into the clinical encounter. A study evaluating SDM among patients with abdominal pain found high rates of provider and patient preference to use SDM for treatment plans. However, providers were rarely observed engaging patients in the decision to order a diagnostic test. Patients who were engaged in analgesic selection had higher satisfaction with pain medication (Ijaz et al., 2018).

SDM has not been widely implemented in EM, and there are several barriers and challenges to its adoption and integration in this setting. Moreover, additional studies are needed to demonstrate its effectiveness and impact in EM, especially on patient outcomes and healthcare utilization. Most of the existing studies on SDM in EM have focused on specific clinical scenarios, such as chest pain, head injury, or anticoagulation, and have used different methods and measures to evaluate SDM. Therefore, there is a need for more systematic and comprehensive research on SDM in EM, using standardized and validated tools and outcome measures and involving diverse and representative populations and settings.

How to most effectively normalize a complex intervention such as a decision aid to facilitate SDM in ED practice is a challenging question that warrants further investigation. SDM, in its essence, requires a clinician to involve a patient in a decision regarding their emergency care and the patient needs to authentically engage in the decision with the degree of support needed to meaningfully participate in the decision. Given the inherent power differential between the clinician and the patient in the emergency care setting, it is our hypothesis that interventions that involve clinicians initiating the SDM discussion are most likely to be effective. If this is the case, then training clinicians to communicate with their patients in ways that they understand, using straightforward language stripped of medical jargon, appropriate for each patient's level of education, numeracy, and cultural background, and equipping clinicians with readily available evidence relevant to the decision at hand are some key elements needed to make SDM a reality in emergency care.

Table 47.1 Examples of SDM in the ED

Topic	Method	Main conclusion
SDM for diagnostic decisions		
Chest pain (Hess et al., 2016)		
Chest pain is a common presenting complaint in the ED. After an initial evaluation, patients at low to moderate risk of acute coronary syndrome have different diagnostic and disposition options	Chest pain choice: multicentre, pragmatic, parallel randomized, controlled trial in 6 EDs comparing SDM to usual care in the choice of admission and further cardiac testing or referral for outpatient evaluation in low-risk chest pain patients	Use of a decision aid increased patient knowledge, engagement, and safely decreased the rate of admission without increasing major adverse cardiac events at 30 days
Head trauma (Hess et al., 2018)		
Children with minor head trauma have a low risk of clinically important traumatic brain injury and might undergo a CT scan of the head or be observed at home	Head CT Choice: cluster randomized trial in 7 EDs comparing a decision aid to usual care in parents of children with minor head trauma. SDM can help communicate the risk of intracranial injury, radiation exposure, costs, benefits, and harms of cranial CT versus observation and elicit parents' preferences and values regarding the management options	The decision aid increased parent knowledge, decreased decisional conflict, and increased involvement in decision making but did not significantly reduce the ED CT rate. It safely decreased healthcare utilization at 7 days without increasing missed intracranial injuries
Thunderclap headache (Marcolini and Hine, 2019)		
Patients with sudden, severe headaches are at risk of subarachnoid haemorrhage (SAH). SAH has a very low prevalence; however, missing the diagnosis has mortality and morbidity implications	Patients and clinicians face the decision of whether to undergo lumbar puncture after a negative CT scan of the head or to be discharged with reassurance	Despite the existence of clinical decision rules, there are no studies testing SDM in practice. It is reported clinicians commonly engage patients in SDM for SAH rule-out
Renal colic (Schoenfeld et al., 2020)		
Patients with flank pain may have a renal colic secondary to kidney stones and can decide to undergo CT scanning or be treated empirically	A decision aid was developed for patients with renal colic. A randomized trial plans to compare SDM with usual care	The decision aid aims to improve patient knowledge, reduce radiation exposure, and enhance patient engagement. The results of the trial have not been published yet
SDM for treatment decisions in the ED		
Otitis media (Anderson et al., 2021)		
Otitis media is a common condition among children treated in the ED and primary care settings	A decision aid was created and refined. A pilot trial was completed using a decision aid to facilitate SDM with parents of children with otitis media	The decision aid helped parents understand the risks and benefits of different treatment options, leading to more informed decision making (**Figure 47.1**)
Musculoskeletal pain (Holland et al., 2016)		
Musculoskeletal pain is one of the most common reasons for ED visits	A study including older adults with acute musculoskeletal pain demonstrated that patients desire to contribute to decisions regarding analgesic selection (16% made the decision by themselves, 37% collaboratively, and 47% let the doctor make the decision)	Patients preferring a more active role were more likely to be college-educated, receive care from a nurse practitioner (as opposed to a physician), and receive care from a female (vs male) provider SDM was not associated with pain reduction or type of pain medication received but was associated with greater patient satisfaction
Goals of care discussions (Walker et al., 2021)		
	A decision aid to facilitate conversations between ED patients, families, and clinicians regarding goals of care in patients with life-limiting illness was developed and refined	This decision aid requires further validation and testing
Intubation/prognosis (Ouchi et al., 2018)		
Unplanned intubation is a common procedure performed in the ED in life-threatening situations	A study of adults 65 years of age and older informed bout prognosis after emergency intubation. One in three older adults dies in the hospital, and only 24% of survivors are discharged home, with most patients going to nursing homes with limited life expectancy	This decision aid requires further validation and testing
SDM for disposition decisions in the ED		
Syncope (Probst et al., 2016)		
Syncope is a transient loss of consciousness, and even after thorough evaluation, syncope may remain unexplained	A decision aid incorporating risk stratification and SDM into syncope care was developed	Clinicians can more confidently engage patients in disposition decisions, including outpatient follow-up, observation, or hospitalization
Dementia (Seidenfeld et al., 2023)		
Persons living with dementia and their care partners want to be involved in care decisions	SDM balances the risks of hospital admission, such as delirium and functional decline, against the risks of discharge, which include return ED visits, falls, worsening morbidity, and mortality	This decision aid is undergoing refinement and validation

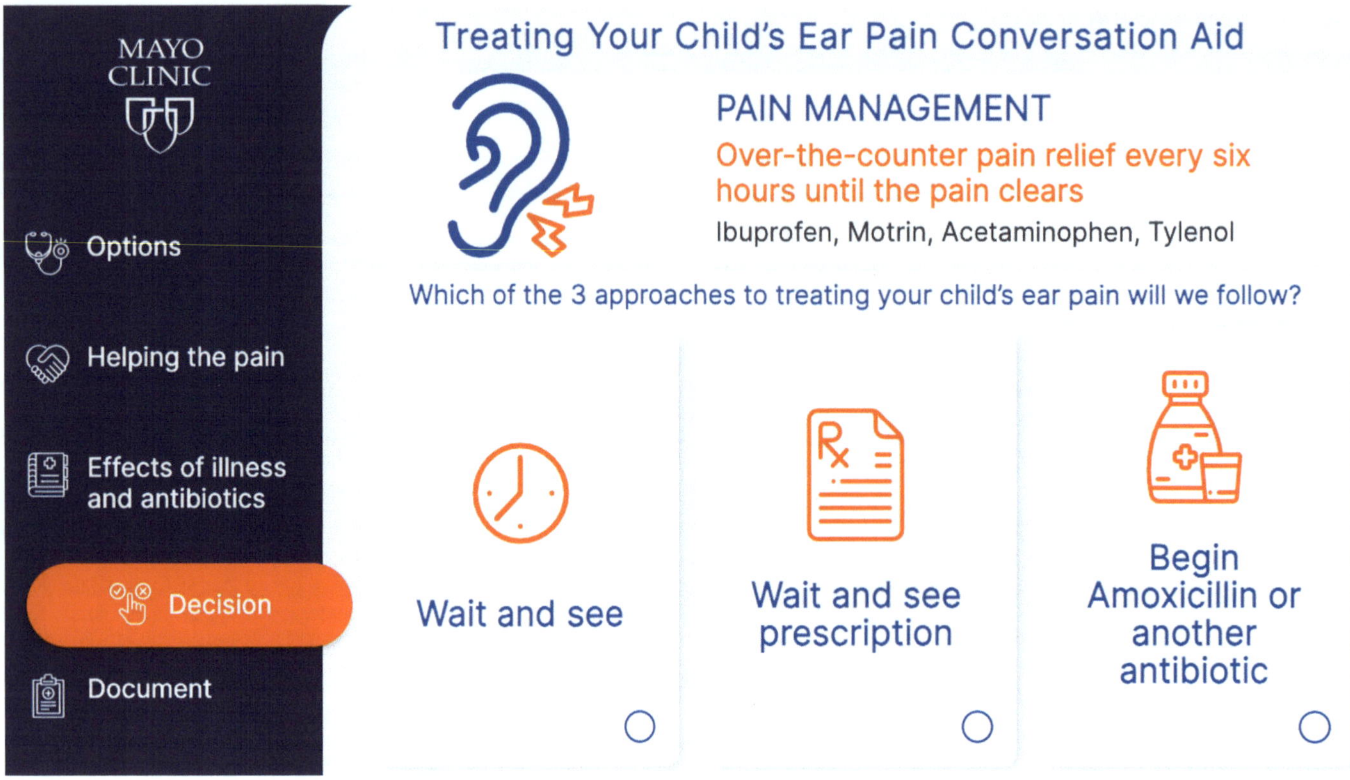

Figure 47.1 Screenshot of the online otitis media decision aid.

Furthermore, the described characteristics presume the one-to-one clinician–patient perspective, not a system perspective. For SDM to become normalized in practice, it will require support at the health system level, with buy-in from hospital and health system leaders, payers to thoughtfully reimburse clinician effort spent engaging patients in SDM, and medicolegal protection for engaging patients in SDM. See Box 47.1 for a patient's perspective.

Unanswered questions remain, including how to assess the impact of SDM on patient outcomes such as satisfaction, trust, adherence, decision regret, quality of life, and health status; how to evaluate the effect of SDM on healthcare utilization, such as rates of diagnostic testing, procedures, admissions, referrals, and costs; how to compare the effectiveness and cost-effectiveness of different SDM interventions and tools, such as decision aids, communication skills training, or decision coaching; and how to identify and address barriers and facilitators to SDM implementation and integration in EM, such as clinician and patient attitudes, knowledge, and skills, organizational and system factors, and ethical and legal issues.

Box 47.1 Patient perspective

Patients and their families typically arrive at the ED at moments of severe and time-sensitive distress and uncertainty, which is often different from the context in the outpatient setting. In contrast to outpatient visits, in the ED, patients do not make appointments or have time to consider and process information regarding diagnoses and treatment before their visits. As a result, fear is high for patients and their families, while the available information to them is low. As such, the ED presents a very different setting for which patients and families try to engage in SDM.

Patients and families most often appreciate being involved in decision making processes in the ED, as it results in improved trust and satisfaction with their care. However, the desire for involvement varies greatly depending on the individual, the decision at hand, and the context. For example, a patient may present at the ED with an injury to the ankle following a sporting event and, in this situation, prefer to be actively engaged in their treatment, planning to return to sport sooner. In another instance, the same patient arrives in the ED in acute anaphylaxis and has no interest in participating in care planning beyond the resolution of the reaction. For some patients, they will prefer to default to the healthcare teams' decisions in all circumstances, whereas others will almost always desire an active role in the decision making. Understanding these preferences is key to implementing SDM effectively.

From the patient and family perspective, several questions need to be explored:

- How do patients perceive and value SDM in EM?
- What are patient preferences and expectations regarding the role of the clinician and their own involvement in the decision making process? Are these unique to specific situations?
- How do patients and families cope with the uncertainty and risk they are faced with while participating in SDM in the ED?
- How do patients and families balance the benefits and harms of different options?
- How do patients and families communicate and collaborate with their healthcare team during ED visits?
- What aspects of communication do they find helpful versus unhelpful or even harmful?

REFERENCES

Anderson, J. L., Oliveira J E Silva, L., Brito, J. P., Hargraves, I. G., Hess, E. P. 2021. Development of an electronic conversation aid to support shared decision making for children with acute otitis media. *JAMIA Open*, **4**, ooab024.

Barrett, T. W., Rising, K. L., Bellolio, M. F., et al. 2016. The 2016 Academic Emergency Medicine Consensus Conference, 'Shared Decision Making in the Emergency Department: Development of a Policy-Relevant Patient-Centered Research Agenda'. Diagnostic testing breakout session report. *Acad Emerg Med*, **23**, 1354–1361.

Carpenter, C. R., Leggett, J., Bellolio, F., et al. 2022. Emergency department communication in persons living with dementia and care partners: a scoping review. *J Am Med Dir Assoc*, **23**, 1313.e15–1313.e46.

Castaneda-Guarderas, A., Glassberg, J., Grudzen, C. R., et al. 2016. Shared decision-making with vulnerable populations in the emergency department. *Acad Emerg Med*, **23**, 1410–1416.

Dodd, K. W., Berman, A., Brown, J., et al. 2016. Funding research in emergency department shared decision making: a summary of the 2016 AEM Consensus Conference panel discussion. *Acad Emerg Med*, **23**, 1340–1345.

Durand, M.-A., Carpenter, L., Dolan, H., et al. 2014. Do interventions designed to support shared decision-making reduce health inequalities? A systematic review and meta-analysis. *PLoS One*, **9**, e94670.

George, N. R., Kryworuchko, J., Hunold, K. M., et al. 2016. Shared decision making to support the provision of palliative and end-of-life care in the emergency department: a consensus statement and research agenda. *Acad Emerg Med*, **23**, 1394–1402.

Griffey, R. T., McNaughton, C. D., McCarthy, D. M., et al. 2016. Shared decision making in the ED among patients with limited health literacy: beyond slower and louder. *Acad Emerg Med*, **23**, 1403–1409.

Grudzen, C. R., Anderson, J. R., Carpenter, C. R., Hess, E. P. 2016. The 2016 AEM Consensus Conference, Shared Decision Making in the Emergency Department: Development of a Policy-Relevant Patient-Centered Research Agenda May 10, 2016, New Orleans, LA. *Acad Emerg Med*, **23**, 1313–1319.

Hess, E. P., Grudzen, C. R., Thomson, R., Raja, A. S., Carpenter, C. R. 2015. Shared decision making in the emergency department: respecting patient autonomy when seconds count. *Acad Emerg Med*, **22**, 856–864.

Hess, E. P., Hollander, J. E., Schaffer, J. T., et al. 2016. Shared decision making in patients with low risk chest pain: prospective randomized pragmatic trial. *BMJ*, **355**, i6165.

Hess, E. P., Homme, J. L., Kharbanda, A. B., et al. 2018. Effect of the Head Computed Tomography Choice decision aid in parents of children with minor head trauma: a cluster randomized trial. *JAMA Netw Open*, **1**, e182430.

Hogan, T. M., Richmond, N. L., Carpenter, C. R., et al. 2016. Shared decision making to improve the emergency care of older adults: a research agenda. *Acad Emerg Med*, **23**, 1386–1393.

Holland, W. C., Hunold, K. M., Mangipudi, S. A., Rittenberg, A. M., Yosipovitch, N., Platts-Mills, T. F. 2016. A prospective evaluation of shared decision making regarding analgesics selection for older emergency department patients with acute musculoskeletal pain. *Acad Emerg Med*, **23**, 306–314.

Ijaz, H., Wong, C., Weaver, J., et al. 2018. Exploring the attitudes & practices of shared decision making for CT scan use in emergency department patients with abdominal pain. *Am J Emerg Med*, **36**, 2263–2267.

Kanzaria, H. K., Booker-Vaughns, J., Itakura, K., et al. 2016. Dissemination and implementation of shared decision making into clinical practice: a research agenda. *Acad Emerg Med*, **23**, 1368–1379.

Marcolini, E., Hine, J. 2019. Approach to the diagnosis and management of subarachnoid hemorrhage. *West J Emerg Med*, **20**, 203–211.

McNaughton, C., Wallston, K. A., Rothman, R. L., Marcovitz, D. E., Storrow, A. 2011. Short, subjective measures of numeracy and general health literacy in an adult emergency department. *Acad Emerg Med*, **18**, 1148–1155.

Ouchi, K., Jambaulikar, G. D., Hohmann, S., et al. 2018. Prognosis after emergency department intubation to inform shared decision making. *J Am Geriatr Soc*, **66**, 1377–1381.

Probst, M. A., Kanzaria, H. K., Frosch, D. L., et al. 2016. Perceived appropriateness of shared decision making in the emergency department: a survey study. *Acad Emerg Med*, **23**, 375–381.

Rising, K. L., Hollander, J. E., Schaffer, J. T., et al. 2018. Effectiveness of a decision aid in potentially vulnerable patients: a secondary analysis of the Chest Pain Choice multicenter randomized trial. *Med Decis Making*, **38**, 69–78.

Schoenfeld, E. M., Houghton, C., Patel, P. M., et al. 2020. Shared decision making in patients with suspected uncomplicated ureterolithiasis: a decision aid development study. *Acad Emerg Med*, **27**, 554–565.

Schoenfeld, E. M., Probst, M. A., Quigley, D. D., et al. 2019. Does shared decision making actually occur in the ED? Looking at it from the patients' perspective. *Acad Emerg Med*, **26**, 1369–1378.

Seidenfeld, J., Bellolio, F., Vashi, A., Van Houtven, C., Hastings, S. 2023. Shared disposition decision-making in the emergency department for persons living with dementia. *J Geriatr Emerg Med*, **4**, 10.17294/2694-4715.1057.

Skains, R. M., Kuppermann, N., Homme, J. L., et al. 2020. What is the effect of a decision aid in potentially vulnerable parents? Insights from the Head CT Choice randomized trial. *Health Expect*, **23**, 63–74.

Walker, L. E., Bellolio, M. F., Dobler, C. C., et al. 2021. Paths of emergency department care: development of a decision aid to facilitate shared decision making in goals of care discussions in the acute setting. *MDM Policy Pract*, **6**, 23814683211058082.

48

Shared decision making interventions for kidney failure treatment and management

Hilary L. Bekker, Jeanette Finderup, Andrew Mooney, Henning Søndergaard, and Anna E. Winterbottom

Introduction

Kidney medicine requires health professionals to manage complex clinical problems and provide personalized care for a chronic disease that worsens over time as people's kidneys fail. As patient populations have got older, people with kidney failure (PwKF) are more likely to have associated comorbidity and frailty issues impacting their clinical, health, and social needs (Bekker et al., 2023). Clinical guidelines recognize the importance of services offering a conservative management pathway alongside established kidney replacement therapies (dialysis and transplant), and signposting to end-of-life care options and plans (National Institute for Health and Care Excellence, 2018). Enabling PwKF to share decision making and plan care with their kidney teams through the use of education, counselling, and patient decision aids (PtDAs) is central to these guidelines (National Institute for Health and Care Excellence, 2018).

PwKF integrate treatments, therapies, dietary changes, and medication regimens into their lives to maintain their kidney function and manage symptoms. They value their kidney teams and care provided, but want more support in making decisions between treatment options and to be informed earlier of the impact of their worsening kidney disease (UK Kidney Association and Kidney Care UK, 2021). Reviews of education programmes, routinely provided leaflets, and PwKF's experiences illustrate variation between services in providing resources enabling PwKF to make informed decisions proactively between options that meet their clinical, health, and social needs (Bekker et al., 2023).

To enhance shared decision making (SDM) processes between PwKF and kidney professionals requires an understanding of the (1) everyday practices biasing, and boosting, their individual reasoning about treatments; (2) interventions known to increase the knowledge and skills of individuals to make reasoned decisions between options, and (3) adaptations to the delivery of kidney care to enhance shared problem-solving about current, and future, kidney failure management. We refer to Bekker's 'Making Informed Decisions Individually and Together' (MIND-IT) framework (Figure 48.1) to represent explicitly the roles of multiple stakeholders making reasoned decisions about treatment and management plans for PwKF, within their healthcare and life contexts (Toft et al., 2022). MIND-IT provides a theoretical structure for those innovating practice to think through the different components needed to impact multiple decision makers at individual (micro), team (meso), and organizational (macro) levels.

There is significant research and improvement literature exploring ways to enhance SDM processes within consultations between PwKF, family, and kidney professionals when planning kidney care (Bekker et al., 2023). This literature reflects the complexity of managing kidney failure as people's health status and daily life needs change, the number of treatment options and health professionals, and the range of interventions supporting staff to involve PwKF in their kidney care. This chapter uses the co-authors' testimonies to identify challenges, and solutions, to enhance SDM process within consultations between stakeholders, drawing on examples from the most investigated decision problems: dialysis modalities (haemodialysis/peritoneal dialysis); conservative management or dialysis; transplant type and dialysis.

See Box 48.1 for our patient perspective.

Specialist kidney nurse (Jeanette Finderup)

For kidney nurses, each decision making encounter with the patient, and their relatives, is unique. Patients are at different stages of their kidney failure, have other health needs and changes in their life that may impact management of their kidney failure at home and in clinic. A patient, their partner, and other relatives all have different decisional needs, knowledge about options, preferences, and support (Finderup et al., 2019). Although health professionals have guidance on kidney failure management and treatment, there is no objective way to judge what the 'best' option is for an individual patient. There is seldom a 'pro' or 'con' for kidney failure options, as what is seen as an advantage for one patient is seen as a disadvantage by another; kidney professionals will have different views about treatment options, and their views may

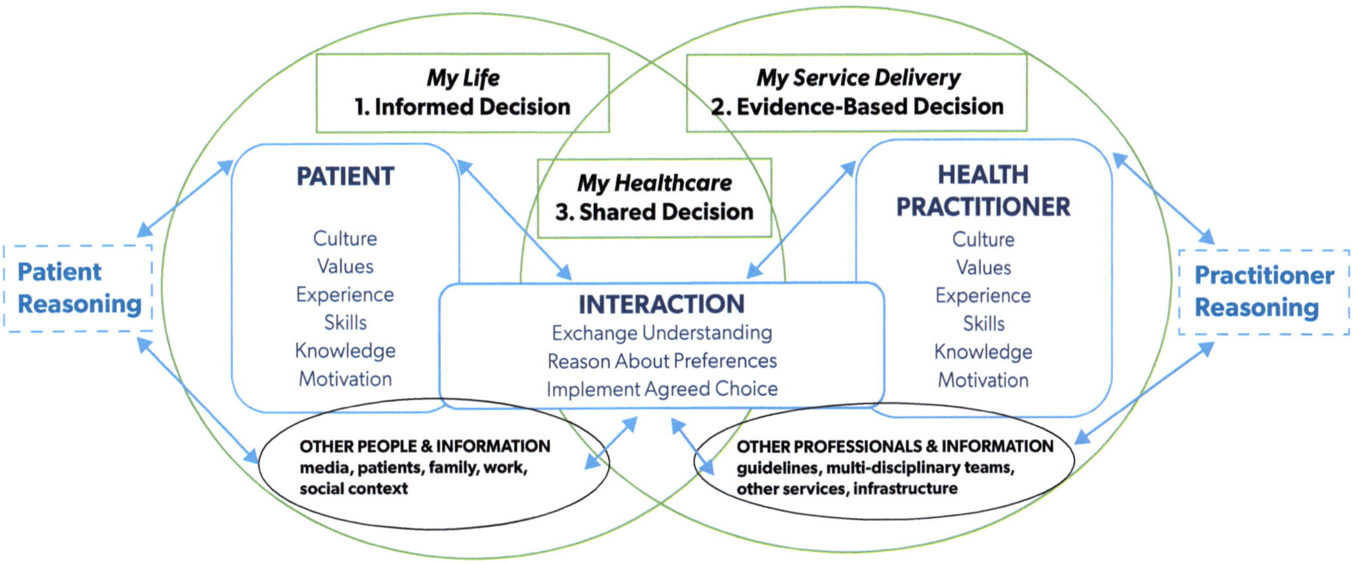

Figure 48.1 Making Informed Decisions Individually and Together (MIND-IT) in healthcare: multiple decision makers intervention development framework.

© Bekker 2021. First published in Breckenridge, K., Bekker, H. L., Gibbons, E., et al. 2015. How to routinely collect data on patient-reported outcome and experience measures in renal registries in Europe: an expert consensus meeting. *Nephrol Dial Transplant*, 30, 1605–1614.

Box 48.1 Patient perspective

Person with kidney failure (Henning Søndergaard)

Having been born with a disability that progressed to me having kidney failure 13 years ago, I learnt two things when managing my health. First, to develop a good working relationship with my kidney team so we can strive together to find the best way possible to benefit my life. Having a good working relationship meant I needed to gain knowledge about my situation, and what is important to me. At times I was like a sponge, gleaning information from other patients, and other health professionals in the country, or world for that matter, and reading books (and now online resources). Second, to be part of relevant patient organizations with patients having similar experiences and to share ideas. I found the best peer support came from these organizations, but I still needed to know what was important for me, what I could use, and also what was not relevant to me, and I could ignore.

I became an active member of the Danish Kidney Association. I identified the need for a PtDA and developed a dialysis decision aid with Jeanette Finderup (Finderup et al., 2020). I wanted to create a PtDA for other patients because I had found one and knew how much it helped my own decision process and preparation to go to my team and ask the right questions before deciding on my treatment choice. I found other patients' experiences differed, and often they had only their kidney team to lean on for advice, and they couldn't know all the aspects of people's lives that might influence their choice.

With the Danish Kidney Association, I continued to work on ideas raised by people going to local kidney clinics around the country (Søndergaard et al., 2023). Most hospitals in Denmark have kidney schools, but we know many patients use them at a time when they are often least able to absorb new knowledge, or 'crash' into kidney failure before they ever get the opportunity to attend their local kidney school. We identified that a set of online modules would support patients to engage with their individual kidney school's education programme (https://www.nyreskole.dk/links-og-oevrigt-materiale/). We worked with kidney teams to find the best way to supplement the clinic-specific curricula with independent and fulfilling learning resources. Our online kidney school resources take the best from peer learning and professional knowledge. It provides a comprehensive teaching resource that is updated regularly when new knowledge becomes available. Both patients and kidney professionals like these resources online so people can go back to, and repeat, learning modules at their own pace.

be different from other team members and PwKF. I have worked on introducing SDM and PtDA guidance to policy (macro level), developed SDM training for health professionals in Denmark (meso level), and provided decision coaching skills training for the integration of our PtDAs across Danish kidney services (micro level).

All kidney professionals are trained to recognize from a range of indicators when an individual patient needs to consider a change to their kidney failure management. Patients, however, are not aware of our clinical reasoning processes and the short- and long-term plans for transitions in kidney care. Many patients, and their relatives, are largely unaware that different options exist along the kidney failure pathway, even if they have had been managing their chronic kidney disease for several years. Many patients do not recognize their symptoms as an indication of their kidney failure getting worse, or that their current treatment is failing to manage their kidney disease.

It is often a shock for patients and their relatives to realize they need to go onto dialysis (Finderup et al., 2019). Even when patients, and relatives, have a lot of information about kidney failure treatment options, have participated in kidney schools, or read about treatment options from other sources, they still need to assimilate this knowledge for use in *their* situation, to navigate *their* daily life, and work with *their* kidney and health professional teams. It is important that partners, carers, and relatives are involved in the decision making processes about treatment so they understand changes in their family member's health and treatment needs, and each other's reasoning. These choices impact the patient's home and their family's lives as management often needs support from relatives at home, or at the hospital.

Kidney service problem-solving (Andrew Mooney and Hilary L. Bekker)

We started collaborating to explore kidney service delivery issues using a medical decision making lens to develop solutions in collaboration with PwKF, kidney professionals, charities, medical companies, and policymakers (Bekker et al., 2023). By drawing on expertise gained from kidney service improvement initiatives, and decision aid interventions, we were able to critique current kidney practice; identify components that boost or hinder people's ability to make reasoned decisions about kidney care; identify solutions known to support people to make informed, value-based decisions between kidney failure management options; and adapt interventions to meet the varied needs of multiple stakeholders across different kidney service pathways. The types of problems explored include:

- Why is there variation by kidney centre between dialysis options, and dialysis and conservative management, home and hospital dialysis, self-managed and supported dialysis, advance care planning, and palliative options?
- How do we enable staff to support PwKF to make informed decisions between treatment options and transitions of care, and peer educators to support PwKF and their families in making dialysis decisions within kidney service pathways?
- How do we support teams to recognize service delivery practices that impair SDM processes, and the means to innovate care within different service infrastructure?

Senior health services researcher in kidney failure (Anna E. Winterbottom)

Our research employs experimental, review and survey methods to investigate patient and health professional experiences of making treatment decisions about kidney failure, and interventions impacting SDM practices (Bekker et al., 2023). Key reflections include:

- Staff want to provide a personalized SDM approach to managing kidney failure but lack skills in what it means to innovate and deliver more SDM practices within their consultations. The advanced kidney care (or low clearance) clinic is where most PwKF receive information about future treatment options, and kidney professionals prepare PwKF to manage their kidney failure. However, there is a lack of consistency in the terms used to describe the clinic, staff roles and titles, pathway options, and how services integrate their education and information resources alongside care planning. Conversations to facilitate informed decision making are difficult to fit into established clinic patterns alongside kidney failure monitoring and care planning as staff have specialist knowledge (e.g. haemodialysis/peritoneal dialysis, home/hospital, geriatric, palliative, etc.) and clinics are organized by specialism. Decisions about changes to care plans are revisited outside standard monitoring systems, but staff lack confidence in talking about options outside their clinical expertise. From our findings, we developed resources supporting kidney professionals' skills when having these difficult conversations with PwKF and their family members (Winterbottom et al., 2022).
- PwKF are less concerned with the technical aspects and medical terminology around treatment than professionals, and more interested in understanding how their kidney failure and experience of symptoms is changing, the impact of treatment on their management regimens, and the consequences for navigating treatment and their daily life. Most information provided by kidney services is used to support professionals' communication about a single option, and local clinic details; most resources are written with little awareness of the negative influence incomplete information, clinical judgements, complex numeric details, pictures, and testimonials have on people's ability to make informed, value-based decisions (Bekker et al., 2023). From our findings, we developed PtDAs to improve people's understanding of kidney failure and treatment over time, and their ability to make reasoned decisions with their kidney teams and family members (Bekker et al., 2020; Winterbottom et al., 2020). Our recent patient and public involvement work on SDM showed PwKF do not feel that decision making is 'shared' but is still based on kidney professionals' judgements of what they consider to be 'best care'. Improving SDM interactions means ensuring a more consistent way for kidney services to support PwKF's engagement with kidney failure options.

Interventions enhancing SDM practices

SDM is seen broadly as the communication process within a consultation between a patient and health professional when making decisions about healthcare; it is often characterized as a two-way exchange of information, values, and preferences, with both parties taking steps to reach an agreement on the choice made, and subsequent management plan (see Chapter 1). A common approach to SDM facilitation within healthcare is training professionals in SDM skills and use of in-consultation prompts summarizing details of options or eliciting preferences (Bekker et al., 2023) (see Chapters 13–15). Although these generic approaches are useful for raising awareness of SDM, they are not sufficient to enable kidney professionals to innovate their practice within the complexities of managing kidney failure (Joseph-Williams et al., 2019). Bekker's MIND-IT framework (Figure 48.1) helps services consider the range of factors impacting PwKF and kidney professionals' reasoning about these decisions, and ways to support SDM processes across healthcare and life contexts. There are many intervention types enabling stakeholders, and organizations, to support effective SDM processes (Bekker et al., 2023).

A focal point of activity for supporting SDM within consultations for kidney failure has been to (1) develop PtDAs supporting PwKF to make informed decisions between healthcare options and prepare them to talk with family and professionals about their reasoning (micro level), (2) enable kidney professionals to integrate PtDAs within existing service pathways (micro level), (3) enhance the communication skills of health professionals to integrate SDM practices with their kidney care (meso level), and (4) innovate policy and service delivery to encourage adoption of SDM practices (macro level). Below, we draw on examples from the authors' experience to illustrate ways to facilitate multiple stakeholders' SDM practices.

PtDAs are evidence-based resources designed to support people to make informed, value-based decisions between healthcare options (see Chapters 17 and 19). Our approach in both UK and Danish settings has been to develop PtDAs from research, and co-designed with stakeholders. Our findings show our PtDAs enhance the health literacy of PwKF by providing the knowledge and skills to (1) think about what matters to them about their kidney disease

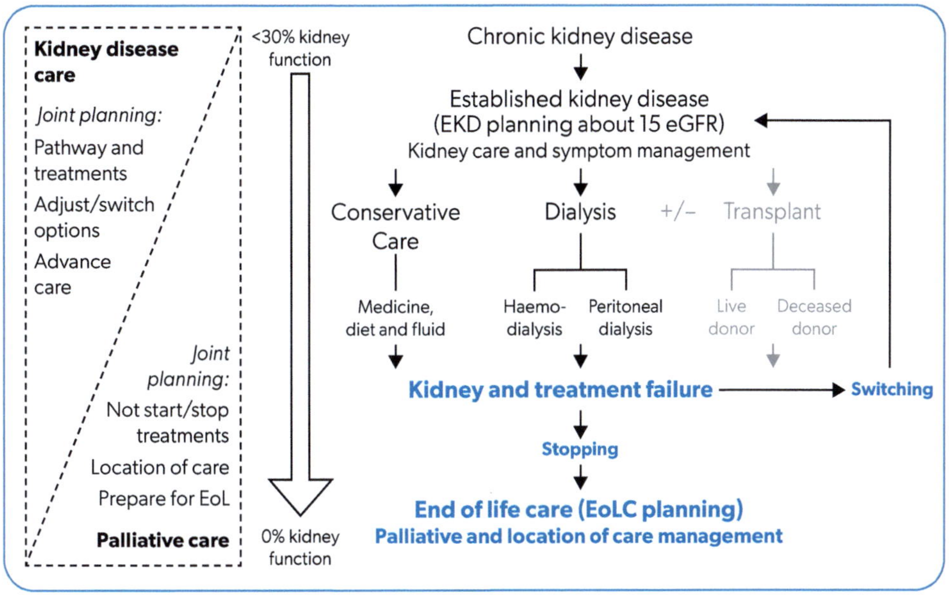

Figure 48.2 Decision map representing options and nested decisions along the kidney failure management pathway.

Reproduced with permission from the University of Leeds, 2020. First published in Winterbottom, A. E., Mooney, A., Russon, L., et al. 2020. Critical review of leaflets about conservative management used in UK renal services. *J Renal Care,* 46, 250–257.

and its management, and (2) engage with kidney teams and plan care that best meets their clinical and daily life needs. They provide accessible, accurate, and balanced information helping PwKF to understand kidney professionals' clinical reasoning when planning care, and guidance to consider what is important to them now, and as their kidney failure and daily life needs may change. These PtDAs are designed to be provided by kidney services and patient-led organizations, and delivered as part of their education packages, or within consultations. Below are components enabling a shared understanding between PwKF and kidney professionals about these decision along the kidney care pathway:

- Decision maps (Figure 48.2): represent the treatment options in the context of managing worsening kidney failure. These maps provide a visual summary of the types of decisions and connections with other choices. The maps prompt PwKF and kidney professionals to share their understanding about other options or pathways and consider their consequences.
- Kidney failure symptoms and management details (Figure 48.3): informed by explanations of how people make sense of illness, helping PwKF recognize the symptoms associated with their kidney failure worsening or management regimens not working. These prompts help PwKF and kidney professionals share an awareness of transition points in care and signpost the need for SDM about sticking, switching, starting, or stopping treatment.
- Framing of options and decision guidance (Figure 48.4): statements explaining kidney professionals' clinical reasoning and prompts encouraging consideration of options about what is important in the daily life of PwKF; these provide a structure to reason about options.
- Interaction prompts (Figure 48.5): support discussions about different aspects of making decisions about kidney failure management and enable an exchange in understanding, reasoning, and values from the different perspectives of those involved in making the decision. These discussions provide a way for kidney professionals to talk explicitly about their tacit knowledge of tailoring care plans for individual needs, and PwKF to talk explicitly about their tacit knowledge of managing kidney failure within their lives.

Decision coaching training provides staff with the non-directive skills needed to guide proactively the decision making process of those making difficult decisions between healthcare options. Within kidney medicine, a decision coach can be any member of the team with responsibility for providing education to PwKF and their families such as kidney and other health professionals, peer educators, service improvement officer, patient organizations, and so on. Training is usually structured with reference to an endorsed PtDA, illustrating the active ingredients boosting people's reasoning, and countering practices impairing people's reasoned decision making. This training provides the decision coach with skills to focus on enabling PwKF to work through a PtDA, evaluate options in accordance with their own beliefs, make trade-offs based on what is important to their lives, and prepare people to engage with kidney professionals. This focus is an important skill to help distance the decision coach from their own judgements informed by their own experiences, goals, and roles within healthcare and life contexts.

Kidney team and service management infrastructure such as multidisciplinary team and service review meetings, organizational improvement initiatives, and staff appraisals are important mechanisms to initiate change in service delivery and innovate practice. These mechanisms allow teams to consider different interventions to address factors that impair or support SDM processes, and address between-service variations in practice. Discussing interventions with defined components (e.g. PtDA, decision coaching, and training manuals), and their integration within clinics, allows services to take ownership of how to innovate their delivery of care to address the needs of their local context.

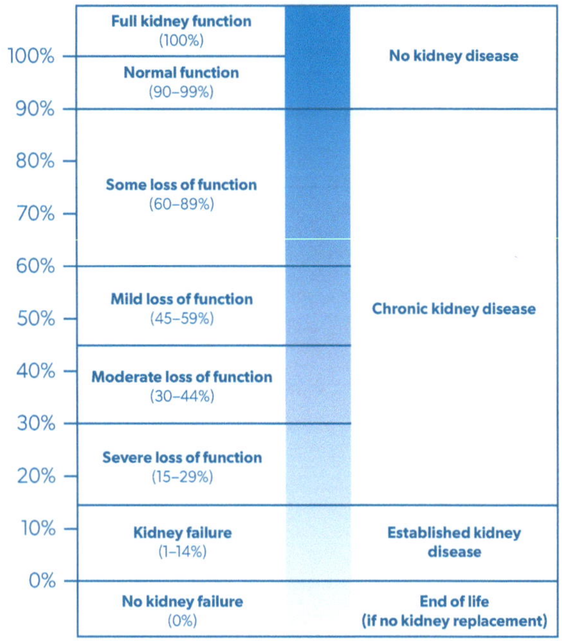

Symptoms	Treatments and therapies
Tiredness, low energy, fatigue, feeling cold	Tablets, injections for iron balance
Itching	Tablets, creams, psychological support
Nausea, vomiting, loss of weight or appetite	Tablets, support with managing protein and nutrients in diet
Swollen legs	Tablets, control of fluid, diet and salt
Memory or concentration loss, sleep problems	Tablets, monitoring, psychological support
Muscle and joint pain	Tablets, psychological support
Leg cramps, restless legs	Tablets, support with diet, psychological support
Back pain	Monitoring, support with fitness, psychological support
Dizziness, visual problems, headaches	Tablets, monitoring, psychological support, expert support for eyes
Shortness of breath	Tablets
Loss of muscle strength	Monitoring, support with fitness
Muscle spasms, stiffness	Tablets, support with fitness and diet
Loss of sex drive	Monitoring, psychological support
Need to urinate more often	Tablets, support with diet and fluid

Figure 48.3 Summaries supporting the link between loss of function, kidney disease stage, symptoms, and management options.

Reproduced with permission from the University of Leeds, 2020. First published in Winterbottom, A. E., Mooney, A., Russon, L., et al. 2020. A dialysis and conservative care decision aid: living with kidney disease. https://www.kidneyresearchyorkshire.org.uk/yorkshire-dialysis-and-conservative-care-decision-aid/

Final reflections from kidney consultant (Andrew Mooney)

These interventions support the SDM process, but there is still a need for clinicians to embrace this way of working. As a consultant facing these decisions daily in kidney clinics for almost 25 years, my frustration is the tendency of doctors to base their interactions with patients on the technicalities of kidney replacement therapies and delivery; this is an approach emphasized throughout our medical training and continuing professional development. I find repeatedly that when I am covering the wards and meeting an inpatient for the first time, I look at clinic letters to determine a patient's circumstance and find it tells me only about blood pressure, haemoglobin levels, and biochemical parameters, which I can look up on their electronic records. Rarely are there details about whether the person can, for example, walk to the shops or needs help getting dressed, let alone their hopes, or beliefs about their treatment. The exchange of information about a patient's circumstances, and their reasoning about kidney failure management, is much more difficult to deliver in any other way than through direct, face-to-face (clinical) encounters. I would prefer doctors are taught skills to make these interactions as productive and mutually rewarding as possible.

The opportunity to meet and talk to patients is a resource-intensive process, and to spend that time talking about anaemia and its treatment, or biochemical derangements and their management, is a waste of that resource. Many aspects of management can, and will, be undertaken by protocol, algorithms, or assisted artificial intelligence applications. There are increasing data telling us it doesn't matter to longevity outcomes whether you have haemodialysis or peritoneal dialysis, or whether your peritoneal dialysis is delivered with a standard or highly permeable membrane, or the haemodialysis machine is dialled to deliver haemodialysis or haemodiafiltration; what does matter is how frail or debilitated you are before you start these treatments. A first step is for clinicians to make assessments about the relationship between frailty, comorbidity, and functional status with likely patient outcomes, and use their clinical expertise when planning care with PwKF in consultations. It is at least, if not more,

My Trade-offs Between Conservative Care and Dialysis Pathways

Managing EKD and its symptoms means people fit daily treatments, visits to kidney units, and changes to diet and fluid routines into their lives. People decide on a pathway by balancing judgements about their kidney function and well-being with their feelings about what is most important in their lives now and for the future. An example of a trade-off might be thinking about what is more important to you in your daily life now, as your kidney disease gets worse:

- The conservative care pathway means a chance to do daily activities (e.g. hobbies, family and pets, leisure and holidays) with fewer regular medical routines, until there is no kidney function left
- The dialysis pathway means fitting an extra set of medical procedures and routines around daily activities (e.g. hobbies, families and pets, leisure and holidays), with a chance of lengthening life when there is no kidney function left.

Given what you know about your EKD, and your reasons for and against each pathway, circle the answer for each option that best matches how you want to manage your EKD:

Table: Thinking about which pathway will suit me best

Conservative care pathway	Yes	No	Unsure
Dialysis pathway	Yes	No	Unsure

Figure 48.4 Statements providing guidance to making trade-offs between options based on individual values.

Reproduced with permission from the University of Leeds, 2020. First published in Winterbottom, A. E., Mooney, A., Russon, L., et al. 2020. A dialysis and conservative care decision aid: living with kidney disease. https://www.kidneyresearchyorkshire.org.uk/yorkshire-dialysis-and-conservative-care-decision-aid/

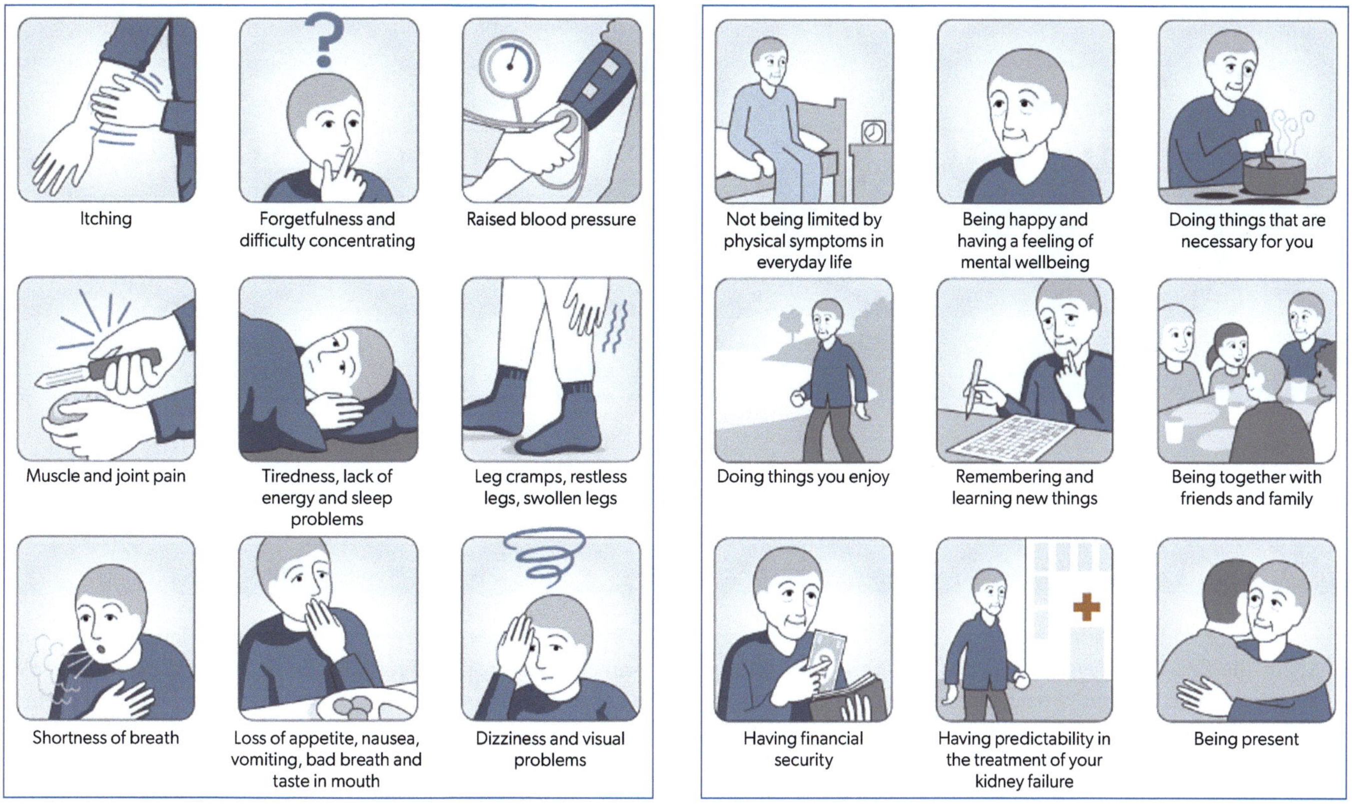
Itching
Forgetfulness and difficulty concentrating
Raised blood pressure
Muscle and joint pain
Tiredness, lack of energy and sleep problems
Leg cramps, restless legs, swollen legs
Shortness of breath
Loss of appetite, nausea, vomiting, bad breath and taste in mouth
Dizziness and visual problems
Not being limited by physical symptoms in everyday life
Being happy and having a feeling of mental wellbeing
Doing things that are necessary for you
Doing things you enjoy
Remembering and learning new things
Being together with friends and family
Having financial security
Having predictability in the treatment of your kidney failure
Being present

Figure 48.5 Symptom and activity prompts to support in-consultation discussions about what is important to PwKF.

Reproduced with permission from Aarhus University Hospital, 2020. First published in Finderup, J., Povlsen, J., Dam Jensen, J., et al. 2020. Dialysis choice. https://e-dok.rm.dk/edok/editor/AAUHNY.nsf/vLookupUpload/ATTACH-RMAP-BT4EF6/$FILE/Dialysis%20Choice%2027082020.pdf

a priority to learn what is important to patients, and recognize it is as useful to kidney failure management as the technical information we invested years in accruing.

REFERENCES

Bekker, H. L., Winterbottom, A., Gavaruzzi, T., et al. 2020. Dialysis: making the right choices for you. The dialysis decision aid booklet (updated 2024). Available at: https://kidneyresearchuk.org/wp-content/uploads/2023/03/KR-decision-Aid-2024-P5-Final-artwork.pdf

Bekker, H. L., Winterbottom, A. E., Gavaruzzi, T., Finderup, J., Mooney, A. 2023. Decision aids to assist patients and professionals in choosing the right treatment for kidney failure. *Clin Kidney J*, **16**, i20–i38.

Finderup, J., Dam Jensen, J., Lomborg, K. 2019. Evaluation of a shared decision-making intervention for dialysis choice at four Danish hospitals: a qualitative study of patient perspective. *BMJ Open*, **9**, e029090.

Finderup, J., Dam Jensen, J., Lomborg, K. 2020. Dialysis choice. Available at: https://e-dok.rm.dk/edok/editor/AAUHNY.nsf/vLookupUpload/ATTACH-RMAP-BT4EF6/$FILE/Dialysis%20Choice%2027082020.pdf

Joseph-Williams, N., Williams, D., Wood, F., et al. 2019. A descriptive model of shared decision making derived from routine implementation in clinical practice ('Implement-SDM'): qualitative study. *Patient Educ Couns*, **102**, 1774–1785.

National Institute for Health and Care Excellence. 2018. Renal replacement therapy and conservative management. NICE guideline [NG107]. Available at: https://www.nice.org.uk/guidance/ng107

Søndergaard, H., Deele, M., Agerskov, H., et al. 2023.The value of partnership in patient-driven as well as in researcher-driven projects. *Res Involv Engagem*, **9**, 20.

Toft, B. S., Rodkjaer, L., Andersen, A. B., et al. 2022. Measures used to assess interventions for increasing patient involvement in Danish healthcare setting: a rapid review *BMJ Open*, **12**, e064067.

UK Kidney Association and Kidney Care UK. 2021. Patient reported experience of kidney care in the UK 2021. Available at: https://www.ukkidney.org/sites/default/files/PREM%20report%202021.pdf

Winterbottom, A., Mooney, A., Hurst, H., et al. 2022. Difficult conversations: talking with people about kidney failure, end of life and advance care planning. Available at: https://kidneycareuk.org/health-professionals/the-difficult-conversations-booklet/

Winterbottom, A. E., Mooney, A., Russon, L., et al. 2020. Critical review of leaflets about conservative management used in UK renal services. *J Renal Care*, **46**, 250–257.

49

Shared decision making in haematology

Paulus A.F. Geerts, Thomas W. LeBlanc, and Wiebe Cnossen

Introduction

This chapter provides a clinical view on shared decision making (SDM) in the field of malignant haematology. This field includes the diagnosis and treatment of haematological cancers, such as the acute and chronic leukaemias, multiple myeloma (MM), and malignant lymphomas, among others. The so-called classical haematological diseases, such as the hemoglobinopathies, autoimmune diseases, congenital diseases, thrombosis, and coagulation, will not be covered. The field includes a wide variety of decision making situations, which will be illustrated by two cases and then discussed. Furthermore, we will discuss decision support tools, including decision aids, and the gaps in evidence and future directions. Finally, a patient's view is given on SDM in the context of malignant haematology.

Case 1

A 66-year-old man with asymptomatic, low-grade myelodysplastic syndrome presented with rapidly progressive pancytopenia and fatigue. A bone marrow examination showed progression to acute myeloid leukaemia (AML), and molecular/cytogenetic studies showed adverse risk abnormalities including loss of chromosome 7, without *TP53* mutation or any targetable mutations in *IDH1*, *IDH2*, or *FLT3* genes. Treatment options are either intensive induction chemotherapy with daunorubicin and cytarabine (the '7 plus 3' regimen), or low-intensity induction with azacitidine and venetoclax. These treatments differ markedly, as intensive induction therapy poses a higher risk of death due to complications of treatment, a more severe symptom burden, and the requirement for prolonged hospitalization. However, it may yield a higher remission rate, and can be part of a curative treatment path with further chemotherapy and allogeneic stem cell transplantation. Low-intensity induction poses less risk of short-term mortality, a less significant symptom burden, and may be administered as an outpatient, but the remission rate may be lower, and is less clearly established as part of a potentially curative treatment path.

Case 2

A 78-year-old lady has received bortezomib, lenalidomide, and dexamethasone treatment for MM for the past 3 years. Besides MM, she has hypertension requiring oral medication. From her chemotherapy, she experienced low-grade polyneuropathy and moderate anaemia, but these do not affect her quality of life. She is independent in daily life and cares for her husband, who uses a wheelchair following a stroke. After an initial very good partial response to treatment with bortezomib, lenalidomide, and dexamethasone, disease progression is now emerging and her haematologist discusses two combination treatment options: either a regimen including an anti-CD38 antibody with pomalidomide or carfilzomib, or an all-oral regimen with pomalidomide, cyclophosphamide, and steroids. In anti-CD38 antibody-naïve patients, greater efficacy is expected with the first option. If the myeloma does progress on this regimen, the all-oral regimen may subsequently be administered. However, the anti-CD38 antibody treatment requires hospital visits for medication administration. Furthermore, the possible side effects differ. For example, daratumumab may increase the chance of infection, carfilzomib may cause hypertension and subsequently cardiovascular events, and pomalidomide and cyclophosphamide may cause cytopenias.

Decision making in haematology: types of decisions and needs from practice

The two cases exemplify the range of different decision making situations in malignant haematology, with various decisional attributes that impact these situations. These attributes are discussed in more detail here.

First, the decisions may widely differ. For example, it may regard acute, 'high-impact' situations, such as deciding about intensive chemotherapy for AML or other acute presentations. In this situation a patient may have to decide within a fairly short period of time about an intensive treatment. Here, emotions and physical discomfort may strongly influence patients' capability to deliberate about a treatment decision. The 'readiness for decision making' may not be optimal.

The decision for second-line therapy for MM in the second case represents a completely different situation. More time is available, and there are more options to choose from, with varying trade-offs; the patient may discuss the decision with relatives or find information on the internet or as provided by the healthcare professionals before making a decision. Furthermore, as this decision regards a more chronic, ongoing treatment, the patient will become experienced with the treatment and may revisit the initial decision as the treatment proceeds. In that context, there would be other options available (Pritlove et al., 2021).

Second, the preferences for involvement in decision making and information may differ between patients, leading to different levels of patient activation, involvement, and empowerment. Over the past 10–15 years most patients with a haematological malignancy have preferred an active or collaborative role in decision making, although still about one-quarter to one-third prefer a more passive role (Rood et al., 2017; Geerts et al., 2020; Bylund et al., 2023). In addition, information needs vary between patients, including cancer-specific, treatment-related, and psychosocial information needs (Rood et al., 2017; Foster et al., 2020). Healthcare providers only variably address these needs.

In more detail, patients may have limited information needs immediately after diagnosis and need additional information later in the disease trajectory when the first shock has been processed (Nissim et al., 2013; LeBlanc et al., 2022; Garvelink et al., 2023). The information backlog at diagnosis may strongly influence patients' decisional role; for example, patients with chronic lymphocytic leukaemia (CLL) preferred a more active role in decision making after becoming more well informed about their situation (Rocque et al., 2018). The typically less urgent context within which CLL decision making takes place may help to facilitate this process, compared with the shorter time frame more typical of decision making about an acute leukaemia.

Third, several factors may affect the intrinsic preferences or priorities for treatment goals or outcomes (Fifer et al., 2020; Jen et al., 2020; Richardson et al., 2020; Auclair et al., 2022; LeBlanc et al., 2022; Garvelink et al., 2023). They may differ between patients but also for one patient over time. The type of disease and its dynamics and treatment milestones may affect the perception of treatment goals and outcomes. For example, patients with AML rank the treatment goal 'reaching a complete remission' very highly (Richardson et al., 2020). This aligns with the dynamics of AML treatment, where reaching a complete remission may make the difference between reaching long-term survival or early death, and the possibility of proceeding to a consolidative and curative-intent allogeneic stem cell transplant. While for patients with MM, on the other hand, side effects are more strongly considered (Auclair et al., 2022). This aligns with MM treatment, which usually is long term and where quality versus length of life is important to consider.

Furthermore, treatment goals may be influenced by experience with prior treatment, such as in the situation of MM or other long-term diseases, where patients often receive several courses and lines of therapy over time. Additionally, preferences or goals may differ between patients and their physicians (Fifer et al., 2020). In general, physicians more highly value survival duration, while patients and caregivers often (also) value quality of life and personal life milestones. Finally, financial impacts of treatment may be considered, also depending on the reimbursement possibilities and patients' insurance and possible own financial contribution (Jen et al., 2020). In the future this may become an increasing problem, considering the enormous rise in costs of targeted therapies.

Fourth, the people interacting with the patient matter, such as the healthcare team and patients' families and friends (Clayman et al., 2017). Patients have a very high regard for their haematologist and strongly value a trusting relationship (Garvelink et al., 2023). They often have a high level of trust in their clinician and may choose to trust them for decisions about the 'right' treatment instead of considering all aspects of treatment decisions themselves (Whitney et al., 2021).

However, as haematologists may not optimally integrate patients' values and preferences in decision making, patients risk agreeing on a treatment proposal by their haematologist that is not optimally aligned with their situation or preferences (Geerts et al., 2020). Furthermore, a large part of the decision making process takes place outside the consultation room. Patients interact with lay people around them, such as family and friends. But nowadays, patients also seek both information and personal contact via patient organizations or online patient communities. This raises additional challenges related to the accuracy of information accessed, and/or its applicability to the particular patient's situation and decision.

Decision aids/tools

SDM is well established in some areas of medicine, with patient decision aids (PtDAs) becoming increasingly available and used. Randomized trials of PtDAs in various other settings show several benefits. For general information about the use and impact of PtDAs, please refer to Chapters 18 to 20. In cancer care, PtDAs are less common and their use is less well established, although still reasonable numbers of PtDAs have been developed (see also Chapter 30). In this setting they generally address the more clearly preference-sensitive decisions without a single standard of care, such as in early-stage prostate cancer. In malignant haematology, however, there have been very few published examples of decision aids, and it is not known how much these are even used in practice.

A recent systematic review found only three randomized trials of PtDAs in haematological malignancies, and six pilot studies (Zhao et al., 2023). Despite this, in modern haematological malignancy practice there are several diagnoses and scenarios that would be very suitable to the development and use of a high-quality decision aid. While published evidence remains limited, the studies identified in the recent systematic review generally showed that decision aids yield improved knowledge and satisfaction, with reduced decisional conflict, across various haematological malignancies including chronic leukaemia (CLL, chronic myelogenous leukaemia), acute leukaemias (AML, acute lymphoblastic leukaemia), various lymphomas, and myeloma, as well as stem cell transplantation.

CLL is one such disease that is quite amenable to decision aids, and wherein SDM is suitable and necessary. This reflects that patients may now face decisions about fixed duration treatments versus continuous therapies, with significant trade-offs in the patient experience of treatment, and no clearly proven differences in outcomes. In the Netherlands, a decision aid for CLL is currently undergoing practical evaluation. This decision aid has been developed in collaboration with haematologists and patients to assist patients and healthcare providers in making treatment choices for CLL. In addition to addressing the clinical/medical situation, patients are specifically guided in determining their personal preferences. Based on the Dutch-approved CLL treatment guideline, all suitable treatment options are clearly presented and compared on criteria relevant to the patient and healthcare provider. This enables patients, haematologists, and nurse specialists to prepare and conduct consultations in a more structured and targeted manner, aiming to improve decision making. The CLL decision aid is available free of charge to all primary care CLL patients and their caregivers (CMyLife, n.d.). The data entered into the PtDA will, with consent, be used for evaluation and informing future patients. These data, combined with clinical data, can contribute to improving guidelines and decision making in the future.

AML is another disease where decision aid development and testing has occurred, and where an increasing number of treatment options are available, with various trade-offs to consider (Hildenbrand et al., 2021). As we developed and tested the decision aid for patients with newly diagnosed AML, we found that many patients did not understand their illness or prognosis adequately at diagnosis, nor did they recognize key features and trade-offs of available treatment paths (e.g. intensive induction vs low-intensity therapy). In a pilot randomized trial testing the feasibility and preliminary efficacy of the PtDA, with a pre–post design, patients had improved knowledge and reduced decisional conflict scores after using the PtDA. The challenge in implementing this PtDA has been that new therapies and practice have changed so rapidly that the PtDA already requires significant revision and updating. This is one of the major challenges in developing and implementing PtDAs in malignant haematology. It is likely that there are also challenges regarding clinicians' willingness and ability to use PtDAs in this setting as well; however, little is known about this in haematology.

Future directions

While SDM has been researched for several decades, SDM research in haematology is still in its infancy.

A first consideration regards the suitability and applicability of the prevailing SDM concept in haematological practice. In our view, the classical concept by Elwyn and colleagues optimally suits patient–physician consultation in an outpatient clinic situation, where enough time is available and the patient has more opportunity for deliberation. As the above two case examples exemplify, the decision making situation in malignant haematology may often not meet these conditions.

Bomhof and colleagues proposed a model for solid tumour oncology that addresses some of these conditions (Bomhof-Roordink et al., 2019). Importantly, this model includes both the consultation and the time outside the consultation, integrating home activities (accessing information, consulting others) into the decision making process. As the decisional attributes of solid and haematological oncology may not be exactly equal, refinement of this model for haematology may further improve applicability to haematology. The aspects of both very acute and dynamic and of chronic recurring decision making situations need to be taken into account. In the latter, for example, a fifth step in decision making may be added, regarding recurrent decision reconsideration.

Subsequently, better understanding of and agreement on SDM in haematology could lead to developing decision support tools that suit the specific situation. Such tools would be different for acute, high impact and for chronic treatment decisions and may build on the distinction of the type 1 (fast, instinctive, and emotional) and type 2 (slower, deliberative, and more logical) thought systems. To develop such tools, more empirical knowledge is needed about the aspects of these specific decisional situations. In the higher urgency situation, the aspect of time needs specific attention in relation to 'readiness for decision making'. Support tools may first need to efficiently clarify the most important information to decide about starting treatment or not. In a second phase, additional information could be provided to and retrieved from the patient, to optimize the patient's situation following starting treatment and to reconsider the initial quick and emotional decision. In the less urgent situation, the aspects of the recurrent chronic decision making processes require further elucidation. Support tools may provide more information and may include more time-consuming value elicitation exercises. Additionally, outcome prioritization should be included in these decision support tools, as the current literature shows very heterogeneous preferences by patients, caregivers, and healthcare professionals.

Finally, to implement SDM in haematology practice, education and guidance are needed for both healthcare professionals and patients. Although campaigns, legal regulations, and financial agreements are currently being worked on to increase knowledge and support implementation, there is a clear need for consciousness and practical application of SDM, along with further education about communication methods and practical use. This requires the haematological decision making culture becoming more patient-centred. Clinicians may not have ever been taught how to elicit preferences and values and may not know how to integrate a PtDA into their clinical practice and therefore may have to re-educate themselves. For further reading about education, implementation, and innovation please refer to chapters in Parts 4, 5, and 8 of this textbook.

See Box 49.1 for our patient perspective.

Box 49.1 Patient perspective

Closing the information gap: a patient's perspective of SDM in MM

As patient emancipation emerged, the importance of SDM increased. For SDM, equality in information between caregiver and patient forms the basis for an effective dialogue. This applies to every stage within the patient journey: diagnosis, treatment, and remission or follow-up. Several knowledge gaps may hinder an effective dialogue in these stages.

In the first stage, following the diagnosis of MM, a patient is confronted with a complex and challenging haematological disease, usually one they have never heard of before. The haematologist may wish to start treatment at relatively short notice following diagnosis. The patient, however, may need some extra time to consider the consequences of the new reality. He or she is struggling to become familiar with the disease and is forced to make the choices that accord with personal wishes and lifestyle. The first knowledge gap is in medical/clinical information and may hinder initial decision making about starting treatment.

A patient-centric information platform which facilities communication with peers may help to close the information gap. MM research is characterized by fast developments in treatment options. Providing access to information about new developments will help patients address information gaps when the disease relapses. Both patient communities and healthcare professional organizations should take roles in tackling this barrier.

During the treatment phase, the medical/clinical information gap between patient and haematologist narrows. The patient becomes familiar with the disease and is informed about the treatment options. Now understanding and considering individual patient goals and preferences becomes a subject of interest. Patients have unique values and priorities, which may significantly impact treatment choices. For example, some may prioritize maintaining quality of life and minimizing treatment-related side effects, while others may prioritize aggressive treatment with the goal of achieving remission. The second knowledge gap is about patients' socio-psychological and economic characteristics. Several factors contribute to this knowledge gap, among others limited available time.

There are some interesting experiments with intelligent and empathic chatbots that have the promise to fill in this second information gap. The data gathered by these chatbots could help enhance the quality of the SDM process.

During the remission or follow-up phase there will be less contact between haematologist and patient, mostly only the regular assessment visits. During this phase the patient is confronted with a lot of questions when they try to pick up their life again. Limitations in physical, cognitive, and emotional conditions raise new questions. In the meantime, other health professionals will be introduced in the patient's journey, professionals who take care of the socio-psychological and economic issues that arise. The third knowledge gap lies within the healthcare system, where cooperation between different types of healthcare providers and knowledge about each other's activities are limited. More integrated healthcare provision will help improve the quality of the patient's journey.

The essence of SDM lies in collaborative conversations between healthcare professionals and the patient. An informed patient and healthcare professional are better equipped to actively participate in decisions regarding a tailor-made patient journey. A collaborative approach not only improves treatment adherence but also empowers patients to face the challenges of picking up their lives with resilience and confidence.

REFERENCES

Auclair, D., Mansfield, C., Fiala, M. A., et al. 2022. Preferences and priorities for relapsed multiple myeloma treatments among patients and caregivers in the United States. *Patient Prefer Adherence*, **16**, 573–585.

Bomhof-Roordink, H., Fischer, M. J., van Duijn-Bakker, N., et al. 2019. Shared decision making in oncology: a model based on patients', health care professionals', and researchers' views. *Psychooncology*, **28**, 139–146.

Bylund, C. L., Eggly, S., LeBlanc, T. W., et al. 2023. Survey of patients and physicians on shared decision-making in treatment selection in relapsed/refractory multiple myeloma. *Transl Behav Med*, **13**, 255–267.

Clayman, M. L., Gulbrandsen, P., Morris, M. A. 2017. A patient in the clinic; a person in the world. Why shared decision making needs to center on the person rather than the medical encounter. *Patient Educ Couns*, **100**, 600–604.

CMyLife. n.d. CLL-keuzehulp [CLL decision aid]. Available at: https://www.cmylife.nl/projecten/cll-keuzehulp

Fifer, S. J., Ho, K. A., Lybrand, S., Axford, L. J., Roach, S. 2020. Alignment of preferences in the treatment of multiple myeloma—a discrete choice experiment of patient, carer, physician, and nurse preferences. *BMC Cancer*, **20**, 546.

Foster, J., Moore, H., Preussler, J. M., et al. 2020. Information needs for treatment decision-making of hematopoietic cell transplant patients 65 years or older and caregivers. *J Cancer Educ*, **35**, 651–660.

Garvelink, M. M., Daniels, K., De Weerdt, O., Van Der Nat, P. B. 2023. Why real world outcome information is indispensable in making treatment decisions for multiple myeloma. *Z Evid Fortbild Qual Gesundhwes*, **176**, 42–50.

Geerts, P. A. F., van der Weijden, T., Bos, G. M. J. 2020. The perception of shared decision-making in hematology by patients and physicians seems satisfactory, but important steps are still ahead of us. *HemaSphere*, **4**, e417.

Hildenbrand, J. D., Davis, D. M., El-Jawahri, A., et al. 2021. A novel decision aid for acute myeloid leukemia: a feasibility and preliminary efficacy trial. *Support Care Cancer*, **29**, 3563–3569.

Jen, W. Y., Yoong, J., Liu, X., Tan, M. S. Y., Chng, W. J., Chee, Y. L. 2020. Qualitative study of factors affecting patient, caregiver and physician preferences for treatment of myeloma and indolent lymphoma. *Patient Prefer Adherence*, **14**, 301–308.

LeBlanc, T. W., Russell, N. H., Hernandez-Aldama, L., et al. 2022. Patient, family member and physician perspectives and experiences with AML treatment decision-making. *Oncol Ther*, **10**, 421–440.

Nissim, R., Zimmermann, C., Minden, M., et al. 2013. Abducted by the illness: a qualitative study of traumatic stress in individuals with acute leukemia. *Leuk Res*, **37**, 496–502.

Pritlove, C., Jassi, M., Burns, B., McCurdy, A. 2021. The work of managing multiple myeloma and its implications for treatment-related decision making: a qualitative study of patient and caregiver experiences. *BMC Cancer*, **21**, 793.

Richardson, D. R., Crossnohere, N. L., Seo, J., et al. 2020. Age at diagnosis and patient preferences for treatment outcomes in AML: a discrete choice experiment to explore meaningful benefits. *Cancer Epidemiol Biomarkers Prev*, **29**, 942–948.

Rocque, G. B., Williams, C. P., Halilova, K. I., et al. 2018. Improving shared decision-making in chronic lymphocytic leukemia through multidisciplinary education. *Transl Behav Med*, **8**, 175–182.

Rood, J. A. J., Nauta, I. H., Witte, B. I., et al. 2017. Shared decision-making and providing information among newly diagnosed patients with hematological malignancies and their informal caregivers: not 'one-size-fits-all'. *Psychooncology*, **26**, 2040–2047.

Whitney, R. L., White, A. E. C., Rosenberg, A. S., Kravitz, R. L., Kim, K. K. 2021. Trust and shared decision-making among individuals with multiple myeloma: a qualitative study. *Cancer Med*, **10**, 8040–8057.

Zhao, J., Abdallah, M., Sanapala, C., et al. 2023. A systematic review of decision aids in hematologic malignancies: what are currently available and what are we missing? *Oncologist*, **28**, 105–115.

50

Shared decision making in plastic surgery

Rakhshan Kamran, Liam J. Peck, Kenny Ardouin, and Jeremy N. Rodrigues

Shared decision making in plastic surgery: the patient–clinician partnership

In recent years, clinical problems can often be addressed by more than just a singular or even binary treatment choice. This poses questions for patients and clinicians in terms of selecting the most appropriate management strategy to achieve satisfactory outcomes. As desired outcomes may differ based on patient preferences, it is necessary for clinicians to have open conversations with patients. In plastic surgery, there are some scenarios which warrant evaluation of shared decision making (SDM) practices. This chapter will review:

- Areas within plastic surgery with good scope for SDM
- Practice and attitudes to SDM in plastic surgery
- The future of SDM in plastic surgery
- Patient perspectives on SDM in plastic surgery.

SDM scenarios and current practice in plastic surgery

Acute/trauma settings

In trauma settings, decision making can be time-sensitive, and dependent on patient preferences, especially when there is a lack of one best treatment option. One potential way to increase effectiveness of SDM in surgical settings is with decision aids (Langbroek et al., 2023); however, attitudes towards these may vary between surgeons, impacting their use and effectiveness.

Woltz and colleagues found a key enabler to SDM was a condition that was not life-threatening, and key barriers included patients wanting surgeons to make the decision for them and SDM being too complex for patients to engage with (Woltz et al., 2018). Key recommendations from this study included increased SDM training built into surgical training programmes and medical curricula, as although trauma surgeons rated SDM as valuable, many felt there were barriers in implementing SDM.

Another study explored patient perceptions of SDM in the facial trauma setting (Liu et al., 2023). This study found that patient decisional conflict and past experiences of discrimination contributed to lower perceptions of SDM taking place, while older age correlated with higher perceived SDM. For facial trauma, SDM was positioned as a way to help reduce healthcare disparities by facilitating patient communication about their preferences (Liu et al., 2023).

Aesthetic surgery

Aesthetic surgery usually presents various treatment options in a setting where the indication for treatment is typically patient request rather than medical necessity. Understanding patient preferences through an SDM process is key to the patient making an informed choice and understanding various treatment options.

The UK General Medical Council, Royal College of Surgeons of England, British Association of Plastic, Reconstructive and Aesthetic Surgeons, and British Association of Aesthetic Plastic Surgeons all publish guidance and codes of conduct for surgeons who perform cosmetic procedures. Each references the concept of SDM, either directly or indirectly, and mandates minimum standards for the process of obtaining consent for elective aesthetic surgery, including relevant information sharing and risk communication, a minimum 2-week 'cooling off' period before the date of procedure as advised by the General Medical Council, and preoperative anaesthetic assessment for procedures involving regional, general, or spinal anaesthesia (General Medical Council, 2016; Royal College of Surgeons of England, 2016; British Association of Plastic, Reconstructive and Aesthetic Surgeons, 2019; British Association of Aesthetic Plastic Surgeons, 2024).

SDM is ideal for breast augmentation decisions, where implants can be inserted through an incision in the axilla, nipple margin, or inframammary fold (Ubbink et al., 2015). Patient preferences for scar location can help guide decision making for surgical incision and approach. Further, patient preferences are important to guide whether to place an implant above or under the pectoral muscle, the implant type (i.e. cohesive or saline, round or anatomically shaped), and the option of an additional procedure to potentially improve outcomes of the procedure (i.e. lipofilling). SDM can be optimized in aesthetic surgery through verbal and graphical tools. Examples of verbal tools include communication of risk through absolute proportions (e.g. '2 out of 100 patients undergoing this aesthetic surgery will develop an infection') (Gigerenzer and Galesic, 2012). Graphical tools include items like pie/bar charts which may provide information on risks and benefits of a procedure for patients who may better understand visual illustrations of data.

Gender-affirming surgery

Gender-affirming surgeries may include facial feminization surgery, feminizing vaginoplasty, phalloplasty, scrotoplasty, metoidioplasty, masculinizing chest surgery, augmentation mammoplasty, and reduction thyrochondroplasty. Studies show that SDM is general best practice in gender-affirming care, yet may face unique challenges (Dewey, 2015). As many patients face discrimination and barriers to accessing high-quality gender-affirming care, there is a need to create a safe environment with patients to engage in effective SDM conversations. To offer SDM more effectively in gender-affirming care, the first step is to clarify the local decisional context, and consider the assumptions, perspectives, and preferences of all key stakeholders involved in the decision making. As gender-affirming care also includes psychosocial and hormonal care, and includes a multidisciplinary team, effective SDM in this area may also include dialogue between clinicians from other specialties (Gerritse et al., 2022).

Hand surgery

In hand surgery, research demonstrates that patients prefer an equal share of decision making responsibility with the surgeon. In general, patients prefer to have increased involvement in decision making tasks (i.e. deciding on treatment), and prefer to have their surgeon more involved in decision making for problem-solving tasks (i.e. diagnosing and comparing risks and benefits) (Cho et al., 2022). Research also shows that the most important consideration for patients in decision making around flap selection is complication risk, followed by scar condition. (Chang et al., 2021). For carpal tunnel syndrome and Dupuytren's contracture, UK National Health Service (NHS) decision aids are available to help patients choose treatment options which best align with their values and preferences (NHS England, 2022a, 2022b).

Breast surgery

Breast surgery, including breast reconstruction, presents several options to patients to choose from (i.e. delayed vs immediate reconstruction). Priorities for patients include avoiding the use of a prosthesis and looking natural without clothes (Lee et al., 2010). These concepts can be used to guide conversations with patients. A widely used decision aid which can be used to aid SDM for breast surgery is BREASTChoice, which provides personalized risk prediction using clinical information from a patient's electronic medical record, and clinician- and patient-relevant components (Politi et al., 2020). BREASTChoice has also been successfully integrated to electronic medical records at some centres, and aided with SDM in deciding on breast reconstructive options after mastectomy.

Paediatric surgery

Paediatrics offers a unique setting for SDM as children have variable abilities and desires to participate in conversations around their healthcare. As various treatment options in paediatric plastic surgery come with their own sets of advantages and disadvantages, it is important to understand patient preferences and decide on a treatment which best aligns with patient needs. For microtia, key components of SDM include understanding psychosocial and functional outcomes following options for microtia reconstruction (Ronde et al., 2024). For craniosynostosis, decision aids have been created for the three major types of single-suture craniosynostosis (sagittal, metopic, unicoronal), and were found to help facilitate discussions around selecting the best treatment which aligns with patient preferences and values (Said et al., 2024). In brachial plexus birth injuries, key facilitators to effective SDM include allowing youth to express their perspectives without external pressures from others during decision making. As youth navigate pressure from parents in decision making around treatment options, and parental experience is impacted from adjusting to having a child with a birth injury, SDM in the context of brachial plexus injury can be challenging to navigate. Decision coaching and decision support tools could help to foster effective SDM in this setting and help youth and their families to decide on the best treatment options which align with their values (Ho et al., 2021).

Future of SDM in plastic surgery

A common clinician-reported barrier to SDM is the perceived lack of time to take part in SDM conversations. However, evidence is lacking on whether SDM consultations take more time than consultations that do not include SDM, with some research demonstrating overall time savings when applying SDM as part of surgical consultations (Veenendaal et al., 2023). The National Institute for health and Care Excellence SDM guideline emphasizes that decision aids are best used in conjunction with other tools and skills to facilitate SDM, such as effective risk communication (National Institute for health and Care Excellence, 2021). Perioperative risk may be assessed in collaboration with tools such as the American Society of Anaesthesiologists physical status classification (Mayhew et al., 2019) *in combination* with other procedure-specific tools, such as the Surgical Outcome Risk Tool (version 2, available at http://www.sortsurgery.com) (Wong et al., 2020).

Online courses exist to train clinicians in SDM principles and risk communication (with specific courses for plastic surgery scenarios), including free resources developed by the Winton Centre for Risk and Evidence Communication in collaboration with the Australian Commission on Safety and Quality in Healthcare, and the Academy of Medical Royal Colleges in the UK (available online via https://moodle.wintoncentre.uk or for NHS staff via the NHS e-learning for health platform, https://www.e-lfh.org.uk/programmes/shared-decision-making/).

SDM in plastic surgery is a *process* rather than a singular event, particularly where time allows in the non-acute setting. This process may be summarized in the form of clinic letters from the surgeon to the patient and their primary care physician (again, especially in an elective setting), but typically this varies by clinician and is not standardized. The culmination of this complex process is formally recognized in the signing of a paper consent form, usually on the day of procedure. There are arguments that the nature and timing of same-day paper consent forms do not promote best practices, with some local healthcare providers adopting digitized consent processes that can be tailored to individual patient needs (St John et al., 2021).

Understanding how best to implement SDM aids for local clinic contexts can be enabled through using guidance from the field of implementation science. Implementation science offers a set of theories, models, and frameworks to conduct implementation studies, which investigate how to improve uptake of an innovation (i.e. decision aids). Through applying methods from implementation science to understand barriers and enablers to the use of decision aids and SDM in various local clinical contexts, evidence-based strategies to maximize SDM can be developed.

See Box 50.1 for our patient perspective.

Box 50.1 Patient perspective

Kenny Ardouin, plastic surgery patient

In recent years, healthcare has evolved towards recognizing patients' expertise as experts by experience. When combined with clinicians' expertise by training, patients and clinicians create a formidable team. Only an individual themselves can understand how it truly *feels* to experience their condition, far more than objective assessment tools are designed to understand.

As both a clinician and patient, I have seen that objectively excellent surgical outcomes do not always improve patient self-perception, and equally a surgically suboptimal outcome can exceed patient expectations. The potential disparity between surgical evaluations of success and patient success criteria demonstrates the importance of SDM to ensure patients and clinicians have the same expectations of what proposed treatments can (and cannot) achieve. Plastic surgery is high stakes, and whether articulated to the treatment team or not, patients certainly have preferences and expectations of surgical procedures. Thorough discussion with the patient around their hopes and goals for treatment is imperative and must occur well in advance of surgery day—it is far better to have an awkward conversation early on, than a potentially litigious one later!

A clinician may have concerns that particular decisions are too complex for patients to evaluate. I would argue that if the level of discussion is too challenging to effectively achieve SDM, it is too complex for fully informed consent. The time required to communicate high-level concepts to patients is often overlooked, but sufficient time spent explaining medical jargon and presenting options using terms that the patient can comprehend is time well spent.

Wherever possible, SDM should include discussion of the risks and benefits of no treatment, to allow the patient to evaluate treatment options relative to each other, and relative to the status quo. In areas like acute/trauma surgery, no treatment may not be an option; however, in elective plastic surgery, this is a valid option—even if patients (and/or their treatment team) have not yet paused to consider it.

It can be difficult to engage in SDM directly with patients, due to co-occurring psychological distress, speech differences, and other human complexities. These alone do not necessitate dismissing SDM, as clinicians in disciplines such as clinical psychology and speech language therapy are well placed to facilitate conversations with patients around treatment goals.

Effective SDM takes time and should not be rushed. While many patients may initially express preference for their surgical team to make the decision for them, such deferral could suggest a lack of autonomy or empowerment—possibly based on previous negative experience where their goals were neither heard nor valued—and could further indicate lack of understanding of the strengths and limitations of the options available. Instead, clinicians are encouraged to reiterate to patients that their perspective is critical to identifying the most appropriate choice, and to provide the time and space for those conversations to occur. When reflecting upon my own consultations as a patient, clinical teams making an effort to address the power dynamic inherent in clinician-patient relationships can highlight that the patient is considered an equal partner in their health. Simple strategies like seating the patient in the same type of (regular) chair for conversational parts of consultations—rather than an examination chair or bed—create a level playing field.

Summary

SDM has particular applicability in plastic surgery due to the wide clinical range of the specialty, and various treatments offered to patients across a range of conditions. SDM contributes to decreased conflict and increased satisfaction with making treatment-related decisions and increases patient knowledge around their condition and treatment options. Future priority areas for SDM in plastic surgery include national surgical associations making calls for increased use of SDM as part of routine clinical practice, increasing clinician knowledge about facilitating effective SDM in plastic surgery, and digitizing and implementing decision aids or consent processes to enable SDM.

REFERENCES

British Association of Aesthetic Plastic Surgeons. 2024. BAAPS code of conduct. Available at: https://baaps.org.uk/_userfiles/pages/files/code_of_conduct_current_1.pdf

British Association of Plastic Reconstructive and Aesthetic Surgeons.2019. BAPRAS code of practice. Available at: http://bapras.org.uk/docs/default-source/default-document-library/code-of-practice-2019_final.pdf

Chang, D. H., Wang, Y. H., Hsieh, C. Y., Chang, C. W., Chang, K. C., Chen, Y. S. 2021. Incorporating patient preferences into a decision-making model of hand trauma reconstruction. *Int J Environ Res Public Health*, **18**, 11081.

Cho, H. E., Baxter, N. B., Billig, J. I., Kotsis, S. V., Haase, S. C., Chung, K. C. 2022. Task-specific patient preferences for shared decision-making in hand surgery. *Plast Reconstr Surg*, **149**, 229E–239E.

Dewey, J. M. 2015. Challenges of implementing collaborative models of decision making with trans-identified patients. *Health Expect*, **18**, 1508–1518.

Gerritse, K., Martens, C., Bremmer, M. A., Kreukels, B. P. C., de Boer, F., Molewijk, B. C. 2022. Sharing decisions amid uncertainties: a qualitative interview study of healthcare professionals' ethical challenges and norms regarding decision-making in gender-affirming medical care. *BMC Med Ethics*, **23**, 1–17.

Gigerenzer, G., Galesic, M. 2012. Why do single event probabilities confuse patients? Statements of frequency are better for communicating risk. *BMJ*, **344**, e245.

General Medical Council. 2016. Guidance for doctors who offer cosmetic interventions—professional standards. Available at: https://www.gmc-uk.org/professional-standards/professional-standards-for-doctors/cosmetic-interventions

Ho, E. S., Parsons, J. A., Davidge, K. M., Clarke, H. M., Wright, F. V. 2021. Shared decision making in youth with brachial plexus birth injuries and their families: a qualitative study. *Patient Educ Couns*, **104**, 2586–2591.

Langbroek, G. B., Ronde, E. M., Lapid, O., et al. 2023. Healthcare professionals' views on shared decision-making in plastic surgery in the Netherlands. *J Plast Reconstr Aesthetic Surg*, **85**, 463–472.

Lee, C. N., Hultman, C. S., Sepucha, K. 2010. Do patients and providers agree about the most important facts and goals for breast reconstruction decisions? *Ann Plast Surg*, **64**, 563–566.

Liu, Y., Wamkpah, N. S., Ballamudi, A., et al. 2023. Shared decision-making in patients seeking surgery for facial trauma: the role of decisional conflict and perceived discrimination. *Facial Plast Surg Aesthet Med*, **26**, 333–338.

Mayhew, D., Mendonca, V., Murthy, B. V. S. 2019. A review of ASA physical status—historical perspectives and modern developments. *Anaesthesia,* **74**, 373–379.

National Institute for health and Care Excellence. 2021. Shared decision making. NICE guideline [NG197]. Available at: https://www.nice.org.uk/guidance/ng197

NHS England. 2022a. Decision support tool: making a decision about carpal tunnel syndrome. Available at: https://www.england.nhs.uk/publication/decision-support-tool-making-a-decision-about-carpal-tunnel-syndrome/

NHS England. 2022b. Decision support tools: making a decision about Dupuytren's contracture. Available at: https://www.england.nhs.uk/publication/decision-support-tools-making-a-decision-about-dupuytrens-contracture/

Politi, M. C., Lee, C. N., Philpott-Streiff, S. E., et al. 2020. A randomized controlled trial evaluating the BREASTChoice tool for personalized decision support about breast reconstruction after mastectomy. *Ann Surg,* **271**, 230–237.

Royal College of Surgeons of England. 2016. Professional standards for cosmetic surgery. Available at: https://www.rcseng.ac.uk/standards-and-research/standards-and-guidance/service-standards/cosmetic-surgery/professional-standards-for-cosmetic-surgery/

Ronde, E. M., van de Lücht, V. A. P., Lachkar, N., Ubbink, D. T., Breugem, C. C. 2024. Stakeholders' views on information needed in a patient decision aid for microtia reconstruction. *Cleft Palate Craniofac J,* **61**, 854–869.

Said, A. M., Zubovic, E., Pfeifauf, K. D., et al. 2024. Shared decision-making: process for design and implementation of a decision aid for patients with craniosynostosis. *Cleft Palate Craniofac J,* **61**, 138–143.

St John, E. R., Bakri, A. C., Johanson, E., et al. 2021. Assessment of the introduction of semi-digital consent into surgical practice. *Br J Surg,* **108**, 342–345.

Ubbink, D. T., Santema, T. B., Lapid, O. 2015. Shared decision-making in cosmetic medicine and aesthetic surgery. *Aesthetic Surg J,* **36**, NP14–NP19.

Veenendaal, H. V., Chernova, G., Bouman, C. M., Etten-Jamaludin, F. S. V., Dieren, S. V., Ubbink, D. T. 2023. Shared decision-making and the duration of medical consultations: a systematic review and meta-analysis. *Patient Educ Couns,* **107**, 107561.

Woltz, S., Krijnen, P., Pieterse, A. H., Schipper, I. B. 2018. Surgeons' perspective on shared decision making in trauma surgery. A national survey. *Patient Educ Couns,* **101**, 1748–1752.

Wong, D. J. N., Harris, S., Sahni, A., et al. 2020. Developing and validating subjective and objective risk-assessment measures for predicting mortality after major surgery: an international prospective cohort study. *PLoS Med,* **17**, e1003253.

51

Shared decision making in palliative and supportive care

Meredith MacMartin, Pola Hahlweg, Joan Collison, and Simon Noble

Background

What is palliative care and what are its components?

Palliative care is an approach that 'improves the quality of life of patients and that of their families who are facing challenges associated with life-threatening illness' (World Health Organization, 2012). According to the World Health Organization, palliative care 'should be provided through person-centred and integrated health services that pay special attention to the specific needs and preferences of individuals' (World Health Organization, n.d.). Improving patients' quality of life is usually done by assessing and treating pain and other physical symptoms, as well as non-physical symptoms such as psychosocial and spiritual distress (Ferrell et al., 2018). Palliative care delivery and nomenclature can vary by practice setting, patient context, and local norms of medical practice. We use palliative care as an umbrella term that may include all of the above, acknowledging that palliative care is a spectrum of services delivered across the course of a serious illness (Box 51.1).

Identifying the goals and values of patients with serious illness, and supporting the creation of treatment plans centred on those goals and values, is at the heart of palliative care, as palliative care practitioners seek to honour patient autonomy (Ferrell et al., 2018; Kuosmanen et al., 2021). Given the focus of palliative care on quality of life as defined by the patient, shared decision making (SDM) practices are ideally suited for palliative care practice. In this chapter we will describe the common processes, distinctive characteristics, and challenges to SDM in palliative care.

Box 51.1 Palliative care alternative nomenclature

Hospice: care directed towards comfort and quality of life specifically towards the end of life (i.e. less than 6 months' life expectancy).

End-of-life care: care for dying patients in the last weeks, days, or hours of life.

Supportive care: care directed towards preventing and managing side effects and consequences of the treatment of serious illness over the course of that illness including into survivorship.

Who provides palliative care?

Interdisciplinary practice is a distinguishing feature of palliative care, which is most often delivered by collaborative teams composed of physicians, nurses, social workers, psychologists, chaplains, other allied health professionals, and those closest to the patients (Ferrell et al., 2018; Sheikh et al., 2022). Palliative care can be delivered across a variety of settings, including in a hospital, in a clinic, and in the community or in-home (Hui and Bruera, 2020; National Institute on Aging, 2021). Palliative care can be delivered by specialized teams, in a clinic, as consulting or assisting teams in a hospital, in a dedicated palliative care unit, or at home. A palliative care approach can also be delivered by non-specialists, such as primary care providers or oncologists. This may be called generalist or primary palliative care (Quill and Abernethy, 2013; Payne et al., 2022).

Who receives palliative care?

The field of palliative care originated from the care of dying patients, and it is patients at the end of life who are most consistently considered appropriate for palliative care. As the specialty has developed and its benefits have been more clearly articulated, more patients have been identified as appropriate to receive palliative care, in many cases alongside disease-directed therapy such as chemotherapy for metastatic cancer. In this chapter we will use the term 'serious illness' or 'seriously ill' to describe patients who receive palliative care. A serious illness is a 'health condition that carries a high risk of mortality, and either negatively impacts a person's daily function or quality of life, or excessively strains their caregivers' (Kelley and Bollens-Lund, 2018).

SDM and palliative care are closely aligned

Assisting or supporting patients with serious illness and their care partners with decision making is explicitly a core component of palliative care as set out by clinical practice and training guidelines (Ferrell et al., 2018; Accreditation Council for Graduate Medical

Education, 2019; Payne et al., 2022). Studies of palliative care practice have likewise identified supporting decision making and care planning as a core part of palliative care practice (Yoong et al., 2013; Hoerger et al., 2018; Khayal and Barnato, 2022). Palliative care expertise in decision making support has been codified in a growing set of formal communication tools designed to facilitate discussions about patient preferences and values, and support the development of patient-centred care plans. The Serious Illness Conversation Guide, developed as part of the Serious Illness Care Program at Ariadne Labs (Boston, Massachusetts, USA) is one example (Bernacki et al., 2015; Paladino et al., 2019, 2020; Baxter et al., 2024).

Integration of palliative care into the care of patients with serious illness has been found to improve a number of patient outcomes, including symptom burden, quality of life, patient and caregiver satisfaction, and healthcare utilization (Temel et al., 2010; Kavalieratos et al., 2016; El-Jawahri et al., 2017; Rogers et al., 2017). Some evidence suggests that support in decision making may be associated specifically with improved outcomes (Hoerger et al., 2018). Given the strong evidence supporting implementation of SDM generally, and the centrality of SDM to palliative care practice, it may be that the decision making support offered by palliative care teams is key to improving the care and experience of seriously ill patients.

Unique characteristics of SDM in palliative care

Timing of decision making support

One of the best-described ways in which palliative care teams engage in SDM is advance care planning, the process of identifying a seriously ill patient's wishes for if or when their condition worsens (Sudore et al., 2017). Advance care planning is done in advance of a decision actually needing to be made, often relatively early in the course of a serious illness. In some health systems, advance care planning may result in the completion of documentation such as an 'advance directive' or 'living will' in the USA or an 'Advance Decision to Refuse Treatment' in the UK (NHS England, 2022). In these types of documents, patients may specify preferences for life-sustaining care such as ventilatory support or cardiopulmonary resuscitation at the end of life. In many countries, advance care planning will embody other proactive processes, including anticipatory prescribing of end-of-life medicines, rationalizing current drug regimens, and facilitating expressions of preferred place for their end-of-life care (Marie Curie, 2022). While advance care planning is done by specialties other than palliative care, it is a key part of the palliative care approach as it seeks to centre patient values.

Palliative care also supports 'real-time' decision making, which is often highly preference sensitive. Ann, whose story is described in Box 51.2, faced a decision about whether to proceed with surgery on a chronic wound. A palliative care approach to this decision might align with the 'three-talk' model of SDM (Elwyn et al., 2017) and include discussion of potential downsides of surgery including the risk of worsening her health status and quality of life ('option talk') and exploration of Ann's hopes and worries about her wound and her future in general ('decision talk'). SDM for real-time decisions may also be used for non-treatment-related decisions, such as options for increased caregiver support or changes in living situation.

Box 51.2 Patient perspective

SDM in palliative care from a patient's and a care partner's perspective

My sister Ann was diagnosed with rheumatoid arthritis in her early twenties, and lived most of her adult life with this chronic debilitating autoimmune disease which eventually left her disabled at age 50. Her disease progressed despite millions of dollars in care that included countless surgeries, hospitalizations and several intensive care unit stays. She spent significant time in institutions, moving between hospitals, rehabilitation centres, and nursing homes. Along the way, she was also diagnosed with psoriasis and acquired a non-healing deep wound which had her tethered to a wound vacuum device for many years, complicated by antibiotic-resistant infections. She was a teacher in the Chicago public school system and had medical insurance coverage through her employer; this kept her in Chicago far longer than was socially, psychologically, and financially beneficial. As a result, the majority of her care was provided hundreds of miles from the support of our family.

In the midst of Ann's struggle, I was introduced to the concept of palliative care by Ira Byock, MD and his wife Yvonne Corbeil, RN, pioneers in the field. At Ann's bedside in the intensive care unit, I requested a palliative care consultation. This request prompted forthright conversations about Ann's prognosis and future medical course, including the likelihood that she would remain highly dependent on the support of others for the rest of her life. Within weeks of starting these discussions, Ann told me, 'This is not living, this is existing'. After examining what was really important to her within the limitations of her illness, Ann relocated to be closer to our family and spent the rest of her life in a nursing home near our parents and brother, who advocated for her medical care to be focused on Ann's quality, not quantity, of life. As a result, she avoided hospitalization for the last 4 years of her life, including choosing not to pursue surgery for her chronic wound when it became clear it would not meaningfully improve her quality of life. She was cared for by an interdisciplinary team who supported her physical, mental, and spiritual well-being. As her health declined, she enrolled in hospice and died a few weeks later just shy of her 61st birthday. Her life was often difficult, but her choice to focus on the quality of her life enabled her to live as well as she could.

Complexity of decisions

Palliative care teams support patients and their care partners with a broad array of decisions across the course of a serious illness (Yoong et al., 2013; Robinson et al., 2014; Hoerger et al., 2018). These decisions are often complex on multiple levels. Patients with serious illness often have multiple medical comorbidities, demanding a holistic approach that considers the impact of any given decision on a variety of conditions. The presence of complex medical illness often leads to a lack of clear evidence-based guidance on anticipated outcomes. Serious illness is often accompanied by psychosocial, emotional, and spiritual concerns—all of which should be accounted for in the process of decision making (Mitchell et al., 2011).

Additionally, many patients with serious illness have care partners who support them and are often involved in the decision making process. The inclusion of care partners, who may have their own perspectives and values, in decision making adds further complexity (Mulcahy Symmons et al., 2023). Furthermore, care partners may increasingly become the primary decision makers when the decision making capacity of a seriously ill patient decreases, posing challenges to traditional SDM models. The complexity of decision making in palliative care leads to different forms of SDM, as teams respond to

Table 51.1 Purposeful palliative care SDM forms

Purposeful SDM form	Palliative care example
Matching preferences	
Patients and clinicians compare available options and match them with patient values, preferences, goals, and priorities	Deciding whether to continue to treat progressive metastatic cancer or cease cancer-directed therapy and transition to hospice
Reconciling conflicts	
The clinician and patient collaborate to articulate differing positions, and reconcile these positions with options	Negotiating caregiving support for a patient with dementia who prioritizes autonomy and privacy but is unsafe at home alone
Problem-solving	
Exploration of potential solutions to address a patient problem	Planning for a hospital discharge with hospice support, determining care needs and support and home
Meaning making	
The patient and clinician develop understanding of the deeper meaning behind patient's situation and options, to identify a path forward	Discussing concerns about withdrawing a ventilator with surrogate decision makers who worry it conflicts with religious teachings

Adapted from Montori, V. M., Ruissen, M. M., Hargraves, I. G., Brito, J. P., Kunneman, M. 2023. Shared decision-making as a method of care. *BMJ Evid Based Med*, 28, 213–217 under the Creative Commons CC-BY-NC 4.0 (https://creativecommons.org/licenses/by-nc/4.0/).

a variety of decision types and settings. These are well reflected in Ian Hargraves and colleagues' understanding of purposeful SDM (Hargraves et al., 2019; Montori et al., 2023) (Table 51.1).

The role of palliative care teams in complex clinical settings

The role of palliative care teams in SDM is not limited to interactions with patients and care partners. As the decisions being made are often complex, palliative care teams must collaborate with other specialists caring for a given patient. This is most often to make sure that they understand treatment options and expected outcomes, and palliative care teams may work collaboratively with primary or referring teams to identify viable options given what is known about patient values. Identifying clear roles and responsibilities for palliative care teams, especially when consulting, helps in developing and maintaining relationships with referring providers (Palliative Care Network of Wisconsin, 2019).

Challenges and opportunities for SDM in palliative care

The complexity of the clinical contexts and decisions encountered in palliative care can pose challenges to implementing SDM. The high degree of uncertainty inherent to multiple comorbidities and advanced illness complicate navigation of treatment choices (Chen et al., 2022). There may be constraints on choices due to financial or regulatory factors, such as lack of resources for caregivers or lack of access to palliative care (Diernberger et al., 2021; Wachterman and Sommers, 2021). Palliative care patients, particularly those with advanced illness, may experience impaired cognition that can limit their decisional capacity, which in turn limits their ability to fully participate in SDM (although does not always fully preclude it) (Elwyn et al., 2023). Finally, patients with serious illness may not prefer to fully participate in decision making, particularly when it involves discussion of end of life or their death (Levinson et al., 2005; Chung et al., 2012). These patients may avoid engaging in decision making or opt out of it entirely, preferring to defer to the judgement of their family, friends, or medical providers. These limits to the participation of palliative care patients in SDM are not always immediately apparent, and identifying them often requires collaboration between the palliative care team and other medical specialists.

Culturally contextualizing SDM in palliative care

Although palliative care has been increasingly integrated into routine medical practice, SDM has not been consistently or identically implemented across palliative care teams and settings. Decision making can be viewed differently across cultural and health system contexts (Cain et al., 2018) and despite being built on the same tenets, palliative care models of service delivery differ globally (Arias-Casais et al., 2019; Connor, 2020). Key drivers for this are complex but are usually a reflection of different funding models, cultural attitudes to death, and the perceived roles of both society and the family in the support of the dying (Morrison, 2013). Cultural and religious values may impact the implementation of SDM in palliative care, as these values may affect patient preferences around information disclosure, discussion of prognosis, and decision making roles (Hurst et al., 2022; Ha et al., 2023). All of these factors should be identified and taken into account by palliative care teams engaging in SDM with patients and their care partners. Financial considerations may also affect utilization of SDM, as systems with constrained resources may provide less treatment options from which to choose. Such challenges, while not insurmountable, must be understood before approaching any aspect of SDM within the context of palliative care.

Summary

SDM in palliative care is highly integrated with routine clinical practice and encompasses a broad range of decisions. Interdisciplinary palliative care teams support complex decision making across care settings and patient populations, and take into account multiple contextual factors to facilitate creation of patient-centred care plans (Figure 51.1).

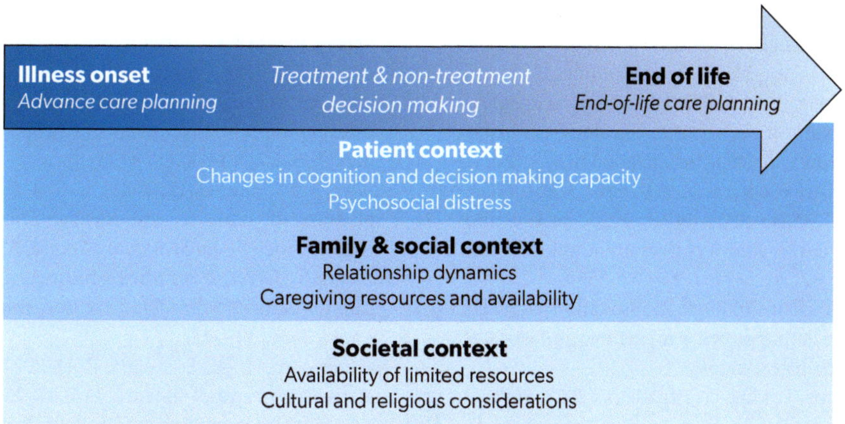
Illness onset
Advance care planning
Treatment & non-treatment decision making
End of life
End-of-life care planning
Patient context
Changes in cognition and decision making capacity
Psychosocial distress
Family & social context
Relationship dynamics
Caregiving resources and availability
Societal context
Availability of limited resources
Cultural and religious considerations

Figure 51.1 Spectrum of decision making and contextual factors for SDM in palliative care.

REFERENCES

Accreditation Council for Graduate Medical Education. 2019. Hospice and palliative medicine milestones. Available at: https://www.acgme.org/globalassets/pdfs/milestones/hospiceandpalliativemedicinemilestones.pdf

Baxter, R., Pusa, S., Andersson, S., et al. 2024. Core elements of serious illness conversations: an integrative systematic review. *BMJ Support Palliat Care,* **14**, e2268–e2279.

Bernacki, R., Hutchings, M., Vick, J., et al. 2015. Development of the Serious Illness Care Program: a randomised controlled trial of a palliative care communication intervention. *BMJ Open,* **5**, e009032.

Cain, C. L., Surbone, A., Elk, R., Kagawa-Singer, M. 2018. Culture and palliative care: preferences, communication, meaning, and mutual decision making. *J Pain Symptom Manage,* **55**, 1408–1419.

Chen, A. T., Tsui, S., Sharma, R. K. 2022. Characterizing uncertainty in goals-of-care discussions among black and white patients: a qualitative study. *BMC Palliat Care,* **21**, 24.

Chung, G. S., Lawrence, R. E., Curlin, F. A., Arora, V., Meltzer, D. O. 2012. Predictors of hospitalised patients' preferences for physician-directed medical decision-making. *J Med Ethics,* **38**, 77–82.

Connor, S. R. (Ed.) 2020. *Global Atlas of Palliative Care*, 2nd edition. Worldwide Hospice Palliative Care Alliance.

Diernberger, K., Shinkins, B., Hall, P., Kaasa, S., Fallon, M. 2021. Incompatible: end-of-life care and health economics. *BMJ Support Palliat Care,* **11**, 296–298.

El-Jawahri, A., Greer, J. A., Pirl, W. F., et al. 2017. Effects of early integrated palliative care on caregivers of patients with lung and gastrointestinal cancer: a randomized clinical trial. *Oncologist,* **22**, 1528–1534.

Elwyn, G., Durand, M. A., Song, J., et al. 2017. A three-talk model for shared decision making: multistage consultation process. *BMJ,* **359**, j4891.

Elwyn, G., Price, A., Franco, J. V. A., Gulbrandsen, P. 2023. The limits of shared decision making. *BMJ Evid Based Med,* **28**, 218–221.

Ferrell, B. R., Twaddle, M. L., Melnick, A., Meier, D. E. 2018. National Consensus Project Clinical Practice Guidelines for Quality Palliative Care Guidelines, 4th Edition. *J Palliat Med,* **21**, 1684–1689.

Ha, J.-H., Lee, C., Yoo, J. 2023. Cultural differences in advance care planning and implications for practice. *Omega,* **87**, 838–855.

Hargraves, I. G., Montori, V. M., Brito, J. P., et al. 2019. Purposeful SDM: a problem-based approach to caring for patients with shared decision making. *Patient Educ Couns,* **102**, 1786–1792.

Hoerger, M., Greer, J. A., Jackson, V. A., et al. 2018. Defining the elements of early palliative care that are associated with patient-reported outcomes and the delivery of end-of-life care. *J Clin Oncol,* **36**, 1096–1102.

Hui, D., Bruera, E. 2020. Models of palliative care delivery for patients with cancer. *J Clin Oncol,* **38**, 852–865.

Hurst, D. J., Potter, J., Naumann, P., et al. 2022. Barriers to patient involvement in decision-making in advanced cancer care: culture as an amplifier. *Narrat Inq Bioethics,* **12**, 77–92.

Kavalieratos, D., Corbelli, J., Zhang, D., et al. 2016. Association between palliative care and patient and caregiver outcomes: a systematic review and meta-analysis. *JAMA,* **316**, 2104–2114.

Kelley, A. S., Bollens-Lund, E. 2018. Identifying the population with serious illness: the 'denominator' challenge. *J Palliat Med,* **21**, S7–S16.

Khayal, I. S., Barnato, A. E. 2022. What is in the palliative care 'syringe'? A systems perspective. *Soc Sci Med,* **305**, 115069.

Kuosmanen, L., Hupli, M., Ahtiluoto, S., Haavisto, E. 2021. Patient participation in shared decision-making in palliative care—an integrative review. *J Clin Nurs,* **30**, 3415–3428.

Levinson, W., Kao, A., Kuby, A., Thisted, R. A. 2005. Not all patients want to participate in decision making. A national study of public preferences. *J Gen Intern Med,* **20**, 531–535.

Arias-Casais, N., Garralda, E., Rhee, J. Y., et al. 2019. EAPC Atlas of Palliative Care in Europe. EAPC Press. Available at: https://view.pagetiger.com/gwirld/1

Marie Curie. 2022. Universal principles for advance care planning. Available at: https://www.mariecurie.org.uk/help/support/terminal-illness/planning-ahead/advance-care-planning

Mitchell, A. J., Chan, M., Bhatti, H., et al. 2011. Prevalence of depression, anxiety, and adjustment disorder in oncological, haematological, and palliative-care settings: a meta-analysis of 94 interview-based studies. *Lancet Oncol,* **12**, 160–174.

Montori, V. M., Ruissen, M. M., Hargraves, I. G., Brito, J. P., Kunneman, M. 2023. Shared decision-making as a method of care. *BMJ Evid Based Med,* **28**, 213–217.

Morrison, R. S. 2013. Models of palliative care delivery in the United States. *Curr Opin Support Palliat Care,* **7**, 201–206.

Mulcahy Symmons, S., Ryan, K., Aoun, S. M., et al. 2023. Decision-making in palliative care: patient and family caregiver concordance and discordance—systematic review and narrative synthesis. *BMJ Support Palliat Care,* **13**, 374–385.

National Institute on Aging. 2021. What are palliative care and hospice care? Available at: https://www.nia.nih.gov/health/hospice-and-palliative-care/what-are-palliative-care-and-hospice-care

NHS England. 2022. Universal principles for advance care planning. Available at: https://www.england.nhs.uk/wp-content/uploads/2022/03/universal-principles-for-advance-care-planning.pdf

Paladino, J., Bernacki, R., Neville, B. A., et al. 2019. Evaluating an intervention to improve communication between oncology clinicians and patients with life-limiting cancer: a cluster randomized clinical trial of the Serious Illness Care Program. *JAMA Oncol,* **5**, 801–809.

Paladino, J., Koritsanszky, L., Nisotel, L., et al. 2020. Patient and clinician experience of a serious illness conversation guide in oncology: a descriptive analysis. *Cancer Med,* **9**, 4550–4560.

Palliative Care Network of Wisconsin. 2019. Consultation etiquette in palliative care. Available at: https://www.mypcnow.org/fast-fact/consultation-etiquette-in-palliative-care/

Payne, S., Harding, A., Williams, T., Ling, J., Ostgathe, C. 2022. Revised recommendations on standards and norms for palliative care in Europe from the European Association for Palliative Care (EAPC): a Delphi study. *Palliat Med,* **36**, 680–697.

Quill T. E., Abernethy, A. P. 2013. Generalist plus specialist palliative care—creating a more sustainable model. *N Engl J Med,* **368**, 1173–1175.

Robinson, J., Gott, M., Ingleton, C. 2014. Patient and family experiences of palliative care in hospital: what do we know? An integrative review. *Palliat Med,* **28**, 18–33.

Rogers, J. G., Patel, C. B., Mentz, R. J., et al. 2017. Palliative care in heart failure: the PAL-HF randomized, controlled clinical trial. *J Am Coll Cardiol,* **70**, 331–341.

Sheikh, M., Sekaran, S., Kochhar, H., et al. 2022. Hospice vs palliative care: a comprehensive review for primary care physician. *J Family Med Prim Care,* **11**, 4168–4173.

Sudore, R. L., Lum, H. D., You, J. J., et al. 2017. Defining advance care planning for adults: a consensus definition from a multidisciplinary Delphi panel. *J Pain Symptom Manage,* **53**, 821–832.e1.

Temel, J. S., Greer, J. A., Muzikansky, A., et al. 2010. Early palliative care for patients with metastatic non-small-cell lung cancer. *N Engl J Med,* **363**, 733–742.

Wachterman, M. W., Sommers, B. D. 2021. Dying poor in the US—disparities in end-of-life care. *JAMA,* **325**, 423–424.

World Health Organization. n.d. Palliative care. Available at: https://www.who.int/health-topics/palliative-care

World Health Organization. 2012. Definition of palliative care. Available at: https://www.who.int/cancer/palliative/definition/en/

Yoong, J., Park, E. R., Greer, J. A., et al. 2013. Early palliative care in advanced lung cancer: a qualitative study. *JAMA Intern Med,* **173**, 283–290.

52

Shared decision making in intensive care and anaesthetics

Mark D. Neuman, Mary C. Politi, May Hua, and Hugo Campos

Introduction and clinical context

Anaesthesia and intensive care are complex, specialized medical domains that have wide impacts on health and patient experiences worldwide. Over 300 million surgical procedures occur annually worldwide, often requiring anaesthesia (Weiser et al., 2015). Conditions requiring intensive care unit (ICU) treatment affect over 20 million individuals globally each year (Adhikari et al., 2010).

Anaesthesia and intensive care both represent high-risk decision making environments. Choices between treatment strategies frequently involve substantial uncertainty. Decisions may occur in time-limited settings, particularly for urgent or emergent surgery or unanticipated critical illnesses. Anaesthesia and intensive care depend extensively on technology for diagnosis, monitoring, and treatment, potentially adding complexity to decisions. Involvement of family members and other caregivers frequently requires integrating multiple (and at times conflicting) perspectives, beliefs, and attitudes.

In this context, important questions exist about which decisions are most amenable to shared decision making (SDM) and how best to support such decisions. The following sections address four key questions about SDM in anaesthesia and intensive care: first, what types of decisions are encountered in anaesthesia and intensive care, and which are most likely to be appropriate for SDM? Second, what is the current extent of SDM around common choices in anaesthesia and intensive care? Third, what interventions have been shown to increase SDM in these contexts? Fourth, what opportunities exist for future research on SDM in anaesthesia and intensive care? Finally, we conclude with a patient perspective, examining potential challenges and opportunities in this context.

What types of decisions are encountered in anaesthesia and intensive care, and which are most likely to be appropriate for SDM?

The modern practice of anaesthesia and intensive care each encompass a broad range of decisions that vary in their urgency, degree of uncertainty, and technical complexity. Certain choices in each domain may additionally be contingent on other upstream treatment decisions. For example, in cases where a certain type of anaesthesia or postoperative intensive care is required for a given surgery to proceed safely, a decision to undergo certain surgical procedures implies a decision also to accept anaesthesia and/or certain critical care services. As such, SDM within these disciplines needs to consider each treatment on its own and the larger treatment context, including implications of upstream decisions to pursue or decline a course of treatment.

Understanding which decisions may or may not be amenable to SDM within anaesthesia and intensive care remains an active discussion area for each discipline. The only contexts in which some degree of SDM is unlikely to be possible at all are those in which (1) the time required to complete SDM would itself potentially compromise stated or implied goals of care (i.e. emergency care where any delay in therapy could lead to death or permanent disability), or (2) upstream decisions dictate a particular course of anaesthesia or critical care to which no safe or feasible alternatives exist. Table 52.1 presents selected examples of such scenarios.

Beyond these specific scenarios, the application of SDM to decisions in anaesthesia and critical care is limited principally by

Table 52.1 Examples in which SDM is unlikely to be possible or not recommended

Reason	Anaesthesia examples	Critical care examples
Unable to delay treatment without risk of harm/disease progression	Endotracheal intubation for rapidly progressing airway compromise Blood transfusion for exsanguination due to multiple trauma	Placement of chest tube for tension pneumothorax Initiation of cardiopulmonary resuscitation for patient in cardiac arrest without a do-not-resuscitate order
Lack of safe alternatives to default treatment	General anaesthesia with positive-pressureventilation for lung resection Central venous access to facilitate volume resuscitation during liver transplantation	Continuation of mechanical ventilation postoperatively following major aortic surgery Invasive neurological monitoring following decompressive craniotomy for stroke

(1) time available within the clinical interaction, (2) preferences of patient and family members regarding involvement in decisions, and (3) clinician attitudes and behaviours. Certain decisions have traditionally been seen as too technical or complex to present to patients—such as the specific selection of drugs for general anaesthesia or choices between different approaches for peripheral nerve block placement (Tylee et al., 2020). Yet recent work has shown that patients may be effectively engaged in decisions regarding not only broad choices between which type of anaesthesia they will receive but also aspects of how anaesthesia will be delivered (Pennington et al., 2023). Moreover, many patients have had past experiences with anaesthesia or critical care or have learned about relevant medications—such as propofol, fentanyl, and ketamine—from the lay press and social media outlets. In these scenarios, patients or their families may express desires to participate in decisions about specific aspects of care, creating potential opportunities for SDM in these contexts.

For patients receiving critical care services, SDM plays an important role due to the inherent uncertainty of survival, the morbidity associated with survival, and the potential for patients to be left in states worse than death. Frequently, clinical decisions must be made related to the initiation, continuation, and withdrawal of life-sustaining therapies (i.e. mechanical ventilation, prolonged mechanical ventilation requiring tracheostomy, dialysis, mechanical circulatory support, vasopressor, and inotropic therapy). The American Thoracic Society and American College of Critical Care Medicine recommend that SDM be the default practice in the ICU and put forward a framework intended to encourage goals-of-care conversations with patients and their families to elicit values that can guide decision making during critical care episodes (Kon et al., 2016). In practice, the use of SDM in determining goals of care is more likely to occur in situations where favourable outcomes with respect to mortality and morbidity (e.g. functional and cognitive ability, health-related quality of life) may not be achievable, as opposed to being routine (Kruser et al., 2019). Barriers to a default practice of SDM, particularly before initiating life-sustaining therapy, relate to issues with the feasibility of implementation. A large number of patients require a temporary course of life-sustaining therapy, and having conversations to facilitate SDM is time-consuming. For most patients with critical illness, at least at the outset, survival is the default goal of care; thus, assuming a course of therapy that prioritizes survival will lead to the provision of goal-concordant care much of the time.

What is the current extent of SDM around common choices in anaesthesia and intensive care?

Evidence suggests a substantial opportunity to increase SDM surrounding common treatment choices in anaesthesia and intensive care. Although most patients express *wanting* to be involved in their anaesthesia decisions, clinicians frequently fail to engage them in decision making (Tylee et al., 2020). In a survey of patients who had previously undergone anaesthesia, only 7.8% reported fully engaging in SDM about anaesthetic options as suggested by low collaboRATE scores (Pennington et al., 2023). Despite these low scores, a majority of respondents stated that their anaesthesia clinicians encouraged them to ask questions, highlighting opportunities to increase SDM over time in this context.

One specific domain in which SDM is actively encouraged within anaesthesia care concerns patients with existing do-not-resuscitate orders who require surgery and anaesthesia. In these settings, national guidelines recommend that clinicians engage patients and families in discussions to assess willingness to permit certain aspects of resuscitative care (e.g. intubation and mechanical ventilation, use of vasoactive medications) during surgery to allow surgery to occur safely. Nonetheless, fewer than 20% of patients with pre-existing do-not-resuscitate orders have a documented discussion of code status before surgery (Hadler et al., 2021).

In the ICU, preference-sensitive decisions are often associated with high stakes. The use of SDM and its principles are well accepted as the ideal mode of communication, but evidence suggests that current practice falls short. Up to 20% of surrogate decision makers (i.e. a family member or other legally designated representative for a patient who cannot make their own decisions due to illness or other factors) report having moderate to strong decision regret, and 50% report mild regret (Andersen et al., 2023). Elements of SDM are often employed during clinical conversations, but several areas may be improved, particularly related to incorporating patient values into decision making. In a study where clinicians were given a scenario and asked to perform a simulated conference discussing the decision to intubate a patient, clinicians commonly shared information and elicited preferences related explicitly to intubation. Still, few explored broader patient or family values (Uy et al., 2013). Similarly, a study of audio-recorded family conferences demonstrated that about 25% of the time, family conferences addressing goals of care did not contain information exchange or value elicitation. Although values were discussed in 68% of conferences, these values were only applied to decisions 44% of the time (Scheunemann et al., 2019). Additionally, there is room to improve clinician skills in addressing emotions and how decisions are framed. Often, intensivists may ask questions regarding treatment using leading phrases that evoke aspirational instead of realistic goals (e.g. 'Would you like us to do everything?' 'What would your loved one want?') and, thus, do not truly promote SDM. While studies have demonstrated gaps in practice, the importance of SDM in the ICU is also clear, as increased use of SDM behaviours has been associated with having increased trust in a physician (Lincoln et al., 2023). As our patient perspective box makes clear, following and respecting patient preferences, even if they are at odds with well-intentioned interventions, lead to good, sometimes unexpected outcomes (Box 52.1).

What interventions have been shown to increase SDM in these contexts?

Supplementing SDM with high-quality patient decision aids is one way to 'level the playing field' for those being seen by care team members who do not always think about patient engagement.

Box 52.1 Patient perspective

'Don't let me die here': Hugo Campos

When Dad experienced severe shortness of breath, his emergency hospital visit led to an unexpected admission. A bedside echocardiogram revealed a large pericardial effusion and a computed tomography scan confirmed a high risk of cardiac tamponade. Despite a pericardiocentesis removing 1.6 litres of fluid from his heart, fluid reaccumulated quickly.

At 91, with many serious health issues, severe hearing loss, and limited cognitive ability, Dad struggled with decision making in his native Portuguese. Since my mother's death, I have been his sole advocate and interpreter, the person who best understands his values and preferences. Despite my own practical knowledge of cardiac issues, coordinating Dad's care and aligning it with his expectations was challenging due to fragmented communication from various doctors.

Navigating the hospital experience was also daunting. The asymmetry of knowledge, power, and lived experiences between doctor and patient puts patients at an enormous disadvantage. Patient portals, mobile health apps, and emerging technologies like generative artificial intelligence may play crucial roles in bridging this gap, enhancing patient literacy, and fostering collaborative doctor–patient relationships.

Dad's worsening condition necessitated a subxiphoid pericardiostomy to drain more fluid from his heart. Dad and I discussed the risks, and despite his fragile health, we consented to the procedure. The pericardiostomy successfully removed an additional 700 millilitres of fluid. Healthcare is inherently uncertain, and despite approaches like SDM, we can never be entirely certain about our choices.

In the ICU, Dad developed severe delirium, and his health declined. He hated it there. I stayed by his side, day after day, sleeping on a couch in a hospital room. During rare moments of lucidity, he begged me to bring him home. He eventually had enough and became adamant about his wishes to leave the hospital. 'I don't care if I die, but I just don't want to die here', he said.

This led to a difficult decision. I informed the hospitalist of our plan to go home and that we no longer consented to further interventions. I requested that the drainage tube be removed and preparations be made for the discharge and transition home. The doctor disagreed with our request but responded with empathy that he would do what he could to make it happen. The following morning, Dad was discharged to hospice care. This experience underscored the importance of empathy and the fact that SDM isn't just about facts—it's about respecting patients' unique lives and stories.

At home, Dad's first meal was a hot bowl of 'canja de galinha', my mother's recipe for Portuguese chicken and rice soup. His mood soon improved and his health followed. Two months later, Dad was discharged from hospice. Two years later, he is still with us.

Decision aids can present information to patients in plain language with balanced information reviewed by end users. They can be less biased than conversations because information can be thoroughly reviewed by end users. However, it is not always possible to develop detailed patient decision aids for use in anaesthesia choices in the context of urgent or emergent surgery or unanticipated critical illness. Thus, conversation aids could address this potential barrier to SDM in this context by creating brief, structured information to enhance discussions without being too prescriptive or detailed. Preliminary evidence suggests that conversation aids that support deliberation could decrease decisional conflict, increase knowledge, and are acceptable to patients considering anaesthesia choices. Table 52.2 summarizes evidence about conversation aids and longer decision aids in this context.

Early-stage evidence also highlights the potential for decision aids to increase SDM in ICU settings. In a recent scoping review of the ICU SDM literature, Lei and colleagues identified nine available decision aids described between 2012 and 2022 (Lei et al., 2023). These decision aids have primarily focused on decisions related to end-of-life care and life-sustaining therapies; specific topics addressed included goals of care, cardiopulmonary resuscitation, use of prolonged mechanical ventilation, and use of renal replacement therapy. Several aids have also focused on supporting surrogate decision makers (e.g. education about the role of a surrogate decision maker, tips for self-care) to aid their participation in the decision making process. Overall, available studies to date have demonstrated that the usability and acceptability of aids are high, and that decision aids have a positive impact on knowledge but do not have a significant effect on prognostic discordance or decision quality. Notably, in one study, surrogates who engaged with a decision aid had worse psychological distress in comparison to usual care at 3 months, suggesting that there also may be potential for harm when aids are used in high-stakes decision making (Muehlschlegel et al., 2022). To help address this possibility, certain interventions currently being studied are designed to provide emotional and psychological support in addition to decisional support for surrogates (Seaman et al., 2018). These interventions acknowledge how stressful and upsetting being a surrogate for a loved one in the ICU can be and the need to help surrogates achieve an emotional state conducive to decision making. Lastly, interventions to improve clinicians' communication skills may also help to increase the likelihood of SDM (Milnes et al., 2023).

What opportunities exist for future research on SDM in anaesthesia and intensive care?

Anaesthesia and critical care team members might worry about SDM increasing the duration of clinical encounters (Elwyn et al., 2013), though conversation aids might not impact encounter length and can be learned quickly (Scalia et al., 2019). Clinicians might also perceive that some patients might not want to engage in SDM (Politi et al., 2013). Training programmes are needed to address these barriers and misperceptions. Although there are numerous SDM guides, data on their effectiveness is limited. International, interdisciplinary experts have agreed on the importance of active listening, plain language terminology, appropriate risk communication, and shared deliberation in SDM training (Légaré et al., 2013). Role play-based training and workshops emphasizing practical skills might lead to more SDM proficiency than didactic theoretical presentations of SDM (Joseph-Williams et al., 2017). More research is needed on ways to enhance anaesthesia and critical care team members' SDM competencies and evaluate the most effective SDM for choices. In the ICU, principles of SDM are much better

Table 52.2 Summary of selected studies of decision aids for anaesthesia care and critical care

Authors, year	Decision scenario	Setting	Study design and sample size	Main findings
Posner et al., 2015	Regional anaesthesia vs alternatives for general/ orthopaedic surgery	Pre-anaesthesia clinic	Pre–post; n = 16	Decision aid use increased discussion of alternatives and patient knowledge about regional anaesthesia
Warner et al., 2015	Smoking cessation vs continuation or reduction prior to surgery	Pre-anaesthesia clinic	Single-centre randomized trial; n = 130	Decision aid use improved decisional quality and patient involvement in decision making but did not affect any aspect of perioperative smoking behaviour
Wilson et al., 2015	Cardiopulmonary resuscitation versus no cardiopulmonary resuscitation	ICU	Single-centre randomized trial; n = 208 patients and surrogates	Video decision aid use improved knowledge and did not change documented resuscitation preferences
Cox et al., 2019	Goals of care for prolonged mechanical ventilation (maximize comfort, aim for survival but avoid prolonged treatment, or maximize survival)	ICU	Multicentre randomized controlled trial; n = 277 patients, 416 surrogates, and 427 clinicians	Decision aid use did not improve prognostic concordance, but was associated with less decisional conflict
Shishido et al., 2020	Epidural analgesia during labour versus no epidural	Labor and delivery service	Pre–post; n = 300	Decision aid use was associated with less decisional conflict, greater knowledge of epidural anaesthesia and satisfaction with decision making, and less uncertainty
Beight et al., 2022	Monitored anaesthesia care for breast surgery vs alternatives	Pre-anaesthesia clinic	Cross-sectional study; n = 32	66% of patients agreed that use of the decision aid increased understanding of options
Muehlschlegel et al., 2022	Goals of care (survival versus comfort care) for patients with acute brain injury	ICU	Multicentre randomized trial; n = 66 surrogates	Decision aid use was associated with fewer changes in code status
Wang et al., 2022	Sugammadex versus neostigmine for operative neuromuscular blockade reversal	Pre-anaesthesia clinic	Multicentre randomized trial; n = 3132	Patients receiving the decision had greater knowledge regarding their options, felt better informed, and felt surer about their choice. Those who received the aid were more likely to choose sugammadex over neostigmine

accepted and incorporated into clinical practice. However, opportunities exist to elicit values and apply them to decision making more consistently. The development of additional decision aids for other value-laden decisions (e.g. tracheostomy) is another area for potential research, although existing decision aids have been limited in their impact. Table 52.3 summarizes barriers to SDM in this context and opportunities to address these in the near and long term.

Table 52.3 Selected barriers to SDM in anaesthesia and critical care and opportunities for future research

Barrier	Opportunities for future research
Lack of research on SDM in anaesthesia	Build on studies in critical care; engage patients and end users in the design, conduct, and evaluation of SDM
Time and resource pressures in both anaesthesia and critical care settings	Use conversation aids rather than longer decision aids; train clinicians in collaborative approaches to conversations in the absence of a written guide; identify situations in which SDM is and is not feasible
Lack of training in SDM in anaesthesia; lack of application of training on goals-of-care conversations in critical care settings	Role play-based training and workshops emphasizing practical skills, focusing on unique contexts in anaesthesia and critical care settings
Lack of evidence-based SDM tools, conversation aids, or decision aids	Design, test, and implement conversation aids or decisions for specific anaesthesia or critical care clinical contexts
Clarity on appropriate SDM decision targets and outcomes for anaesthesiology and critical care settings	Build consensus on appropriate outcomes such as decisional conflict, decision regret, and level of desired individual and family engagement, some of which overlap with standard decision outcomes in other contexts, others of which might be unique

REFERENCES

Adhikari, N. K., Fowler, R. A., Bhagwanjee, S., Rubenfeld, G. D. 2010. Critical care and the global burden of critical illness in adults. *Lancet,* **376**, 1339–1346.

Andersen, S. K., Butler, R. A., Chang, C. H., Arnold, R., Angus, D. C., White, D. B. 2023. Prevalence of long-term decision regret and associated risk factors in a large cohort of ICU surrogate decision makers. *Crit Care,* **27**, 61.

Beight, L., Pardo, J., McCarthy, K., et al. 2022. An electronic monitored anesthesia care (MAC) decision aid for breast conserving surgery. *J Clinical Anesth,* **78**, 110648.

Cox, C. E., White, D. B., Hough, C. L., et al. 2019. Effects of a personalized web-based decision aid for surrogate decision makers of patients with prolonged mechanical ventilation: a randomized clinical trial. *Ann Intern Med,* **170**, 285–297.

Elwyn, G., Scholl, I., Tietbohl, C., et al. 2013. 'Many miles to go ...': a systematic review of the implementation of patient decision support interventions into routine clinical practice. *BMC Med Inform Decis Mak,* **13**, S14.

Hadler, R. A., Fatuzzo, M., Sahota, G., Neuman, M. D. 2021. Perioperative management of do-not-resuscitate orders at a large academic health system. *JAMA Surg,* **156**, 1175–1177.

Joseph-Williams, N., Lloyd, A., Edwards, A., et al. 2017. Implementing shared decision making in the NHS: lessons from the MAGIC programme. *BMJ,* **357**, j1744.

Kon, A. A., Davidson, J. E., Morrison, W., Danis, M., White, D. B. 2016. Shared decision-making in intensive care units. Executive summary of the American College of Critical Care Medicine and American Thoracic Society policy statement. *Am J Respir Crit Care Med,* **193**, 1334–1336.

Kruser, J. M., Benjamin, B. T., Gordon, E. J., et al. 2019. Patient and family engagement during treatment decisions in an ICU: a discourse analysis of the electronic health record. *Crit Care Med,* **47**, 784–791.

Légaré, F., Moumjid-Ferdjaoui, N., Drolet, R., et al. 2013. Core competencies for shared decision making training programs: insights from an international, interdisciplinary working group. *J Contin Educ Health Prof,* **33**, 267–273.

Lei, Y., Zhou, Q., Tao, Y. 2023. Decision aids in the ICU: a scoping review. *BMJ Open,* **13**, e075239.

Lincoln, T. E., Buddadhumaruk, P., Arnold, R. M., et al. 2023. Association between shared decision-making during family meetings and surrogates' trust in their ICU physician. *Chest,* **163**, 1214–1224.

Milnes, S. L., Kerr, D. C., Hutchinson, A., et al. 2023. Effect of communication skills training on documentation of shared decision-making for patients with life-limiting illness: an observational study in an intensive care unit. *Crit Care Resusc,* **25**, 20–26.

Muehlschlegel, S., Goostrey, K., Flahive, J., Zhang, Q., Pach, J. J., Hwang, D. Y. 2022. A pilot randomized clinical trial of a goals-of-care decision aid for surrogates of severe acute brain injury patients. *Neurology,* **99**, e1446–e1455.

Pennington, B. R. T., Politi, M. C., Abdallah, A. B., et al. 2023. A survey of surgical patients' perspectives and preferences towards general anesthesia techniques and shared-decision making. *BMC Anesthesiol,* **23**, 277.

Politi, M. C., Dizon, D. S., Frosch, D. L., Kuzemchak, M. D., Stiggelbout, A. M. 2013. Importance of clarifying patients' desired role in shared decision making to match their level of engagement with their preferences. *BMJ,* **347**, f7066.

Posner, K., Mincer, S. L., Harvey, A. E., Xue, A. H., Van Norman, G. A., Domino, K. B. 2015. Regional anesthesia decision aids in the pre-anesthesia clinic improve patient engagement and knowledge. In: The Anesthesiology Annual Meeting, American Society of Anesthesiologists. Abstract A2211.

Scalia, P., Durand, M. A., Berkowitz, J. L., et al. 2019. The impact and utility of encounter patient decision aids: systematic review, meta-analysis and narrative synthesis. *Patient Educ Couns,* **102**, 817–841.

Scheunemann, L. P., Ernecoff, N. C., Buddadhumaruk, P., et al. 2019. Clinician-family communication about patients' values and preferences in intensive care units. *JAMA Intern Med,* **179**, 676–684.

Seaman, J. B., Arnold, R. M., Buddadhumaruk, P., et al. 2018. Protocol and fidelity monitoring plan for four supports. a multicenter trial of an intervention to support surrogate decision makers in intensive care units. *Ann Am Thorac Soc,* **15**, 1083–1091.

Shishido, E., Osaka, W., Henna, A., Motomura, Y., Horiuchi, S. 2020. Effect of a decision aid on the choice of pregnant women whether to have epidural anesthesia or not during labor. *PLoS One,* **15**, e0242351.

Tylee, M. J., Rubenfeld, G. D., Wijeysundera, D., Sklar, M. C., Hussain, S., Adhikari, N. K. J. 2020. Anesthesiologist to patient communication: a systematic review. *JAMA Netw Open,* **3**, e2023503.

Uy, J., White, D. B., Mohan, D., Arnold, R. M., Barnato, A. E. 2013. Physicians' decision-making roles for an acutely unstable critically and terminally ill patient. *Crit Care Med,* **41**, 1511–1517.

Wang, L. K., Lin, Y. T., Chen, J. T., et al. 2023. Effect of patient decision aids on choice between sugammadex and neostigmine in surgeries under general anesthesia: a multicenter randomized controlled trial. *Korean J Anesthesiol,* **76**, 280–289.

Warner, D. O., LeBlanc, A., Kadimpati, S., Vickers, K. S., Shi, Y., Montori, V. M. 2015. Decision aid for cigarette smokers scheduled for elective surgery. *Anesthesiology,* **123**, 18–28.

Weiser, T. G., Haynes, A. B., Molina, G., et al. 2015. Estimate of the global volume of surgery in 2012: an assessment supporting improved health outcomes. *Lancet,* **385**, S11.

Wilson, M. E., Krupa, A., Hinds, R. F., et al. 2015. A video to improve patient and surrogate understanding of cardiopulmonary resuscitation choices in the ICU: a randomized controlled trial. *Crit Care Med,* **43**, 621–629.

53

Shared decision making in psychosomatic conditions

Yaara Zisman-Ilani, Wiebke Frerichs, Scout Silverstein, and Martin Härter

Introduction

Shared decision making (SDM) has traditionally focused on improving decision making processes and promoting person-centred care in medical settings involving specific medical decisions and focusing primarily on somatic conditions. In the last two decades, an expansion of SDM to mental health conditions has evolved, addressing primarily pharmacological decisions (Zisman-Ilani et al., 2017). Yet, SDM has been less often applied in conditions where psychosocial factors in the aetiology, course, and adaption to those conditions play a major role. This chapter discusses how SDM can be better applied to psychosomatic conditions, by describing examples of efforts to promote SDM in this field, considering existing challenges, and pointing out evolving opportunities.

Psychosomatic medicine and conditions: working definition

Modern medicine acknowledges that most health conditions, somatic and mental, are affected by genetics and biology, but also by the environment as well as psychological and social factors. Such a holistic view of health is rooted in the biopsychosocial model (Engel, 1977) and is also represented by modern psychological approaches and public health frameworks such as the social determinants of health, where individuals are viewed in the context of their psychosocial environment. Psychosomatic medicine, a specialty of medicine, focuses on the health conditions where a mind–body connection is of important clinical significance.

Psychosomatic medicine initially evolved in Western Europe, Germany in particular, between the two world wars, as a branch of psychiatry heavily influenced by the psychoanalytical lens and Freudian ideas (Zipfel et al., 2016; Deter et al., 2018). Early conceptions of psychosomatic medicine believed in the mind–body relationship, and understood and treated somatic conditions as the results of psychological states (Theorell, 2007). The rise of the Nazis in Germany in 1933 led to a swift exodus and emigration of many psychosomatic practitioners to the USA and the UK. Here psychosomatic medicine thought leaders, and practitioners, were influenced by new ideas about group and family impacts on health, or where the context and environments play roles in an individual's health (Deter et al., 2018). This emerging holistic perception of the coexistent influences of somatic, or biological, factors, along with psychological and social/environmental factors has led to an updated perception of psychosomatic conditions, also known as the biopsychosocial model (Theorell, 2007; Zipfel et al., 2016; Deter et al., 2018).

Today, psychosomatic conditions encompass patients with different, often long-term conditions with medical and psychological impacts on patients' health, functioning, and quality of life. Psychosomatic conditions include mental-focused disorders such as somatoform disorders (e.g. pain disorder, conversion disorder), headaches, sexual dysfunction, and eating disorders, but also physical conditions such as cancer, coronary heart disease, asthma, and diabetes, where emotional and psychological conditions result in and/or increase physiological impacts on the body. Many of the psychosomatic conditions are characterized by increased levels of depression and anxiety.

Putting theory into practice—examples of SDM research in fibromyalgia, psoriasis, and eating disorders

Not many studies exist demonstrating the use of SDM in psychosomatic conditions. For example, in psoriasis, a long-term inflammatory skin disorder, psychological stressors can trigger flare-ups due to intricate nervous, immune, and endocrine system interactions. Yet, most SDM studies are mainly focused on pharmacological options (Larsen et al., 2019). Tan and Wolfe developed and explored a patient decision aid (PtDA) for psoriasis treatment selection (Figure 53.1) (Tan and Wolfe, 2012, 2014). While limited by sample size and lacking a control group, their pilot study yielded promising results. The PtDA demonstrably reduced decisional conflict, increased preparedness

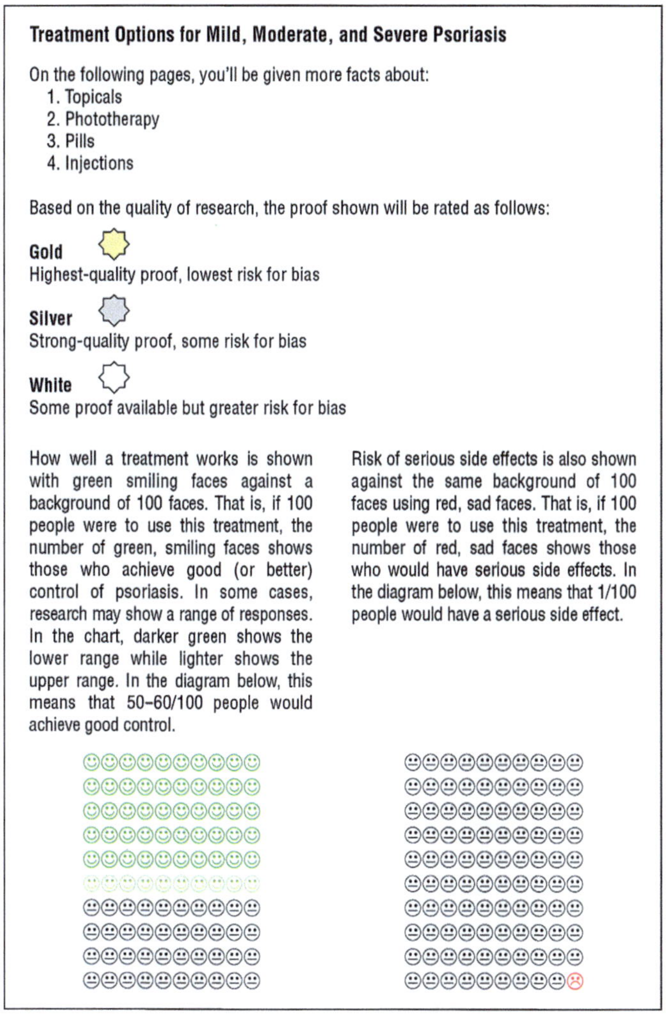

Figure 53.1 Example of the patient decision aid treatment options for mild, moderate, and severe psoriasis.

Reproduced with permission from Tan, J., Wolfe, B. 2012. A patient decision aid for psoriasis based on current clinical practice guidelines. *Arch Dermatol*, 148, 718–723.

for decision making, and improved knowledge and confidence in discussing pharmacological options with dermatologists. The PtDA also influenced treatment preferences: patients shifted towards less intensive options (topicals and phototherapy) after PtDA use, aligning with SDM principles and potentially leading to more cost-effective and patient-centred care. Further analysis revealed a personalized approach: people with milder cases opted for less intensive treatments, while people with severe cases chose stronger options. This could benefit both patients and dermatologists by streamlining consultations and improving treatment adherence. Positive feedback on the tool suggests its potential for wider patient use.

Tan and Wolfe's study sheds light on PtDA application in psoriasis management (Tan and Wolfe, 2014). The observed reduction in decisional conflict and improved preparedness highlights the PtDA's potential to empower patients in navigating psoriasis treatment decisions. As the first intervention study exploring SDM in psoriasis, further research with larger and controlled study designs is crucial to confirm these promising findings and establish the PtDA's role in optimizing SDM for individuals with psoriasis. Inclusion of psychological and psychosocial factors and treatment options into existing medical-based psoriasis PtDAs or in addition to existing psoriasis PtDAs can improve SDM (Larsen et al., 2019), making it more relevant to the patient's daily experiences (e.g. addressing stigma, shame, and so on).

Fibromyalgia syndrome (FMS) is another psychosomatic condition, which exemplifies applied SDM research, with patient-centred communication and collaborative decision making, and SDM emerges as a promising strategy to improve treatment and satisfaction in FMS management. The condition is marked by widespread pain and potential psychological complexities and challenges. Bieber and colleagues studied an SDM intervention for physicians treating patients with FMS (Bieber et al., 2008). This intervention, involving patient education about common symptoms, diagnosis, pathogenesis, treatment options, and prognosis, and physician communication training, led to significantly better patient-reported communication compared to a control group. This suggests SDM training can enhance communication and potentially improve patient experience. However, limitations existed, mainly regarding the study setting and potential bias. Further research was needed to explore the long-term impact and broader applicability of SDM in FMS care.

Addressing these limitations, Bieber and colleagues conducted a 1-year follow-up study (Bieber et al., 2006). The study confirmed the sustained positive effects of SDM on communication and revealed improved coping skills in the SDM group, suggesting a potential benefit for patient well-being. While direct health-related outcomes remained unchanged, these findings solidify SDM's value in improving communication and patient experience in FMS management. These studies demonstrate the potential of SDM to enhance communication, empower patients, and potentially improve coping skills in FMS management. These findings warrant further research on the broader applicability and long-term impact of SDM interventions, paving the way for its potential inclusion as standard practice in FMS care.

There is limited research on SDM in eating disorders, although there are many opportunities where SDM could be integrated, as exemplified by the patient's perspective (Box 53.1) (Himmerich et al., 2019). Eating disorders are characterized by disordered eating and weight-control behaviours that impair physical health and psychosocial functioning. Klein and colleagues described a decision tool for treating athletes with eating disorders to determine safety risks for return to sport (Klein et al., 2021). The decision tool presents several risk factors and describes the magnitude of risk for each risk category (weight status, caloric intake, eating disorder behaviour frequency, menstrual status, and bone health). Developing SDM tools for drug-related treatments for eating disorders, discussing psychopharmacological treatments, potential comorbid mental disorders, and pharmacological strategies to alleviate the health consequences of an eating disorder may be further avenues to develop SDM in eating disorders (Himmerich et al., 2019).

Challenges for SDM in psychosomatic conditions

The power of the 'classical' SDM approach is in addressing specific and defined decisions with clear treatment options from which to choose. However, in psychosomatic conditions as well as chronic diseases, when a myriad of symptoms and complaints co-occur and

Box 53.1 Patient perspective

I was diagnosed with an eating disorder (not otherwise specified) when I was 19. At the age of 28, under the setting of increased stress, I first met the criteria for anorexia nervosa. This led to my first admission to an eating disorder unit, as my condition escalated rapidly and the physical consequences required more intensive care than outpatient treatment could provide. During this time, I tried to leave the medical hospital to avoid transfer to a specialized eating disorder facility. Consequently, I was involuntarily committed to a facility where I experienced callous, unhelpful care. Over the following years, I remained quite ill. My illness severity was due, in part, to being underinsured and the resulting inaccessibility of high-quality care. However, the length and intensity of my illness were also attributed to my treatment providers neglecting to ask me what I knew about my illness, how I understood its function, and what language felt the most salient to describe my experience.

Four years later, still struggling with anorexia nervosa, I found myself once more in intensive medical care. Fortunately, this time I was incredibly lucky to have a team of providers who approached my care collaboratively, with me, for the first time, at the centre of the decision making process, emphasizing my autonomy and choice. They asked to learn more about my preferences and needs and discussed the next steps. For example, they let me choose where to order food from, a critical element in the treatment of anorexia nervosa, and when to walk outside. I often walked to a nearby park to enjoy fresh air, and I even took a cab home to pack a bag for the inevitable transfer to an eating disorder unit. Most importantly, the team let me direct them to where I would like to be sent for care. They listened to my experiences and perspectives and even asked me questions to learn from my narrative. I was offered this SDM process, complete with liberties and boundaries, which increased my resilience for the next step in my care. I was able to be admitted to the eating disorder treatment service I chose, where I stayed for an additional 6 weeks. I'm thrilled to say that this was my last inpatient admission to date, and I believe it is in large part due to the collaborative approach, as no decision about me was made without me.

I believe strongly in a person's right to choose how and when to receive treatment and which treatment they prefer. From my experience, I believe that SDM is beneficial not just in allowing for a less harmful experience of inpatient hospitalization but also in thinking expansively about what alternatives exist in deciding the next steps for care. Is community respite an option? Equine therapy? A psychosocial clubhouse? I imagine achieving SDM is not just life-changing for individuals with anorexia nervosa and other eating disorders but can be life-saving.

different health professionals should be involved, current, specified SDM tools and interventions are often not easily applicable and relevant and raise questions. For example, for a patient with a somatic condition, cancer, and a resulting psychological condition, depression, which decision aid should be used and by whom? Should it be a decision aid for a specific cancer type and a decision aid for depression? Should these decision aids be used creatively to encompass the co-occurring comorbid condition? Often, cancer is treated as the primary health condition, and the SDM focus is dedicated to choosing oncological therapy. Depression treatment decisions are viewed as secondary and are often led by oncologists with no specific training in depression care, which affects the quality of the depression-related SDM.

These questions arise in response to the long-term and complex nature of psychosomatic conditions, involving co-occurring symptoms and requiring different providers for different conditions and treatment plans, and where the focus is more about 'planning' than decision making (Joseph-Williams et al., 2019). However, psychosomatic conditions are also characterized by situations with no clear-cut simple solutions. Often patients with psychosomatic conditions are required to choose between different types of behavioural therapies, psychosocial interventions, and recovery or rehabilitation programmes. These are comprehensive interventions, including multicomponent elements, making a core principle of SDM, a comparison of options between nutritional rehabilitation and psychological therapies for a person with anorexia nervosa, for example, challenging. Behavioural and psychosocial intervention often cannot simply fit into a decision aid structure of pros and cons, and often these types of usually combined interventions do not have simple evidence-based power or effect, making a comparative option discussion less effective.

Recommendation for the SDM field

It is time to expand the 'classic' SDM model and tools that primarily focus on symptoms and medical treatments to psychosomatic conditions that are often longer term by nature, affected by psychosocial factors, and require multidisciplinary teams and treatments. When applying SDM in psychosomatic conditions, psychosocial factors should take centre stage, which aligns with the person-centred care approach and the biopsychosocial model of care. Current PtDA formats may be less relevant for many psychosomatic decisions.

New SDM tools and interventions are needed to account for the complex treatments and nature of psychosomatic conditions. We recommend that such interventions and tools will include educating providers, not just patients, on the nature of psychosomatic conditions, emphasizing that these conditions require long-term care and involve many decisions over time. Importantly, several treatment approaches should be combined instead of one (apparently) straightforward procedure as is often the case with 'classical' SDM. For example, SDM interventions that focus on shared care planning and preference elicitation that are common in the field of SDM in mental health (Zisman-Ilani et al., 2017) can be borrowed or used to inspire the development of a new line of SDM tools and interventions. These interventions do not involve PtDAs to weigh options, but instead focus on eliciting patient preferences and discussing patients' values. Goal-setting can also be integrated into the 'classical' SDM model. Goals play a central role in guiding decisions in long-term and/or psychosomatic conditions, although the clinician and the patient has to judge when and how often to focus on goals. Bringing goals into clearer focus changes how potential interventions are considered. A goal-based approach will strengthen the person-centred care being offered because it is more aligned to personal priorities, while also paying attention to what might be practical and realistic (Elwyn and Vermunt, 2020).

REFERENCES

Bieber, C., Müller, K. G., Blumenstiel, K., et al. 2006. Long-term effects of a shared decision-making intervention on physician–patient interaction and outcome in fibromyalgia. A qualitative and quantitative 1 year follow-up of a randomized controlled trial. *Patient Educ Couns*, **63**, 357–366.

Bieber, C., Müller, K. G., Blumenstiel, K., et al. 2008. A shared decision-making communication training program for physicians treating fibromyalgia patients: effects of a randomized controlled trial. *J Psychosom Res,* **64,** 13–20.

Deter, H. C., Kruse, J., Zipfel, S. 2018. History, aims and present structure of psychosomatic medicine in Germany. *Biopsychosoc Med,* **12,** 1.

Elwyn, G., Vermunt, N. P. C. A. 2020. Goal-based shared decision-making: developing an integrated model. *J Patient Exp,* **7,** 688–696.

Engel, G. L. 1977. The need for a new medical model: a challenge for biomedicine. *Science,* **196,** 129–136.

Himmerich, H., Bentley, J., Lichtblau, N., Brennan, C., Au, K. 2019. Facets of shared decision-making on drug treatment for adults with an eating disorder. *Int Rev Psychiatry,* **31,** 332–346.

Joseph-Williams, N., Williams, D., Wood, F., et al. 2019. A descriptive model of shared decision making derived from routine implementation in clinical practice ('Implement-SDM'): qualitative study. *Patient Educ Couns,* **102,** 1774–1785.

Klein, D. A., Sylvester, J. E., Schvey, N. A. 2021. Eating disorders in primary care: diagnosis and management. *Am Family Physician,* **103,** 22–32.

Larsen, M. H., Hagen, K. B., Krogstad, A. L., Wahl, A. K. 2019. Shared decision making in psoriasis: a systematic review of quantitative and qualitative studies. *Am J Clin Dermatol,* **20,** 13–29.

Tan, J., Wolfe, B. 2012. A patient decision aid for psoriasis based on current clinical practice guidelines. *Arch Dermatol,* **148,** 718–723.

Tan, J., Wolfe, B. 2014. Improved decisional conflict and preparedness for decision making using a patient decision aid for treatment selection in psoriasis: a pilot study. *J Cutaneous Med Surg,* **18,** 114–118.

Theorell, T. 2007. Psychosomatic medicine. In: Fink, G. Ed. Encyclopedia *of Stress,* 2nd edition, pp. 296–301. Academic Press.

Zipfel, S., Herzog, W., Kruse, J., Henningsen, P. 2016. Psychosomatic medicine in Germany: more timely than ever. *Psychother Psychosom,* **85,** 262–269.

Zisman-Ilani, Y., Barnett, E., Harik, J., Pavlo, A., O'Connell, M. 2017. Expanding the concept of shared decision making for mental health: systematic search and scoping review of interventions. *Ment Health Rev J,* **22,** 191–213.

54

Shared decision making in rheumatology

Namrata Singh, Eileen Davidson, Cheryl Crow, and Jennifer L. Barton

History and status of shared decision making in rheumatology

Despite the concept of shared decision making (SDM) being first introduced in 1972, its relevance to the clinical practice of rheumatology long predates the official definition (Morrison et al., 2022). Advances in understanding the pathophysiology of rheumatic diseases and an explosion of novel therapeutics and enhanced treatment strategies over the past quarter century have improved outcomes yet also introduced more complexity around decision making. With a greater understanding of disease processes and integration of patient experience into measuring response to therapy through patient-reported outcomes, the practice of rheumatology calls for a truly collaborative approach to ensure safe, high-quality care. This change is clearly stated in the perspective of our patient representative's comments (Box 54.1).

This shift from paternalism towards SDM has been acknowledged by persons living with rheumatic diseases and rheumatology professional societies and is reflected in clinical practice guidelines across multiple conditions, including rheumatoid arthritis (RA) (Conley et al., 2023), systemic lupus erythematosus, and psoriatic arthritis. Despite these calls to action, the question remains: what is the actual status of SDM in rheumatology?

A scoping review of the literature reporting on SDM in rheumatology identified 63 studies that included 13,767 patients and 396 clinicians, with just over half conducted in the USA (Morrison et al., 2022). The majority of studies focused on RA (68%), followed by lupus (17%), psoriatic arthritis (8%), and ankylosing spondylitis (8%). Thirteen decision aids (DAs) were identified, the majority of which focused on RA. SDM was associated with improvement in patient satisfaction, knowledge, self-efficacy, and improved trust with clinicians. Additional impacts of SDM included improved adherence to treatment plans and lower medication costs compared with patients who did not report SDM. Studies reported variation by patient characteristics with lower education, lower socioeconomic status, limited health literacy, and language barriers associated with reports of poor SDM communication. Clinician behaviours, such as being patient-centred, respectful, and sensitive, correlated with greater success in facilitating SDM.

In an attempt to understand why SDM may not be implemented in rheumatology clinical practice, the review uncovered several barriers. Rheumatologists voiced concern about adding time to a

Box 54.1 Patient perspective

SDM for a patient with a rheumatic disease

I actively strive to be involved in the decision making process, particularly when it comes to managing my rheumatic disease. It's not just about finding the right medications but also about choosing the best way of living with rheumatoid arthritis (RA).

RA affects so many areas of my life, much more than what can be covered in a short visit to my rheumatologist. By actively participating in decision making, I can better find solutions for managing my condition.

Having my rheumatologist lay out three pages of information about different medications was really helpful. The information came from someone I trusted. The visuals also helped more than reading a block of words. Appointments can cause a lot of anxiety and fear, making it difficult to concentrate and take in new information.

As I understood my illness more, I found that making decisions became less daunting. The more I learned about the likely consequences of leaving my condition untreated and the ineffectiveness of various medications in achieving remission, the more confident I became in my choices. I read more and found resources that have guided me. Engaging with my care team has become easier.

To understand social media, I had to experience it first-hand. I soon realized that only some of the information on social media is reliable. There are many misconceptions about treating diseases like RA online, and many can be dangerous.

The long gaps between appointments with the rheumatology clinic can be frustrating, especially when flare-ups happen, and I desperately need relief. My impulse is to turn to Google for answers. Unfortunately, the information we stumble upon can create anxiety. This is especially true when social media groups talk about medication, so it's crucial for me to have access to other resources beyond my appointments with rheumatologists. Speaking to others with RA can be comforting, and I learn a lot from someone who has already dealt with RA. But if online communities are not regulated, you don't know who you are talking to. I am learning to become a better judge of reliable information that I then discuss with my clinician. It is becoming more of a collaboration.

Table 54.1 Patient DAs developed for rheumatological conditions

Source	Name	Population	Format	Purpose
Barton et al., 2014b	RA Choice	RA	Print	Exploring and choosing between options for treatment
Fraenkel et al., 2012	RA-Guide	RA	Website	Communicating risks and benefits about biological therapy
Hazlewood et al., 2020	None	RA	Website	Discrete-choice experiment to choose between triple therapy and methotrexate
Li et al., 2013, 2014	Animated, Self-serve, Web-based Research tool (ANSWER)	RA	Website	Considering methotrexate as a therapy
Li et al., 2018	Animated, Self-serve, Web-based Research tool (ANSWER-2)	RA	Website	Considering changing to a biological treatment
Lopez-Olivo et al., 2018, 2021	None	RA	Video	'Edutainment' model video tool to help patients learn about treatment options
Martin et al., 2017	None	RA	Print	Choosing between treatments for RA
Meade et al., 2015	Motherhood choices: decision aid for women with rheumatoid arthritis	RA	Print	Considering having children
De Abreu et al., 2009	None	Lupus nephritis	Print	Choosing between cyclophosphamide and mycophenolate
Meyappan et al., 2021	None	Gout	Print	Choosing between non-steroidal anti-inflammatory drugs, allopurinol, febuxostat, and probenecid
Nota et al., 2017	None	RA, ankylosing spondylitis, psoriatic arthritis	Website	Initiating or changing between disease-modifying anti-rheumatic drugs
Qu et al., 2019	Shared decision-making in lupus electronic tool (SMILE)	Systemic lupus erythematosus	Website	Educating patients about treatments for lupus
J. A. Singh et al., 2019	Individualized decision aid for diverse women with lupus nephritis (IDEA-WON)	Lupus nephritis	Website	Choosing between treatments for lupus nephritis

visit, difficulties communicating risk and scientific information to patients, and lack of knowledge about available DAs and lack of training in SDM. Patients reported technical barriers when navigating online formats, lack of clear invitations to participate in SDM from their clinicians, and cultural barriers. Patients also expressed concern about delays in treatment due to SDM. Additionally, a study by Mathijssen et al. (2020) of audio-recorded, routine RA visits in the Netherlands found the level of SDM to be very low, reinforcing a need for training and tools.

Treatment of rheumatic conditions often focuses on the achievement of a target or goal of low disease activity or remission. In SDM, goal elicitation and an alignment of goals have been identified as key components (Elwyn and Vermunt, 2020). Do patients with RA and clinicians discuss treatment goals? Are they aligned? In a study of over 900 adults with RA, the majority (63%) reported they did not discuss RA treatment goals with their clinicians. Those patients who did discuss goals were three times more likely to report being satisfied with their treatment plans, more likely to have improved disease activity, and 68% more likely to reach remission (O'Neill et al., 2021). In another study examining goal concordance between patients with RA and their clinicians, goal concordance was associated with higher adherence to therapy (Barton et al., 2023). Goal discussions are critical to high-quality SDM, and tools to elicit goals in RA have been developed but need wider testing (Kahler et al., 2022).

Interventions to implement SDM in rheumatology include DAs, clinician training, and patient activation. Of the DAs identified by Morrison et al. (2022) in the scoping review, eight focused on RA, one on gout, three on lupus, and one each on medication initiation across multiple conditions including RA, psoriatic arthritis, and ankylosing spondylitis. Table 54.1 outlines the details of each intervention study.

While SDM is embedded in many rheumatology guidelines, barriers to implementation exist. Given the inconsistency in the measurement of outcomes across SDM studies, gaps in uptake, and quality, the Outcome Measures in Rheumatology (OMERACT) working group on SDM convened in 2014 to identify and later publish proposed core outcome domains for studies of SDM interventions (Toupin-April et al., 2021). The OMERACT SDM Working Group is developing a core outcome measurement set (Naye et al., 2024), leading to a potential pathway to uniformly measure and compare results across studies of SDM interventions in rheumatology.

SDM and rheumatology—unique contexts

What are the conversations like for persons with RA and cancer?

In the 2021 RA treatment guidelines, the American College of Rheumatology outlined overarching principles for managing patients with RA in various scenarios, such as in disease-modifying antirheumatic drug-naïve patients with low or moderate disease activity, those with persistent disease activity despite the use of conventional synthetic disease-modifying anti-rheumatic drugs, and medication tapering or discontinuation among those at target (Fraenkel et al., 2021). Guidelines addressed specific populations such as patients with RA and pulmonary disease or infections. However, for patients with RA and solid malignancies, the guideline panel could not provide recommendations given the constantly evolving research on this topic. This highlights unique issues in the management of patients with rheumatic and musculoskeletal diseases (RMDs) and cancer, where the principle of SDM is so important.

Conversations around treatment among patients with RMDs and a recent cancer diagnosis (within 5 years of diagnosis) are complicated by several factors: heterogeneity across cancers and between various stages of the same cancer, lack of evidence around the comparative safety of various disease-modifying anti-rheumatic drugs after a cancer diagnosis, how to best communicate across specialists, and lastly, how to uphold what matters most to the patient (N. Singh et al., 2023). Better evidence, and more collaboration among the patients, their caregivers, and the involved specialists are all needed to support the development of tools to facilitate SDM for people with RMDs and cancer.

Reproductive health and SDM in rheumatology

Rheumatologists not only help RMD patients manage their disease activity, they also have a unique opportunity to initiate discussions about family planning and pregnancy with patients who face difficult discussions about the use of teratogenic therapies, impacts of pregnancy on disease outcomes, potential lower fertility levels, and risk of poorer pregnancy outcomes. Recognizing this, the American College of Rheumatology published guidelines for managing reproductive health in RMD (Sammaritano et al., 2020). In contrast to SDM for patients with RMDs and cancer, a much stronger evidence base exists to support SDM among rheumatologists and patients regarding reproductive health. A key component of SDM around reproductive health in rheumatology is open communication and dialogue not only between rheumatologist and patient but also with other healthcare professionals in maternal–fetal medicine and obstetrics/gynaecology.

Little is known about rheumatologists' perspectives on family planning counselling. Talabi et al. (2020) found that rheumatologists' apprehensions about managing complicated pregnancies may negatively influence their discussions with patients about pregnancy planning or avoidance. Talabi et al. also found that rheumatologists do not prescribe contraception and rarely refer patients to gynaecologists for contraceptive care. In another study assessing barriers experienced by dermatologists and rheumatologists in engaging women of reproductive age in SDM before, during, and after pregnancy, Murray et al. (2021) identified gaps in knowledge, skill, and confidence in reproductive healthcare discussions. Despite this, women with RMDs of childbearing age want rheumatologists to play an active role in their reproductive healthcare and coordinate directly with their gynaecologists. Meade et al. (2015) developed a DA for women with RA as a resource to support women and their partners around family planning. In a randomized controlled trial, women who received the DA had a 13% increase in knowledge scores and decreased decisional conflict compared with the control group. Future work to facilitate SDM around reproductive care among RMD patients is needed.

Barriers to communication and SDM in rheumatology (health literacy, language proficiency)

Despite advances in therapy for various rheumatic diseases, variation exists among outcomes for different patient populations. Disparities in outcomes and processes of care in lupus and RA are documented but remain less well studied among other RMDs. Besides system- and access-related issues contributing to disparities, health literacy and language proficiency are likely additional disparity drivers. Barton et al. (2011) found that patients with RA who were non-White, immigrants, or with limited English language proficiency had higher disease activity and poorer function despite having access to effective therapies. A later study showed that limited health literacy and English language proficiency were associated with suboptimal SDM communication among persons with RA (Barton et al., 2014a). Can SDM reduce disparities for persons with barriers to communication? To address this knowledge gap, Barton et al. (2014b) developed a low-literacy decision aid (RA Choice) in three languages. In a pilot trial of RA Choice, the intervention was acceptable, improved knowledge, and reduced decisional conflict among vulnerable patients (Barton et al., 2016).

Interprofessional SDM in rheumatology

Since most RMDs are chronic, the interprofessional team is critical in providing patient education and supporting decisions regarding daily self-management behaviours, medications, and potential surgeries. The rheumatology interprofessional team comprises rheumatologists, nurses, physician's assistants, occupational and physical therapists, mental health clinicians (such as social workers, psychologists, and psychiatrists), pharmacists, registered dietitians, massage therapists, and more. Additional team members might include non-licensed professionals such as complementary medicine practitioners (e.g. acupuncturists), health coaches, and personal trainers. Family and caregivers also constitute important team members who support the patient's goals and desired health outcomes. Clinical members of the interprofessional team often perform an in-depth evaluation of the patient's functional strengths, barriers, and needs. They actively collaborate with the patient (and caregivers if applicable) to determine patient-centred goals and evidence-based methods to achieve them.

In addition to SDM around pharmacological treatment, SDM is often utilized when patients contemplate lifestyle-based self-management behaviours such as exercise, nutrition, and mind–body approaches to minimize pain, fatigue, and other symptoms. The 2022 American College of Rheumatology guidelines for non-pharmacological treatments for RA strongly recommended consistent engagement in exercise (England et al., 2023). Knowing this evidence-based recommendation, an occupational therapist might collaborate with a patient with RA to determine ways to integrate cardiovascular exercise, stretching, and strengthening into their daily routine. The interprofessional team member's job is not only to recommend the intervention but to collaboratively support the patient so they can incorporate the intervention into their life through modifications to the patient's context and environment. Put plainly: many patients know 'what' to do regarding nutrition and exercise, but they lack the 'how'. The interprofessional team member helps the patient to identify environmental supports and sustainable routines. They put together a plan of action, encouraging movement and exercise, and continually re-evaluate how the plan is working.

Rheumatology interprofessional team members often educate patients on medication management and ways to cope with stressors that accompany rheumatic disease. A physical therapist working with a patient with osteoarthritis in the thumb might educate the patient on ways to modify daily activities to protect their joints. They might also instruct the patient on how to apply modalities such as heat and cold to reduce pain and inflammation and how and when to deploy these methods.

As part of SDM, a pharmacist or nurse might provide education about the medication routine, answer questions, and help the patient understand the purpose of their medication plan. Along with the rheumatologist, they might also help the patient make difficult decisions about which medications to try and for how long.

Additionally, a social worker or other mental health clinician might assist with the patient's psychosocial functioning by utilizing evidence-based therapeutic interventions such as cognitive behaviour therapy or acceptance and commitment therapy. These can improve the quality of life and self-efficacy for people with chronic pain and chronic health conditions such as those often seen in rheumatology (Johnston et al., 2010; DiRenzo and Finan, 2019).

Due to the chronic, fluctuating nature of RMDs, rheumatology is a ripe environment for interprofessional collaboration.

Future SDM in rheumatology

Advances in treatment and strategies for persons with rheumatic disease present opportunities for improved outcomes and, for some, remission. The complexity of options for treatment and the need for clear communication to establish a diagnosis, assess treatment response, and safely prescribe therapies underscore the importance of SDM in rheumatology. This is reflected in the inclusion of SDM as an overarching principle in treatment guidelines across many rheumatic conditions, the development of tools to facilitate SDM, and the evaluation of the quality of SDM in unique contexts, such as patients with RA and cancer or those considering pregnancy. Despite SDM being a crucial component of high-quality care in rheumatology, the uptake and broad implementation of SDM still need improvement. Focus on populations at risk for disparities in outcomes and access is needed, as certain groups may benefit more from true collaborative care, elicitation of goals, and preferences. A research agenda for SDM in rheumatology should include ongoing efforts to develop interventions to facilitate SDM with input from diverse populations of patients with RMD (including those with limited health literacy, lower socioeconomic status, and racial and ethnic minority populations), systematic evaluation of interventions, and broad implementation of effective interventions. Interprofessional team approaches to care may decrease burden on rheumatology clinicians and increase patient capacity for self-management and self-efficacy, leading to enhanced outcomes for all persons with rheumatic disease.

REFERENCES

Barton, J. L., Koenig, C. J., Evans-Young, G., et al. 2014b. The design of a low literacy decision aid about rheumatoid arthritis medications developed in three languages for use during the clinical encounter. *BMC Med Inform Decis Mak,* **14,** 104.

Barton, J. L., Markwardt, S., Niederhausen, M., et al. 2023. Are we on the same page? A cross-sectional study of patient–clinician goal concordance in rheumatoid arthritis. *Arthritis Care Res,* **75,** 625–633.

Barton, J. L., Trupin, L., Schillinger, D., et al. 2011. Racial and ethnic disparities in disease activity and function among persons with rheumatoid arthritis from university-affiliated clinics. *Arthritis Care Res,* **63,** 1238–1246.

Barton, J. L., Trupin, L., Schillinger, D., et al. 2016. Use of low-literacy decision aid to enhance knowledge and reduce decisional conflict among a diverse population of adults with rheumatoid arthritis: results of a pilot study. *Arthritis Care Res,* **68,** 889–898.

Barton, J. L., Trupin, L., Tonner, C., et al. 2014a. English language proficiency, health literacy, and trust in physician are associated with shared decision making in rheumatoid arthritis. *J Rheumatol,* **41,** 1290–1297.

Conley, B., Bunzli, S., Bullen, J., et al. 2023. What are the core recommendations for rheumatoid arthritis care? Systematic review of clinical practice guidelines. *Clin Rheumatol,* **42,** 2267–2278.

De Abreu, M. M., Gafni, A., Ferraz, M. B. 2009. Development and testing of a decision board to help clinicians present treatment options to lupus nephritis patients in Brazil. *Arthritis Rheum,* **61,** 37–45.

DiRenzo, D., Finan, P. H. 2019. Self-efficacy and the role of non-pharmacologic treatment strategies to improve pain and affect in arthritis. *Curr Treatm Opt Rheumatol,* **5,** 168–178.

Elwyn, G., Vermunt, N. P. C. A. 2020. Goal-based shared decision-making: developing an integrated model. *J Patient Exp,* **7,** 688–696.

England, B. R., Smith, B. J., Baker, N. A., et al. 2023. 2022 American College of Rheumatology guideline for exercise, rehabilitation, diet, and additional integrative interventions for rheumatoid arthritis. *Arthritis Care Res,* **75,** 1603–1615.

Fraenkel, L., Bathon, J. M., England, B. R., et al. 2021. 2021 American College of Rheumatology guideline for the treatment of rheumatoid arthritis. *Arthritis Care Res,* **73,** 924–939.

Fraenkel, L., Peters, E., Charpentier, P., et al. 2012. Decision tool to improve the quality of care in rheumatoid arthritis. *Arthritis Care Res,* **64,** 977–985.

Johnston, M. R., Foster, M., Shennan, J., Starkey, N. J., Johnson, A. 2010. The effectiveness of an acceptance and commitment therapy self-help intervention for chronic pain. *Clin J Pain,* **26,** 393–402.

Hazlewood, G. S., Marshall, D. A., Barber, C. E. H., et al. 2020. Using a discrete-choice experiment in a decision aid to nudge patients towards value-concordant treatment choices in rheumatoid arthritis: a proof-of-concept study. *Patient Prefer Adherence,* **14,** 829–838.

Kahler, J., Mastarone, G., Matsumoto, R., ZuZero, D., Dougherty, J., Barton, J. L. 2022. 'It may help you to know . . .': the early-phase qualitative development of a rheumatoid arthritis goal elicitation tool. *J Rheumatol,* **49,** 142–149.

Li, L. C., Adam, P. M., Backman, C. L., et al. 2014. Proof-of-concept study of a Web-based methotrexate decision aid for patients with rheumatoid arthritis. *Arthritis Care Res,* **66,** 1472–1481.

Li, L. C., Adam, P. M., Townsend, A. F., et al. 2013. Usability testing of ANSWER: a web-based methotrexate decision aid for patients with rheumatoid arthritis. *BMC Med Inform Decis Making,* **13,** 131.

Li, L. C., Shaw, C. D., Lacaille, D., et al. 2018. Effects of a web-based patient decision aid on biologic and small-molecule agents for rheumatoid arthritis: results from a proof-of-concept study. *Arthritis Care Res,* **70**, 343–352.

Lopez-Olivo, M. A., Ingleshwar, A., Volk, R. J., et al. 2018. Development and pilot testing of multimedia patient education tools for patients with knee osteoarthritis, osteoporosis, and rheumatoid arthritis. *Arthritis Care Res,* **70**, 213–220.

Lopez-Olivo, M. A., Lin, H., Rizvi, T., et al. 2021. Randomized controlled trial of patient education tools for patients with rheumatoid arthritis. *Arthritis Care Res,* **73**, 1470–1478.

Martin, R. W., Enck, R. D., Tellinghuisen, D. J., et al. 2017. Comparison of the effects of a pharmaceutical industry decision guide and decision aids on patient choice to intensify therapy in rheumatoid arthritis. *Med Decis Making,* **37**, 577–588.

Mathijssen, E., Vriezekolk, J. E., Popa, C. D., van den Bemt, B. J. F. 2020. Shared decision making in routine clinical care of patients with rheumatoid arthritis: an assessment of audio-recorded consultations. *Ann Rheumat Dis,* **79**, 170–175.

Meade, T., Dowswell, E., Manolios, N., Sharpe, L. 2015. The motherhood choices decision aid for women with rheumatoid arthritis increases knowledge and reduces decisional conflict: a randomized controlled trial. *BMC Musculoskelet Disord,* **16**, 260.

Meyappan, M., Loh, W. S. A., Tan, L. Y., et al. 2021. Development of a novel gout treatment patient decision aid by patient and physician: a qualitative research study. *Health Expect,* **24**, 431–443.

Morrison, T., Foster, E., Dougherty, J., Barton, J. 2022. Shared decision making in rheumatology: a scoping review. *Semin Arthritis Rheum,* **56**, 152041.

Murray, S., Augustyniak, M., Murase, J. E., et al. 2021. Barriers to shared decision-making with women of reproductive age affected by a chronic inflammatory disease: a mixed-methods needs assessment of dermatologists and rheumatologists. *BMJ Open,* **11**, e043960.

Naye, F., Toupin-April, K., de Wit, M., et al. 2024. OMERACT Core outcome measurement set for shared decision making in rheumatic and musculoskeletal conditions: a scoping review to identify candidate instruments. *Semin Arthritis Rheum,* **65**, 152344.

Nota, I., Drossaert, C. H. C., Melissant, H. C., et al. 2017. Development of a web-based patient decision aid for initiating disease modifying anti-rheumatic drugs using user-centred design methods. *BMC Med Inform Decis Mak,* **17**, 51.

O'Neill, K., Marks, K. E., Sinicrope, P. S., et al. 2021. Importance of shared treatment goal discussions in rheumatoid arthritis—a cross-sectional survey: patients report providers seldom discuss treatment goals and outcomes improve when goals are discussed. *ACR Open Rheumatol,* **3**, 870–878.

Qu, H., Hu, X., Singh, J. A. 2019. Factors influencing implementation of a computerized, individualized, culturally tailored lupus decision aid in lupus clinics: a qualitative semi-structured interview study. *Clin Rheumatol,* **38**, 2793–2801.

Sammaritano, L. R., Bermas, B. L., Chakravarty, E. E., et al. 2020. 2020 American College of Rheumatology guideline for the management of reproductive health in rheumatic and musculoskeletal diseases. *Arthritis Rheumatol,* **72**, 529–556.

Singh, J. A., Fraenkel, L., Green, C., et al. 2019. Individualized decision aid for diverse women with lupus nephritis (IDEA-WON): a randomized controlled trial. *PLoS Med,* **16**, e1002800.

Singh, N., Grivas, P., Makris, U. E., Suarez-Almazor, M. E., O'Hare, A. M., Barton, J. L. 2023. Use of disease-modifying antirheumatic drugs in rheumatoid arthritis: supporting shared decision-making between patients with cancer and clinicians. *ACR Open Rheumatol,* **5**, 305–307.

Talabi, M. B., Clowse, M. E. B., Blalock, S. J., Hamm, M., Borrero, S. 2020. Perspectives of adult rheumatologists regarding family planning counseling and care: a qualitative study. *Arthritis Care Res,* **72**, 452–458.

Toupin-April, K., Décary, S., de Wit, M., et al. 2021. Endorsement of the OMERACT core domain set for shared decision making interventions in rheumatology trials: results from a multi-stepped consensus-building approach. *Semin Arthritis Rheum,* **51**, 593–600.

PART 7
The view from allied disciplines

55

Shared decision making in midwifery

Deirdre Daly, Valerie Smith, Marianne Nieuwenhuijze, and Ellen McEvoy

Contextualizing shared decision making in midwifery care

Shared decision making (SDM), although promoted for decisions where evidence shows more or less similar outcomes and side effects between options, is also applicable for other healthcare decisions. Most women in maternity care wish to be involved in decision making or want to exercise their autonomy (Alruwaili et al., 2023). SDM can contribute to a greater mutual understanding through the exchange of information and dialogue, with the woman making the final decision (Nieuwenhuijze and Low, 2013).

Understanding SDM in midwifery

As a concept, defining SDM in midwifery is complex, given that various other terms and concepts convey similar philosophical approaches to care and practice. These include informed decision making (Goldberg and Shorten, 2014), informed choice (O'Brien et al., 2018), autonomy-supportive decision making (Joyce et al., 2022), decision making autonomy (Vogels-Broeke et al., 2023), empowerment, and woman-centred care (O'Brien et al., 2021; Hall et al., 2023). Although all are laudable concepts within midwifery practice and the woman–midwife relationship, they do not include the core essential elements that make SDM unique and different. SDM is also not informed consent (Begley et al., 2019). Informed consent requires the fulfilment of three conditions: that the woman is competent, that she has been given the necessary information about treatment or care and understands this information, and that giving consent is her free choice. What makes SDM different is that it includes symmetry in power relations with the midwife and woman discussing and deciding *together* upon a course of care, the midwife offering evidence-based and expert knowledge free from the influence of personal biases (Begley et al., 2019, 2021), and an explicit acknowledgement that the woman's knowledge is a necessary prerequisite (Begley et al., 2021). Implicit within these core elements is respect for each woman's autonomy and right to self-determination. There are other factors that make SDM in midwifery, and opportunities for achieving SDM, distinctive. The longitudinal nature of a woman's pregnancy, labour, birth, and postpartum experience is unique and lends itself to establishing continuity of midwife carer throughout. Continuity of carer can facilitate and enhance the development of trust, which takes time. The woman needs time to develop trust in the midwife, and until such trust develops, there may be an asymmetry in power in a woman–midwife relationship (Begley et al., 2019). A woman's experiences of being or not being involved in decisions about what happens to her can have a profound impact on how she reflects on her birth experiences, as exemplified by the perspective offered by one woman in Box 55.1.

Box 55.1 Patient perspective

An individual woman describes her perspective of SDM in midwifery

As a woman who has had two children, I rarely encountered SDM during my care. I completed birth preparation courses and wrote birth plans, but both my labours needed to be induced and once that process started, I felt that there was no time for my preferences.

Reflecting on my pregnancies, I trusted my body to develop a healthy baby. But when it came to childbirth, there seemed to be a shift from being a baby–mother partnership to one that was a baby–midwife partnership. I felt like I was a bystander, not in control of what was happening to my body.

Birth is a moment that lies between growing a baby and the start of a lifetime of parenting, and those moments remain vivid memories for me. I was so focused on the responsibility of nurturing and delivering my baby that I didn't factor my own needs into my questions, and on the rare occasion that I did, I felt selfish. After my first birth, I was left with regrets and questions. Yet, when I became pregnant again, my focus instantly switched to the baby and away from my own needs. No two experiences are the same; while my care provider in my second pregnancy did answer my questions about my first pregnancy and birth, the second birth brought fresh challenges. I wish I knew how to have had a deeper involvement in my care.

I remember feeling defeated and deflated as my second baby had to be helped into the world with forceps. Happy, of course, that he was safe but broken and exhausted. I'll never forget the lines of the midwife's face, her brown hair in a ponytail, blue mask on her face. My husband declined to cut the cord, and her brown eyes looked straight into mine as she asked if I would like to do it instead. Despite my second birth being more traumatic for me than the first, I always felt that, in some way, it was better. Reflecting now, I connect with that moment. I felt involved in my care.

The feeling of being offered a genuine choice is powerful. For me, it was healing. Whenever a care provider took a moment to explain something to me in more detail or ask me very specific questions about my experience, it made me feel like I was important. It helped me understand, and ultimately, though those moments were few, they helped me heal.

My births had similar points of progression, but I felt that the course was predefined for me and not with me and that the professionals were in a rush to get to those points. Had I been given time and opportunity for discussion, I may have ultimately reached those points of progression in the same way, but I think that I would feel differently now. Simply being included in the process at the end of my second birth was so healing, and I can only imagine how powerful a woman would feel if she was included in all decisions about her care.

Circumstances and complexities for SDM

Achieving SDM in midwifery can be facilitated or hindered by myriad circumstances within the wider maternity care structures and services. Structurally, maternity care systems in many countries are organized into antenatal, intrapartum, and postpartum departments, all staffed by different professionals. Although such organization does not prevent SDM from occurring, fragmentation and compartmentalization of care make it more difficult to develop an equitable woman–midwife trusting relationship and balance of power, with free and open dialogue. The necessity for some women to require care from multiple professionals within the multidisciplinary care team because of medical, obstetric, or social complexities can also hinder SDM. This may be because multidisciplinary team members do not have a shared philosophical approach to offering care and may offer conflicting advice. Overcoming these structural complex impediments to SDM requires having a shared approach to care, mutual multidisciplinary team member respect, and shared evidenced-based practice and treatment guidelines that multidisciplinary team members agree to follow.

SDM in midwifery policy and practice guidance globally

The World Health Organization's (WHO) report on patient engagement (WHO, 2016a), although not referring specifically to SDM in midwifery, does reference how healthcare providers' perceptions of a patient's (woman's) ability to communicate influence their style of interactions. Healthcare professionals (HCPs) held more patient-focused interactions with patients whom they perceived to be better communicators (WHO, 2016a). Targeting the attitudes and behaviour of HCPs through education was identified as important in supporting SDM. The WHO's three documents that provide recommendations for positive antenatal (WHO, 2016b), intrapartum (WHO, 2018), and postnatal maternity care (WHO, 2022), refer to promoting and facilitating women's choices, women's autonomy in decision making, and women having a sense of personal achievement and control through involvement in decision making. However, the recommendations for positive postnatal care are from the only document that refers specifically to SDM, stating: 'communication strategies, using culturally acceptable methods that respect and facilitate shared decision-making, are integral to the assessment of discharge criteria' (WHO, 2022, p. 165).

The International Confederation of Midwives' definition of the midwife does not refer to SDM but does state that the midwife 'works in partnership with women' (International Confederation of Midwives, 2023, p. 2). Their 'Philosophy and model of midwifery care' document further acknowledges that 'midwifery care takes place in partnership with women, recognising the right to self determination, and is respectful, personalised, continuous and non-authoritarian' (International Confederation of Midwives, 2014, p. 2). While SDM is not identified explicitly, 'partnership' and 'non-authoritarian' imply a balance of power within the woman–midwife relationship, and the '*right to self-determination*' suggests an acknowledgement of the woman's autonomy and her right to decide what is best for her.

Guidance on decision making by the International Federation of Gynecology and Obstetrics (FIGO) is presented in relation to human rights and an ethical framework for respectful care (FIGO, 2020, 2021). The framework for respectful care, for example, presented under the four ethical principles of beneficence, non-maleficence, justice, and autonomy, does not describe SDM explicitly but does refer to decision making as 'a collaborative effort between the pregnant woman, her family and her health care providers' (FIGO, 2021, p. 2).

Operationalizing SDM in midwifery care

The way in which SDM in midwifery occurs is often guided by the circumstances surrounding the decisions that need to be made. Decision making during antenatal care without time pressure is substantially different from decision making during birth when circumstances are, more often, time-pressured. For example, in situations of suspected fetal compromise where urgent action might be needed. Still, respectful behaviour, which includes expressing empathy, giving information about the situation, even when time is limited to discuss possible options, and explicitly seeking women's consent, is essential in all circumstances (International Confederation of Midwives, 2014; FIGO, 2021).

In non-pressing circumstances, the conversation (*team talk*) begins with creating ground for respectful collaboration and working towards a trusting relationship (Elwyn et al., 2017). Trust is something that is built by showing trustworthiness and reliability (O'Neill, 2013). It is an important value for women in midwifery care but is challenging when a midwife meets the woman for the first time, for example, during labour and birth (International Confederation of Midwives, 2014; Smythe et al., 2016). In this conversation, it must be made clear to the woman that the midwife, and other HCPs, will support her in the decision making process and respect her autonomy in making the final decision.

In progressing the conversation (*option talk*), options relevant to the decision that needs to be made are discussed. This also includes an exploration of the woman's wishes and values. This conversation, therefore, should not involve a one-way flow of information; rather, it should be a dialogue between those directly involved in the decision. The BRAINS acronym (Table 55.1) is a helpful guide for ensuring that all aspects in decision making are discussed (College Perinatale Zorg (CPZ) [Perinatal Care Board], 2020, p. 16).

The benefits and risks associated with the decision should be discussed, as well as implications related to any procedures that might

Table 55.1 The BRAINS decision making acronym

Benefits	The benefits of the procedure, aim to achieve
Risks	The risks and side effects, other interventions that go along with it
Alternatives	Other options
Intuition	Resonation of the information
Nothing	What if we do nothing and wait
'Scuse me	Time to sink in, think, discuss (with others), decide

Source: data from College Perinatale Zorg (CPZ) [Perinatal Care Board]. 2020. Zorgstandaard Integrale Geboortezorg versie 1.2 [Care standard integrated maternity care version 1.2], p. 16. Available at: https://www.zorginzicht.nl/binaries/content/assets/zorginzicht/kwaliteitsinstrumenten/zorgstandaard-integrale-geboortezorg.pdf

be performed. Decision aids can be helpful but do not replace the conversation between the woman and her care provider (Stacey et al., 2024). After discussing all options, the woman and her partner need (some) time to process the information to come to a decision. Even if time is limited, a few minutes alone for the woman and her partner is valuable.

Concluding the conversation, a better-informed decision can be made that meets the woman's needs and values. In principle, the woman's preference is always leading; however, women may decline to lead and may choose to defer the final decision to the HCP, which should equally be respected. In such situations, striving for informed consent is a minimal requirement. Alternatively, if a woman's choice is to wait (should circumstances allow), further follow-up and contact information should be provided. Throughout the decision making conversation, the woman's partner (or primary support person), should, where possible, be closely involved, with the woman's agreement.

In more urgent circumstances, it remains important that the midwife or other HCP verbalizes what is happening and what actions are essential. A conversation after actions have been taken, where the care provider explains what has happened and why certain choices were made, and that then allows the woman, and her partner, to express their experiences and opinions, is of critical importance (Nieuwenhuijze et al., 2014). This conversation allows for reflection and promotes understanding, especially in emergency or intense time-pressured decision making situations. In such cases, it is helpful to start the conversation with the parents' experience and then move to discussions on the assumed desire by all to achieve the best outcome for the mother and baby.

Birth plan

Birth plans can facilitate SDM and women's sense of autonomy and control during birth (Shareef et al., 2023). In a birth plan, pregnant women can express their childbirth expectations, preferences, and values. In subsequent conversations, different scenarios can be explored to prepare women for unforeseen circumstances and SDM when the expected birth course is not being fulfilled.

Informed refusal

Circumstances where a woman makes an informed refusal to follow midwifery or other HCP advice can create a situation where the autonomy and the best interests of those involved need to find balance. The risk of coercion can be minimized by having an open and honest conversation without placing undue pressure on the woman. Supported by good communication skills, empathy, and acceptance of vulnerability, the SDM framework allows women and midwives to have meaningful conversations without sacrificing a woman's autonomy or the midwife's capacity to practise their profession with integrity (Megregian and Nieuwenhuijze, 2018).

Women's and clinicians' perspectives of SDM in midwifery

Studies on SDM from the perspectives of women and maternity clinicians, albeit largely explored in the context of high-income countries (Alruwaili et al., 2023), offer valuable insight and understanding of SDM in midwifery. For instance, studies have shown how some women are unaware of the concept of SDM (Asah-Opoku et al., 2023), how others prefer not to engage in SDM, and how the degree to which women wish to engage varies (Nieuwenhuijze and Low, 2013; López-Toribio et al., 2021; Alruwaili et al., 2023). Conversely, some women have described having to 'fight' to be involved in SDM (López-Toribio et al., 2021, p. 5), requiring more information, greater support, and time for SDM processes (Schwarz et al., 2016; Coates et al., 2020a; Johansson and Thies-Lagergren, 2022). Maternity clinicians, although committed to SDM (Kennedy et al., 2013) are equally challenged by insufficient time for effective SDM, especially in emergency situations (Asah-Opoku et al., 2023), or may lack the skills needed for supportive SDM (Hamilton et al., 2023). In this regard, clinicians themselves recognize that the process of SDM can be 'poor' (Kenyon et al.., 2016, p. 1), with discussions often limited or persuasive towards women accepting clinician preferences rather than being respectful of informed choice (Munro et al., 2017).

Effective SDM is associated with higher maternal satisfaction scores, positive birth experiences (Say et al., 2011; Hall et al., 2023; Shahveisi et al., 2023), and reduced maternal anxiety (Say et al., 2011). Optimizing SDM in midwifery is, therefore, critically important. Educational interventions and decision aids are showing promise (Coates et al., 2020b). However, further research involving the development and evaluation of SDM interventions in midwifery is required.

REFERENCES

Alruwaili, T. A., Crawford, K., Jahanfar, S., Hampton, K., Fooladi, E. 2023. Pregnant persons and birth partners' experiences of shared decision-making during pregnancy and childbirth: an umbrella review. *Patient Educ Couns,* **114**, 107832.

Asah-Opoku, K., Onisarotu, A. N., Nuamah, M. A., et al. 2023. Exploring the shared decision making process of caesarean sections at a teaching hospital in Ghana: a mixed methods study. *BMC Pregnancy Childbirth,* **23**, 426.

Begley, K., Begley, C., Smith, V. 2021. Shared decision-making and maternity care in the deep learning age: acknowledging and overcoming inherited defeaters. *J Eval Clin Pract,* **27**, 497–503.

Begley, K., Daly, D., Panda, S., Begley, C. 2019. Shared decision-making in maternity care: acknowledging and overcoming epistemic defeaters. *J Eval Clin Pract,* **25**, 1113–1120.

Coates, D., Goodfellow, A., Sinclair, L. 2020a. Induction of labour: experiences of care and decision-making of women and clinicians. *Women Birth,* **33**, e1–e14.

Coates, D., Thirukumar, P., Henry, A. 2020b. Making shared decisions in relation to planned caesarean sections: what are we up to? *Patient Educ Couns,* **103**, 1176–1190.

College Perinatale Zorg (CPZ) [Perinatal Care Board]. 2020. Zorgstandaard Integrale Geboortezorg versie 1.2 [Care standard integrated maternity care version 1.2]. Available at: https://www.zorginzicht.nl/binaries/content/assets/zorginzicht/kwaliteitsinstrumenten/zorgstandaard-integrale-geboortezorg.pdf

Elwyn, G., Durand, M. A., Song, J., et al. 2017. A three-talk model for shared decision making: multistage consultation process. *BMJ,* **359**, j4891.

International Federation of Gynecology and Obstetrics. 2020. Integrating human rights and women's health competencies for practice. Available at: https://www.figo.org/news/integrating-human-rights-and-womens-health-competencies-practice

International Federation of Gynecology and Obstetrics. 2021. Ethical framework for respectful maternity care during pregnancy and childbirth. Available at: https://www.figo.org/sites/default/files/2021-09/FIGO_Statement_Ethical-Framework-Respectful-Maternity-Care-During-Pregnancy-Childbirth_0.pdf

Goldberg, H. B., Shorten, A. 2014. Differences between patient and provider perceptions of informed decision making about epidural analgesia use during childbirth. *J Perinat Educ,* **23**, 104–112.

Hall, H., Fooladi, E., Kloester, J., et al. 2023. Factors that promote a positive childbearing experience: a qualitative study. *J Midwifery Womens Health,* **68**, 44–51.

Hamilton, E. L., McLaughlin, K., Mollart, L. 2023. Factors that influence women's decision on the mode of birth after a previous caesarean section: a meta-ethnography. *Int J Community Based Nurs Midwifery,* **11**, 152–168.

International Confederation of Midwives. 2014. Philosophy and model of midwifery care. Available at: https://www.internationalmidwives.org/our-work/policy-and-practice/philosophy-and-model-of-midwifery-care.html

International Confederation of Midwives. 2023. International definition of the midwife. Available at: https://www.internationalmidwives.org/assets/files/definitions-files/2023/07/08l_en_international-definition-of-the-midwife.pdf

Johansson, M., Thies-Lagergren, L. 2022. Women's experience of the decision-making process for home-based postnatal midwifery care when discharged early from hospital: a Swedish interview study. *Eur J Midwifery,* **6**, 60.

Joyce, K., Anne de la, C., Linda, M., et al. 2022. Autonomy-supportive decision-making in maternity care during prenatal consultations: a qualitative interaction analysis. *BMJ Open,* **12**, e063463.

Kennedy, H. P., Grant, J., Walton, C., Sandall, J. 2013. Elective caesarean delivery: a mixed method qualitative investigation. *Midwifery,* **29**, e138–e144.

Kenyon, S. L., Johns, N., Duggal, S., Hewston, R., Gale, N. 2016. Improving the care pathway for women who request Caesarean section: an experience-based co-design study. *BMC Pregnancy Childbirth,* **16**, 348.

López-Toribio, M., Bravo, P., Llupià, A. 2021. Exploring women's experiences of participation in shared decision-making during childbirth: a qualitative study at a reference hospital in Spain. *BMC Pregnancy Childbirth,* **21**, 631.

Megregian, M., Nieuwenhuijze, M. 2018. Choosing to decline: finding common ground through the perspective of shared decision making. *J Midwifery Womens Health,* **63**, 340–346.

Munro, S., Kornelsen, J., Corbett, K., Wilcox, E., Bansback, N., Janssen, P. 2017. Do women have a choice? care providers' and decision makers' perspectives on barriers to access of health services for birth after a previous Cesarean. *Birth,* **44**, 153–160.

Nieuwenhuijze, M., Low, L. K. 2013. Facilitating women's choice in maternity care. *J Clin Ethics,* **24**, 276–282.

Nieuwenhuijze, M. J., Korstjens, I., de Jonge, A., de Vries, R., Lagro-Janssen, A. 2014. On speaking terms: a Delphi study on shared decision-making in maternity care. *BMC Pregnancy Childbirth,* **14**, 223.

O'Brien, D., Butler, M. M., Casey, M. 2021. The importance of nurturing trusting relationships to embed shared decision-making during pregnancy and childbirth. *Midwifery,* **98**, 102987.

O'Brien, D., Casey, M., Butler, M. M. 2018. Women's experiences of exercising informed choices as expressed through their sense of self and relationships with others in Ireland: a participatory action research study. *Midwifery,* **65**, 58–66.

O'Neill, O. 2013. What we don't understand about trust. TED Talk. Available at: https://www.ted.com/speakers/onora_o_neill

Say, R., Robson, S., Thomson, R. 2011. Helping pregnant women make better decisions: a systematic review of the benefits of patient decision aids in obstetrics. *BMJ Open,* **1**, e000261.

Schwarz, C., Gross, M. M., Heusser, P., Berger, B. 2016. Women's perceptions of induction of labour outcomes: results of an online-survey in Germany. *Midwifery,* **35**, 3–10.

Shahveisi, M., Nourizadeh, R., Mehrabi, E. 2023. The effect of shared decision-making in choosing the method of labor analgesia on childbirth experience among primiparous women. *PLoS One,* **18**, e0274559.

Shareef, N., Scholten, N., Nieuwenhuijze, M., Stramrood, C., de Vries, M., van Dillen, J. 2023. The role of birth plans for shared decision-making around birth choices of pregnant women in maternity care: a scoping review. *Women Birth,* **36**, 327–333.

Smythe, E., Hunter, M., Gunn, J., et al. 2016. Midwifing the notion of a 'good' birth: a philosophical analysis. *Midwifery,* **37**, 25–31.

Stacey, D., Lewis, K. B., Smith, M., et al. 2024. Decision aids for people facing health treatment or screening decisions. *Cochrane Database Syst Rev,* **1**, CD001431.

Vogels-Broeke, M., Cellissen, E., Daemers, D., Budé, L., de Vries, R., Nieuwenhuijze, M. 2023. Women's decision-making autonomy in Dutch maternity care. *Birth,* **50**, 384–395.

World Health Organization. 2016a. *Patient Engagement: Technical Series on Safer Primary Care.* World Health Organization. Available at: https://www.who.int/publications/i/item/9789241511629

World Health Organization. 2016b. *WHO Recommendations on Antenatal Care for a Positive Pregnancy Experience.* World Health Organization. Available at: https://www.who.int/publications/i/item/9789241549912

World Health Organization. 2018. *Intrapartum Care for a Positive Childbirth Experience.* World Health Organization. Available at: https://www.who.int/publications/i/item/9789241550215

World Health Organization. 2022. *WHO Recommendations on Maternal and Newborn Care for a Positive Postnatal Experience.* World Health Organization. Available at: https://www.who.int/publications/i/item/9789240045989

56

Shared decision making in physiotherapy

Rob Letchford, Elaine Taylor, Martin Dando, and Zoe Silsbury

SDM in physiotherapy: from rhetoric to reality

Preparing this chapter has afforded us a rare opportunity to take time to reflect, consider, and share learning from our experience of embedding shared decision making (SDM) in musculoskeletal (MSK) physiotherapy practice and beyond. The recently published National Institute for Health and Care Excellence (NICE) SDM guideline in the UK (NICE, 2021) provides a structured lens for us to present our case study, to celebrate and share our success, and make proposals for future directions. We hope that sharing this reflection will prove as valuable to you, as creating it has been for us.

The rhetoric

SDM has been discussed in national policy, the physiotherapy literature, and clinical practice for many years. Physiotherapy is one of 13 allied health professions in Wales, whose work is informed by 'A Healthier Wales' (Welsh Government, 2018, 2019)—a long-term 'whole systems' plan that emphasizes personalized care and empowering people to manage their health and well-being. Further, the National Clinical Framework (Welsh Government, 2021), The Health and Social Care (Quality and Engagement) Wales Act (Welsh Government, 2023), and the All Wales Rehabilitation Framework (Welsh Government, 2022) are all underpinned by principles of involving people and working collaboratively through practices such as SDM. Working in partnership and involving service users and carers in decisions about their care is recognized in the standards of conduct, performance, and ethics set out by our regulators (Health and Care Professions Council), while our education and trade union body (Chartered Society of Physiotherapy) regards SDM as a 'non-negotiable ethos' that impacts practice across all sectors and specialisms.

Alongside the political drivers and governing bodies, physiotherapy researchers have taken up the challenge to explore, develop, communicate, and debate SDM's value in clinical practice. In their debate article, Hoffmann and colleagues argue that SDM should be an integral part of physiotherapy practice, but numerous factors continue to hinder widespread and effective implementation (Hoffmann et al., 2020). Décary and co-workers agree that SDM has a bright future in MSK practice, portraying it as the 'Excalibur' in the fight against overuse in MSK healthcare (Décary et al., 2021).

Despite the rhetoric towards SDM in physiotherapy, systematic reviews of patient experiences (Grenfell and Soundy, 2022; Barker et al., 2023), national and international observations (Dierckx et al., 2013; Jones et al., 2014; Ogawa et al., 2023), and chronic MSK pain decision aid effectiveness studies (Bowen et al., 2020) show that this rhetoric is not yet reality, its impacts on relevant health outcomes are unclear, and we are not fully realizing the potential benefits of SDM.

This dissonance is not unique to the discipline of physiotherapy, or the topic of SDM. Reassuringly, researchers and healthcare champions continue to consider the barriers and facilitators unique to physiotherapy and propose SDM strategies and models that could support more sustainable and meaningful change in practice (Zadro et al., 2021; Hoffmann et al., 2022).

We will summarize our journey towards enabling a meaningful change that started with MSK physiotherapy services in the South East of Wales, UK, that is beginning to gain traction and spread nationally. We will then share our success, challenges, learning, and proposals for the future.

Our recent reality

Shifting from paradigm, theory, knowledge, and skills into core business is a complex journey (Figure 56.1). In 2012, a small group of passionate clinicians formed a partnership with local academics to explore and grow their use of SDM. Local developments were boosted in 2016 by a centrally funded 'Making Choices Together' SDM train the trainer programme. This enabled the group to build on their developing knowledge, skills, and resources and to produce a local profession and speciality specific training and implementation plan (described in Table 56.1).

Initially, this spread across the local profession and specialities, and then to teams in neighbouring health boards. As momentum and support grew, a systematic dissemination and spread approach was facilitated in 2023 by the Dragon's Heart Institute 'Spread and Scale Academy'.

The uptake of the train the trainer package continues to spread across Wales, reaching many allied health professional staff who

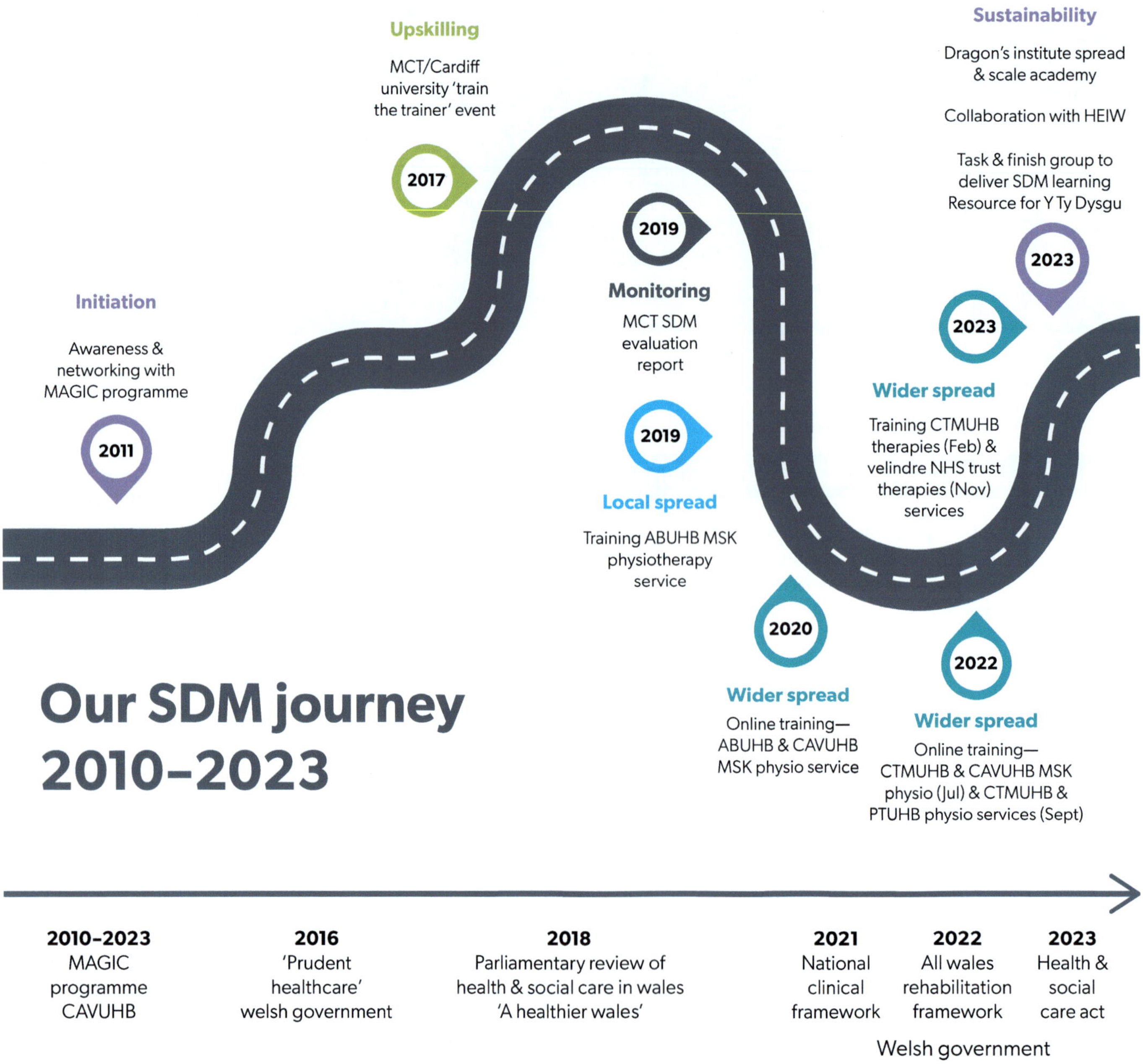

Figure 56.1 Our SDM implementation journey 2010–2023. ABUHB, Aneurin Bevan University Health Board; CAVUHB, Cardiff and Vale University Health Board; CTMUHC, Cwn Taf Morgannwg University Health Board; HEIW, Health Education and Improvement Wales; MCT, Making Choices Together; PTUHB, Powys Teaching University Health Board.

Table 56.1 Our package of SDM training and implementation

The training package	The package consists of up to two short training session (3 hours) with prereading and reflective practice. The sessions are aligned to the three-talk model, focusing on developing the desire, knowledge, and skills to perform SDM, with opportunity for practical rehearsal in familiar case studies with peer feedback
The quality improvement package	Participants are encouraged to implement a personal development plan including observed practice with reflection logs and feedback tools. The Collaborate and OPTION tools are encouraged to gain feedback from lived experience

are now equipped to deliver the SDM training and support implementation planning across all Welsh health boards and trusts (Figure 56.2).

Further, it is now linked to a national programme at Health Education and Improvement Wales—the strategic workforce and continuing professional education body in Wales. The initial profession (physiotherapy) and speciality (MSK) specific training has been adapted so that it provides a consistent framework, but with local adaptability to meet different professional, speciality, and multiprofessional team's needs. Additionally, it is being adapted for the national e-learning platform, 'Y Ty Dysgu'. This signifies a move towards sustainability, regular update, validation, and quality assurance of the resources against evolving knowledge and guidelines.

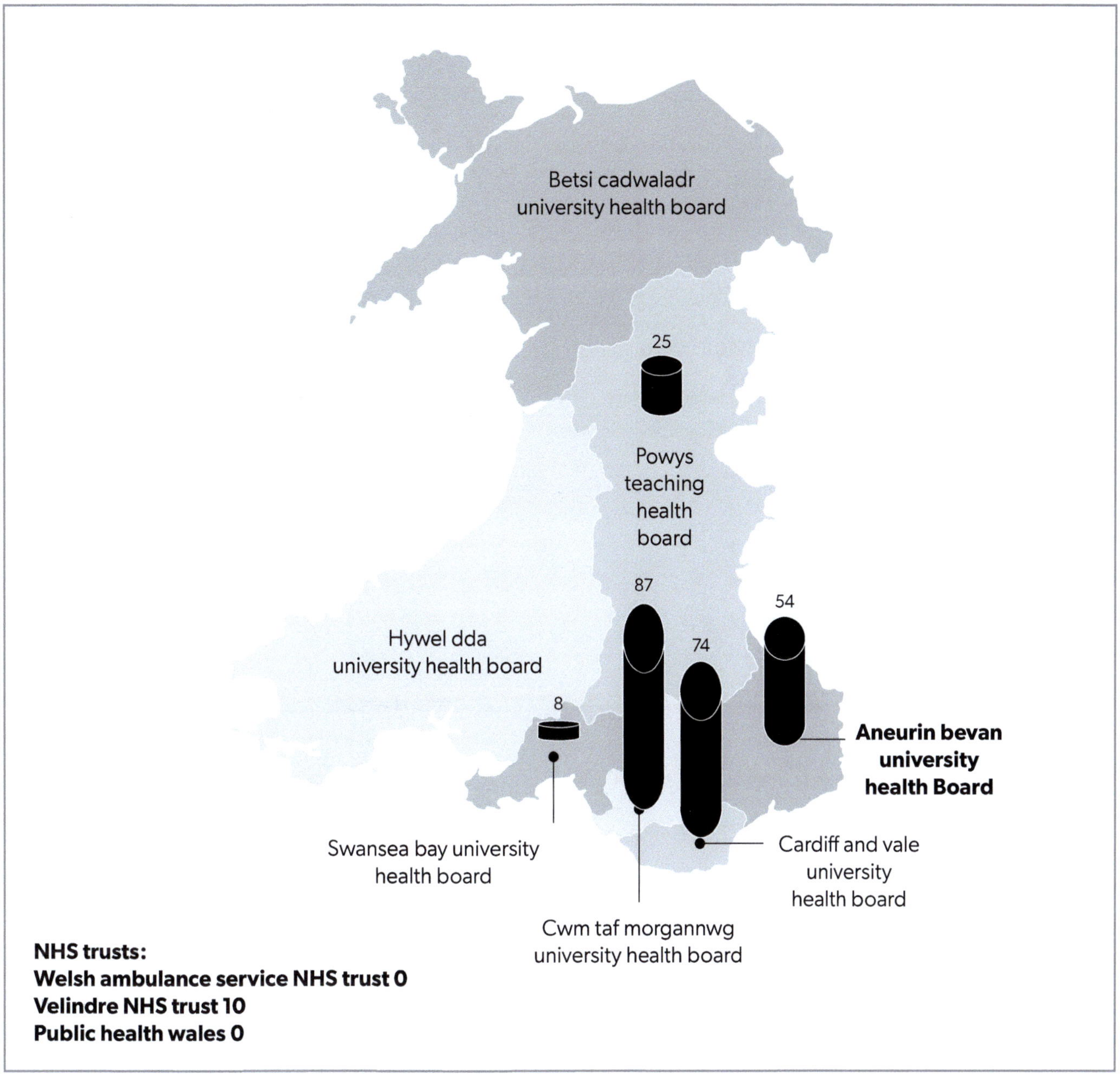

Figure 56.2 Scale and spread of our SDM train the trainer programme. Number of attendees 2019–2023.
Adapted from the NHS Wales Shared Services Partnership (NWSSP) website. Available at: https://nwssp.nhs.wales/a-wp/governance-e-manual/knowing-who-does-what-why/organisation-structure-of-nhs-wales/

This sustainable delivery model enabling further spread and scale, alongside consistent evaluation of the training, will allow further learning of the challenges of and facilitators to closing the gap between rhetoric and reality.

Our reflections and learning

We have reflected on our experiences against the NICE SDM guideline recommendations (NICE, 2021), covering what has gone well, what areas need more work, and key learning (summarized in Table 56.2).

NICE recommendations 1 and 2: embedding SDM at the organization level and putting SDM into practice

What has gone well

The inclusion of person-centred care in multiple national and local health board policy and strategic documents, and the prioritization and support from senior leadership, has been a significant facilitator. It has led to the expectation that SDM is included throughout our quality statements and clinical pathways and has released a small investment for training and quality improvement.

Our journey has been motivated and led by a growing community of clinical leaders, who have empowered the growth of a clinical

Table 56.2 Our progress and learning against the NICE SDM guideline (2021) recommendations

NICE recommendations		What has gone well	What could we do better
1. Embedding SDM at organizational level	High-level leadership	National and local policy and strategy Senior clinical leadership	Coproduction with lived experience
	Planning and implementing	Organic and emergent improvement plan built on: • Academic collaboration • Train the trainer system • Spread and scale • Opportunism • Collaborative working • Spread of existing good practice • Targeted in speciality/profession • Spread and scale across specialities • Identification of learning needs	Consistent and complete quality improvement Electronic measure collection Audit cycles for quality assurance
	Sharing information	National pathways Electronic data and information resources	Sharing with the public Consistency across headboards
	Supporting healthcare professionals skills and competencies	Embedding in therapy skills supplementary skills including: • Communication • Self-management • Complexity and uncertainty • Person-centred care Embed three talk model Practical training Focus on speciality/profession	Higher priority in practice-based learning Higher priority alongside speciality 'clinical skills' Lived experience training facilitators
	Promoting to service user	Inclusion in routine practice	Awareness in population Knowledge and skills in population
2. SDM into practice	Before	Inclusion in education and triage interventions	Lack of reliable high-quality resources
	During	Core component of some consultations Some 'what matters' conversations 'What matters to me' within some clinical records Some 'chunk and check' and 'teach back' Some use of decision aids Some letters to the person	Core component of all consultations Consistent 'what matters' conversations Consistent recording of 'what matters to me' Consistent 'chunk and check' and 'teach back' Consistent use of decision aids in practice All letters to the person Unified patient record to document what matters, values, and preferences
	After or between	Time to consider and reflect when not time critical decision	Greater flexibility in system to enable time Greater resources to assist
3. Patient decision aids	Healthcare professionals	Included in community health pathways Included in condition-specific therapy pathways	Used in consultation Developed for more conditions Develop for accessibility, e.g. literacy, language Developed for complex participatory interventions There was more appropriate data about what matters most
4. Communicating risk to patients	Discussing numerical information	Some personalized risk/benefits conversations Some 'do nothing' options	More personalized risk/benefit conversations More 'do nothing' options Meaningful data/information in relation to: • What really matters to people • Risks and benefits of participatory complex interventions Uncertainty in clinical practice

community of practice, which crosses professional and organizational boundaries through coordinated and collaborative working. The team has been able to focus the journey on the goal of addressing quality of care through a person-centred and value-based lens. Our improvement plan has been organic and evolving; taking advantage of opportunities as they arise, its adaptable design has allowed for diversification and sharing resources to other professions and specialities. The consistent use of the 'three-talk model' of SDM has enabled SDM to become embedded in the local language and facilitated its use.

SDM has become a key component of triage interventions and processes, and also our group education interventions—supporting individuals to find the way that works best for them. During consultations it is 'nudged' by the inclusion of 'what matters to me' prompts in clinical records, and the skills of 'chunk and check' and 'teach back' are regularly used when agreeing care plans with patients. Importantly, there is an increased understanding of the time required for deliberation and the use of appropriate supporting resources (e.g. printed and online information resources).

Local evaluation shows increased knowledge, theory, skills, competence, and capability in SDM among the teams, and it is now seen as a 'golden thread' that runs through all our training and development programmes. There is considerable progress with valuing the unique expertise of individuals, their experiences, beliefs, values, and preferences; this is now a core part of many consultations. The process has also highlighted the importance of developing advanced skills in communication, which has enabled the implementation of complementary formal training packages.

What we could do better

While we have well-established forums for co-production, it remains a challenge to bring the lived experience voice into training and delivery environments. We are yet to create the level of involvement of the population that will be crucial if SDM is to be an expected and participatory part of clinical practice. Inclusion of information prior to appointments has had limited impact on people using our services. As such, we are particularly interested and have initiated research to investigate how we assess the capabilities required to engage in SDM and use that knowledge to facilitate participation where it is wanted.

Attempts to formalize and standardize our evaluation and improvement processes have only been partially successful. As is often the case in pressured clinical environments, this vital part of the change process is often not given the priority it deserves. As such, while there are plans to use outcome and experience measures, observed practice, and reflective logs, most sites have only achieved a partial data set. The digitization of this type of work into electronic patient records will be a big step towards being more robust and complete in this improvement work.

The most consistent challenge, and one common to all change practices, has been personal attitudinal change within physiotherapy professionals. It has highlighted that as a profession we need to become more comfortable with being vulnerable to the unknown, complexity, risk, and uncertainty in human healthcare systems, and the limitations of the currently available evidence. As healthcare professionals there can be a desire to have all the answers, and therapists are particularly prone to the 'righting response' and 'fixer' mentality. However, it is essential for SDM that we share uncertainty, and some change is needed so that professionals see the benefit of doing so. This speaks directly to our ability to effectively communicate risk, benefits, and consequences, which are the topics of the next two NICE recommendations.

NICE recommendations 3 and 4: patient decision aids and communicating risk, benefits, and consequences

What has gone well

We have seen growth in the skills and capabilities to have better conversations, and are seeing a rise in compliments and experience, which appear linked to listening, understanding, and choice.

SDM offers a tool through which we can have better conversations about the uncertainty in healthcare, which in turn enables the consideration of complexity that is so often minimized by reductive scientific methods. Through the SDM lens, clinicians are experiencing the sharing of uncertainty, both with the people they work with and colleagues. Many are feeling the well-evidenced positive impact of this on their resilience, their ability to thrive in an uncertain world. The experience builds evidence and passion for the further implementation of other person-centred methods of delivering healthcare, in particular self-management.

The clinical leadership team are growing influence at local and national forums, enabling the increasing inclusion of patient decision aids in clinical pathways. While this could be a significant enabler for the spread and embedding of SDM in clinical practice, it will not guarantee it.

What we could do better

Unfortunately, despite several national and international clinical guidelines, the evidence base that we are currently working with is limited and often remains poorly communicated (Zadro et al., 2021), which is a significant challenge when communicating information about outcomes to patients.

Within therapies, we often deal with complex interventions—a combination of treatments and management strategies based on individual needs and preferences. It is challenging to capture the data for this through 'gold standard' randomized controlled trials, and more appropriate methods such as realistic evaluations are unfortunately seen as less scientifically robust. Quite simply, we do not currently have the scientific evidence base to know what combination of interventions works for the unique individual, and often base the options and decision much more on previous clinical experiences and on the patient's values and preferences. Hence the vital need for SDM in therapeutic practice.

Current methods and guidelines for the development and implementation of patient decision aids do not account for this complexity and lack of scientific evidence base (Zadro et al., 2021). The work of the International Patient Decision Aid Standards Collaboration (Witteman et al., 2021) and clinical academics will be central to designing aids that can be applied across complex decisions. It is vital that people using these tools are involved throughout this process to create a product and recommendations that are usable and fit for purpose. There will need to be clarity and transparency about what the data mean to the unique individual person.

For complex interventions there is a need for associated decision aids and conversations to capture the complex effects of combining interventions, and the relative risks and benefits of including or excluding certain components. For example, participating in exercise interventions for low back pain without the education and psychologically informed components. These data may be better informed from data registries, populated from routine daily practice. The pooling of 'big data' could enable the types of analysis needed to understand relationships between components of care, which can be included in decision aids and/or conversations. This will of course still need applying to the unique individual person with appropriate understanding of uncertainty.

Underpinning all of this will be making sure we capture data that matters to people: what outcomes, benefits, and risks of rehabilitation interventions matter to them? While symptom resolution or improvement can be a goal, it is often not this simple and people have other priorities. For many, preventing or slowing a deterioration is the goal, and these benefits reach across the biopsychosocial spectrum. Participating in an element of social, family, or work life are things that are highly valued by individuals, for example.

The physical and biological risks that are relatively easy to describe for medicines and surgery are often minimal in rehabilitation. However, the psychological (such as failure, self-efficacy, and hope) and sociological risks (such as identity, employment, lifestyle, and social networks) are less quantifiable, and alternative methods to enable conversations regarding these are required.

We must be mindful of the changing nature, volume, and complexity of the population's health needs. As infectious diseases become less prevalent and we see increasing success of interventions for other common sources of mortality, we are increasingly challenged by multiple morbidity from combinations of long-term conditions. Increasingly, therapy will necessitate a holistic approach targeted at a whole person with multiple comorbidities, and will require different SDM conversations, interventions, and data to support choice.

Key learning

Through our implementation journey (Figure 56.1), the following key learning themes emerged:

1. *Simple to teach, complex to embed.* Our experience has shown that SDM has well-defined knowledge and skills that can be simple both to teach and learn. However, application within clinical practice as a business-as-usual activity is a different prospect. There is a need to invest in teaching SDM in both undergraduate and postgraduate training, and in the quality improvement mechanisms that embed it in daily practice. There is a need to invest population health education to create more active participants in healthcare. Enabling this across diverse societies with variance in health, risk, language, literacy, and capability will require considerable work.
2. *Information that's important, studies that are relevant.* It has become clear that the information that people need to share decisions is often not available. Data from randomized controlled studies describe outcomes for the average individual in a well-defined population undergoing a well-defined intervention. However, in the unique world of multiple morbidity, person-centred care, and participatory complex interventions, we simply do not have the data to predict outcome in this way. It is challenging to describe the myriad of risks and benefits that may impact health and other parts of the person's life, such as their work, social, self-identity, self-worth, etc. There is a need to consider alternative research methods such as realistic evaluation, and the use of local 'big data' that captures outcomes that matter to patients is advantageous and needed.
3. *Know yourself and embrace uncertainty.* Healthcare professionals need to embrace the uncertainty and complexity in modern healthcare. They need to be willing and able to be vulnerable to the unknown and feel comfortable sharing and communicating that uncertainty with patients. We need to be open about what is predictable and what is not, and what the risks of participatory interventions are. For many therapists this will mean learning to overcome the 'righting reflex', to enable people to explore solutions rather than provide them. This will mean addressing the perceived risk to self and system.
4. *What matters? Get to know others.* Communication has always been and remains a core skill that needs to be honed and practised. Despite this, it often does not receive equal priority on the curriculum as 'clinical' knowledge and skills. This need to be addressed; communication must be a 'golden thread' of clinical practice. We need to use these skills to understand the people that we interact with, value their expertise and strengths, prioritize their stories, and understand what matters in the context of their beliefs and preferences. This is the foundation for exploring options and supporting people to make the best decisions for them.

See Box 56.1 for our patient perspective.

Box 56.1 Patient perspective

I'm Elaine, a 64-year-old widow, from a middle-income background and of white European ethnicity. My background is in health and well-being; I have studied and taught yoga and several complementary therapies for most of my life. I am recovering from sepsis and a subsequent total hip replacement and would like to share my experience of SDM in my rehabilitation.

My experience began in May 2021, when I was admitted to hospital with acute sepsis. It was on discharge from critical care that I was first supported to set a long-term goal that matters to me; this was to regain the use of my legs and to walk unaided on the farm with my dog.

The physiotherapy team were helpful in reducing my anxieties; there was no rush, no obligation. Everyone seemed to care and take time to understand how I felt, what mattered to me, and to discuss and agree what we would work together. I was asked how much I wanted to do, how strong I was feeling, and how my confidence was. Every visit was about my needs, my feelings, and my well-being. I felt cared for, safe, and listened to.

After a long period of anxiety and feeling loss, grief, confusion, and helplessness, my confidence returned in September, and I went home.

A year later, I'd progressed enough to consider total hip replacement. SDM was evident in many conversations; the whole team got on board with my goal to walk with my dog on the farm unaided. Prior to surgery, conversations led me to choose to attend the ESCAPE hip pain programme, to research nutrition, cut out inflammatory food, and attend a mindfulness course.

In February 2023 I had my total hip replacement. On the ward and in rehab after, I felt listened to, cared for, and focused on my goal to walk independently with my dog on the farm. We discussed timescales for regaining strength, flexibility, and endurance. The news was that recovery would likely be longer than most, however I felt no disappointment; rather I was more determined.

Time is never an issue with the physio team. It is often challenging for me to admit to my weaknesses and fears. They were meticulous in reviewing my history, listening to my goals and desires, and advising timescales for regaining a lifestyle I had thought was gone.

I began to establish friendships, to go out, and drive an automatic car. Recently I applied to work as a volunteer catering assistant in the local hospice and I've been on a yoga retreat. I am free of pain and I can walk on the farm again with my dog—on windy days and in muddy weather I use a walking frame for stability.

My journey continues, I work with my health providers and my own body to regain a life I thought was lost forever.

Conclusion

The supportive rhetoric around SDM in physiotherapy continues to grow through evidence, regulations, and policy. Through securing leadership and building skills and capabilities, our profession and multiprofessional colleagues are moving closer to a reality where SDM is a consistent part of 'business as usual'. There is, however, a need for us to reflect individually and as a profession about how we achieve a more person-centred way of working within a health-care system that is in transformation. Four challenges for the future seem clear: (1) taking SDM from a teachable system to a fully implemented business as usual, through enabling professionals to experience the mastery experience of benefits to both person and professional. (2) Collecting and presenting the appropriate information, through appropriate methods, to make it useful and meaningful to the person that is making the decision. (3) Professionals need to look inside themselves to understand and be vulnerable about mental models and biases that prevent person-centred methods. (4) Finally, the skill of listening, being genuinely curious to understand the people we serve, and to use all of this to fully inform a shared decision.

REFERENCES

Barker, K., Toye, F., Seer, K. 2023. A synthesis of qualitative research to understand the complexity behind treatment decision-making for osteoarthritis. *Osteoarth Cartil Open*, **5**, 100355.

Bowen, E., Nayfe, R., Milburn, N., et al. 2020. Do decision aids benefit patients with chronic musculoskeletal pain? A systematic review. *Pain Med*, **21**, 951–969.

Décary, S., Zadro, J., O'Keefe, M., et al. 2021. Overcoming overuse part 5: is shared decision making our Excalibur? *J Orthop Sports Phys Ther*, **51**, 53–56.

Dierckx, K., Deveugele, M., Roosen, P., et al. 2013. Implementation of shared decision making in physical therapy: observed level of involvement and patient preference. *Phys Ther*, **93**, 1321–1330.

Grenfell, J., Soundy, A. 2022. People's experience of shared decision making in musculoskeletal physiotherapy: a systematic review and thematic synthesis. *Behav Sci (Basel)*, **12**, 12.

Hoffmann, T., Bakhit, M., Michaleff, Z. 2022. Shared decision making and physical therapy: what, when, how, and why? *Braz J Phys Ther*, **26**, 100382.

Hoffmann, T., Lewis, J., Maher, C. 2020. Shared decision making should be an integral part of physiotherapy practice. *Physiotherapy*, **107**, 43–49.

Jones, L., Roberts, L., Little, P., et al. 2014. Shared decision-making in back pain consultations: an illusion or reality? *Eur Spine J*, **23**, S13–S19.

National Institute for Health and Care Excellence. 2021. Shared decision making. NICE guideline [NG197]. Available at: https://www.nice.org.uk/guidance/ng197

Ogawa, T., Fujimoto, S., Omon, K., et al. 2023. Shared decision-making in physiotherapy: a cross-sectional study of patient involvement factors and issues in Japan. *BMC Med Inform Decis Mak*, **23**, 135.

Welsh Government. 2018. A healthier Wales: our plan for health and social care. Available at: https://www.gov.wales/healthier-wales-long-term-plan-health-and-social-care

Welsh Government. 2019. Allied health professions framework: look forward together. Available at: https://www.gov.wales/allied-health-professions-ahp-framework

Welsh Government. 2021. National clinical framework: a learning health and care system. Available at: https://www.gov.wales/national-clinical-framework-learning-health-and-care-system

Welsh Government. 2022. All Wales rehabilitation framework: principles to achieve a person-centred value-based approach. Available at: https://www.gov.wales/health-and-social-care-services-rehabilitation-framework

Welsh Government. 2023. The Health and Social Care (Quality and Engagement) Wales Act. Available at: https://www.gov.wales/health-and-social-care-quality-and-engagement-wales-act-summary

Witteman, H. O., Maki, K. G., Vaisson, G., et al. 2021. Systematic development of patient decision aids: an update from the IPDAS Collaboration. *Med Decis Making*, **41**, 736–754.

Zadro, J., Traeger, A., Décary, S., et al. 2021. Problem with patient decision aids. *BMJ Evid Based Med*, **26**, 180–183.

57

Shared decision making in nursing and advanced practice nursing

Kirsten Lomborg, Jeanette Finderup, Sally Thorne, and Henning Søndergaard

Introduction

'Not my best day', nurse Irene thought as she changed into home clothes after work at the hospital. Mrs Jones, aged 86, had received haemodialysis in her clinic three times a week for several years. For the past month Mrs Jones had seemed increasingly disengaged, and this morning she had concluded their conversation by saying 'I really can't take it anymore'. Thinking back on Mrs Jones' comment, Irene realized that Mrs Jones might have been signalling a need to talk about her thoughts and values surrounding quality of life and end-of-life care. Perhaps she should be offered an opportunity to discuss possible options if she no longer wanted to continue dialysis? Irene had not found a way to start the conversation today, even though she thought Mrs Jones had been trying to invite it. 'Did I fail?', Irene asked herself. She knew about shared decision making as a concept, but in a situation such as this with Mrs Jones, her skills didn't match up to her ideals, and for that matter neither did those of her colleagues who all tended to avoid such sensitive conversations. Reflecting on her disappointment in her own confidence and competence in this regard, Irene began to consider how she could prepare herself to be proactive in that area of patient care and ultimately improve the overall level of service within her clinic. She wondered if advanced practice nursing studies might help her develop her capability in this area and began to explore further education as a possibility.

Shared decision making (SDM) is a crucial element in person-centred care and should be enacted as interdisciplinary teamworking in partnership with patients. This has long been recognized among policymakers and researchers, but evidence shows that experiences with implementation are mixed and efforts to improve practice have generally been sluggish. Thus, transformative changes are needed and engaging the exceptional potential of care provided by nurses and advanced practice nurses (APNs) may be vital to achieve 'routine' SDM.

All nurses contribute to SDM, but some find themselves in more suitable environments and with stronger competencies than others to improve SDM in clinical practice. Growing evidence shows that higher-level nurse education improves patient outcomes (Hafsteinsdóttir et al., 2019). A further education option is APN education which is a practice-oriented academic postgraduate opportunity. Many think that APNs within a care system can improve SDM development and implementation processes towards better patient outcomes. Because this contention has not yet been supported by the development of a robust evidence base, we approach the issue through consideration of what exists in the form of experiences and discussion and draw on an example case from a hospital's kidney department (Box 57.1).

Box 57.1 Patient perspective

I have had kidney failure for 14 years and have been on home haemodialysis for 12 years. Back in 2014 and inspired by the USA, I searched for funding and developed a Danish patient decision aid in app format to help with the choice of dialysis organized by the Danish Kidney Association, Nyreforeningen. When the app was ready, I faced a challenging time in my illness trajectory and teamed up with an advanced practitioner nurse who assisted with further funding and the content of the patient decision aid. This patient decision aid app has been scientifically evaluated (Therkildsen et al., 2019) and has been running for 8 years. I did this because I believed that as a patient with kidney failure on dialysis, the decision about dialysis choice should be made as a shared decision, rather than solely the patient's own choice.

I am most likely considered a strong patient due to my ability to self-manage a complex treatment for several hours, multiple times a week, as well as search for funding and develop a patient decision aid in app format. However, I also have tough times where my illness trajectory makes me vulnerable, and I question whether I live to dialyse or dialyse to live. I have many thoughts about decisions regarding end-of-life care. I have attempted to discuss these issues with my healthcare professionals, but sometimes I have encountered nurses like Nurse Irene who do not respond to patients' requests to talk about end-of-life care decisions.

Therefore, when I was asked to be a patient partner in a PhD project where a nurse was developing and testing a SDM intervention about end-of-life care, I immediately agreed. I have personal experiences with this situation, and through my work in the national kidney association, I knew that a SDM intervention in this area was needed.

The decision needs of patients, relatives, and clinicians were investigated (Buur et al., 2024). Here are some quotations from this investigation that align with my own experiences and what I have heard from members of our patient organization:

> But there are also many times when healthcare professionals are stressed, and I hold back my thoughts about something because I do not get the opportunity to express them. They do not have time to listen, and this sometimes frustrates me because I cannot share my thoughts. (Patient)
>
> But I also want to say that when it came down to it, he [the patient] was more open than I was, but he was also the one who was ill. He quickly realized that there was an end date to this, and he wanted us to talk about it, but I couldn't at first. (Relative)
>
> They [healthcare professionals] only tell you that everything is fine, and then the next day, you are admitted. (Patient)

Based on the data and through workshops with patients, relatives, and clinicians, we developed this SDM intervention, which includes training for healthcare professionals, a patient decision aid, and conversations between patients, relatives, and healthcare professionals. The intervention has been evaluated, but the results have not yet been published. However, the results from prototyping some parts of the intervention have shown promising results (Buur et al., 2023a):

> And a nice patient decision aid. It has definitely provided more nuances. It has offered broader perspectives than I had before. (Participant)
>
> It might very well lead to us discussing some of these elements [benefits and harms of the decision options] over a glass of red wine tonight. It cannot be ruled out. (Participant)
>
> Then you would be better able to weigh the benefits and harms, because what does life-saving treatment really entail? (Participant)

As a patient with many ups and downs in my illness trajectory, being a part of this work has meant a lot to me. It gives me a sense of purpose and helps me consider my options. Most importantly, it allows me to contribute to something that benefits all patients with kidney failure, their relatives, and healthcare professionals.

The contribution of nursing knowledge to SDM

SDM among patients and healthcare professionals about choices related to care and treatment puts different logics into play. First, there is the patient's desire for well-being and an underlying layperson's logic about health and illness. Second, there is the physician's ideal of curing disease and an underlying biomedical logic. In addition, there is the nurse's positioning, which includes both an ideal of care and an underlying biomedical logic. It has been argued that the standpoint of nursing knowledge, situated between the physician and the patient logics, constitutes a more holistic understanding of human health than the common disease-and-dysfunction views in current healthcare (Risjord, 2010). This places the nurse in a favourable position for SDM and for the transformative changes needed to shift from episodic care and treatment to team-based person-centred care.

Healthcare choices of concern to patients involve a wide range of decisions about care and care planning, aspects in which the nursing profession can engage independently, team practice notwithstanding. The conditions of the nursing standpoint are rooted in clinical practice, where in most settings nurses have more frequent and close contact with patients than other healthcare professionals, giving them optimal opportunities to get to know patients as more than just a person with a symptom, an injury, or a diagnosed disease.

Decisions about care and care planning include such elements as self-management support and what, how, when, and where patients will meet their basic needs of food and fluid, movement, sleep and rest, hygiene, and skin care (Rosca et al., 2023). Nurses bring education, knowledge, and experience to these core aspects of patient health and illness experience and nursing knowledge should be recognized as a specialized and valuable contribution to achieving SDM based on understanding what is most important to the patient(s). Enhancing the nursing contribution to SDM in general could strengthen a healthcare system's capacity for person-centred care and its overall resilience, especially for patients with long-term conditions and in circumstances where healthcare systems are challenged by such factors as ageing populations, mental health issues, chronic disease management, health inequality, rising costs, and shortages or imbalances in healthcare workforce.

Advanced practice nursing competencies

In 2020, the World Health Organization called for the expansion and greater recognition of nursing roles, including APNs, to better meet patient care needs (World Health Organization, 2020). The APN term has been known for more than 60 years and the APN workforce is growing, although with varying prevalence globally and in different roles and job titles. The International Council of Nurses defines an APN as 'a generalist or specialized nurse who has acquired, through additional graduate education (minimum of a master's degree), the expert knowledge base, complex decision making skills, and clinical competencies for advanced nursing practice' (International Council of Nurses, 2020). There is, however, no uniform understanding of the APN role worldwide and there are variations among jurisdictions with respect to the regulation of APNs and their education, licensing, and accreditation requirements. In some countries, APNs function autonomously based on a special prescribing licence. In others, licences to prescribe specific treatments that are traditionally assigned to physicians can be delegated to APNs. The specific scope of diagnostic and prescriptive rights is of considerable importance in determining the extent to which APNs can actively participate in or lead SDM. Clearly, where APNs have prescriptive authority, whether in a general or a specific and specialized context, they will be more appropriately positioned to independently support SDM in the contexts that are the typical focus of the evolving SDM evidence base.

The manner in which APN roles and activities develop in different healthcare systems may be driven not only by health-related aspirations but also financial and social interests (R. Lewis, 2022). APNs can serve as substitutes in performing tasks that may have been formerly carried out by physicians or others on the interprofessional healthcare team, and they can supplement existing healthcare services with new initiatives that enhance the continuity and quality of care. The two most common APN roles internationally are nurse practitioners, who function with a wider scope of diagnostic and treatment autonomy than is the case for registered nurses, and clinical nurse specialists, whose expanded competencies are used at the level of systems of nursing and healthcare delivery (International Council of Nurses, 2020). Both APN roles are frequently engaged in care settings for persons with acute, chronic, or complex conditions.

There is no international standard for APN curricular requirements. Typically, a training programme targets advanced clinical practice competency, excellence, and leadership to enhance complex patient processes across sectors and specialties. These professional learners develop skills in advancing evidence-based care, and they develop knowledge around coordination of care and treatment within and across primary health, community, and hospital services. For example, Canadian programmes aim at training nurse practitioners in the primary sector to 'assess, diagnose and treat acute and chronic conditions experienced across the lifespan' and 'to initiate interventions in urgent, emergent, and life-threatening situations' (Canadian Nurses Association, 2024). This emphasis towards more autonomous practice is similar to the scope in the USA. In Australia, the APN's autonomous field of activity is clearly defined to include a licence to prescribe medications, make referrals, request diagnostic and pathology investigations in acute hospital departments, mental health, community and primary healthcare, or chronic condition management in both the public and private healthcare system (Bonner et al., 2019).

The contribution of advanced practice nursing to SDM

Soliciting preferences and tailoring information are two of the most important mechanisms in SDM. Based on an integrative review, a framework to specifically depict SDM in nursing emphasizes the phase *before* working towards a shared decision (Truglio-Londrigan and Slyer, 2018). Here the nurse's holistic knowledge of the patient's condition and situation, combined with the nurse's communicative skills, create a respectful and trust-based relationship. According to another review that sought to explain differences in the degree of patient involvement in SDM, nurses play an important role through explaining (and reiterating) information and in supporting the patient to express preferences, values, and needs (Zagt et al., 2024). Nurses often draw on the mechanisms of non-directive decision coaching to solicit preferences and support patients to actively participate in a health decision. Decision coaching can be provided before the SDM or as a part of SDM process. Nurses have well-developed and specific skills in providing decision coaching and are therefore an important part of the wider SDM commitment. They use critical reflection and analysis in support of diagnosing the problem, providing options, screening for decisional needs, providing support to address decisional needs, monitoring progress in decision making, and screening for factors influencing implementation (K. B. Lewis et al., 2016).

Where physicians are prepared to delegate the responsibility for certain treatment decisions, the role of nursing can become considerably more prominent. For example, in Denmark, nephrologists have delegated the choice of dialysis modality to nurses (Finderup et al., 2020) and new clinical pathways have been developed with evidence-based communicative tools and patient decision aids for SDM with a clinical nursing specialist as the driver and with the overall purpose of empowering patients with kidney failure to engage in decisions, such as on advance care planning.

Advance care planning and SDM are often seen as two different concepts, but they can be integrated in one enhanced process of patient-informed choice (Rosca et al., 2023). Advance care planning engages patients in decision making about everyday nursing care decisions, treatment-related medical decisions, and end-of-life decisions, best applied by all members of an interdisciplinary team, but typically with nurses taking a lead. For example, a recent PhD project, conducted by a nurse, aimed to develop an SDM intervention to support people with kidney failure, their relatives, and healthcare professionals in planning and deciding about end-of-life care together (Buur et al., 2022). It included a complex intervention developed from a scoping review of the relevant literature, semi-structured interviews describing multiple stakeholder experiences of involvement in SDM towards end-of-life care, a mixed methods study to develop a prototype SDM intervention, and an acceptability and feasibility test of the intervention (Buur et al., 2023b). This work shows that these types of interventions can be delivered within hospital-based kidney services. The interventions meaningfully engage nurses in SDM with patients and show how nursing knowledge acts as a driver for hospital and clinic system-level interdisciplinary practice change.

Summary

In this chapter, we have highlighted the special position of knowledge that enables nurses to form strong professional relationships with patients who are faced with small and large treatment choices. We have broadly described the education and roles of APNs and have advocated for their relevance in SDM—both for the patients themselves and to enhance healthcare systems moving towards truly person-centred approaches.

SDM involves holistic thinking with an understanding of the individual's life situation. But understanding is not enough. The most important health professional competencies needed for SDM include effective communication skills, empathy, cultural competence, critical thinking, and the ability to translate complex medical information into understandable language for patients. Close contact and engagement with patients over time is essential to enacting fulsome collaboration in exploring their treatment options and integrating their values and sense of autonomy into decisions. Both structural and health professional transformations are needed to spread SDM, and the nurses' professional positioning, training, and knowledge base are excellent resources in this process. APNs are specialized nurses who, in addition to their professional expertise, have the skills to initiate and implement team-based change projects. They are also trained to lead the continuous quality assurance of new initiatives such as SDM.

There are excellent examples of SDM change projects driven by APNs. From these, we know that the degree of success depends not only on the skill of the APNs, but also on their access to formal authority within the healthcare team to truly engage patient collaboration.

'Oh boy! A lot has happened to our care of the most seriously ill patients', Irene thought, as she reflected on her work in the hospital's dialysis clinic this morning. It was a year since she had graduated as an APN, and it had really paid off. She had learned so much that helped her apply her expanded knowledge to her ideals of patient-centred care. Irene was particularly proud that, based on skills gained during her programme, she had successfully initiated and, together with her team and its patient representatives, implemented an interdisciplinary strategy to ensure better options for patients with kidney failure around their treatment options. Based on her enhanced system leadership understanding, Irene had assumed responsibility for further developing the SDM being used and the clarification of essential SDM competencies across the kidney failure healthcare team.

It was highly satisfying to see how dialogue with the patients had become not only more efficient but also more caring. 'It will be interesting to see how much further we can develop this', she thought. 'Will we see changes over time in the proportion of patients who prefer conservative kidney management over dialysis? And what might we learn if we track the characteristics of those patients?' Based on these successes, Irene was convinced that there were many other decisions that could be usefully supported by nurses with evidence-based and value-clarifying tools, and she was happy that she was beginning to establish a network for SDM across the hospital's professional pillars. By expanding her own expertise, she was playing a major role in advancing the system's capacity to respond in a meaningful way to the SDM support available to all patients and professionals.

REFERENCES

Bonner, A., Havas, K., Tam, V., et al. 2019. An integrated chronic disease nurse practitioner clinic: service model description and patient profile. *Collegian,* **26**, 227–234.

Buur, L. E., Bekker, H. L., Madsen, J. K., et al. 2023a. Patient involvement interventions for patients with kidney failure making end-of-life care decisions: a scoping review. *JBI Evid Synth,* **21**, 1582–1623.

Buur, L. E., Bekker, H. L., Mathiesen, C. L., et al. 2023b. Decision coaching for people with kidney failure: a case study. *J Ren Care,* **49**, 220–228.

Buur, L. E., Bekker, H. L., Rodkjaer, L. Ø., et al. 2024. Decisional needs in people with kidney failure, their relatives and health professionals about end-of-life care options: a qualitative interview study. *J Adv Nurs,* **80**, 3345–3358.

Buur, L. E., Finderup, J., Søndergaard, H., Kannegaard, M., Madsen, J. K., Bekker, H. L. 2022. Shared decision-making and planning end-of-life care for patients with end-stage kidney disease: a protocol for developing and testing a complex intervention. *Pilot Feasibil Stud,* **8**, 226.

Canadian Nurses Association. 2024. Nurse practitioners. Available at: https://www.cna-aiic.ca/en/nursing/advanced-nursing-practice/nurse-practitioners

Finderup, J., Lomborg, K., Jensen, J. D., Stacey, D. 2020. Choice of dialysis modality: patients' experiences and quality of decision after shared decision-making. *BMC Nephrol,* **21**, 330.

Hafsteinsdóttir, T. B., Jónsdóttir, H., Kirkevold, M., Leino-Kilpi, H., Lomborg, K., Hallberg, I. R. 2019. *Leadership in Nursing: Experiences from the European Nordic Countries.* Springer Nature.

International Council of Nurses. 2020. *Guidelines on Advanced Practice Nursing 2020.* International Council of Nurses.

Lewis, K. B., Stacey, D., Squires, J. E., Carroll, S. 2016. Shared decision-making models acknowledging an interprofessional approach: a theory analysis to inform nursing practice. *Res Theory Nurs Pract,* **30**, 26–43.

Lewis, R. 2022. The evolution of advanced nursing practice: gender, identity, power and patriarchy. *Nurs Inq,* **29**, e12489.

Risjord, M. 2010. *Nursing Knowledge: Science, Practice, and Philosophy.* Wiley-Blackwell.

Rosca, A., Karzig-Roduner, I., Kasper, J., Rogger, N., Drewniak, D., Krones, T. 2023. Shared decision making and advance care planning: a systematic literature review and novel decision-making model. *BMC Med Ethics,* **24**, 64.

Therkildsen, S. B., Handen, L. H., Jensen, L. E. D., Finderup, J. 2019. A patient decision aid app for patients with chronic kidney disease: questionnaire study. *JMIR Form Res,* **3**, e13786.

Truglio-Londrigan, M., Slyer, J. T. 2018. Shared decision-making for nursing practice: an integrative review. *Open Nurs J,* **12**, 1–14.

World Health Organization. 2020. *State of the World's Nursing Report: Investing in Education, Jobs and Leadership.* World Health Organization. Available at: https://www.who.int/publications/i/item/9789240003279

Zagt, A. C., Bos, N., Bakker, M., et al. 2024. A scoping review into the explanations for differences in the degrees of shared decision making experienced by patients. *Patient Educ Couns,* **118**, 108030.

58

Shared decision making in pharmacy

Jonathan Underhill, Steven D. Williams, Carole Pitkeathley, and Neal Maskrey

From safe and efficient medicine supply to person-centred prescribing—a short history of the pharmacy profession

The practice of pharmacy began with medieval apothecaries who were responsible for diagnosing disease as well as formulating, dispensing, and administering medicines to the public. Since the seventeenth century, pharmacy professionals in the UK have been regulated, currently by the General Pharmaceutical Council. Other countries have similar mechanisms. Moving into the twentieth century, the Pharmacy Act of 1954 gave full prescribing rights and responsibilities to UK pharmacists for medicines supplied 'over the counter' in a community retail pharmacy setting. In more recent times, pharmacists who have attained a further qualification to become a pharmacist independent prescriber can also prescribe any medicine within their scope of practice, in a similar way to medical doctors. Other countries continue to explore the clinical roles of pharmacists and the option of pharmacist prescribing, but it is not yet mainstream anywhere other than in the UK.

As the focus of pharmacy has evolved over the last century from safe and efficient supply of medicines to delivering a clinical service where the most appropriate medicine is prescribed for the individual, so too has the skill set required and the education provided. Person-centred care approaches and shared decision making (SDM) should ensure a person's values and preferences about medicines are considered when reaching an agreed decision. SDM is now included in recent updates to the General Pharmaceutical Council's 'Standards for Pharmacy Professionals' (General Pharmaceutical Council, 2024) and the prescribing competency framework (Royal Pharmaceutical Society, 2024), and should always be an important part of a pharmacist's everyday practice. However, as we will see from the patient perspective box later in this chapter, pharmacy practice has not always lived up to these ideals.

In this chapter we will describe the various opportunities for SDM in pharmacy, reflect on key challenges, describe current initiatives to support SDM, and consider the patient perspective.

Embracing uncertainty to support SDM in pharmacy

Delivering healthcare is a complex activity involving human-to-human interaction, where clinicians respond to changing scenarios and apply the best available scientific evidence to an individual situation. As a science-based profession, elements of undergraduate pharmacy teaching have historically focused on the chemistry and pharmacology/mechanism of action of medicines and how they are formulated. This contrasts with everyday clinical practice, where there is often no single 'right' answer. Pharmacists must progress from *novice* (can make simple decisions) to *expert* (can use clinical reasoning) in a methodical way while navigating the messy uncertainty of clinical practice. Key elements include accessing and processing the best available evidence, understanding the likely risks and benefits of treatment options, communicating with people to ascertain 'what matters to them', and then applying that to the individual situation, often with incomplete information.

However, for SDM to be fully embedded in pharmacy, pharmacists must strive to become more comfortable working in the 'grey' (uncertainty) (e.g. where diagnosis is unclear and/or evidence is uncertain), and not solely in the theoretical 'black and white', where certainty is assumed (e.g. where a clear diagnosis has been made and there is strong agreement on the best treatment option, using data from large clinical trials). Where there is high uncertainty about which option is best on a population level, the need to account for the person's individual values and preferences becomes even more important—as discussed elsewhere within this textbook, this is the essence of SDM.

Benefits of SDM in pharmacy

Studies have explored how pharmacists have integrated SDM into their clinical practice, within hospital (Fitzpatrick et al., 2023), primary care (Rosenberg-Yunger et al., 2018), and community settings (Baqir et al., 2017). The evidence from these studies suggests that attempting to engage in true SDM results in better relationships between the person and the clinical pharmacist, with improved communication and medication adherence (where medicines are taken in line with the regimen agreed between person and clinician). In addition, patients report being more actively engaged in consultations, especially in discussions about their treatment plans, and are better motivated to self-manage their chronic illnesses (Basger et al., 2023).

Done well, SDM can transform patients' care and experience. However, improvement of SDM skills rests on four factors:

1. Knowledge acquisition.
2. Observation of good practice.
3. Practice of the skill and feedback in a safe environment.
4. Assessment of the skill.

While improving SDM knowledge can be easily achieved through transactional education, it is more difficult and time-consuming to improve skills via clinical supervision, getting feedback on practice, and assessment of how well a clinician conducts a SDM consultation. While the study of human decision making is a well-established area of cognitive psychology, it is still not widely taught to pharmacy professionals.

In the UK, education resources are freely available to enable pharmacists, and other healthcare professionals, to improve their knowledge in this area. The National Institute for Health and Care Excellence SDM guideline (National Institute for Health and Care Excellence, 2021a) included an e-learning package based around the following modules (National Institute for Health and Care Excellence, 2021b):

- Orientation and background.
- Cognitive psychology: the science of how we all make decisions.
- Evidence-based medicine.
- Probability and uncertainty.
- Consultation skills.
- Practising SDM, staying up to date.

Challenges for implementing SDM in pharmacy

Many barriers to SDM between pharmacists and individuals are present in healthcare systems. Most will be common to other healthcare professionals and clinical settings, as identified by the MAGIC SDM implementation programme (The Health Foundation, n.d.). Within community pharmacy, ease of pharmacist accessibility without an appointment increases access to SDM discussions. However, the busy commercial environment also poses time restraints, and acts as a key barrier. Limited availability of private consultation areas is another barrier specific to SDM for the pharmacy profession, as well as lack of easy access to the patient's clinical notes, particularly in the community pharmacy setting. Further, there might be a perceived lack of authority or mandate to challenge treatment/management decisions made by other healthcare professionals, particularly if the pharmacist is not an independent prescriber themselves.

In the UK, many of these barriers are being addressed through initiatives such as 'Pharmacy First' launched by NHS England in January 2024 (NHS England 2024). However, they still provide a significant obstacle for the pharmacy profession to fully implement SDM in the UK and internationally, and more work is needed to identify solutions.

See Box 58.1 for our patient perspective.

Box 58.1 Patient perspective

Patient and public perspective on SDM with pharmacy professionals—a personal story of how pharmacy is changing

My elderly mother lived alone and struggled with a range of conditions, including high blood pressure, for which she had been prescribed ramipril (an ACE inhibitor). At her annual check-up at the general practice, she was found to be dehydrated and with some damage to her kidney. I received a call later that day from the clinical pharmacist attached to the practice. This interaction completely changed my perception of pharmacists based on my previous experience from a few years ago.

We discussed my mother's various conditions—her lifestyle, her cognitive function, and her everyday circumstances. The pharmacist explained clearly, patiently, and simply, the importance of good hydration and how this may impact some of her medicines. It was a breath of fresh air.

My mother always prefers coffee to any other drink, so we discussed ways of helping her drink more water, helping her to understand the problems if she didn't drink enough, and also what could be done about the combination of medicines she was taking for her many different conditions. He asked me, 'What do you think really matters to your mother?' Based on my response, we discussed options and together made a plan for how I could help my mother help herself. After discussion, we agreed to adjust the dose of ramipril, try to implement a plan to encourage and remind her to drink more water, alter certain foods to reduce salt and sugar, etc. and to speak again in a couple of weeks. It was one of the best healthcare discussions I have had—I felt listened to, understood, and, for the first time in my interactions with the NHS, in partnership for my mother's care.

When my mother's blood pressure was taken after a couple of weeks, the results were not good. She hadn't stuck to the 'one coffee, one water' plan, nor had she reduced her salt/sugar intake. The pharmacist understood this, we had both agreed that, in her mid-eighties, my mother was unlikely to change her habits quickly—indeed, she might not want to. We agreed to keep up with the plan for another 4 weeks and then regroup.

After 4 weeks, the pharmacist rang me again. This time the results were marginally better, but my mother was still resisting drinking water—I was devastated given the effort we had made. Still, the pharmacist helped me understand we could find some middle ground, adjust the medication again, and try different techniques with my mother's fluid intake. Over the next few months, we chatted a few more times, and, slowly but surely, my mother's blood pressure improved. She was still not drinking enough, but her hydration levels did improve a little. Throughout, the pharmacist was keen that I was in agreement with the plan, was able to manage it, and explain it to my mother while making sure it would not impact me too much. I always felt involved, that I had shared in developing the plan and reaching decisions about my mother's care and that he was as invested in reaching the best outcome for my mother as I was.

My previous experience with pharmacists had not been so positive. Growing up in the 1970s and 1980s, you went to the community pharmacist or 'chemist' to pick up a prescription from an intermediary who was the only person allowed to speak to the faceless pharmacist behind the closed dispensary door. Occasionally, advice was given about different medications or minor ailments, but this was rarely a two-way discussion. Rather, advice was dispensed and expected to be followed in a paternalistic fashion. Decisions were made *for you* rather than *with you*, and there was rarely that sense of feeling listened to or valued. Even in the 1990s and 2000s, when visiting a pharmacy, I never really felt included in discussions/decisions about my care; it still felt like an imbalance of knowledge and power. As time and resource pressures increased on pharmacies, if anything, I felt less able to engage or share.

As patients we want access to services in a way that works for us, or our loved ones, and in a way that we can understand. We want to be involved in discussions and decisions about our care, with just enough information provided to enable us to consider it at the time and afterwards at our convenience. My experience with the pharmacist who helped with my mother's care gave me all of those things. It gave me confidence in the service and encouragement to engage and ask questions. It was exactly what I would have described had someone asked me what I wanted. The shared discussions and agreements helped me at a time when I was not sure where to turn, when getting an appointment with a GP would have taken too long and would probably not have made me feel like decisions were shared. It was the right thing at the right time and helped achieve the best result we could.

The role of SDM in structured medication reviews

The use of innovative medicines in higher-income countries has transformed healthcare and, arguably, helped to increase life expectancy. However, as people are living longer, this means more people develop multiple conditions in older age—also known as multimorbidity. In the UK, more than 50% of people over the age of 75 years have two long-term conditions (Department of Health and Social Care, 2023) and 15% of patients take five or more regular medicines a day (Department of Health and Social Care, 2021); there is a similar picture in other high-income countries worldwide.

A recent UK study found that adverse drug reactions contributed to 16.5% of hospital admissions, those patients took more medicines and had more comorbidities, and 40% of the medical admissions were avoidable or possibly avoidable. Medicines most involved were water tablets (diuretics), blood thinners, blood pressure medicines, stomach acid suppressants, chemotherapy drugs, and steroid inhalers (Osanlou et al., 2022). So-called problematic polypharmacy is one of the major challenges to healthcare in the UK and other high-income countries, and one that the pharmacy profession must engage with as a priority.

The most recent UK Chief Medical Officer's report highlighted the importance of helping people with multiple long-term conditions (multimorbidity) in older age:

> Much of the medical profession and healthcare services in the UK is organised around single diseases or single organ systems in a way that is ill-suited to a future of increasing multimorbidity. People can spend their time going to multiple unrelated specialist clinics, be on several care pathways and are prescribed multiple medications (polypharmacy). (Department of Health and Social Care, 2023)

As highlighted in the patient perspective (Box 58.1), the care of older people with multimorbidity and polypharmacy requires the successful involvement of different health and care professionals. Pharmacists as generalist medicines experts will play an increasingly important role in ensuring patients' values and preferences are fully considered when a person chooses to use medicines. This is particularly the case when considering the nexus between quality and quantity of life. In England, pharmacist independent prescribers are now common and provide one way to address polypharmacy and improve the optimization of people's medication regimens (Croke et al., 2023).

In April 2020, NHS England issued guidance that general practitioner (GP) practices use appropriate tools to identify and prioritize patients who would benefit from a structured medication review by clinical pharmacists—particularly those in care homes and with complex and problematic polypharmacy on ten or more medications (NHS England, 2020). Patients (and families and carers) are offered 30-minute appointments where, through a process that aligns with SDM, they are encouraged to ask questions about their medicines. This is to help them get the most benefit from medications, and even reduce or stop some (known as deprescribing). This can be daunting for patients. However, national campaigns can help to promote this behavioural change, for example, 'When it comes to getting the best from our medicines, we all need to know: it's OK to ask . . .' (Me and My Medicines, n.d.).

Pharmacists or GPs undertaking such reviews also need the confidence to listen and act upon patient's wishes. A series of polypharmacy action learning sets have been shown to significantly improve awareness, confidence, and management of inappropriate polypharmacy, and SDM about stopping medicines with these health professionals (Brooks et al., 2022).

These discussions are especially important where there may be medico-legal concerns about stopping medicines started by a specialist that no longer suit the individual's lifestyle, or where they are doing more harm than good (Brown et al., 2022).

Pharmacist prescribers can use a simple acronym 'PLAN' as way of remembering how to structure a medication review consultation, which incorporates principles of SDM (Table 58.1).

Pharmacists must be able to both understand and communicate uncertainty to patients, utilize evidence-based decision aids for commonly prescribed medicines to help with 'BRAN' (Benefits of the medicine; Risks of the medicine; Alternatives to the medicine; No change from current management) discussions (GP Evidence, n.d.), and trust and support patients in their decision making. Educational programmes (Health Innovation Wessex, n.d.) and public-facing resources exist to aid this (Prestwich, 2023).

All UK pharmacists who qualify from 2026 onwards will have the legal right and responsibility to prescribe within their scope of practice. This represents a paradigm shift in how medicines are prescribed, especially for community pharmacists who are a regular point of contact for patients with multiple long-term conditions and increasingly deal with common self-limiting conditions (e.g. sinusitis/sore throat/urinary tract infection) to reduce the burden on GP practices (NHS England, 2024). Pharmacists will need to be aware,

Table 58.1 The 'PLAN' approach to medication review consultations

Prepare	Assess the clinical notes before the patient enters the consultation regarding why medicines were first started etc.
Listen	Listen to what matters to the patient about their medicines in relation to their health and day-to-day life
Agree	Use the BRAN (Academy of Royal Colleges, n.d.) and three-talk models of SDM
Notes	Record in the clinical notes what the treatment discussions were, if another health professional was consulted, and the monitoring, worsening advice guidance, and follow-up agreed

knowledgeable, and comfortable with using PLAN and BRAN to ensure the best person-centred care through SDM; importantly, these discussions may ultimately result in not prescribing a medication for self-limiting conditions.

Requirements for SDM in pharmacy

Whether it involves pharmacist prescribers conducting formal medication reviews using PLAN and BRAN (as in the UK) or pharmacists who are engaging in discussions to ensure the best medication outcomes for patients with polypharmacy (Lenander et al., 2014; iSIMPATHY, 2023), we propose several prerequisites to improve the quantity and quality of good SDM by pharmacists:

Private consultation area

Healthcare is, by definition, personal, so conversations about people's medicines may be difficult in a busy shop within a traditional community pharmacy setting or at a bedside within a hospital ward. Privacy is often impossible in such situations. Telephone or video consultations can remove this obstacle and work well for some people, but can be very transactional, and are less good for in-depth conversations about medicines.

Access to the patient's clinical notes

If pharmacists do not have ready access to the patient's clinical notes, this hampers safe and effective conversations about, or prescribing of, medicines outside the management of very simple self-limiting conditions. Access to notes enables a more holistic view of what is going on, over and above what a person is able to communicate to you (which relies on good memory, health literacy, etc.).

Acceptance of the pharmacist as a medicines expert

Pharmacists in the UK undertake 5 years of study and must pass a registration exam to join the General Pharmaceutical Council's register. During their undergraduate course, they will spend thousands of hours studying the effects of medicines on the body, as well as the myriad other aspects of medicines use. This is in contrast with other healthcare professionals whose courses have a far wider ranging curriculum. Despite this expertise, there remains a reluctance by some to recognize pharmacists as the medicines experts and there remains resistance from other healthcare professionals and the public to fully utilize the pharmacy workforce. The same is true in many other countries.

In addressing this, it is clear that medical colleagues gain confidence in pharmacists' ability to perform SDM as they work more closely together, thus trusting their real medicines expertise, and through gaining feedback from their patients about good consultation experiences. Service evaluation or research into new services provided by pharmacists will help with this nationally and internationally (Elliott et al., 2016).

Consultation skills

Patients open up about their true medicine-taking habits when put at ease and when they are confident in the abilities of pharmacists. Key to this is an understanding of their medical history, asking about what matters most to them, displaying knowledge and experience of the medication within the context of their medical conditions, and knowing when to discuss the matter with another healthcare professional.

Confidence working in the grey

As discussed earlier in this chapter, this is crucial for pharmacists and is improved by access to the patient's clinical notes, acceptance as a medicines expert, and systems in place to develop evidence-based practice, clinical supervision, and communities of practice (Gabbay and Le May, 2016).

Summary

Overall, despite the challenges outlined in this chapter, the future opportunities for SDM in pharmacy are exciting and important. There is the prospect of more appropriate skill mix within healthcare, where the expertise of pharmacy is better utilized to facilitate SDM and person-centred optimization of medicines. As confidence grows within the pharmacy profession to hone these skills, the public and other healthcare professionals will continue to grow to trust pharmacy teams to improve the use of medicines. The near future is one where all newly qualified pharmacists in the UK can prescribe independently within their scope of practice, with SDM a routine part of this process.

REFERENCES

Academy of Royal Colleges. n.d. Choosing Wisely UK: shared decision making using BRAN. Available at: https://www.aomrc.org.uk/projects-and-programmes/choosing-wisely/

Basger, B. J., Moles, R. J., Chen, T. F. 2023. Uptake of pharmacist recommendations by patients after discharge: implementation study of a patient-centered medicines review service. *BMC Geriatr,* **23,** 183.

Baqir, W., Hughes, J., Jones, T., et al. 2017. Impact of medication review, within a shared decision-making framework, on deprescribing in people living in care homes. *Eur J Hosp Pharm,* **24,** 30–33.

Brooks, C. F., Argyropoulos, A., Matheson-Monnet, C. B., Kryl, D. 2022. Evaluating the impact of a polypharmacy action learning sets tool on healthcare practitioners' confidence, perceptions and experiences of stopping inappropriate medicines. *BMC Med Educ,* **22,** 499.

Brown, E. L., Poltawski, L., Pitchforth, E., et al. 2022. Shared decision making between older people with multimorbidity and GPs: a qualitative study. *Br J Gen Pract,* **72,** e609–e618.

Croke, A., Cardwell, K., Clyne, B., et al. 2023. The effectiveness and cost of integrating pharmacists within general practice to optimize prescribing and health outcomes in primary care patients with polypharmacy: a systematic review. *BMC Prim Care,* **24,** 41.

Department of Health and Social Care. 2021. Good for you, good for us, good for everybody: a plan to reduce overprescribing to make patient care better and safer, support the NHS, and reduce carbon emissions. Available at: https://www.gov.uk/government/publications/national-overprescribing-review-report

Department of Health and Social Care. 2023. Chief Medical Officer's annual report 2023: health in an ageing society. Available at: https://www.gov.uk/government/publications/chief-medical-officers-annual-report-2023-health-in-an-ageing-society

Elliott, R. A., Boyd, M. J., Salema, S., et al. 2016. Supporting adherence for people starting a new medication for a long-term condition through community pharmacies: a pragmatic randomised controlled trial of the New Medicine Service. *BMJ Qual Safe*, **25**, 747–758.

Fitzpatrick, K., Addie, K., Shaw, M., et al. 2023. Implementing an innovative, patient-centred approach to day case arthroplasty: improving patient outcomes through remote preoperative pharmacist consultations. *Eur J Hosp Pharm*, **31**, 321–326.

Gabbay, J., Le May, A. 2016. Mindlines: making sense of evidence in practice. *Br J Gen Pract*, **66**, 402–403.

General Pharmaceutical Council. Standards for pharmacy professionals. Available at: https://www.pharmacyregulation.org/standards/standards-for-pharmacy-professionals

GP Evidence. n.d. Summaries of the evidence on the benefits and harms of treatments for long term conditions. Nuffield Department of Primary Care Health Sciences, University of Oxford. Available at: https://gpevidence.org/

Health Innovation Wessex. n. d. Polypharmacy masterclasses. Available at: https://healthinnovationwessex.org.uk/projects/610/polypharmacy-masterclasses

iSIMPATHY. 2023. Stimulating innovation management of polypharmacy and adherence in the elderly evaluation report. Available at: https://www.isimpathy.eu/uploads/iSIMPATHY_Evaluation_report_ver8_online.pdf

Lenander, C., Elfsson, B., Danielsson, B., et al. 2014. Effects of a pharmacist-led structured medication review in primary care on drug-related problems and hospital admission rates: a randomized controlled trial. *Scand J Prim Health Care*, **32**, 180–186.

Me and My Medicines. n.d. When it comes to getting the best from our medicines, we all need to know: it's OK to ask. Available at: https://meandmymedicines.org.uk/

National Institute for Health and Care Excellence. 2021a. Shared decision making. NICE guideline [NG197]. Available at: https://www.nice.org.uk/guidance/ng197

National Institute for Health and Care Excellence. 2021b. Shared decision making learning package. Available at: https://www.nice.org.uk/guidance/ng197/resources/shared-decision-making-learning-package-9142488109

NHS England. 2020. Network contract directed enhanced service contract specification 2020/21—PCN requirements and entitlements. Available at: https://www.england.nhs.uk/publication/des-contract-specification-2020-21-pcn-entitlements-and-requirements/

NHS England. 2024. Launch of NHS Pharmacy First advanced service. Available at: https://www.england.nhs.uk/long-read/launch-of-nhs-pharmacy-first-advanced-service/

Osanlou, R., Walker, L., Hughes, D. A., et al. 2022. Adverse drug reactions, multimorbidity and polypharmacy: a prospective analysis of 1 month of medical admissions. *BMJ Open*, **12**, e055551.

Prestwich, G. 2023. The patient as a project manager [Podcast]. Available at https://www.theauralapothecary.com/51-graham-prestwich-the-patient-as-a-project-manager/

Rosenberg-Yunger, Z. R. S., Verweel, L., Gionfriddo, M. R., et al. 2018. Community pharmacists' perspectives on shared decision-making in diabetes management. *Int J Pharm Pract*, **26**, 414–422.

Royal Pharmaceutical Society. A competency framework for all prescribers. Available at: https://www.rpharms.com/resources/frameworks/prescribing-competency-framework/competency-framework

The Health Foundation. n.d. MAGIC: shared decision making. Available at: https://www.health.org.uk/funding-and-partnerships/programme/magic-shared-decision-making

59

Shared decision making in dentistry

Anwen Cope, Ivor G. Chestnutt, and Jennifer Wilson

Introduction

The World Health Organization's 2022 *Global Oral Health Status Report* estimated that oral diseases affect close to 3.5 billion people worldwide. The most common oral diseases are dental caries ('tooth decay'), periodontal disease ('gum disease'), and oral cancer. As with other non-communicable long-term conditions, poor diets high in sugar, tobacco use, and excessive alcohol consumption are significant risk factors.

Oral diseases disproportionally affect the poor and socially disadvantaged. There is a strong and consistent gradient between socio-economic status (income, employment, and educational level) and the prevalence and severity of oral diseases. This association exists from early childhood to older age and across populations in high-, middle-, and low-income countries.

Despite the societal burden associated with oral diseases, oral health services are often under-resourced. Countries with universal dental care are global exceptions, rather than the norm. Only one-fifth of countries provide state-funded dental care for children and adolescents, and such systems are rare in low-income countries, where there are also lower numbers of dentists per capita (Petersen et al., 2020).

Oral healthcare systems often require patients to make payments towards their care, either fully or in part. Out-of-pocket payments for essential oral healthcare can result in catastrophic health expenditures, leading to economic hardship.

Shared decision making in dentistry

How are patients involved in their dental care?

Discussion about shared decision making (SDM) began in the dental literature in the mid-2000s. Early work focused on decisions about operative treatment options, such as root canal treatment versus extraction of a tooth (Johnson et al., 2006). However, to consider patient involvement in its fullest sense, we should not be limited simply to the appraisal and selection of treatment options. We also need to reflect on the role that patients play in their wider dental care journey, from recognition and conceptualization of their dental problem, through to the evaluation of the success of treatment. To isolate discrete decisions from the wider dynamic of the patient–clinician relationship is an artificial distinction. These decisions occur within established (often long-standing) relationships. Clinicians and patients enter a consultation with pre-existing feelings and views that will influence their trust and willingness to engage in SDM. Each will have attitudes about their role in the decision making process, constructed from previous encounters and wider health-related beliefs. These will influence how the decision making process unfolds. In a new dentist–patient relationship, particularly where patients are in pain, or are dentally phobic, it may be particularly challenging for clinicians to establish patients' preferences and expectations regarding their involvement in the decision making process (Hayer and Wassif, 2022).

How are decisions made in dentistry?

Although SDM is gaining increasing attention in dentistry, its use is not ubiquitous. While patients report a desire to be involved in decisions about their dental care, there is a widespread misunderstanding of what constitutes SDM among dental practitioners. Discussions around treatment options are typically focused more on information provision and gaining (apparent) informed consent rather than collaboration (Hayer and Wassif, 2022; Scott et al., 2022).

Given the dental professional's position of knowledge and power in the consultation, the onus is on them to have the skills to engage the patient and to elicit their goals and preferences. Clinicians must be able to gauge the degree to which patients want to be involved in various decisions about their care, so-called optional autonomy, and how best to achieve this (Hayer and Wassif, 2022).

However, there is evidence that dentists may misjudge their patients' desire for involvement in decision making (Scott et al., 2022). As a result, patients can experience a mismatch between the level of involvement they desire, versus what they experience (Chapple et al., 2003). Furthermore, even when engaged in a collaborative decision making process, the information prioritized by dental professionals may not be that which is most important or useful to patients (Tonogai et al., 2024). An important example of this is discussion about the cost of care. Evidence from both the medical and dental literature is that cost of treatment options is often not prioritized for discussion by clinicians. This may be due to discomfort addressing patients' financial status. However, these are often important issues for patients, who may be responsible for some or all of the cost of care.

What decisions are there?

Within an episode of dental care there may be several individual decisions. Some of these will be diagnostic ('Should a radiograph ["X-ray"] be taken?'), some clinical ('What material should be used to restore this cavity?'), some relating to aspects of patient care ('When should the next dental appointment be scheduled?'). Some decisions relate to the single consultation ('Should additional sedative techniques be used for an anxious patient?') while others are longer-term behavioural commitments ('What is the best tool to clean between the teeth?'). Some decisions may result in irreversible action, such as the extraction of a tooth, whereas others, such as the duration of the dental recall interval, can be reviewed and changed at a later stage.

What becomes clear is that the comparative 'stakes' of these decisions will vary. Dental practitioners are more likely to recognize the role of SDM in decisions they perceive to be higher stakes, such as those involving irreversible, operative, or expensive procedures, or where there is likely to be an aesthetic impact (Scott et al., 2022). Conversely, studies have revealed a reluctance to engage in SDM for lower-stakes decisions, such as the length of dental recall interval (the time between 'check-ups') or whether to have a scale and polish (Scott et al., 2022; Verdugo et al., 2024). This may be driven by pragmatism; it is inefficient to have in-depth discussions about the pros and cons of every decision that arises during a clinical encounter, particularly in a dental practice environment where time is short and there is an imperative to maintain a high patient throughput.

Similarly, prolonged discussion about relatively minor issues is unlikely to provide patients with a satisfying experience. In practice, clinicians must therefore be able to rapidly and accurately ascertain patient preferences for involvement in specific decisions. This in itself can be challenging, since the values underlying patient preferences vary between individuals. For example, most patients will readily accept the benefit versus risk of having a radiograph taken, but a small proportion of patients hold strong preferences regarding exposure to X-rays.

Why does SDM matter in dentistry?

Patients wanting to be involved in decisions about their dental care is in itself sufficient reason for dental professionals to use collaborative decision making. However, the wider medical literature also tells us that patients whose practitioners use SDM can demonstrate improved health outcomes, are more confident managing their conditions, and may be more likely to engage in health-promoting behaviours. While dental studies are scarcer, patients engaged in SDM may be more knowledgeable and have greater satisfaction with their dental care (Johnson et al., 2006; Brandt et al., 2023). SDM is not just appropriate for patients with high health literacy. There is evidence of improved outcomes in disadvantaged groups and even a narrowing of inequalities.

In addition to improved patient outcomes and the effect on inequalities, policymakers in several countries have provided a clear mandate to use SDM in dental consultations. Similarly, dental indemnity or malpractice insurance providers are also widely supportive, since using SDM in clinical consultations may reduce the likelihood of litigation in situations where patients suffer adverse clinical outcomes (Schoenfeld et al., 2019).

What are the limits of SDM?

SDM can be applied to a wide range of decisions about dental care. In particular, when there is no evidence of superiority of one management option over another reasonable option, then SDM could be viewed as a necessary approach. One concern cited by dental practitioners as a barrier to using SDM, is the risk of patients selecting an 'unwise' treatment option (Scott et al., 2022). An example of this would be a patient requesting antibiotics for pulpitis, a painful inflammatory condition of the dental pulp where there is evidence that antibiotics do not confer improved outcomes. Selection of an antibiotic as the preferred treatment strategy in this situation may indeed lead to poorer clinical outcomes compared to root canal treatment or extraction of the tooth. However, SDM is not about patients selecting any treatment they desire, it is a collaboration that blends evidence, professional expertise, and patient perspectives. It is about the patient being supported so that they may be involved in making a decision between a number of *reasonable* treatment options. Since evidence would suggest that antibiotics are not a reasonable option in this scenario, they should not be part of the menu of options presented by the practitioner. Instead, the dentist should focus on eliciting patient values and preferences for root canal treatment, extraction, or a 'watchful waiting' approach.

See Box 59.1 for our patient perspective.

Box 59.1 Patient perspective

Jennifer Wilson, patient contributor

Can you briefly outline the decision that you were making about your clinical care?

I had an abscess around a molar tooth. This tooth had previously undergone a root canal and crown treatment around 24 months earlier. This initial procedure had been in Canada, via emergency dental travel insurance.

This appointment was now back in the UK with my long-standing National Health Service (NHS) dentist. They explained that I had two treatment options. The first was to attempt a further root canal treatment. The second was to extract the tooth and either leave a gap or replace it with an implant. I was very concerned that without an implant to replace a large molar, I would experience further problems with teeth moving in the upper jaw. Therefore, an extraction without an implant was not an acceptable option to me.

What was your experience with making this decision?

It was a difficult decision. The first root canal treatment had been traumatic, needing substantial time in the chair over three visits. I had trusted the Canadian dentist and recalled their explanation of the complexity of the treatment—more roots than average, running deep and close to the nerve.

The NHS dentist was willing to briefly discuss the pros and cons of each treatment option, but I felt that their time was constrained. They said the previous treatment looked exemplary and, while a second root canal treatment could succeed, there was at least a 50/50 chance it would fail given the resources put into the previous treatment. They explained that they could extract the tooth, but an implant would require referral to a private specialist.

Ultimately, I decided to go straight for the implant route. My gut feeling was that the second root canal treatment would not work and therefore I would pay for treatment twice over, dealing with the anxiety and pain of two procedures. When I saw the surgeon at the implant clinic, they recognized that I was facing a difficult decision regarding the probability of treatment success, pain, and cost. This provided some reassurance they were not pushing an implant for their own financial benefit.

My perception was that my regular dentist thought I should have an implant but did not want to push me towards that option due to the cost pressures. When I next saw them, they expressed satisfaction with the implant, which I took to be an implicit approval of my choice.

What was the hardest part about deciding?

The hardest parts were knowing that I did not have any medical comprehension about the probability of a second root canal treatment succeeding and feeling like there was no unbiased adviser or statistics available.

If all treatments had been free at the point of delivery, I suspect I would have felt more comfortable about the advice I received from both dentists. I was concerned about paying for a second root canal treatment. My perception was that my dentist had little confidence it would work, and I knew from experience that they had limited time for each appointment. However, an implant would be expensive and an invasive treatment. I also felt that I should try to preserve my natural tooth for as long as possible.

The memory of the earlier root canal treatment also distorted my decision making ability as, in all honesty, knowing I would be awake during either procedure reduced my willingness to risk two treatments!

Thinking back to your choice, how do you feel about your decision now?

I have never doubted the decision. The extraction was very difficult—more than 2.5 hours—even when undertaken by a highly qualified and regarded surgeon. My recollection is that they found a root twisted around a nerve, which had not been visible on X-ray scans. Consequently, I am convinced a second root canal treatment would have failed.

As most patients have limited medical knowledge, information is crucial and the financial model for delivering dentistry in the UK makes it hard to trust the independence of the advice being received.

The future for SDM in dentistry

Education and training

The widespread misunderstanding of SDM in dentistry signals a substantial unmet educational need among the dental profession. SDM goes beyond the traditional informed consent model commonly taught during healthcare professional education as it requires clinicians to offer evidence-based alternatives and then actively engage with a patient regarding their values and preferences. Clinicians therefore need appropriate training to ensure they can adequately facilitate the process. Only a minority of dental undergraduates currently receive teaching in SDM (Sin et al., 2021). More opportunities for training at undergraduate and postgraduate level are required if SDM is to become widely adopted in dentistry.

Policy and practice

Although SDM occurs between patients and clinicians, it is unlikely to occur in the absence of supportive healthcare systems (for fuller discussion see Chapter 17). Firstly, policymakers, dental regulators, and leaderships of clinical organizations need to actively support SDM. Secondly, the conditions for SDM also need to be supported. This requires identification and removal of any barriers to its implementation. There should also be a recognition that successful application of sharing decision making often requires longer appointments and that clinical care provision needs to be designed accordingly (Hayer and Wassif, 2022; Scott et al., 2022). In some cases, this will also involve appropriately rewarding dental teams who engage in SDM. Thirdly, SDM resources are needed. The use of decision aids, for example, facilitates greater involvement in decision making (see also Chapters 18 and 19). These aids, of which there are a few in dentistry (Johnson et al., 2006; Kupke et al., 2013; Brandt et al., 2023), need to be evidence-based, appropriate for the patient group, and acceptable to clinicians. Finally, measures of patient experience and outcome, and specifically decisional quality, that act as key indicators of the extent of the implementation of SDM are needed to close the feedback loop to support practice change.

Skill mix in dentistry

While most global dental care is provided by dentists, there is a growing number of mid-level providers (also called dental therapists, dental hygienists, or dental auxiliaries). These are dental professionals who provide clinical care but typically have a narrower scope of practice than dentists. Depending on the setting, they may work under the supervision or prescription of a dentist or as an independent clinician. There are many calls to increase skill mix in dentistry by expanding the training, scope of practice, and use of mid-level providers, particularly in countries where there are high levels of unmet dental need.

If skill mix is implemented to its full potential, patients will likely see several dental professionals during a single course of treatment—a dentist for an oral examination and treatment planning, a hygienist for a scale and polish, a therapist for a filling, before returning to the dentist for complex restorative treatment such as a crown. Feasibly, a preference-sensitive decision could arise at any one of these encounters and therefore the whole dental team needs to have the necessary skills to involve patients in decisions about their care.

Research priorities

Focusing on SDM training for dental teams and decision aids would neglect a larger issue relating to SDM research in dentistry. Dentistry is a discipline which has been described as an 'orphaned field of medicine' in which there is a large 'evidence-void' (Sellars and Wassif, 2019). As an illustration, of the 45 Cochrane systematic reviews on dental caries, a condition experienced by 2 billion people worldwide, 25 report low- or very low-quality evidence and a further four could identify no relevant trials. In reality, this may be a problem of focus, with comparatively greater research effort devoted to the investigation of the minutiae of complex restorative procedures, but less to everyday dentistry such as the management of acute conditions. Until there are robust studies about the relative rates of success, failure, and other outcomes of common treatment options, discussions of risk during SDM will continue to be based on substandard evidence. The current situation serves neither patient nor clinician.

Conclusion

The opportunities for SDM in dentistry are substantial. Many patients want to be involved in decisions about their care. Those that are, are often more satisfied and knowledgeable as a result. There is also evidence that patients may experience better health outcomes and that SDM may even contribute to the flattening the social gradient in oral health. The barriers, however, are considerable: unmet educational needs among the dental team; a mismatch between patient and practitioner priorities; and oral healthcare systems which are not conducive to its application. Balancing the additional resources needed for SDM against the huge number of patients worldwide who cannot access affordable dental care is a challenge for policymakers. In a world where resources are stretched, do you give the best service to the few, a little for the many, or even less to the rest?

REFERENCES

Brandt, S., Lauer, H. C., Güth, J. F., et al. 2023. Impact of two different patient decision aids in prosthodontic consultations: a prospective randomized controlled study. *Clin Oral Investig*, **27**, 7841–7849.

Chapple, H., Shah, S., Caress, A. L., Kay, E. J. 2003. Exploring dental patients' preferred roles in treatment decision making—a novel approach. *Br Dent J*, **194**, 321–327.

Hayer, N., Wassif, H. S. 2022. General dental practitioners' perceptions of shared decision making: a qualitative study. *Br Dent J*, **232**, 227–231.

Johnson, B. R., Schwartz, A., Goldberg, J., Koerber, A. 2006. A chairside aid for shared decision making in dentistry: a randomized controlled trial. *J Dent Educ*, **70**, 133–141.

Kupke, J., Wicht, M. J., Stützer, H., Derman, S. H., Lichtenstein, N. V., Noack, M. J. 2013. Does the use of a visualised decision board by undergraduate students during shared decision making enhance patients' knowledge and satisfaction?—a randomised controlled trial. *Eur J Dent Educ*, **17**, 19–25.

Petersen, P. E., Baez, R. J., Ogawa, H. 2020. Global application of oral disease prevention and health promotion as measured 10 years after the 2007 World Health Assembly statement on oral health. *Community Dent Oral Epidemiol*, **48**, 338–348.

Schoenfeld, E. M., Mader, S., Houghton, C., et al. 2019. The effect of shared decision making on patients' likelihood of filing a complaint or lawsuit: a simulation study. *Ann Emerg Med*, **74**, 126–136.

Scott, H., Cope, A. L., Wood, F., et al. 2022. A qualitative exploration of decisions about dental recall intervals—part 2: perspectives of dentists and patients on the role of shared decision making in dental recall decisions. *Br Dent J*, **232**, 327–331.

Sellars, S., Wassif, H. S. 2019. Is dentistry the orphaned field of medicine? Ethical consideration for evidence-based dentistry. *Br Dent J*, **226**, 177–179.

Sin, M., Butt, S., Barber, S. K. 2021. Assessing dentist and dental student knowledge of and attitudes towards shared decision making in the United Kingdom. *Eur J Dent Educ*, **25**, 768–777.

Tonogai, J., von Bergmann, H., Chvartszaid, D., Dempster, L. 2024. Patient and clinician perspectives on implant dentistry decision aid content: results from an enhanced Delphi study. *J Prosthodont*, **33**, 18–26.

Verdugo, J., Laughter, L., Chambers, D. W. 2024. Shared decision making in scaling and root planing. *Eur J Dent Educ*, **28**, 184–190.

60

Shared decision making for people living with multimorbidity

Perspectives from psychology, physiotherapy, occupational therapy, and lived experience

Darren Flynn, Katherine Baker, Gemma Bradley, Craig Craggs, and Jason Scott

Introduction

The person living with a long-term condition and their family are the only continuous entity in a largely discontinuous health and social care system. This statement applies across different health and social care systems and its veracity becomes more apparent when applied to people living with multiple long-term conditions, referred to as multimorbidity (MM). Shared decision making (SDM) has important implications for supporting people living with MM, which we will discuss in this chapter.

MM is conceptually different from comorbidity. Comorbidity focuses on an index condition (that takes precedence over any additional 'comorbid' conditions), whereas MM relates to a person living with two or more somatic or mental health conditions, including learning disability, substance misuse, sensory impairment, and symptom complexes, where one condition does not take precedence over another (National Institute for Health and Care Excellence, 2016). The literature has described clusters or patterns of somatic MM (respiratory, painful/gastrointestinal, cardio-cerebrovascular, and cardiometabolic) associated with new/persisting depression and anxiety (Ronaldson et al., 2021). Increased prevalence of MM is associated with age, deprivation, reduced life expectancy, poor health-related quality of life (HRQoL), and increased use of healthcare (e.g. Barnett et al., 2012).

A vignette of a person living with MM is described in Box 60.1; this will be used as an exemplar throughout this chapter, with reference to an actual lived experience perspective of MM, written by our patient co-author (Box 60.2).

Box 60.1 Scenario—John

John, age 53, male, is living with the following long-term conditions:

- Type 2 diabetes.
- Mild/moderate depression and anxiety.
- Elevated lipids.
- Obstructive sleep apnoea managed with continuous positive airway pressure therapy.
- Shoulder and low-back pain:
  - Obesity (body mass index >40 kg/m^2).
  - Medications: type 2 diabetes (metformin); depression and anxiety (citalopram); atorvastatin (statin).
  - Sedentary (low-active) lifestyle.
  - Employed as a delivery driver (zero-hours contract).
  - Married with one child (age 15).

Theoretical perspectives of SDM

From an applied health psychology perspective, SDM can be viewed as a series of behaviours associated with specific competencies, which 'permits the development and evaluation of interventions that target modifiable variables that are antecedents of intentions to engage in SDM and actual SDM behaviour' (Flynn, 2012, p. 76).

In England, 43% and 61% of adults (aged 18–65 years) do not have adequate literacy and numeracy skills, respectively, to allow them to routinely understand health information (Rowlands et al., 2015). Health literacy is conceptually linked to behaviours that are required to actively engage in SDM with health professionals: communicate

Box 60.2 Patient perspective

Lived experience perspective on MM

As a young child, I suffered from a severe head injury which affected my ability to process sensory information and utilize my motor functions. I had repeated bouts of unipolar depression throughout primary school and was taken into hospital on several occasions. Furthermore, because of nutritional deprivation, I developed arthritis that has persisted throughout my adult life. I never engaged in SDM with any therapists for these conditions. I accept that as a child SDM may not have been possible, but as an adult I feel I have been neglected by the medical system, perhaps because of lack of information exchange and consultation. It may be the case that there is a lack of treatment options available for arthritis and child mental health difficulties, at least certainly at the time when I developed these conditions.

In early 2001, in adulthood, I had a bout of severe depression and consulted a general practitioner and was prescribed venlafaxine. I took time out of my biomedical degree against my tutor's advice, and this made my condition significantly worse, because I withdrew from productive degree activities and came close to jeopardizing my career that I greatly valued. I was reassured by my family that I could complete my degree after taking time out, which was the only effective engagement of SDM I received.

I was later diagnosed with bipolar disorder. I was able to complete my degree, but my career was very much hampered. I was placed on sodium valproate, which caused joint pains as the therapist was not informed of my arthritis. During the COVID-19 pandemic I was hospitalized and had a bout of catatonia that lasted 5 weeks. After experiencing partial recovery, I did engage in SDM to manage my daily life and leisure activities. I currently engage with a care coordinator to manage negative thinking and engage in occupational therapy for work-related activity, further education, and training.

I consulted a clinical psychologist to establish the root causes of my mental health difficulties and difficulties forming productive relationships with people. I feel this experience has contributed to persistent depressive thoughts and distrust towards people. It became apparent to the psychologist that I was neurodivergent, and my occupational therapist guided me to improved self-awareness and understanding of how this limits my ability to function properly. I practise mindfulness to help focus on and manage challenging tasks in my everyday life.

I feel that self-management is greatly improved by SDM with therapists; although their engagement with me is temporary, this had a beneficial effect as it empowered me to feel I could improve the quality of my life. I currently go out when I can and maintain hygiene, have a healthy diet without alcohol, get exercise, and keep my blood cholesterol levels down. This multifaceted approach has been supported by SDM and networking between my general practitioner and therapists. I am happy with the progression of SDM practice that has occurred throughout my lifetime. There is certainly room for improvement and therapists should recognize that patients like me require SDM as a lifelong process.

effectively and share information; access, understand, and act on information about the nature of their condition(s) and the services available; and confidence and skills to express their personal priorities, preferences, and values to clinicians (Muscat et al., 2021).

As such, health literacy is an important prerequisite for effective engagement in SDM and to realize the positive outcomes from SDM interventions, particularly for people living with MM. Muscat and colleagues proposed an integrated model of SDM and health literacy (Muscat et al., 2021), drawing on Nutbeam's hierarchy of functional (basic reading/writing skills) and communicative/interactive health literacy skills (advanced cognitive, literacy, and social skills needed to actively engage in daily activities, and derive meaning from health communication, and application of this information to dynamic circumstances) (Nutbeam, 2000). The highest level in Nutbeam's hierarchy is critical health literacy. These are transferable social and cognitive skills that enable people to critically assess the relevance and trustworthiness of health information for them as individuals, and to use these assessments to achieve empowerment and greater autonomy *across* health decisions and decision making contexts (Muscat et al., 2021). For John, acquisition of critical health literacy skills is particularly important as he is faced with making multiple preference-sensitive decisions (with complex interactions—discussed later) across a range of different contexts (e.g. appointments with clinicians in primary and secondary care, employment, and family life) and over time.

Physiotherapy perspective

Person-centred care is a requirement for physiotherapists in the UK, with professional regulatory standards emphasizing the need to 'facilitate' peoples' preferred role in decision making. Pacheco-Brousseau and colleagues analysed three models of SDM and their relevance to physiotherapy, with all models including collaboration, prioritization, continuous dialogue, and a focus on peoples' goals and values (Pacheco-Brousseau et al., 2022). The dual-layer SDM model (Ng et al., 2019) highlights the importance of prioritizing the conditions and symptoms that are most important to the person as a first step—acknowledging these are likely to change and discouraging physiotherapists from making assumptions about what should take priority.

Despite efforts to embed SDM in physiotherapy, there are discrepancies between these goals and what is observed and experienced in practice (Stenner et al., 2016). This has been attributed to the profession's roots in the medical model, which, until recently, has failed to acknowledge the importance of integrating evidence into a collaborative discussion (Hoffman et al., 2020).

For John, it would be important to understand the impact and relative importance of his back and shoulder pain, before any further physical assessment or diagnosis is made. People often struggle to clearly convey pain and John may need support with this. It may be helpful to provide information to John about the impact of musculoskeletal pain on his other conditions (and vice versa). For example, John may not feel that pain is a priority, but it is likely a factor contributing to sedentary behaviour (i.e. avoiding pain), and he may not know how it could be exacerbating some of his other symptoms such as anxiety/depression.

Occupational therapy perspective

Person-centred care SDM is considered a central tenet of occupational therapy, with roots in humanistic philosophy that places high value on the quality of the partnership between person and therapist. For occupational therapists, this partnership is a key vehicle to understanding the meaning attributed to occupation and how occupation-focused approaches can facilitate change.

SDM principles are included in occupational therapy models. One example is the Canadian Model of Occupational Performance and Engagement, which denotes the concept of spirituality at the centre of understanding occupation, with spirituality representing uniqueness and essence of the person, driving meaning and purpose of occupations (Townsend and Polatajko, 2007). Nevertheless, research has shown dissonance between theories of SDM and enactment in occupational therapy practice. With John, there is a need to consider his strengths, capabilities, values, and motivation. But for John to be engaged and involved in these conversations, they need to be posited using curious questions about everyday life, noticing where he gets 'stuck', the things he frequently returns to, and observing non-verbal cues.

Occupational therapy assessments can inherently focus on symptoms and bodily functions, identifying deficits, dysfunctions, and deviations from an individual's normal (Aas and Bonsaksen, 2023). For John, these assessments risk focusing on reductionist components of dysfunction, such as rating scores related to anxiety, or goals that focus on changing bodily functions and structures, such as achieving weight loss. Returning to what matters most is again significant (Hammell, 2023). It may be important for him to do a valued activity himself and without help. Or it may be more important that the person helping him is not experiencing undue stress.

Challenges of SDM in the context of MM

SDM would involve eliciting John's personal preferences for treatment/management from the available options, eliciting his personal values towards the different balance of benefits, risks, and consequences for each available option (including doing nothing), and engaging John in a SDM discussion to identify the optimal decision for him.

This SDM process is complicated in John's case. Evidence from randomized controlled trials and associated guidelines are predominately based on single conditions. Application of multiple 'single-condition' guidelines increases risk of conflicting advice, safety concerns (due to polypharmacy) and excessive treatment burden in terms of attendance at multiple appointments, adherence to multiple medications, and self-management advice (Hughes et al., 2013). This is also reflected in the lived experience account (Box 60.2). There are complex interactions between John's conditions and symptoms, which also interact with the benefits, risks, and consequences of his current treatments, and other options available to him both now and in the future. This complexity of applying SDM to people living with MM is shown in Figure 60.1.

The distinction noted above between MM and comorbidity is important for SDM. Taking a MM viewpoint, no single condition takes precedence over the others. Therefore, SDM in MM has an additional first step that is not required for SDM with comorbidities or single conditions.

A key initial task would be to engage John in a discussion about his priorities in terms of which condition(s) or symptom(s), including his current treatments, are having the greatest negative impact on his HRQoL. This will provide valuable insights into which symptoms or conditions are most important for John. However, he (and the multiple clinicians involved in his care) may not be aware of the complex interactions conveyed in Figure 60.1, which would complicate the SDM process and prevent John from making truly informed decisions. For example:

1. *Drug treatment-condition interactions*: e.g. the potential interaction between citalopram, diabetes, and depression.
2. *Condition-condition interactions*: depression and anxiety may exacerbate shoulder and lower back pain and vice versa.
3. (1) and (2) above may result in reduced motivation to engage in protective health behaviours such as attendance at routine appointments, and adherence to medication, physical activity, and dietary behaviour change, which in turn impact across all John's conditions.

Alternatively, John may prefer to discuss how well he is managing his current treatment load, taking the focus away from conditions and helping to reduce cognitive overload.

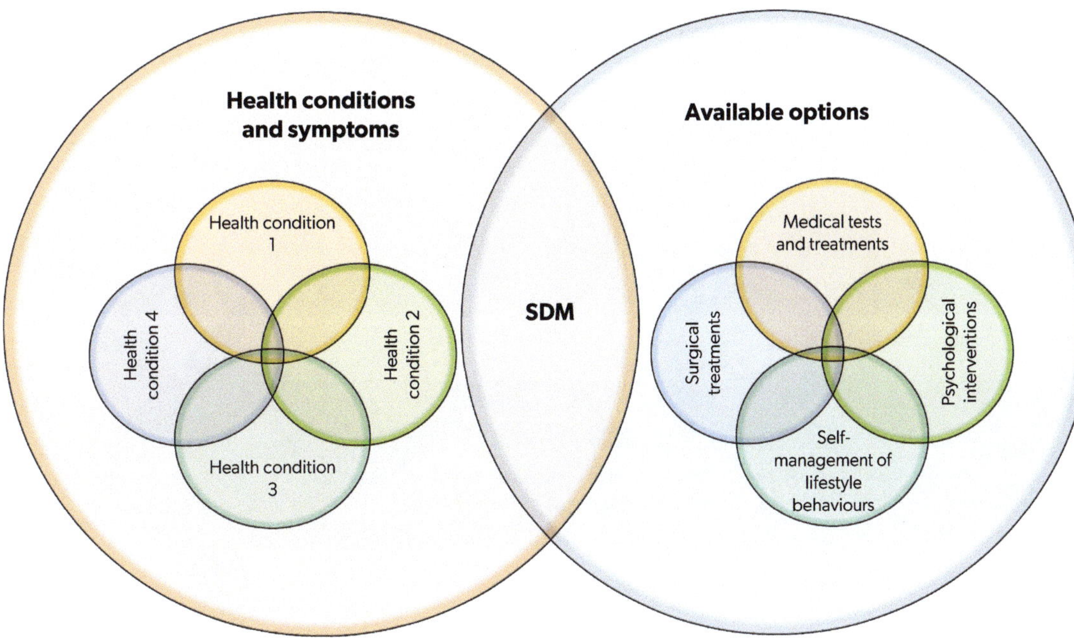

Figure 60.1 Complexity of condition and treatment interactions in the context of multimorbidity.

SDM and the HRQoL gap

There is general consensus that the optimal approach to MM is delivering patient-centred care (via an SDM process) within a primary care setting (along with robust clinical systems to identify people with MM, individualized management plans, medication reviews, and coordination of care), which will lead to improved HRQoL and other positive health outcomes (National Institute for Health and Care Excellence, 2016). Some of these elements are reflected in the example of lived experience (Box 60.2).

A systematic review of 16 randomized controlled trials of interventions in primary/community care for people with MM (eight care coordination/self-management support studies, four self-management support studies, and four medicines management studies) reported limited or no effectiveness for improving HRQoL (Smith et al., 2021). These authors posited three foci of future research: patient experience of care, optimizing medicines management, and targeting health behaviour change.

One study included in the systematic review (Smith et al., 2021), the 3D (dimensions of health, depression, and drugs) approach pragmatic trial (Salisbury et al., 2018), focused on individual priorities and SDM with adults with three or more long-term conditions. No improvements were reported for HRQoL (EQ-5D-5L), perceived illness, or treatment burden. A related cost-effectiveness analysis was equivocal (Thorn et al., 2020). However, compared with usual care, significant improvements were reported across all six measures of patient experience: Patient Assessment of Chronic

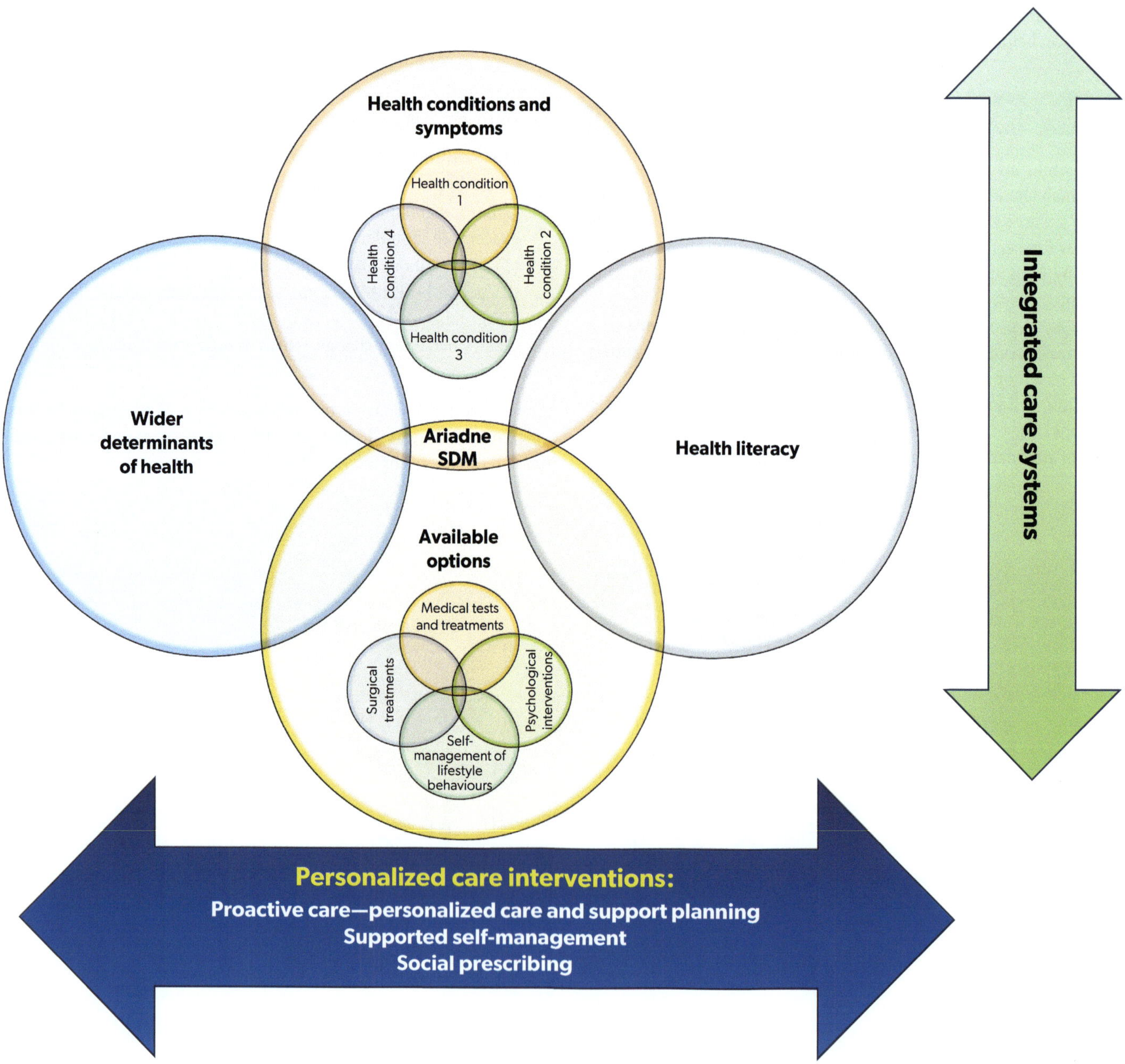

Figure 60.2 Framework for SDM research.

Illness Care measure (patient activation, delivery system design, goal-setting, problem-solving, and follow-up/coordination); relational empathy; care related to their priorities; experiencing their care as joined up; having written care plans; and overall satisfaction with care. Improved patient experience is consistent with the wider SDM literature, although these findings highlight important issues with implementation of SDM interventions for MM, and avenues to address the SDM–HRQoL gap.

Improved patient experience from SDM needs to be considered alongside effectiveness and cost-effectiveness. These, as well as measures of patient safety were comparable with usual care in the 3D approach pragmatic trial. Therefore, SDM interventions for MM that improve patient experience, which are cost-neutral with comparable cost-effectiveness and safety, should be considered sufficient evidence for implementation. As discussed in a commentary on the 3D approach pragmatic trial (Dowrick, 2018), 'The core components of the intervention could have been insufficient to treat deep-rooted health problems, especially since only 49% of the intervention participants attended both appointments' (p. 5). The lack of impact on HRQoL is also a feature of interventions targeting high users of care (associated with MM) such as 'hot-spotting (cost-containment strategies) aimed at individual 'high-cost patients', but as with the 3D approach pragmatic trial they do not address wider determinants of health or health inequities (Lantz, 2020).

Solutions to the SDM and HRQoL gap

Dowrick proposed the development of 'multi-modal approaches, linking patient-centred primary care with public health policy level interventions addressing behavioural, environmental, and occupational determinants of long-term illness and inequity' (Dowrick, 2018, p. 5). This highlights the wider determinants of health and personalized care interventions such as social prescribing, personalized care and support planning, and supported self-management.

Application of the Ariadne principles, which aim to lessen the burden of conditions and treatment (Muth et al., 2014) involve elucidating the complex interactions between conditions, medical and non-medical treatments, and their consequences, including overall treatment burden (medications, appointments for screening, monitoring and receipt of treatment, and self-management of health behaviours, as well as clinical disciplines involved in John's management) with a focus on developing realistic collaborative treatment goals to address John's priorities (Hoffmann et al., 2018). For example, a SDM process may lead to a personalized goal for John to improve his levels of physical activity (with multiple preference-sensitive options), which were identified as a management option that would likely positively impact all his health conditions. This may include other decisions such as de-prescribing as part of medications management and development of a personalized care plan. This should also be a life-long process (Box 60.2).

We propose a revised framework to guide research on the SDM–HRQoL gap (Figure 60.2). This framework emphasizes the need for better integration of care across primary care and community services that address the wider determinants of health and health inequities, alongside health literacy, with SDM at its core based on Ariadne principles.

Summary

At the start of this chapter, we wrote that the person living with a long-term condition and their family are the only continuous entity in a largely discontinuous health and social care system, which is reflected by an example of lived experience in Box 60.2. There is a pressing need to evaluate the impact of SDM interventions for MM in the context of 'better' integrated care (health and social care and community organizations) to address the wider determinants of health, and truly position the person with MM at the centre of their care and empower them to improve their HRQoL.

REFERENCES

Aas, M. H., Bonsaksen, T. 2023. Exploring occupation-based practice among occupational therapists in hospitals and rehabilitation institutions. *Scand J Occup Ther,* **30**, 1074–1084.

Barnett, K., Mercer, S. V., Norbury, M., et al. 2012. Epidemiology of multi-morbidity and implications for health care, research and medical education. *Lancet,* **380**, 37–43.

Dowrick, C. 2018. Comment: patient-centred care for multimorbidity: an end in itself? *Lancet,* **392**, 4–5.

Flynn, D. 2012. Shared decision making. In: Forshaw, M., Sheffield, D., Eds. *Health Psychology in Action*, pp. 69–83. Wiley-Blackwell.

Hammell, K. W. 2023. Focusing on 'what matters': the occupation, capability and wellbeing framework for occupational therapy. *Cad Bras Ter Ocup,* **31**, e3509.

Hoffmann, T., Jansen, J., Glasziou, P. 2018. The importance and challenges of shared decision making in older people with multimorbidity. *PLoS Med,* **15**, e1002530.

Hoffmann, T. C., Lewis, J., Maher, C. G. 2020. Shared decision making should be an integral part of physiotherapy practice. *Physiotherapy,* **107**, 43–49.

Hughes, L. D., McMurdo, M. E. T., Guthrie, B. 2013. Guidelines for people not for diseases: the challenges of applying UK clinical guidelines to people with multimorbidity. *Age Ageing,* **43**, 62–69.

Lantz, P. M. 2020. 'Super-utilizer' interventions: what they reveal about evaluation research, wishful thinking, and health equity. *Milbank Q,* **98**, 31–34.

Muscat, D. M., Shepherd, H. L., Nutbeam, D., et al. 2021. Health literacy and shared decision-making: exploring the relationship to enable meaningful patient engagement in healthcare. *J Gen Intern Med,* **36**, 521–524.

Muth, C., van den Akker, M., Blom, J. W., et al. 2014. The Ariadne principles: how to handle multimorbidity in primary care consultations. *BMC Med,* **12**, 223.

National Institute for Health and Care Excellence. 2016. Multimorbidity: clinical assessment and management. NICE guideline [NG56]. Available at: https://www.nice.org.uk/guidance/ng56

Ng, C. J., Lee, Y. K., Abdullah, A., et al. 2019. Shared decision making: a dual-layer model to tackling multimorbidity in primary care. *J Eval Clin Pract,* **25**, 1074–1079.

Nutbeam, D. 2000. Health literacy as a public health goal: a challenge for contemporary health education and communication strategies into the 21st century. *Health Promot Int,* **15**, 259–267.

Pacheco-Brousseau, L., Stacey, D., Ben Amor, S., Poitras, S. 2022. Shared decision-making conceptual models for physiotherapy: a theory analysis. *Physiotherapy,* **115**, 111–118.

Rowlands, G., Protheroe, J., Winkley, J., et al. 2015. A mismatch between population health literacy and the complexity of health information: an observational study. *Br J Gen Pract,* **65**, e379–e386.

Ronaldson, A., Arias de la Torre, J., Prina, M., et al. 2021. Associations between physical multimorbidity patterns and common mental health disorders in middle-aged adults: a prospective analysis using data from the UK Biobank. *Lancet Reg Health Eur,* **8**, 100149.

Salisbury, C., Man, M. S., Bower, P., et al. 2018. Management of multimorbidity using a patient-centred care model: a pragmatic cluster-randomised trial of the 3D approach. *Lancet,* **392**, 41–50.

Smith, S. M., Wallace, E., Clyne, B., et al. 2021 Interventions for improving outcomes in patients with multimorbidity in primary care and community setting: a systematic review. *Syst Rev,* **10**, 271.

Stenner, R., Swinkels, A., Mitchell, T., Palmer, S. 2016. Exercise prescription for patients with non-specific chronic low back pain: a qualitative exploration of decision making in physiotherapy practice. *Physiotherapy,* **102**, 332–338.

Thorn, J., Man, M.-S., Chaplin, K., et al. 2020. Cost-effectiveness of a patient-centred approach to managing multimorbidity in primary care: a pragmatic cluster randomised controlled trial. *BMJ Open,* **10**, e030110.

Townsend, E. A., Polatajko, H. J. 2007. *Enabling Occupation II: Advancing an Occupational Therapy Vision for Health, Well-Being, & Justice Through Occupation.* Canadian Association of Occupational Therapists.

PART 8
The way forward

61

Ten pillars of AI-enabled shared decision making

A practical guide

Samira Abbasgholizadeh Rahimi, Dan Poenaru, Glyn Elwyn, and Karina Prévost

Introduction

Artificial intelligence (AI) refers to computer systems that can do complex tasks such as making decisions or solving problems that historically only a human could do (Xu et al., 2021). AI has many subfields including machine learning. There are two different types of AI: 'narrow AI', which comprises systems designed for specific tasks like chatbots or recommendation algorithms, and 'general AI', which are hypothetical systems with human-like intelligence, capable of understanding and accomplishing complex intellectual tasks.

Recent years have witnessed significant technological advancements in the field of AI and its subfield, machine learning, leading to a new era of innovation across many domains, including healthcare. General AI, sometimes referred to as artificial general intelligence, is a form of AI with the capacity to understand, learn, and apply knowledge in various contexts—much like human cognitive abilities. This incorporates the ability to reason, plan, learn from experience, communicate in natural language, and integrate all these skills towards completing the defined tasks across a breadth of domains. Unlike narrow AI, which is designed for specific tasks, general AI can perform a wide range of tasks and solve problems for which it has not been specifically programmed. Some AI experts believe that general AI already exists in the latest generation of large language models (Bubeck et al., 2023), and others predict AI will outperform humans within the next decade (Bengio et al., 2024).

AI can facilitate shared decision making (SDM) at various points in the process. However, a recent review (Abbasgholizadeh Rahimi et al., 2022) shows that using AI in SDM remains in its infancy. Further efforts are required to strengthen and standardize its use in SDM, and to evaluate its impact on the process in various populations and settings. The application of AI in medicine shows promise and is expected to enhance SDM in different ways including offering predictions and risk assessments that could inform both patients and clinicians during the SDM process. This process could potentially lead to more nuanced and holistic decisions in complex medical scenarios (Abbasgholizadeh Rahimi et al., 2022). However, the integration of AI in SDM must carefully consider the ethical implications and the need to balance technology's input with the irreplaceable value of human judgement and patient autonomy (Gould et al., 2023). The aim of this chapter is to shed light on the potential uses of AI for facilitating SDM, for the benefit of both patients and clinicians.

Application of digital technologies and AI in SDM

Digital health technologies are already being used to support SDM. For instance, studies showed (mobile) 'mHealth' technologies have the potential to facilitate and support SDM in diagnostic and treatment decisions (Abbasgholizadeh Rahimi et al., 2017). Such digital platforms can facilitate the exchange of information, discussion of treatment options, and mutual decision making between patients and healthcare providers. These platforms typically feature tools for information dissemination, communication, and the documentation of patient preferences and treatment plans.

The integration of AI in SDM could leverage its capacity for pattern recognition and predictive analytics to provide personalized risk assessments and treatment recommendations. This is shown by various applications where AI supports the prediction of medical outcomes, thus contributing to more informed and personalized care (Abbasgholizadeh Rahimi et al., 2022). For instance Twiggs and colleagues created a predictive tool designed to evaluate the potential outcomes of total knee replacement in patients suffering from severe osteoarthritis, to assist them in making the decision (i.e. whether or not have surgery) tailored to the specific needs of each patient (Twiggs et al., 2019). AI's role in SDM processes is expected to grow, with potential uses including enhancing risk communication (about treatment or screening options), recognizing patterns in specific patients' health data (e.g. to prompt discussion of risk and risk factors), and recommending personalized treatment or screening. This will help streamline the decision making process by providing comprehensive data analysis to support clinicians and patients to make decisions based on better informed preferences.

AI can enhance various aspects of clinical care, including diagnosis, treatment planning, and treatment delivery, by providing additional options and evidence for clinicians and patients to consider (Sloane and Silva, 2020; Macri and Roberts, 2023). AI-driven clinical prediction tools use patient data to predict specific outcomes, risk stratify patients, or suggest personalized diagnostic or therapeutic options. One such example is our team's (SAR, DP) ongoing study of the use of AI to move the prediction of the severity of acute appendicitis from the operating room to the emergency room, hence enabling personalized SDM in this disease before a commitment to operative treatment is made. Machine learning's advancements have led to an increase in such clinical prediction tools, and which compare favourably with traditional methods in both validity and clinical efficacy (Neporent, 2023). In SDM, AI can inform decision making and allow healthcare providers to focus more on patient interaction, thus fostering a patient-centred approach (Abbasgholizadeh Rahimi et al., 2022; Macri and Roberts, 2023).

AI-based decision support systems are being developed to improve therapeutic decisions and patient care. These systems can promote patient self-determination and enhance the SDM process, although medical staff must retain control over these systems and maintain their relationship with patients (Sloane and Silva, 2020; Giordano et al., 2021). Moreover, AI can improve patient engagement by providing healthcare virtual assistants, self-service portals, and risk assessments, which support personalized and data-driven approaches to patient care (Davenport and Kalakota, 2019; Subramaniam, 2023). AI can also assist in the process of developing SDM materials for the patient–provider interaction, ensuring that these materials are written in easily understandable language and in the patient's preferred language. One such example is the use of an AI robot facilitating weight-loss management by supporting SDM about choice of weight-loss plans among overweight or obese participants (Chu et al., 2022).

A recent systematic review of AI applications in SDM only identified six such applications, equally divided between generalist and specialist clinical care. Despite proposed development, none of them has yet reached implementation in practice (Abbasgholizadeh Rahimi et al., 2022). Of note, however, while most studies included healthcare providers and patients in the validation stages of the AI solutions, none had included either group in the actual design and development of the AI solutions (Abbasgholizadeh Rahimi et al., 2022).

Ten pillars of AI-enabled shared decision making

In the near future, AI and generative AI will facilitate SDM in different ways. An early example of these recent efforts is exemplified by *Chat-Orthopedist*, a retrieval-augmented large language model facilitating SDM for adolescent idiopathic scoliosis patients (Shi et al., 2023). We introduce a forward-looking AI-SDM guide in Figure 61.1 with ten innovative ways AI could facilitate SDM in the future. This includes aspects on patients' education and empowerment, risk prediction and management, preference elicitation, development of tailored options, analysing patient-generated data, improving accessibility and health literacy, clinical documentation during clinical encounters, SDM tools, measurement, and training.

Challenges and considerations

Microsoft launched *Tay*, an AI chatbot, on Twitter (now X) in March 2016. It was designed to learn from user interactions. However, a significant issue arose when some users began sending offensive tweets to *Tay* and the chatbot began to mimic the language. This led to responses that were racist and sexist in nature. This troubling development transformed *Tay* into an echo chamber full of hate speech. Within less than 24 hours of its debut, Microsoft had to deactivate *Tay* and issue an apology for the bot's offensive output. The *Tay* incident highlights one of several instances where AI has deviated from its presumed intended purpose, demonstrating the challenges and risks associated with AI development and deployment in public domains. However, the advancements in AI that we witness today with generative pre-trained transformers (GPTs), the large language model upon which popular chatbots like *ChatGPT* is based, evolved largely from the early stages of AI models that were in *Tay*, which Microsoft had pursued before the emergence of transformer-based models.

This example among others highlights the need to ensure the responsible use of AI and be constantly aware of the ethical implications, which although important in all domains, remain critically important in healthcare and during a SDM process. These underlie the concerns noted in the patient's perspective (Box 61.1).

Responsible AI

Responsible AI refers to the practice of using AI in a manner that is ethical, safe, and reliable (Microsoft, 2024). Responsible AI could encompass several key principles. Microsoft outlines six key principles for responsible AI as follows: accountability, inclusiveness, reliability and safety, fairness, transparency, and privacy and security (Microsoft, 2024). Different principles are defined by various frameworks. For instance, a recent systematic review in this area (Siala and Wang, 2022) synthesized relevant knowledge from AI governance and ethics, and proposed a responsible AI framework—that is, 'SHIFTing AI'—that encompasses five core themes for AI solution developers, healthcare professionals, and policymakers. These five core themes are sustainability, human-centredness, inclusiveness, fairness, and transparency (Siala and Wang, 2022).

In the SDM process, AI should be seen as a tool that assists patients and clinicians in the SDM process, rather than being the sole decision maker. This ensures that AI complements patients' and clinicians' judgement and expertise in the SDM process. The clarity of roles in patient–clinician–AI collaboration could enhance the acceptance of AI as a collaborative partner, rather than being seen as a replacement. Such collaboration can lead to more informed, data- and value-driven decision making processes. By combining AI's ability with clinicians' knowledge and patients' values and ethical considerations, a more holistic approach to SDM can be achieved. This is especially important as it will ensure that decisions are not only data-driven but also human-centred and ethically sound.

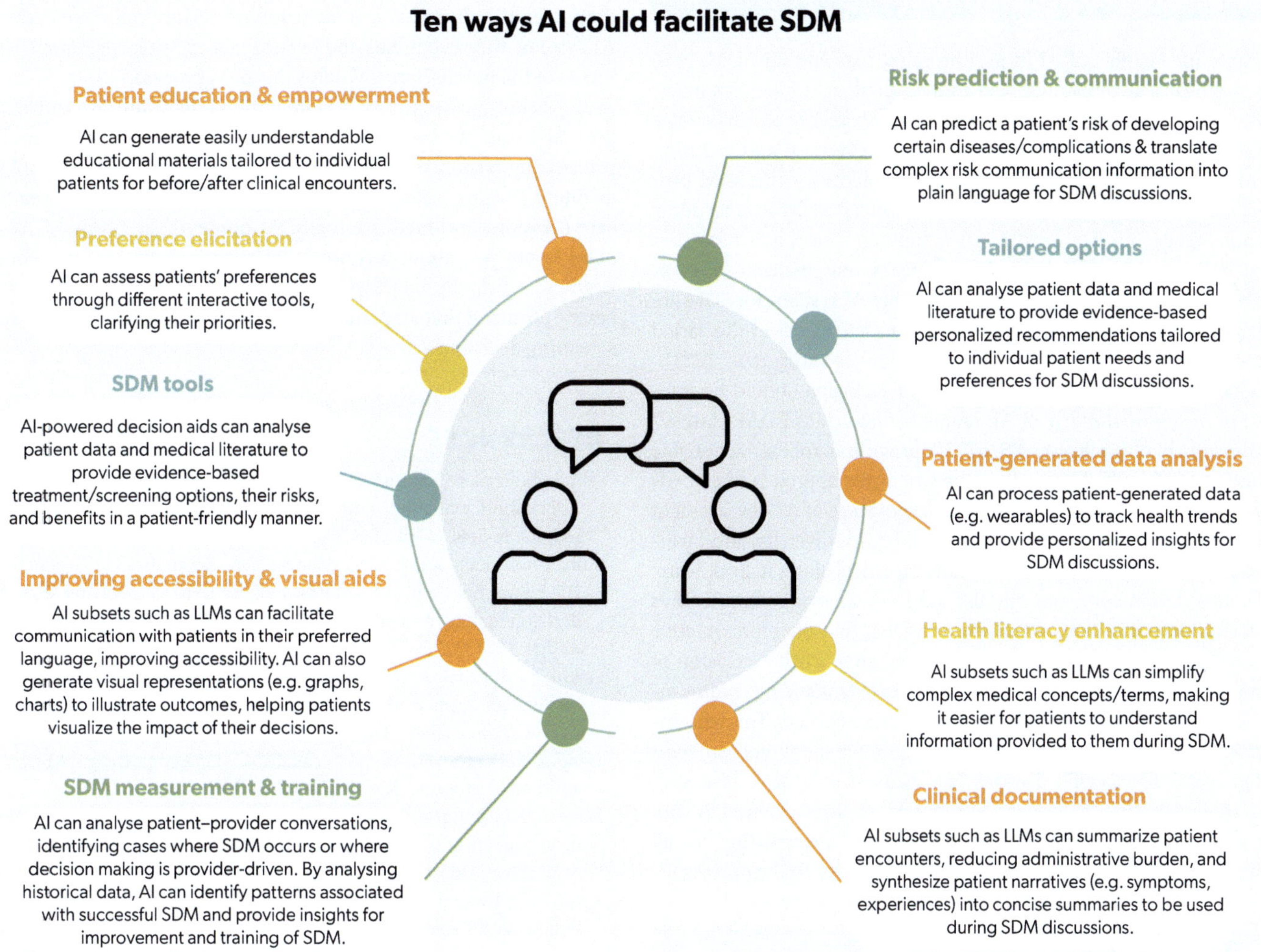

Figure 61.1 AI-SDM guide highlighting ten Pillars of AI-enabled shared decision making.

Box 61.1 Patient perspective

Digital technology, AI, and SDM

SDM has played a significant role in my extensive journey as a patient within the hospital system. Some experiences were positive, while others were fraught with challenges. Over time, I've come to understand that, for me, the benefit of SDM lies in the quality of the therapeutic relationship between patients and caregivers. It is a human-to-human bond. When done properly, SDM can give hope, satisfaction, and empower patients and their family. When SDM doesn't work, it can lead to profound traumas. Patients facing SDM are often worried, tired, and scared, and these need to be taken into consideration.

As patients, the arrival of AI in SDM puts us at a crossroads. I'm convinced that many changes will be beneficial: I cannot, and do not want to, ignore the potential of AI. These include more efficient training for professionals (which enhances proper SDM for patients), and more personalized care for patients that better aligns with their values and specific needs. It all sounds like good news to me. However, I am also worried because this is a major change. I'm not convinced that we understand how this will affect us. We need to be cautious because the arrival of AI in SDM will affect things in ways that we can't even imagine.

As a patient, I think AI will shift the conversation. I will not be alone with my doctor anymore, there will be a stranger in the house. Someone I am not familiar with: our AI newcomer will be there. Will this newcomer have the potential to increase the power imbalance in a SDM conversation? I think it may. Patients are not all alike; we have different backgrounds, different values, needs, trust issues, and variable digital literacy. I hope we learn to understand the limitations of AI and I am convinced that more efforts need to be put into this area.

The arrival of AI means that SDM is venturing into new territories. The challenge lies in finding a delicate balance between the capacity of technologies and the definite need for a human-to-human approach. That balance may be hard to reach, but preserving a therapeutic relationship will remain a crucial part of SDM. We will need to navigate these new technological territories with caution and respect to preserve what is, for me, the essence of SDM: a human-to-human conversation that arrives at a good solution. AI must remain a tool that only supports that process rather than replaces it.

Inclusion, diversity, and equity

Despite the benefits of AI in healthcare settings and for SDM, both AI and health systems must also address challenges in equity, diversity, and inclusion principles and practices to realize those benefits (Nyariro et al., 2023). The absence of equity, diversity, and inclusion concepts, principles, and practices in AI systems for the SDM process can introduce bias and discrimination especially against some population groups. The most at-risk groups often belong to minorities that have been historically and systemically marginalized (Seyyed-Kalantari et al., 2021). It is vital to ensure that AI systems for SDM are designed with diverse perspectives and datasets to reflect the varied experiences and needs of different populations (Nyariro et al., 2023).

Consideration of equity, diversity, and inclusion should be integral to the entire lifecycle of AI. Frameworks such as EDAI (https://pubmed.ncbi.nlm.nih.gov/39546793/) provide a robust, actionable solution for this challenge, offering a structured approach to embedding equity, diversity, and inclusion at every stage of AI development and deployment. AI could even promote equity, diversity, and inclusion in healthcare by helping to identify historical biases in healthcare. AI's data-driven approach can also aid in diversifying clinical trials and studies (Askin et al., 2023), ensuring that they are representative of the entire population. Moreover, AI can support the inclusion of people with different languages and abilities by enhancing communication methods, such as direct translation in encounters. This will empower patients and facilitate SDM processes for those with different language skills, specific diseases (e.g. neurodegenerative diseases), and other variations in learning and interaction styles. In brief, AI can be a powerful tool in the SDM process in healthcare, ensuring that all patients have a voice and are meaningfully involved in the process.

Conclusion

The integration of AI and machine learning into healthcare has led to a new era of innovation, with much potential for facilitating SDM. Generative AI systems such as large language models represent a significant leap forward, offering the potential for AI systems to perform a wider range of tasks such as generating and analysing big complex clinical datasets including images, videos, texts, and help in solving complex problems. The application of AI in SDM is still emerging, with potential uses that are explained in our AI-SDM guide. However, AI should be responsibly developed and used in the SDM process. Some potential challenges we might face include ethical concerns particularly regarding the 'black box' nature of advanced machine learning methods, their safety and fairness, and patients' and healthcare providers' trust in these AI tools. Moreover, transparency about using these systems in communication with patients is important. Patients need to be fully aware of how these systems impact their care experience and decision making process, and understand the privacy concerns associated with consenting to using AI tools to facilitate their SDM experience.

To use the full potential of AI in SDM, joint efforts are needed from AI experts and engineers, healthcare professionals, policymakers, patients, and the public. This includes strengthening and standardizing the use of AI in SDM; ensuring the responsible use of AI in and for SDM by adhering to ethical principles such as accountability, inclusiveness, and transparency; and finally incorporating equity, diversity, and inclusion principles in the life cycle of AI systems to prevent bias and ensure that AI tools benefit all segments of the population and helps the SDM process.

As AI continues to evolve, its integration into healthcare and SDM processes presents both immense opportunities and challenges. By prioritizing responsible use of AI, it can become a valuable tool in facilitating more informed, personalized, and equitable healthcare decisions and facilitate the SDM process. The future of AI in SDM is not just about technological advancement but also about augmenting the human aspects of care and decision making processes, ensuring that all patients have a voice in their treatment and screening decisions.

REFERENCES

Abbasgholizadeh Rahimi, S., Cwintal, M., Huang, Y., et al. 2022. Application of artificial intelligence in shared decision making: scoping review. *JMIR Med Inform*, **10**, e36199.

Abbasgholizadeh Rahimi, S., Menear, M., Robitaille, H., Légaré, F. 2017. Are mobile health applications useful for supporting shared decision making in diagnostic and treatment decisions? *Glob Health Action*, **10**, 1332259.

Askin, S., Burkhalter, D., Calado, G., El Dakrouni, S. 2023. Artificial intelligence applied to clinical trials: opportunities and challenges. *Health Technol (Berl)*, **13**, 203–213.

Bengio, Y., Hinton, G., Yao, A., et al. 2024. Managing extreme AI risks amid rapid progress. *Science*, **384**, 842–845.

Bubeck, S., Chandrasekaran, V., Eldan, R., et al. 2023. Sparks of artificial general intelligence: early experiments with gpt-4. arXiv preprint arXiv:2303.12712.

Chu, Y.-T., Huang, R.-Y., Chen, T. T.-W., et al. 2022. Effect of health literacy and shared decision-making on choice of weight-loss plan among overweight or obese participants receiving a prototype artificial intelligence robot intervention facilitating weight-loss management decisions. *Digit Health*, **8**, 20552076221136372.

Davenport, T., Kalakota, R. 2019. The potential for artificial intelligence in healthcare. *Future Healthc J*, **6**, 94–98.

Giordano, C., Brennan, M., Mohamed, B., Rashidi, P., Modave, F., Tighe, P. 2021. Accessing artificial intelligence for clinical decision-making. *Front Digit Health*, **3**, 645232.

Gould, D. J., Dowsey, M. M., Glanville-Hearst, M., et al. 2023. Patients' views on AI for risk prediction in shared decision-making for knee replacement surgery: qualitative interview study. *J Med Internet Res*, **25**, e43632.

Macri, R., Roberts, S. L. 2023. The use of artificial intelligence in clinical care: a values-based guide for shared decision making. *Curr Oncol*, **30**, 2178–2186.

Microsoft. 2024. What is responsible AI? Available at: https://learn.microsoft.com/en-us/azure/machine-learning/concept-responsible-ai?view=azureml-api-2

Neporent, L. 2023. 5 AI tools every doctor should know about. Available at: https://www.psychiatrist.com/news/5-ai-tools-every-doctor-should-know-about/

Nyariro, M., Emami, E., Caidor, P., Abbasgholizadeh Rahimi, S. 2023. Integrating equity, diversity and inclusion throughout the lifecycle of AI within healthcare: a scoping review protocol. *BMJ Open*, **13**, e072069.

Seyyed-Kalantari, L., Zhang, H., Mcdermott, M. B. A., Chen, I. Y., Ghassemi, M. 2021. Underdiagnosis bias of artificial intelligence algorithms applied to chest radiographs in under-served patient populations. *Nat Med,* **27**, 2176–2182.

Shi, W., Zhuang, Y., Zhu, Y., Iwinski, H., Wattenbarger, M., Wang, M. D. 2023. Retrieval-augmented large language models for adolescent idiopathic scoliosis patients in shared decision-making. In: *Proceedings of the 14th ACM International Conference on Bioinformatics, Computational Biology, and Health Informatics*, Article 14, pp. 1–10. Association for Computing Machinery.

Siala, H., Wang, Y. 2022. SHIFTing artificial intelligence to be responsible in healthcare: a systematic review. *Soc Sci Med,* **296**, 114782.

Sloane, E. B., Silva, R. J. 2020. Artificial intelligence in medical devices and clinical decision support systems. In: Iadanza, E. Ed. *Clinical Engineering Handbook*, pp. 556–568. Academic Press.

Subramaniam, A. 2023. Top 5 AI use cases for driving patient engagement in healthcare. Available at: https://kanini.com/blog/how-is-artificial-intelligence-ai-transforming-patient-engagement/

Twiggs, J. G., Wakelin, E. A., Fritsch, B. A., et al. 2019. Clinical and statistical validation of a probabilistic prediction tool of total knee arthroplasty outcome. *J Arthroplasty,* **34**, 2624–2631.

Xu, Y., Liu, X., Cao, X., et al. 2021. Artificial intelligence: a powerful paradigm for scientific research. *Innovation (Camb),* **2**, 100179.

62

Shared decision making

A patient perspective

Sara Riggare, Amy Price, Dawn P. Richards, Valerie C. Cates, and Glen Hazlewood

Patients' roles in shared decision making

My neurologist doesn't even know if I take my medications or not. Shared decision making is a 'healthcare setting' thing. In my everyday life, I am the decision maker.

Sara Riggare

Autonomy is a fundamental human value that includes being able and allowed to make decisions for ourselves. The same applies in healthcare through shared decision making (SDM). SDM has been described as 'a method of care' and that 'anytime a patient and clinician figure out together what to do about the patient's situation, they are doing SDM' (Montori et al., 2023). Nevertheless, a recent Cochrane review concluded that even though a wide variety of activities have been developed to increase SDM, it is difficult to state which activity is best in different contexts (Légaré et al., 2018). Enacting effective SDM is not without challenges and barriers related to communication, logistics, epistemology, costs, legal implications, and time—which can all limit clinicians' and patients' capabilities and involvement (Waddell et al., 2021; Elwyn et al., 2023).

When it comes to patients' roles in SDM 'no matter how much the patient wants to participate, if the physician is not willing, then shared decision making will not occur' (Charles et al., 1997). There are several potential reasons for this, most of them related to fundamentally different perspectives. For clinicians, treatment decisions are 'just' part of their job; but for patients, the process of making decisions and the decision itself can profoundly affect all aspects of their lives.

Patient preference in the healthcare system and beyond

Indeed, each patient is unique, and even the same individual may exhibit varying preferences depending on the circumstances or timing. Sometimes patients value additional support with decision making due to feeling overwhelmed, such as when they experience mental or physical barriers or when health system constraints may limit choice due to cost-control, legal or political complications—and this too is a preference (Elwyn et al., 2023). Importantly, not all patients want the same level of involvement in healthcare decisions. Studies using the Control Preferences Scale (Degner et al., 1997) demonstrate this. For example, a study with cancer patients in Germany found that around one-third of patients wanted equal responsibility with clinicians in treatment decisions, one-third wanted more say in the decisions, and one-third wanted less (Hahlweg et al., 2020). Less than 5% preferred to leave decisions completely in the hands of clinicians, showing most patients want some degree of involvement, but there is still variability in preferred levels of involvement (Hahlweg et al., 2020).

Factors influencing level of patient involvement—a collaborative perspective

Traditionally, categorizations of patient level of involvement are described from healthcare professional and researcher perspectives. One example is the Patient Activation Measure (PAM), which is an instrument for assessing 'an individual's knowledge, skills, and confidence for managing their health and healthcare' on four levels (Hibbard et al., 2004). Patients on the lowest level are described as being passive, overwhelmed, and possibly naïve to their health management and healthcare role. On the highest level, patients are described as competent in their healthcare behaviours, but may need assistance in stressful situations (Rademakers et al., 2016).

Another example is the categorization of patients by levels of health literacy and psychological empowerment suggested by Schulz and Nakamoto. They propose four categories: (1) *high-needs patients* (low health literacy, low psychological empowerment); (2) *needlessly dependent patients* (high health literacy, low psychological empowerment); (3) *dangerous self-managers* (low health literacy, high psychological empowerment); and (4) *effective self-managers* (high health literacy, high psychological empowerment) (Schulz and Nakamoto, 2013).

These above examples of categorizations have certainly contributed to the field of patient involvement, though we believe they would have benefited from a more nuanced approach. In both examples, the onus is almost entirely on patients to be involved. Given our collaborative perspectives as patients and a clinician with long-term and varied experiences with different healthcare systems and providers, we want to offer an alternative way to categorize levels of patient involvement and propose factors that make SDM more or less likely to take place. This approach considers *individuals* (i.e. patients, clinicians, and caregivers—including their attitudes, values, skills, and knowledge), the *situation* (i.e. if this is a familiar or new situation for the patient and/or clinician), and the *healthcare system* in which the individuals are situated (i.e. if it supports patients as active partners in their care and decision-making or not).

Figure 62.1 presents an overview of the main factors we see as influencing levels of patient involvement in SDM:

- Institutions (top left) are the largest overarching element and most slow to change. Institutions can either support or resist SDM.
- The situation is the second largest overarching element (middle left) and is dynamic in nature. Situations can be familiar or unfamiliar.
- The clinicians (middle right) are the third largest element and can be progressive or more conservative. Clinicians are quicker to change than the institution but are also at the behest of the system they work within.
- The patients (bottom right) are most impacted by the above-listed overarching elements and can either have high or low skills and knowledge.

These levels can influence other levels in a top-down (institution to patient) or bottom-up (patient to institution) manner. Below we describe each one in turn.

Individual patient characteristics

People who have lived with chronic conditions for some time can become experiential and knowledge experts in their condition, and may know more about the clinical presentations and suitable treatments than healthcare professionals (Snow et al., 2013). They are experts in living with these conditions, irrespective of whether they effectively manage them or not.

Individual patient characteristics are important for SDM. A qualitative interview-based study of patients and healthcare professionals identified five elements of patient readiness for SDM: (1) understanding of and attitude towards SDM; (2) health literacy; (3) skills in communicating and claiming space; (4) self-awareness; and (5) consideration skills (Keij et al., 2021). Further, a patient's level of readiness for SDM can be influenced by factors like age, health literacy, cultural and educational backgrounds, support from family members or others, and whether or not they have accepted their diagnosis (Keij et al., 2021).

In Figure 62.2 we describe two levels of individual patient characteristics influencing level of SDM involvement: high and low levels of skills and knowledge. Patients with high levels of skills and knowledge would correspond to PAM level 4, reported to be 31–54% of people with chronic conditions (Rademakers et al., 2016). These 'self-empowered' patients can add to the clinicians' knowledge of their conditions, ask insightful questions, and proactively seek collaborations with healthcare professionals to ensure their care aligns with their lifestyle, needs, values, and preferences. Further, they are often seen as leaders by their peers and others in their community. Patients with less advanced levels of skills and knowledge may need additional support to fully participate in SDM.

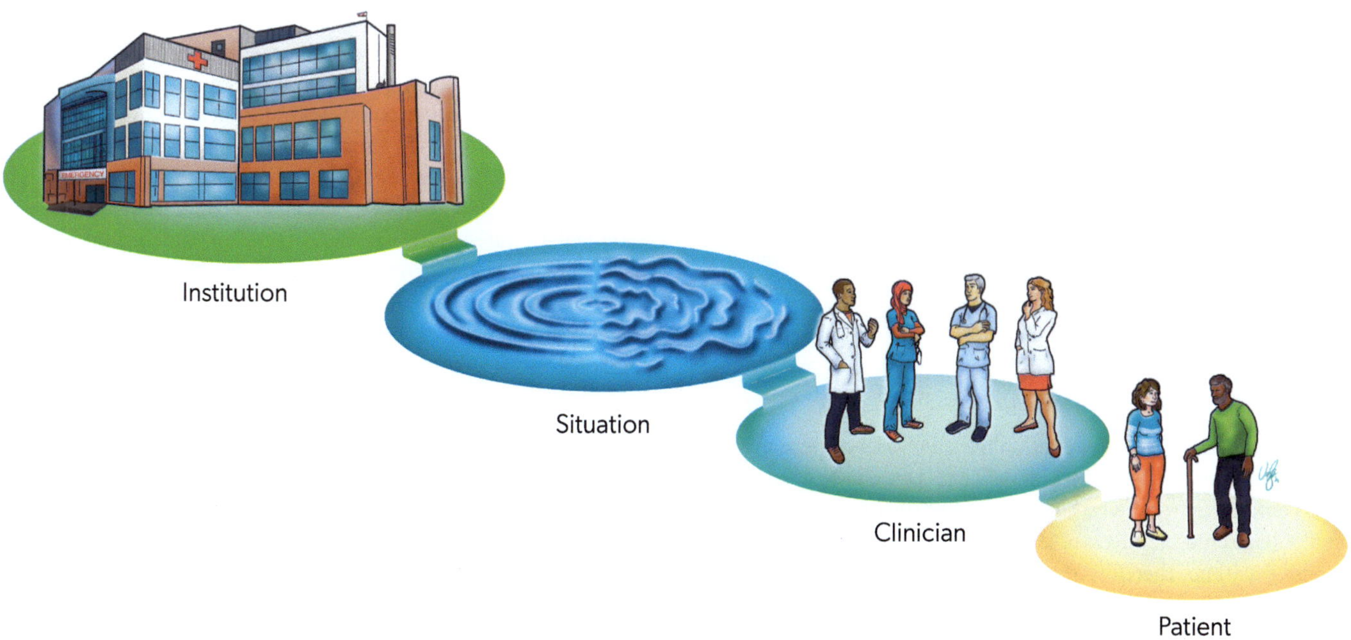

Figure 62.1 Institutions have the largest influence on SDM, followed by the situation, the clinician, and finally, the patient. However, all influence one another to some degree.

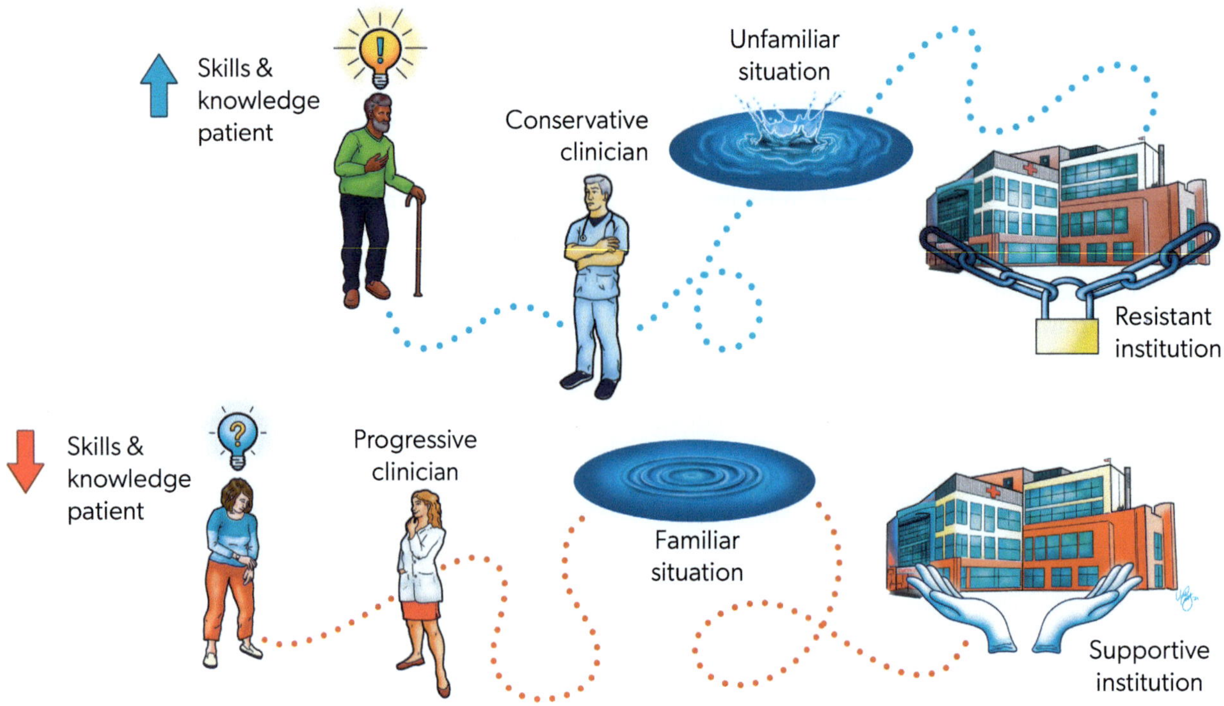

Figure 62.2 Different combinations of a high- or low-skill/knowledge patient, progressive or conservative clinician, familiar or unfamiliar situation, and supportive or resistant institution can shape the SDM process.

Individual clinician characteristics

SDM is dependent on the patient–clinician relationship (Keij et al., 2021) and the ever-present power imbalance can make it difficult for patients to express their needs, values, and preferences clearly in the consultation room. There are several reasons why a patient would feel unable to or choose not to assert themselves in a clinical situation. Studies have shown that clinicians have different attitudes towards different conditions, meaning that conditions such as myocardial infarction, leukaemia, and brain tumours are seen as more 'prestigious' than conditions with less distinct symptoms such as fibromyalgia, for example (Album and Westin, 2008; Scoles and Nicodemo, 2022). Clinicians' perceptions of patients' behaviours are also important. Patients who are perceived as 'disruptive' or 'difficult' can face authoritarian clinician behaviours and even suffer diagnostic errors (Frosch et al., 2012; Mamede et al., 2016). In other cases, SDM may not occur because a clinician simply chooses a treatment for the patient without suggesting or presenting other alternatives that may be available.

In Figure 62.2, individual clinician characteristics are exemplified by the two levels: conservative and progressive, referring primarily to communication and interaction style.

Characteristics of the healthcare decision

Every healthcare decision depends on the situational context. For example, some situations will be unfamiliar to a patient (e.g. an unexpected emergency room visit), whereas other situations will be more familiar (e.g. a routine check-up). Moreover, familiarity is not static; it changes over time. Therefore, the familiarity with a given situation can impact the decisions people make in healthcare. We define this as 'unfamiliar' or 'familiar' situational characteristics (Figures 62.1 and 62.2).

People living with chronic or long-term conditions become familiar with the mysterious ways in which healthcare works. They become familiar with how their condition presents over time and may feel they need less help in making decisions for that condition. However, even patients who are self-management experts can find the situation overwhelming if they have to seek urgent care for an acute injury or condition (Snow et al., 2013).

Characteristics of healthcare system

The last characteristic we propose that influences the patient experience in SDM is the healthcare system itself. The healthcare system can be designed to facilitate rather than hinder SDM. This involves creating pathways that enable patients to access their medical information easily, understand their health conditions, and feel empowered to engage in constructive discussions with healthcare providers. A supportive system can provide time, training, and reimbursement for healthcare professionals to use communication and SDM techniques, ensuring they are equipped to partner effectively with patients in care. Unfortunately, the reality is that many clinicians feel unsupported by the work environment (Scott Duncan et al., 2023) with understaffing and workload pressures leading to compromised time with patients. This can also lead patients to become fearful about 'doctor-bothering' or encroaching on doctors' time (Llanwarne et al., 2017).

Patients can contribute to all levels of the healthcare system

While SDM is focused on the individual patient–clinician encounter, important co-production tasks can take place at multiple levels to support SDM.

One example is the active involvement of patients in SDM implementation, planning, and roll-out. The UK National Institute for Health and Care Excellence SDM guideline recommends including patients and their informal caregivers at the systems level by involving them in SDM implementation (NICE National Institute for Health and Care Excellence, 2021). To achieve this, the guidelines recommend:

> Consider appointing a patient director (from a healthcare service user background) to work with the senior leader and be responsible for raising the profile of the service user voice in planning, implementing, and monitoring SDM, especially from those in under-served populations supporting the embedding of shared decision making at the highest level of the organisation.

Another example is patient involvement in clinical practice guidelines. Treatment recommendations should consider patient input and preferences for the trade-offs involved (Montori et al., 2013). Our own experience (authors DPR, GH) of rapid guideline development that included multiple perspectives (i.e. patients, rheumatologists, researchers) is shared here. COVID-19 vaccines were approved in Canada in autumn 2021. This represented a remarkable achievement particularly for vulnerable populations such as people with autoimmune rheumatic diseases who are immunosuppressed due to their medications, and who have been shown to have worse outcomes from COVID-19 infection.

Initially, recommendations in Canada for the vaccine were against providing it to people with autoimmune rheumatic diseases. In response, rheumatology clinicians and patient communities across Canada mobilized in 2022 to develop guidelines for people with autoimmune rheumatic diseases (Hazlewood et al., 2021). Patient partners from the Canadian Arthritis Patient Alliance were engaged in all stages of developing this guideline as panel members. They were provided with training, compensation, and a safe space to engage at all meetings. The guidelines aligned with patient values and best evidence, finding that the potential benefits of vaccination outweighed the small theoretical risk of disease flare (Canadian Rheumatology Association, 2022). A decision tool was co-developed about the vaccine to support SDM (Canadian Rheumatology Association, 2021). A separate patient-preference study co-developed with patient partners later confirmed patients' preferences (Hazlewood et al., 2023), illustrating how patients can contribute to field of SDM in healthcare.

The patient of the future is already here!

As Charles and colleagues stated in 1997, it really does take two to tango (Charles et al., 1997)—and a lot has happened since 1997. Patients today have access to an immense amount of information, literally in the palm of their hands. Smartphones, generative artificial intelligence, and 'Dr Google' have created an information revolution that enables patients to know as much about the literature on their conditions as their clinicians. In addition, up to 50% of people living with chronic conditions are willing and able to take a lot of responsibility for managing their health and healthcare (Rademakers et al., 2016).

Today's autonomous patients approach healthcare with confidence, embracing the role of 'active contributor' rather than 'passive recipient'. They are often self-empowered, well informed about their condition(s), and prepared to engage in purposeful dialogue with their healthcare providers. They have even organized their own care teams (Riggare and Unruh, 2015). This shift requires a corresponding change in the healthcare delivery model, one that recognizes and values the contributions patients make to their own care.

When a self-empowered patient encounters a conservative clinician, they may choose a 'clinician-centred' approach. This refers to a dynamic where patients consciously minimize their own knowledge and refrain from asking informed questions to avoid intimidating or challenging the clinician. Patients can adopt this approach when they have previously encountered clinicians who appeared threatened by their well-informed queries, thus generating an unproductive power struggle. In order to navigate the healthcare system effectively, these patients in subsequent healthcare encounters may choose to play by the unspoken rules of the medical establishment, which could mean deferring to the clinician's authority.

It is a priority to respect variation across circumstances, conditions, and values. We recognize that the same patient may want to be as autonomous as possible and prefer minimally disruptive medicine in one instance (May et al., 2009), yet may also look for maximally supportive medicine in another instance. As such, patients can choose to promote SDM while remembering that deferring the decision to a trusted clinician is also an available choice. Actively listening and respecting the patient as an individual with values and preferences even in uncertainty promotes SDM as a standard of care.

Knowledge in the palm of patients' hands is not going away any time soon. Neither is the attitude that patients should be able to participate as much or as little as they wish to in their care based on their knowledge and circumstances. We would argue that patients, as a whole, have changed over time, and with that, healthcare systems and providers must also do the same. The patient of the future is already here—it is time for healthcare systems and providers of the future to step up.

See Box 62.1 for our clinician perspective.

Box 62.1 Clinician perspective

At its core, SDM is about supporting patients to make informed healthcare choices that are the right ones for them. From the patient's perspective, SDM means being heard and understood, and having a collaborative relationship with their healthcare provider. People make decisions all the time in their day-to-day lives, so it must seem jarring when it comes to their healthcare choices, where the stakes are very high, to accept a paternalistic model that ignores their preferences. As outlined in this chapter, nearly all patients want some degree of SDM. It is clinicians' responsibility to ensure that patients are fully informed of the available options and to support patients in choosing the option that aligns with their values.

The authors discuss four pillars that need to be considered for optimal SDM from the patient perspective: characteristics of the patient, clinician, situation (i.e. decision being made), and system. As the authors outline, the empowerment or activation of patients should be encouraged and supported within health systems. However, this doesn't mean the onus for SDM should fall entirely on the patient. Patients differ in their health literacy and skills to engage in SDM with healthcare providers. Clinicians should be aware of this and adapt approaches accordingly. Clinicians can also help identify the decisions where SDM is especially important. These will be the decisions where there are important risk/benefit trade-offs without a clearly superior option. From a systems perspective, it is essential that SDM is considered and supported throughout healthcare systems. Clinical practice guidelines and policy decisions need to consider patient preferences when weighing the risks and benefits of treatment alternatives, help identify preference-sensitive decisions, and support SDM models. While critical aspects of SDM happen in the patient–clinician encounter, there is a lot that can be done outside of the encounter, and health systems can support this. Patients now have access to an unprecedented amount of information online, and health systems should support patients by providing trustworthy information and decision aids to support their decision-making. As noted in this chapter, the patient of the future is here, and clinicians and healthcare systems need to adapt!

REFERENCES

Album, D., Westin, S. 2008. Do diseases have a prestige hierarchy? A survey among physicians and medical students. *Soc Sci Med,* **66**, 182–188.

Canadian Rheumatology Association. 2021. Decision tool for COVID-19 vaccination. Available at: https://rheum.ca/decision-tool/

Canadian Rheumatology Association. 2022. Canadian Rheumatology Association position statement on COVID-19 vaccination. Available at: https://rheum.ca/wp-content/uploads/2022/03/FINAL-Updated-PS-on-COVID-19-Vacc-March-25_2022_for-publication.pdf

Charles, C., Gafni, A., Whelan, T. 1997. Shared decision-making in the medical encounter: what does it mean? (Or it takes at least two to tango). *Soc Sci Med,* **44**, 681–692.

Degner, L. F., Sloan, J. A., Venkatesh, P. 1997. The Control Preferences Scale. *Can J Nurs Res,* **29**, 21–43.

Elwyn, G., Price, A., Franco, J. V. A., Gulbrandsen, P. 2023. The limits of shared decision making. *BMJ Evid Based Med,* **28**, 218–221.

Frosch, D. L., May, S. G., Rendle, K. A., Tietbohl, C., Elwyn, G. 2012. Authoritarian physicians and patients' fear of being labeled 'difficult' among key obstacles to shared decision making. *Health Aff (Millwood),* **31**, 1030–1038.

Hahlweg, P., Kriston, L., Scholl, I., et al. 2020. Cancer patients' preferred and perceived level of involvement in treatment decision-making: an epidemiological study. *Acta Oncol,* **59**, 967–974.

Hazlewood, G. S., Pardo, J. P., Barnabe, C., et al. 2021. Canadian Rheumatology Association recommendation for the use of covid-19 vaccination for patients with autoimmune rheumatic diseases. *J Rheumatol,* **48**, 1330–1339.

Hazlewood, G. S., Colmegna, I., Hitchon, C., et al. 2023. Preferences for COVID-19 vaccination in people with chronic immune-mediated inflammatory diseases. *J Rheumatol,* **50**, 949–957.

Hibbard, J. H., Stockard, J., Mahoney, E. R., Tusler, M. 2004. Development of the Patient Activation Measure (PAM): conceptualizing and measuring activation in patients and consumers. *Health Serv Res,* **39**, 1005–1026.

Keij, S. M., van Duijn-Bakker, N., Stiggelbout, A. M., Pieterse, A. H. 2021. What makes a patient ready for shared decision making? A qualitative study. *Patient Educ Couns,* **104**, 571–577.

Légaré, F., Adekpedjou, R., Stacey, D., et al. 2018. Interventions for increasing the use of shared decision making by healthcare professionals. *Cochrane Database Syst Rev,* **7**, CD006732.

Llanwarne, N., Newbould, J., Burt, J., Campbell, J. L., Roland, M. 2017. Wasting the doctor's time? A video-elicitation interview study with patients in primary care. *Soc Sci Med,* **176**, 113–122.

Mamede, S., Van Gog, T., Schuit, S. C., et al. 2016. Why patients' disruptive behaviours impair diagnostic reasoning: a randomised experiment. *BMJ Qual Safe,* **11**, 1–6.

May, C., Montori, V. M., Mair, F. S. 2009. We need minimally disruptive medicine. *Br Med J,* **339**, b2803.

Montori, V. M., Ruissen, M. M., Hargraves, I. G., Brito, J. P., Kunneman, M. 2023. Shared decision-making as a method of care. *BMJ Evid Based Med,* **28**, 213–217.

Montori, V. M., Brito, J. P., Murad, M. H. 2013. The optimal practice of evidence-based medicine: incorporating patient preferences in practice guidelines. *JAMA,* **310**, 2503.

NICE National Institute for Health and Care Excellence. 2021. Shared decision making. NICE guideline [NG197]. Available at: https://www.nice.org.uk/guidance/ng197

Rademakers, J., Maindal, H. T., Steinsbekk, A., Gensichen, J., Brenk-Franz, K., Hendriks, M. 2016. Patient activation in Europe: an international comparison of psychometric properties and patients' scores on the short form Patient Activation Measure (PAM-13). *BMC Health Serv Res,* **16**, 570.

Riggare, S., Unruh, K.T. 2015. Patients organise and train doctors to provide better care. *BMJ,* **351**, h6318.

Schulz, P. J., Nakamoto, K. 2013. Health literacy and patient empowerment in health communication: the importance of separating conjoined twins. *Patient Educ Couns,* **90**, 4–11.

Scoles, B., Nicodemo, C. 2022. Doctors' attitudes toward specific medical conditions. *J Econ Behav Organ,* **204**, 182–199.

Scott Duncan, T., Riggare, S., Bylund, A., et al. 2023. Empowered patients and informal care-givers as partners?—a survey study of healthcare professionals' perceptions. *BMC Health Serv Res,* **23**, 404.

Snow, R., Humphrey, C., Sandall, J. 2013. What happens when patients know more than their doctors? Experiences of health interactions after diabetes patient education: a qualitative patient-led study. *BMJ Open,* **3**, e003583.

Waddell, A., Lennox, A., Spassova, G., Bragge, P. 2021. Barriers and facilitators to shared decision-making in hospitals from policy to practice: a systematic review. *Implement Sci,* **16**, 74.

63

The importance of cost conversations as part of shared decision making

Mary C. Politi, Carrie C. Coughlin, Lindsay M. Kuroki, and Jessica Miller

Overview

Costs of healthcare are rising worldwide (Schoen et al., 2013; Gordon et al., 2018; Organisation for Economic Cooperation and Development, 2023). In addition to costs to the healthcare system, in the USA, patients are increasingly responsible for higher out-of-pocket expenses for healthcare visits, procedures, and medications, before insurance benefits are applied (Abdus et al., 2016; Claxton et al., 2019). The burden of costs on patients contributes to what many refer to as *financial toxicity*, or the psychosocial and behavioural responses to financial hardship from care costs (Altice et al., 2017; Jones et al., 2020; Lyman and Kuderer, 2020; Bradley et al., 2021). One participant described the difficulty managing financial aspects of care on top of her illness (George et al., 2021): 'The billing was extremely daunting. I kept a three-ring binder that was three inches thick [to make sense of the bills] . . . It was a mess.'

Care costs directly affect patients' choices and adherence to clinical recommendations. Many patients describe delaying or forgoing care deemed necessary because of its cost, or skipping or rationing prescribed medications (Knight et al., 2018; Smith et al., 2018; Thomas et al., 2021). Patients overwhelmingly want to discuss costs with clinicians to prepare for what to expect. When the care team does not acknowledge costs when discussing treatment options, the burden falls on the patient to navigate through the cost-related consequences of care (Politi et al., 2023). In addition, current payor systems obscure costs and patients' responsibility for those costs (George et al., 2021).

In this chapter, we will characterize cost complexity from the patient, clinician, and system levels and call for more transparency to support health decisions and reduce financial toxicity. We will focus on the US healthcare system; although costs affect patients worldwide, the unique aspects of the US healthcare system increase the burden on patients.

Cost complexity for the patient

Patients and caregivers often incur high costs when seeking care, which can result in financial distress and/or toxicity (Kahn-Boesel et al., 2023). Costs affect both insured and uninsured patients, and can discourage needed care and/or create debt. This section discusses examples of *direct costs* (costs of care itself), *indirect costs* (costs of secondary aspects of care such as time off work, reduced wages, transportation), and their financial impacts on patients.

Direct costs

Estimating care costs is challenging because of the uncertainty about which services might be needed. For patients with health insurance, outpatient visit co-payments are typically listed on insurance documents and can often be estimated in advance. Co-insurance is more difficult to estimate, as patients pay a percentage of a visit, which is often unknown upfront. Outpatient visits are billed based on their medical complexity or length. Patients may also incur unexpected costs during a visit, such as for an unplanned procedure, blood tests, or imaging. For more advanced or inpatient care, estimating out-of-pocket costs can be very complicated, preventing patients and families from making financially informed decisions prior to deciding on treatment. Estimates can be provided based on diagnostic and procedure codes, but the duration of a procedure, required medications used, length of hospital stay, and more can modify costs. For patients without insurance, navigating negotiations for payment plans and rates can be daunting, and costs can be quite high and opaque (Montero et al., 2022). Billing can also be delayed by months, making it hard for patients to anticipate when costs will be due.

Prescription medication costs also contribute to patients' burden. Different pharmacies can charge different amounts for the same medication, and many patients and clinicians do not know which pharmacy has the best price for a particular drug. Additionally, patients might not know what a 'reasonable' medication price might be, and what price should prompt seeking another pharmacy, replacement medication, or co-payment support. Some patients and families worry about being judged for questioning medication costs or admitting costs are high (Meisenberg et al., 2015; Harrington et al., 2020). Patients might not have transportation to less expensive pharmacies and have difficulty filling prescriptions at new locations. Unfortunately, searching for lower prices can delay or complicate care and increase patient and caregiver anxiety and frustration (Etteldorf et al., 2022).

Indirect costs

Indirect costs such as parking/transportation, meals, time off work, supplies not covered by insurance, and childcare can increase expenses well beyond what direct costs would suggest. Moreover, absenteeism (time off work) and presenteeism (being at work without functioning to full capacity) both contribute to lost wages and productivity (Kahn-Boesel et al., 2023). Indirect costs of follow-up visits and care after major procedures also increase the financial burden on patients.

Consequences of cost and financial toxicity

Many patients self-ration care or medication as a result of this complexity and unaffordability, worsening disparities in health outcomes (Knight et al., 2018; Thomas et al., 2021). Economic reserves, diagnosis severity, and insurance type can influence financial burden and can contribute to age- and race-based health disparities (Everson et al., 2023). Patients might try to adjust the timing of care-seeking based on their insurance or personal needs; scheduling of care relative to the calendar year, the start of a new billing cycle, or a change of insurance plan can directly affect costs. Clinicians should consider these contextual factors when collaborating on care plans. See one pertinent example of timing of care and its associated cost consequences in the patient perspective box (Box 63.1).

Most patients want to have conversations about cost, but few are willing to raise the subject and engage in these discussions with clinicians (Everson et al., 2023). The complexities noted above both contribute to a care gap and provide opportunities for intervention.

Cost transparency for the clinical team

While clinicians agree that addressing costs is important, many hesitate to discuss the topic with patients. Barriers to cost conversations include insufficient training, uncertainty about cost data, lack of resources to offset such costs, and concerns about compromising the patient–physician relationship (Zafar et al., 2014). Many clinicians never receive formal education on cost-effectiveness analyses, cost strategies, or shared decision making (Patel et al., 2011; Zafar et al., 2014). Even when clinicians overcome barriers to discussing costs, unconscious biases likely inhibit these conversations. For example, many oncologists report discomfort discussing costs with patients, and acknowledge that they may omit treatment options (ration care) based on their perceptions of patients' ability to afford it (Schrag and Hanger, 2007). Some overestimate patients' level of difficulty paying medical bills, particularly among those with less education or lower socioeconomic status (Garcia-Bautista et al., 2023). Clinicians can paradoxically overestimate the importance of cost discussions with patients who are White, with higher income and education, yet costs disproportionately affect patients who are Black and Hispanic with fewer financial resources (Montero et al., 2022).

Uncertainty about patients' out-of-pocket costs and resources to offset these costs hinders the quality and value of cost conversations. For example, for private insurance plans, clinicians might not know how much of a patient's yearly deductible has been met, what their insurance plan charges, and which pharmacy has the best price for a medication. Clinicians worry about being perceived as basing treatment decisions on cost if they ask about these details, even though

Box 63.1 Patient perspective

Exemplifying costs of care challenges

Blake was born with large congenital melanocytic nevi ('moles') on her scalp, face, and multiple areas of her body. She had her first appointment with a paediatric dermatologist at 6 weeks old. Blake had her congenital melanocytic nevi documented and photographed. A biopsy of one nevus showed that it was 'atypical', and that the area needed to be fully removed by a plastic surgeon. Additionally, due to her number of nevi, we were told that a magnetic resonance imaging scan of her brain was needed.

The surgery and magnetic resonance imaging were scheduled for December 2022. However, the surgeon was called to an emergency and we were told that the planned surgery for Blake had to be rescheduled. Family who had taken time off work to be there with us, even flying out from other states, were then unable to offer support. And what was particularly upsetting was the impact on our out-of-pocket costs. Each year, our insurance requires us to pay out-of-pocket until we reach a $3750 deductible, after which they start sharing care costs until we reach a $7500 out-of-pocket maximum. Because we had reached the maximum in 2022, the surgery would have been fully covered in December. However, when surgery was rescheduled to January 2023, we then needed to reach these out-of-pocket limits in the new year. A 2-week delay significantly affected our surgery costs.

A year and a half later, Blake had another area of concern on her large scalp nevus, and we decided to move forward with more extensive removal. We wanted to schedule the procedures at the beginning of the calendar year so that we could try to get as much done and covered without paying our annual out-of-pocket for 2 years. Part of the preparation was tissue expansion, but instead of taking 3 months, it took 6 months and added to the expenses. Blake finally had surgery, and then we faced additional costs for needed dressing removal which required another visit, and more anaesthesia. Unfortunately, the skin graft disintegrated and we had to use creams and medicine to keep infections out of her open wound. After waiting a year, we scheduled her for her first fat graft, knowing she would have to wait another 6 months for the next procedure. We tried to schedule it all in the same calendar year to help with out-of-pocket costs, but it wasn't possible due to unexpected complications and delays.

Costs really added up. In addition to the costs of the surgeries and travel to the medical centre, I missed work for many months to take care of her since she wasn't allowed to go to daycare. My husband also frequently missed work since we had to travel 2 hours to the surgeries and appointments, and someone needed to take care of her in the car. We also had to find help with our other two daughters. In addition to these indirect costs, never once were we given an estimate of what the direct costs would be for treatments. Cost transparency could have helped us prepare for what to expect from this long journey.

patients overwhelmingly want to discuss costs at the place in which they are receiving care. As one patient told us (George et al., 2021): 'I would rather hear it [costs of care] from somebody at the medical facility ... I wanna talk to the people ... where I'm actually getting treatment.'

While not all cost conversations result in cost-reducing outcomes, they can help clinicians and patients plan for what to expect and consider alternative treatments or schedules (Espinoza Suarez et al., 2020; Espinoza Suarez et al., 2021). These discussions can enhance the patient–clinician relationship. As many as 57% of patients who discuss costs with their physicians report lower out-of-pocket costs as a result, mostly without changing their core treatment decision (Zafar et al., 2015). They receive referrals to financial assistance programmes, help with insurance approval/coverage, less expensive prescription medications, fewer tests, and/or fewer clinician visits. Therefore, several national organizations, including Costs of Care and the American Society of Clinical Oncology, have developed concrete strategies to reduce out-of-pocket costs and financial toxicity through collaborative discussions and shared-decision making (Meropol et al., 2009; Gupta et al., 2022).

Potential approaches to system-level cost transparency

Increasing price transparency might reduce financial toxicity (e.g. by providing public access to charges and/or patient expenses for care) (Sinaiko and Rosenthal, 2011). Hospitals, health centres, professional societies, insurance companies, and/or government entities should develop more transparent cost information about healthcare procedures and supplies (Centers for Medicare and Medicaid Services, n.d.; Henrikson et al., 2019; Sloan et al., 2022). When patients know in advance about a healthcare need, clear price lists, ranges, or algorithmic predictions of expenses can help them gather, analyse, and organize their finances; tools or individual financial navigators could then provide more personalized estimates of costs based on specific insurance and clinical details (Henrikson et al., 2019; Sloan et al., 2022). Financial navigation programmes could also support patients as they weigh options for treatment when there are multiple options available, or direct them toward resources or hospital payment plans to offset costs when there are no lower-cost alternatives (de Moor et al., 2021; Henrikson et al., 2022). To date, though, patients continue to report difficulty understanding what costs will be covered and how to optimize their insurance to pay for chosen care. As one patient told us (George et al., 2021): 'I don't know if there are any hospitals or even insurance companies that will quote you how much something will cost ... You just don't know until you receive the bill.'

With more regulation at the government level mandating cost transparency, hospitals and care facilities could meet patients where they are receiving care, in places they trust, rather than having patients seek this information from outside sources.

Conclusion

As the compelling story in Box 63.1 exemplifies, patients/families can incur thousands of dollars in care costs, often unexpectedly. Even when patients prepare in advance, timing shifts and complications can delay care and/or add a cost-related burden. Clinicians and health systems, should consider affordability as a measure of care quality, as not all patients will be able to receive needed care without significant sacrifices and life adjustments. More than 18% of US households carry medical debt, and this debt impacts their ability to pay for food, housing, and social needs (Himmelstein et al., 2022). As the clinician section describes, discussing costs can lower the financial burden on patients in many instances. This chapter only scratches the surface of the numerous cost-related challenges to care and the importance of discussing costs openly and ahead of time when collaborating on health decisions.

REFERENCES

Abdus, S., Selden, T. M., Keenan, P. 2016. The financial burdens of high-deductible plans. *Health Aff (Millwood)*, **35**, 2297–2301.

Altice, C. K., Banegas, M. P., Tucker-Seeley, R. D., Yabroff, K. R. 2017. Financial hardships experienced by cancer survivors: a systematic review. *J Natl Cancer Inst*, **109**, djw205.

Bradley, C. J., Yabroff, K. R., Shih, Y. T. 2021. A coordinated policy approach to address medical financial toxicity. *JAMA Oncol*, **7**, 1761–1762.

Centers for Medicare and Medicaid Services. n.d. Hospital price transparency. Available at: https://www.cms.gov/priorities/key-initiatives/hospital-price-transparency

Claxton, G., Rae, M., Damico, A., Young, G., Mcdermott, D., Whitmore, H. 2019. Health benefits in 2019: premiums inch higher, employers respond to federal policy. *Health Aff (Millwood)*, **38**, 1752–1761.

De Moor, J. S., Mollica, M., Sampson, A., et al. 2021. Delivery of financial navigation services within National Cancer Institute-designated cancer centers. *JNCI Cancer Spectr*, **5**, pkab033.

Espinoza Suarez, N. R., Lavecchia, C. M., Fischer, K. M., Kamath, C. C., Brito, J. P. 2021. Impact of cost conversation on decision-making outcomes. *Mayo Clin Proc Innov Qual Outcomes*, **5**, 802–810.

Espinoza Suarez, N. R., Lavecchia, C. M., Ponce, O. J., et al. 2020. Using shared decision-making tools and patient–clinician conversations about costs. *Mayo Clin Proc Innov Qual Outcomes*, **4**, 416–423.

Etteldorf, A., Rotolo, S., Sedhom, R., et al. 2022. Finding the lowest-cost pharmacy for cancer supportive care medications: not so easy. *JCO Oncol Pract*, **18**, e1342–e1349.

Everson, J., Henderson, S. C., Cheng, A., Senft, N., Whitmore, C., Dusetzina, S. B. 2023. Demand for and occurrence of medication cost conversations: a narrative review. *Med Care Res Rev*, **80**, 16–29.

Garcia-Bautista, A., Kamath, C., Ayala, N., et al. 2023. Financial toxicity in the clinical encounter: a paired survey of patient and clinician perceptions. *Mayo Clin Proc Innov Qual Outcomes*, **7**, 248–255.

George, N., Grant, R., James, A., Mir, N., Politi, M. C. 2021. Burden associated with selecting and using health insurance to manage care costs: results of a qualitative study of nonelderly cancer survivors. *Med Care Res Rev*, **78**, 48–56.

Gordon, N., Stemmer, S. M., Greenberg, D., Goldstein, D. A. 2018. Trajectories of injectable cancer drug costs after launch in the United States. *J Clin Oncol*, **36**, 319–325.

Gupta, R., Harmon, J., Wallingford, S., Petrilli, C., Chino, F. 2022. The affordability accelerator: a road map to improve patient out-of-pocket costs and trustworthiness in health care. *NEJM Catalyst*, **3**, 20 May.

Harrington, N. G., Scott, A. M., Spencer, E. A. 2020. Working toward evidence-based guidelines for cost-of-care conversations between patients and physicians: a systematic review of the literature. *Soc Sci Med,* **258**, 113084.

Henrikson, N. B., Anderson, M. L., Dickerson, J., et al. 2022. The Cancer Financial Experience (CAFÉ) study: randomized controlled trial of a financial navigation intervention to address cancer-related financial hardship. *Trials,* **23**, 402.

Henrikson, N. B., Banegas, M. P., Tuzzio, L., et al. 2019. Workflow requirements for cost-of-care conversations in outpatient settings providing oncology or primary care: a qualitative, human-centered design study. *Ann Intern Med,* **170**, S70–S78.

Himmelstein, D. U., Dickman, S. L., McCormick, D., Bor, D. H., Gaffney, A., Woolhandler, S. 2022. Prevalence and risk factors for medical debt and subsequent changes in social determinants of health in the US. *JAMA Network Open,* **5**, e2231898.

Jones, S. M., Henrikson, N. B., Panattoni, L., Syrjala, K. L., Shankaran, V. 2020. A theoretical model of financial burden after cancer diagnosis. *Future Oncol,* **16**, 3095–3105.

Kahn-Boesel, O., Cautha, S., Ufere, N. N., Ananthakrishnan, A. N., Kochar, B. 2023. A narrative review of financial burden, distress, and toxicity of inflammatory bowel diseases in the United States. *Am J Gastroenterol,* **118**, 1545–1553.

Knight, T. G., Deal, A. M., Dusetzina, S. B., et al. 2018. Financial toxicity in adults with cancer: adverse outcomes and noncompliance. *J Oncol Pract,* **14**, Jop1800120.

Lyman, G. H., Kuderer, N. 2020. Financial toxicity, financial abuse, or financial torture: let's call it what it is! *Cancer Invest,* **38**, 139–142.

Meisenberg, B. R., Varner, A., Ellis, E., et al. 2015. Patient attitudes regarding the cost of illness in cancer care. *Oncologist,* **20**, 1199–1204.

Meropol, N. J., Schrag, D., Smith, T. J., et al. 2009. American Society of Clinical Oncology guidance statement: the cost of cancer care. *J Clin Oncol,* **27**, 3868–3874.

Montero, A., Kearney, A., Hamel, L., Brodie, M. 2022. *Americans' Challenges with Health Care Costs.* Kaiser Family Foundation.

Organisation for Economic Cooperation and Development. 2023. Health at a glance 2023. OECD Publishing. Available at: https://www.oecd.org/en/publications/2023/11/health-at-a-glance-2023_e04f8239.html

Patel, M. S., Davis, M. M., Lypson, M. L. 2011. Advancing medical education by teaching health policy. *N Engl J Med,* **364**, 695–697.

Politi, M. C., Housten, A. J., Forcino, R. C., Jansen, J., Elwyn, G. 2023. Discussing cost and value in patient decision aids and shared decision making: a call to action. *MDM Policy Pract,* **8**, 23814683221148651.

Schoen, C., Osborn, R., Squires, D., Doty, M. M. 2013. Access, affordability, and insurance complexity are often worse in the United States compared to ten other countries. *Health Aff (Millwood),* **32**, 2205–15.

Schrag, D., Hanger, M. 2007. Medical oncologists' views on communicating with patients about chemotherapy costs: a pilot survey. *J Clin Oncol,* **25**, 233–237.

Sinaiko, A. D., Rosenthal, M. B. 2011. Increased price transparency in health care—challenges and potential effects. *N Engl J Med,* **364**, 891–894.

Sloan, C. E., Gutterman, S., Davis, J. K., et al. 2022. How can healthcare organizations improve cost-of-care conversations? A qualitative exploration of clinicians' perspectives. *Patient Educ Couns,* **105**, 2708–2714.

Smith, K. T., Monti, D., Mir, N., Peters, E., Tipirneni, R., Politi, M. C. 2018. Access is necessary but not sufficient: factors influencing delay and avoidance of health care services. *MDM Policy Pract,* **3**, 2381468318760298.

Thomas, A., Valero-Elizondo, J., Khera, R., et al. 2021. Forgone medical care associated with increased health care costs among the U.S. heart failure population. *JACC Heart Fail,* **9**, 710–719.

Zafar, S. Y., Chino, F., Ubel, P. A., et al. 2015. The utility of cost discussions between patients with cancer and oncologists. *Am J Manag Care,* **21**, 607–615.

Zafar, S. Y., Tulsky, J. A., Abernethy, A. P. 2014. It's time to have 'the talk': cost communication and patient-centered care. *Oncology (Williston Park),* **28**, 479–480.

64

Increasing equity in shared decision making

Marie-Anne Durand, Julie Ayre, Catherine H. Saunders, Christine M. Marx, and Kirsten J. McCaffery

Can shared decision making reduce health inequities?

Socially disadvantaged populations often experience more disease burden and less healthcare access than more advantaged groups. Those widening health inequalities are often described through the social gradient of health (Marmot, 2005). The more disadvantaged a person is (income, race or ethnicity, educational attainment, disability, and so on), the worse their health will be. Addressing this challenge should be a priority.

A disadvantage may involve one or more specific attributes, contexts, or group types. We define a social disadvantage in light of the PROGRESS-Plus framework (O'Neill et al., 2014). Socially disadvantaged populations are less likely to engage in shared decision making (SDM) than more advantaged groups (Thomson et al., 2005). This may be exacerbated by language barriers, physical impairments, or lower educational attainment. Younger patients, women, and people from higher socioeconomic groups are more likely to assume active roles in medical decision making (Thomson et al., 2005). There is a risk that SDM increases health inequities between those who are naturally able to engage in SDM and those who find it more challenging. See key terms and definitions in Box 64.1.

Box 64.1 Key terms and definitions

What are health inequalities?
Differences in the health status and achievements of individuals and groups experienced within and between countries.

What are health inequities?
Systematic differences in the health status of different population groups with significant social and economic costs to individuals and societies.

What is a disadvantage?
Relative social, cultural, physical, educational, geographical, or financial disparities that have engendered environmental, historical-structural, or social restrictions to opportunities for health (Kilbourne et al., 2006; Commission on Social Determinants of Health, 2008; Sydor, 2013).

Over the past decade, many have advocated for SDM as an approach to address and potentially reduce health inequalities and inequities (King et al., 2011). Several systematic reviews have assessed the impact of patient decision aids (PtDAs) and other SDM interventions on socially disadvantaged populations (Durand et al., 2014; Enard et al., 2016; Yen et al., 2021).

Findings from the most recent review and meta-analysis suggested that PtDAs improved knowledge and patient–clinician communication, and reduced decisional conflict and the proportion undecided among socially disadvantaged populations (Yen et al., 2021). PtDAs did not affect anxiety. These findings were held when all SDM interventions (that did not meet the definition of a PtDA) were included. There was limited information on the interventions' effects on clinical outcomes. There were no differences in satisfaction, attitudes, or self-efficacy. Only five out of the twelve PtDA studies that compared outcomes by disadvantaged standing found that outcomes improved more for socially disadvantaged participants. There was significant heterogeneity, and no specific features led to improved outcomes for socially disadvantaged populations. The authors of the 2021 review concluded that while most outcomes of interest were improved among socially disadvantaged populations, there was no evidence of a reduction in health inequalities. Further research is needed.

How can we increase equity in SDM?

Equity is a complex construct. It is related to social justice and fairness (Braveman and Gruskin, 2003). It is an ethical principle closely related to human rights. It is inherently normative and value-based (Braveman et al., 2001). Inequities are seen as unfair, while inequalities may not always be (Braveman and Gruskin, 2003). According to Braveman and Gruskin, equity can be defined as the absence of disparities systematically associated with a social advantage or disadvantage (Braveman and Gruskin, 2003). We define health equity in Box 64.2.

Box 64.2 Health equity definition

The US Centers for Disease Control and Prevention defines equity in health as 'the state in which everyone has a fair and just opportunity to attain their highest level of health' (Centers for Disease Control and Prevention, 2024).

Achieving health equity necessitates efforts to address current and historical injustices, tackle economic, social, physical, and other obstacles to healthcare and health, and ideally eliminate preventable health disparities (Braveman and Gruskin, 2003). Accordingly, promoting equity in SDM entails enabling everyone, irrespective of their socioeconomic position, educational attainment, physical or mental impairments, or health literacy levels, to engage in medical decision making in situations of clinical equipoise. Increasing equity in SDM means making the necessary adaptations before, during, and after medical visits to enable a dialogue about available treatment or screening options between health professionals and *all* individuals.

Scholars and policymakers have long advocated for an approach that makes information, interventions, and services accessible and understandable to all people and is proportional to the level of disadvantage. In 2010, the principle of 'proportionate universalism' was introduced as a solution to reduce health inequities: 'Actions should be universal but with an intensity and a scale that is proportional to the level of disadvantage' (Francis-Oliviero et al., 2020). The big idea behind it is simple: if you make healthcare globally, and SDM interventions specifically, as easily accessible and understandable as possible, you are more likely to increase equity. See Box 64.3.

Beyond this broad principle, there are approaches to help researchers, healthcare professionals, and others expand their perspectives and increase equity and inclusion. Training healthcare and allied healthcare professionals and providing tools to more effectively engage socially disadvantaged patients can improve outcomes and potentially reduce inequities (Durand et al., 2021; Yen et al., 2021). We know, however, from our efforts to implement SDM, that education and tools are difficult to integrate in routine clinical practice (Elwyn et al., 2013). We do not yet know whether brief health professional training and patient-facing resources are enough to durably improve health equity. There are very few longitudinal studies of SDM interventions and even fewer among socially disadvantaged populations.

The need for more accessible and understandable SDM interventions has been clearly articulated in the literature. A recent systematic review reported that only 25 of 213 decision aids (11.7%) considered the needs of people with lower health literacy or people from socially disadvantaged communities (Muscat et al., 2021). None of the decision aids included in this review met the grade 8 (or below) readability level recommended in decision aid guidelines and health literacy guidance for clear communication. Ten were assessed as easy to understand, and only five were considered sufficiently easy to act on, using an established and widely used health literacy assessment tool (the PEMAT: Patient Education Materials Assessment Tool).

Box 64.3 Health literacy definition

The term health literacy first appeared in the 1970s. It designates *people's capacities to meet the complex demands of health in a modern society* (Sørensen et al., 2012). Having sufficient health literacy means placing one's own health and that of one's family and community into context, understanding which factors are influencing it, and knowing how to address them. Clinicians and health organizations can support this goal.

Further, no reviews have investigated the extent to which PtDAs adhere to accessibility guidelines to support uptake by people with disability. The Mayo Clinic has, for example, created several decision aids on various topics, written at grade 6–8 reading level and adhering to the 'Web Content Accessibility Guidelines' (World Wide Web Consortium, n.d.). Though these guidelines do not guarantee the needs of people with disability are met, they provide a promising starting point. In addition, co-designed, person-centred resources already exist to support communication with people with disability (Noorlandt et al., 2020). These could be integrated or further adapted to develop, adapt, evaluate, and implement SDM interventions accessible to all.

Beyond being understandable for all, SDM approaches may need to be adapted to relevant cultural contexts. The first step in culturally appropriate SDM is ensuring clear communication. Practitioners should ensure—whenever possible—they are using qualified or certified medical interpreters (Niven, n.d.). The US Agency for Healthcare Research and Quality has a 'Universal Health Literacy Precautions' toolkit with more information on patients' rights to interpreter services (Brega et al., 2015). It is also essential to ask patients about their communication preferences: written or verbal information, how much detail they would like, and to what extent they value being involved in decision making.

If high-quality written materials are available with vetted, culturally competent content relevant to the particular patient at hand, those materials can enhance culturally relevant SDM. For instance, a culturally tailored PtDA that also scores well on the IPDAS Collaboration Criteria Checklist with good readability would help address equity. Although the practice is burgeoning, there are efforts to codify processes for cultural adaptations of PtDAs (Chenel et al., 2018). Beyond culturally relevant translation, this can include practices like using pictures or videos of people from the target cultural group in the PtDAs, adapting the delivery mechanism, or revising the content (Chenel et al., 2018). A more radical approach to equity in SDM may also challenge a Western worldview of health and medicine. In the face of the COVID-19 pandemic, Australian health services collaborated with Aboriginal health workers and community members to develop a holistic and culturally responsive resource for SDM that could support discussion about COVID-19 vaccines (Dimopoulos-Bick et al., 2023). The resource depicts SDM in the context of 'yarning' (storytelling) that encourages discussion about community, family, and kinship; culture and connections to land and sea; personal experiences; and physical/spiritual connections.

Further, health literacy and accessibility guidelines provide useful foundational advice for more equitable SDM interventions. The Centers for Disease Control and Prevention has, for example, developed multiple resources to promote the development of visual health information (Centers for Disease Control and Prevention, 2023). The 'Do no harm guide' aims to apply equity awareness in data visualization (Urban Institute, 2024). However, in isolation, these guidelines are unlikely to fully meet the needs of the target users. Partnering with relevant communities (also called patient and public involvement in research (PPIR)) is needed to improve the quality, acceptability, and implementation of health interventions

(Greenhalgh et al., 2019). The benefits of PPIR have been demonstrated across the research timeline (Brett et al., 2014). PPIR increases research relevance, feasibility, rigour, and quality (Forsythe et al., 2019). It can also improve recruitment, collection, analysis, and dissemination of data (Crocker et al., 2018).

However, not all stakeholders are equally engaged in PPIR (Dawson et al., 2018; Reynolds et al., 2021). It has traditionally involved more advantaged and empowered partners who have the time, financial flexibility, confidence, and self-efficacy to engage in research. Taking the voices and needs of socially disadvantaged populations into account will help ensure that the study's measures, interventions, methods, dissemination, and implementation strategies are accessible and acceptable to them (Dawson et al., 2018). To promote equity in research and in health, researchers should strive to engage the full range of stakeholders affected by health and social care research, who may feel overlooked or ignored by mainstream society (Loignon et al., 2023).

Frameworks for achieving PPIR are highly variable and will depend on specific project needs and parameters. For example, over 60 frameworks for patient and public involvement exist, each with a varying focus on addressing power differentials, setting patient priorities, engaging the public in programme development, reporting transparency, and project governance (Greenhalgh et al., 2019). Patient and public involvement can also range temporally (e.g. from the earliest conceptual stages through to dissemination of study findings) and in depth (e.g. from tokenistic 'box-ticking' through to genuine and enduring partnerships that establish trust between the project team and community). Establishing trust is particularly important when working with disadvantaged groups. This is illustrated by the '4M Model,' a framework for health communication with multicultural populations (Zachariah et al., 2022).

Figure 64.1 summarizes ways of increasing equity in SDM while integrating the perspective of a patient partner and co-author of this chapter.

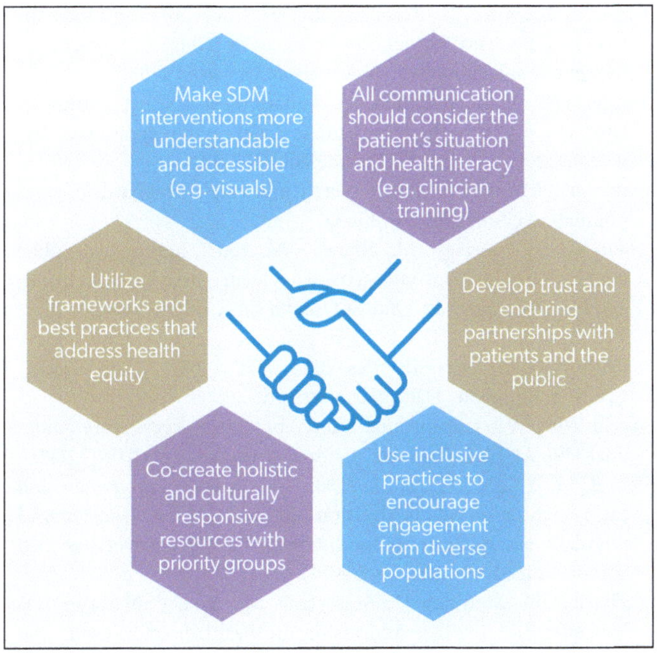

Figure 64.1 Patient perspective. Increasing equity in SDM.

Ongoing challenges

While many strategies exist and continue to be tested to increase equity, several ongoing challenges must be considered. We know that existing SDM resources are unlikely to meet the needs of socially disadvantaged groups. This is in part because research and implementation have not consistently focused on making SDM resources accessible and inclusive. It is typically more time and resource intensive to develop or make adaptations to interventions to meet accessibility guidelines, be readable, and be culturally appropriate. It is also possible that a higher proportion of people in socially disadvantaged communities have other priorities (food security, shelter, basic health needs) that render SDM more superfluous and something they are potentially less interested in. Until accessible and widely acceptable interventions are routinely available, it is difficult to determine whether this is the case.

If we seek to improve equity in SDM by developing more inclusive and accessible resources, it is crucial that we listen to the needs of socially disadvantaged people in these communities. This includes considering time commitments, translation, patient navigation, peer support, and financial reimbursement adapted to socially disadvantaged populations. This is thus likely to impact research and implementation scopes, timelines, as well as budgets. PPIR initiatives must also seek to test and refine strategies to create research environments that actively foster community members' knowledge, skills, and confidence to engage in research.

Advances in digital technology and artificial intelligence could potentially increase inequities. They may also provide innovative strategies to support better communication for diverse groups. Digital technology is rapidly evolving to play a significant future role in assisting communication across communities (Hwang et al., 2022). If implemented wisely, could it facilitate communication across diverse and socially underserved populations? Machine learning and artificial intelligence are already available to help with translations with variable accuracy. Artificial intelligence-assisted technology could, in time, create accurate and reliable simplified health texts and translations with pictorial content (Parsons, 2022). However, there is growing recognition of the inequities and bias associated with digital technology and the need for processes and regulations to ensure access, safety, and quality across diverse populations (Lutz, 2019).

Conclusion

Increasing equity in SDM is both an ethical imperative and a potentially powerful lever to improve outcomes for all across countries and populations. Growing evidence suggests that PtDAs and other SDM interventions improve outcomes for socially disadvantaged populations. However, evidence remains mixed regarding a potential reduction in health inequities through the use of these interventions. Further research is needed.

This chapter provides an overview of approaches to increase equity in SDM while discussing likely challenges. Sustainably increasing equity in SDM requires more systematic efforts to use equitable methods, promote implementation and dissemination strategies that address equity, and for funding bodies and policymakers to make adaptations accordingly. More detailed expectations and necessary adjustments should also be made to foster equitable, participatory engagement in SDM research. Adaptations may include changes to scopes, budgets, timelines, the use of translation, patient/peer navigation, peer support, and financial reimbursement adapted to socially disadvantaged populations' needs.

REFERENCES

Braveman, P., Gruskin, S. 2003. Defining equity in health. *J Epidemiol Community Health,* **57**, 254–258.

Braveman, P., Starfield, B., Geiger, H. J. 2001. World Health Report 2000: how it removes equity from the agenda for public health monitoring and policy. *BMJ,* **323**, 678–681.

Brega, A. G., Freedman, M. A. G., LeBlanc, W. G., et al. 2015. Using the health literacy universal precautions toolkit to improve the quality of patient materials. *J Health Commun,* **20**, 69–76.

Brett, J., Staniszewska, S., Mockford, C., et al. 2014. Mapping the impact of patient and public involvement on health and social care research: a systematic review. *Health Expect,* **17**, 637–650.

Centers for Disease Control and Prevention. 2023. Guidance & tools. Available at: https://www.cdc.gov/healthliteracy/developmaterials/guidancestandards.html

Centers for Disease Control and Prevention. 2024. What is health equity? Available at: https://www.cdc.gov/health-equity/what-is/index.html

Chenel, V., Mortenson, W. B., Guay, M., Jutai, J. W., Auger, C. 2018. Cultural adaptation and validation of patient decision aids: a scoping review. *Patient Prefer Adherence,* **12**, 321–332.

Commission on Social Determinants of Health. 2008. *Closing the Gap in a Generation: Health Equity Through Action on the Social Determinants of Health: Commission on Social Determinants of Health Final Report.* World Health Organization.

Crocker, J. C., Ricci-Cabello, I., Parker, A., et al. 2018. Impact of patient and public involvement on enrolment and retention in clinical trials: systematic review and meta-analysis. *BMJ,* **363**, k4738.

Dawson, S., Campbell, S. M., Giles, S. J., Morris, R. L., Cheraghi-Sohi, S. 2018. Black and minority ethnic group involvement in health and social care research: a systematic review. *Health Expect,* **21**, 3–22.

Dimopoulos-Bick, T., Follent, D., Kostovski, C., et al. 2023. Finding Your Way—a shared decision making resource developed by and for Aboriginal people in Australia: perceived acceptability, usability, and feasibility. *Patient Educ Couns,* **115**, 107920.

Durand, M.-A., Carpenter, L., Dolan, H., et al. 2014. Do interventions designed to support shared decision-making reduce health inequalities? A systematic review and meta-analysis. *PLoS One,* **9**, e94670.

Durand, M.-A., Yen, R. W., O'Malley, A. J., et al. 2021. What matters most: randomized controlled trial of breast cancer surgery conversation aids across socioeconomic strata. *Cancer,* **127**, 422–436.

Elwyn, G., Scholl, I., Tietbohl, C., et al. 2013. 'Many miles to go ...': a systematic review of the implementation of patient decision support interventions into routine clinical practice. *BMC Med Inform Decis Mak,* **13**, S14.

Enard, K. R., Dolan Mullen, P., Kamath, G. R., Dixon, N. M., Volk, R. J. 2016. Are cancer-related decision aids appropriate for socially disadvantaged patients? A systematic review of US randomized controlled trials. *BMC Med Inform Decis Mak,* **16**, 64.

Forsythe, L. P., Carman, K. L., Szydlowski, V., et al. 2019. Patient engagement in research: early findings from the Patient-Centered Outcomes Research Institute. *Health Aff (Millwood),* **38**, 359–367.

Francis-Oliviero, F., Cambon, L., Wittwer, J., Marmot, M., Alla, F. 2020. Theoretical and practical challenges of proportionate universalism: a review. *Rev Panam Salud Publica,* **44**, e110.

Greenhalgh, T., Hinton, L., Finlay, T., et al. 2019. Frameworks for supporting patient and public involvement in research: systematic review and co-design pilot. *Health Expect,* **22**, 785–801.

Hwang, K., Williams, S., Zucchi, E., et al. 2022. Testing the use of translation apps to overcome everyday healthcare communication in Australian aged-care hospital wards—an exploratory study. *Nurs Open,* **9**, 578–585.

Kilbourne, A. M., Switzer, G., Hyman, K., Crowley-Matoka, M., Fine, M. J. 2006. Advancing health disparities research within the health care system: a conceptual framework. *Am J Public Health,* **96**, 2113–2121.

King, J. S., Eckman, M. H., Moulton, B. W. 2011. The potential of shared decision making to reduce health disparities. *J Law Med Ethics,* **39**, 30–33.

Loignon, C., Alunni-Menichini, K., Leblanc, C., Wilson, I., Foisy, J., ENGAGE committee. n.d. Inclusive practices in participatory or partnership-based research with socially excluded persons. Available at: https://ssaquebec.ca/wp-content/uploads/2023/04/Loignon-et-al.-2022-Inclusive-practices-in-PPR-with-socially-excluded-persons.pdf

Lutz, C. 2019. Digital inequalities in the age of artificial intelligence and big data. *Hum Behav Emerg Technol,* **1**, 141–148.

Marmot, M. 2005. Social determinants of health inequalities. *Lancet,* **365**, 1099–1104.

Muscat, D. M., Smith, J., Mac, O., et al. 2021. Addressing health literacy in patient decision aids: an update from the International Patient Decision Aid Standards. *Med Decis Making,* **41**, 848–869.

Niven, A. n.d. FAQs—translators and interpreters. Available at: https://www.ncihc.org/faq-translators-and-interpreters

Noorlandt, H. W., Echteld, M. A., Tuffrey-Wijne, I., et al. 2020. Shared decision-making with people with intellectual disabilities in the last phase of life: a scoping review. *J Intellect Disabil Res,* **64**, 881–894.

O'Neill, J., Tabish, H., Welch, V., et al. 2014. Applying an equity lens to interventions: using PROGRESS ensures consideration of socially stratifying factors to illuminate inequities in health. *J Clin Epidemiol,* **67**, 56–64.

Parsons, T. 2022. The promise and peril of ChatGPT, a remarkably powerful AI chatbot. *The Hub,* 16 Dec. Available at: https://hub.jhu.edu/2022/12/16/what-is-chatgpt-artificial-intelligence-tinglong-dai/

Reynolds, J., Ogden, M., Beresford, R. 2021. Conceptualising and constructing 'diversity' through experiences of public and patient involvement in health research. *Res Involv Engagem,* **7**, 53.

Sørensen, K., Van den Broucke, S., Fullam, J., et al. 2012. Health literacy and public health: a systematic review and integration of definitions and models. *BMC Public Health,* **12**, 80.

Sydor, A. 2013. Conducting research into hidden or hard-to-reach populations. *Nurse Res,* **20**, 33–37.

Thomson, R., Murtagh, M., Khaw, F.-M. 2005. Tensions in public health policy: patient engagement, evidence-based public health and health inequalities. *Qual Saf Health Care,* **14**, 398–400.

Urban Institute. 2024. Do no harm guide. Available at: https://www.urban.org/sites/default/files/2024-04/Do_No_Harm_Guide_Crafting_Equitable_Data_Narratives.pdf

World Wide Web Consortium. n.d. Web content accessibility guidelines (WCAG) 2.1. Available at: https://www.w3.org/TR/WCAG21/

Yen, R. W., Smith, J., Engel, J., et al. 2021. A systematic review and meta-analysis of patient decision aids for socially disadvantaged populations: update from the International Patient Decision Aid Standards (IDPAS). *Med Decis Making,* **41**, 870–896.

Zachariah, D., Mouwad, D., Muscat, D. M., Ayre, J., Nutbeam, D., McCaffery, K. J. 2022. Addressing the health literacy needs and experiences of culturally and linguistically diverse populations in Australia during COVID-19: a research embedded participatory approach. *J Health Commun,* **27**, 439–449.

65

The law and shared decision making

Recent developments

Thaddeus Mason Pope, Valerie Gutmann Koch, and Nadine Montgomery Allam

Introduction

This chapter examines how the law is helping to bridge the persistent gap between robust study-based research into, and sparse clinical practice of, shared decision making (SDM). Because the law is an important lever that can help reduce and eliminate barriers to wider adoption, policymakers are using legislation, regulation, and medical malpractice liability to promote wider uptake of SDM and patient decision aids (PtDAs) in healthcare delivery.

While the law is a key tool for promoting wider uptake of SDM, it is not sufficient by itself. We need varied tools to drive and expand clinical adoption (Coulter, 2018; Ryan and Hill, 2024). Other chapters in this volume illustrate the need for a range of implementation strategies like healthcare provider education and professional society leadership. But the law offers two strategic benefits. First, law has a powerful symbolic value and function. It helps create a culture that is receptive to new ideas and new ways of working. Public affirmation of a norm through law and government action expresses its public worth (Gusfield, 1967; Lamb, 2017). Second, the law has an instrumental function. It provides meaningful incentives that motivate change (Pope, 2017).

Given space limitations, we have not comprehensively reviewed SDM legal developments across the world. We recognize that they exist, and are aware of developments in Australia and the UK (General Medical Council, 2020; Australian Commission on Safety and Quality in Health Care, 2021). In this chapter, we focus on recent legal developments in the USA. This concentration is appropriate for three reasons. First, the USA is the most populous jurisdiction to meaningfully espouse SDM (Bravo et al., 2022). Second, it is widely perceived as a worldwide leader in SDM (Elwyn et al., 2018; Légaré et al., 2020; Lu et al., 2022). Third, as many studies on SDM were conducted in the USA as all other countries combined (Stacey et al., 2024).

The USA is a federal system with 56 jurisdictions. While most aspects of healthcare like liability and licensure/registration, are regulated at the state level, there have been significant SDM initiatives at both the state and federal levels. These current and emerging legal incentives and penalties are helping to drive the evolution from a one-way, disclosure-oriented informed consent to a two-way, participation-oriented SDM process. This chapter describes three types of legal tools that have been deployed: (1) mandates, (2) payment incentives, and (3) medical malpractice liability incentives. But first, it is important to distinguish SDM from the more familiar, traditional legal doctrine of informed consent.

Distinguishing SDM from the traditional legal doctrine of informed consent

While there is renewed and growing attention on SDM, many of its basic tenets were enshrined into the law more than 60 years ago. Between the 1960s and 1980s, courts increasingly recognized the legal doctrine of informed consent (Beauchamp, 2011; Pope, 2017). Dozens of appellate courts across the USA (and worldwide) held that clinicians owe a legal duty to apprise patients about certain risks, benefits, and alternatives to proposed treatment. These courts further held that failing to make these disclosures is negligence that exposes the clinician to medical malpractice liability if the patient is injured (Natanson v. Kline, 1960; Canterbury v. Spence, 1972; Sidaway v. Board of Governors of the Bethlem Royal Hospital and the Maudsley Hospital, 1985). Today, the doctrine of informed consent 'has become firmly entrenched in American tort law' (Cruzan v. Director, Missouri Department of Health, 1990).

Legal recognition of informed consent was an important improvement in patient safety and self-determination. Unlike the simple 'authorization' still required for organ donation or release of protected health information, the law of informed consent requires clinicians to convey information about the risks, benefits, and alternatives of a proposed intervention. Thereby, the doctrine of informed consent shifted the paradigm of healthcare communication towards a more patient-centred approach to medical decision making.

But this shift was limited. Informed consent moved the model only so far. Today, clinicians must obtain permission to treat and make certain disclosures prior to obtaining that permission. This is informed consent. It is narrower than and materially different from SDM. In two respects, SDM requires more: both in 'what' clinicians must discuss with patients and in 'how' they must discuss it.

Informed consent disclosure duties are constricted

Under the doctrine of informed consent, the scope of information that clinicians must discuss with patients is narrowly circumscribed and confined. For example, in many jurisdictions, clinicians must disclose only the information that a reasonably prudent physician would disclose under the same circumstances. In these 'standard of care' jurisdictions, legal duty is measured by the norms of the medical profession, not by the patient's need for information. So, this disclosure duty retains some of the paternalism of the pre-1970s. After this time, approximately half of US jurisdictions adopted a standard that requires clinicians to provide information that a reasonable patient would consider material in making a treatment decision (American Law Institute, 2023; Rozovsky, 2024). This shift, at least in those jurisdictions, represents a move away from physician paternalism and towards patient autonomy. The UK made a similar move far more recently (Montgomery v. Lanarkshire Health Board, 2015).

Both legislatures and regulatory agencies have addressed some of the gaps in clinician disclosure obligations by enacting ad hoc mandates. As evidence or media stories spotlight how patients are under-informed about a particular healthcare intervention, policymakers sometimes respond by enacting a law requiring certain disclosures in that situation. To better assure that patients are engaged in the decision making process and that they understand their medical treatment choices, legislatures and regulatory agencies have increasingly enacted statutory disclosure mandates for various diagnostic and treatment situations.

For example, in the late 1970s and early 1980s, physicians were not disclosing less invasive treatment options to their breast cancer patients. In response, states enacted statutes that require physicians to present the advantages, disadvantages, and risks of all medically viable alternative therapies. Some of these statutes even require the use of 'standardized written information' (Pope and Hexum, 2014). Similarly, a growing number of states have enacted statutes requiring physicians to provide terminally ill patients with 'comprehensive information and counselling regarding end-of-life options' (Pope and Hexum, 2014). And states with authorized medical aid in dying specify detailed disclosure and counselling requirements (Vermont, 2013). Most recently, many states and the Food and Drug Administration require screening mammography providers both to notify women whether they have dense breasts and to explain the significance of breast density (Food and Drug Administration, 2023).

However, these situation-specific solutions to the problems of informed consent may be limited. Legislation or regulation is hardly workable for the broad range of medical interventions that patients receive every day. Rulemaking processes can be slow and cumbersome in addressing more than a handful of treatments, much less keeping them updated. And some of these mandates (e.g. regarding abortion and gender-affirming care) are politically motivated and not evidence-based (Sawicki, 2023). Moreover, these mandates focus on only the 'content' of disclosures and not on the 'way' the information is conveyed.

Informed consent requires only one-way communication

In addition to requiring only a narrow scope of disclosure, the doctrine of informed consent is limited and constrained in a second way. Even patient-oriented formulations focus on mere disclosure rather than on patient understanding (Pope 2019; Koch, 2024a, 2024b). The physician's duty is only to 'deliver' certain information to the patient, not to ensure that it is communicated clearly or that the patient understands and appreciates it. Indeed, while the UK recently adopted a 'reasonable patient' standard, commentators suggest it might 'best be seen as an evolution rather than a revolution' (Le Gallez et al., 2022). In any case, the courts subsequently constrained the scope of the required disclosure (Montgomery v. Lanarkshire Health Board, 2015; McCulloch v. Forth Valley Health Board, 2023).

Despite its name, 'informed consent' fails to ensure the patient's consent is 'informed'. While physicians might make legally sufficient disclosures, the 'message' is often not meaningfully received by the patients for whose benefit the disclosure is made. Informed consent does not require the clinician either to tailor information for patients or to include their goals, preferences, or preferences in the decision process (Himmelfarb et al., 2023).

For these reasons, the legal doctrine of informed consent has largely failed to meaningfully empower patients to make medical diagnostic and treatment decisions that match their preferences (Pope, 2017). If patients do not understand their options, they cannot form or express relevant preferences about those options. As practised, informed consent has become a 'ritualistic signature' on a form that does not reflect complete or bidirectional communication between provider and patient about relevant risks, benefits, and alternatives. It is like clicking a box agreeing to terms and conditions. However, change is afoot, especially in the USA, which has been a trailblazer in this area.

See Box 65.1 for our patient perspective.

Box 65.1 Patient perspective

On 1 October 1999, my son, Sam Montgomery, was delivered stillborn, weighing 9 lb 6 oz, requiring cardiopulmonary resuscitation and adrenaline to restore his heartbeat. During his delivery, an obstetric emergency called shoulder dystocia arose for a period of 12 minutes. Various desperate measures to deliver his shoulders failed, including attempts to break his clavicles and an attempt to push his head back inside to perform a caesarean section. Finally, clinicians tried to sever my pubis symphysis but were unsuccessful. My obstetrician stated that with one final surge of adrenaline on her part and sheer force, she pulled him out by his left arm. I was told he was likely deprived of oxygen for the full 12 minutes.

Sam spent 6 weeks in the Special Care Baby Unit. He had his lungs ventilated, suffered seizures due to hypoxic encephalopathy, and had trauma to his face, head, and neck with subdural haematomas. He was diagnosed with left-sided Erb's palsy and cerebral palsy.

My concerns dismissed and my questions unanswered

Looking back, I couldn't understand why it all went so wrong. During my pregnancy, I was told that I was 'high risk' due to my type 1 diabetes. So, I attended a joint diabetic–obstetric clinic fortnightly for ultrasounds and appointments with both diabetic and obstetric consultants. From 32 weeks, I saw from my centile chart that my baby was large and gaining weight rapidly, reaching the 95th centile. This worried me, so I raised my concerns repeatedly with my consultant, particularly about my ability to deliver my baby vaginally, given his large size and my small stature at only five feet. I was continually met with reassurances that I was being monitored closely. I was told I would be induced at 38+5 weeks. But I still felt that my questions had not been addressed, nor options for delivery discussed.

The labour was long, requiring augmentation with oxytocin. Because it was not progressing by the following evening, I was advised to proceed to the theatre for a trial of forceps. At this point, I was asked to sign a consent form, but I had no real understanding of the procedure being proposed or the potential complications that could arise. The subsequent tragic events need no further elaboration.

After my long recovery, I wanted to understand more about Sam's tragic outcome. Despite a basic explanation of events by my consultant, nobody explained why this had happened and if it could have been predicted or prevented. My sister, through her training in anaesthetics, which included the fact that doctors have a duty to inform patients and discuss options and significant risks fully, supported me in finding answers.

Undisclosed risks were material

We researched what the risk of shoulder dystocia in my circumstance might be. After looking through General Medical Council and obstetric college guidelines, and many scientific papers, it became clear that my care regarding the explanation of risks, options for delivery, and informed consent had been substandard. I discovered I had a 9–10% risk of shoulder dystocia with the risk factor of diabetes alone, which increased further by my small stature. My prolonged labour, use of oxytocin, and rotational forceps all increased that risk further.

I was devastated that these crucial risk factors had not been disclosed to me despite my requests antenatally. I had not been given the information I was entitled to, nor been allowed to be a partner in the decision making process regarding the delivery of my child. Decisions with potentially far-reaching consequences were being made for me without my knowledge or involvement. It is, after all, Sam and I that live with the consequences of those decisions.

Providers offered no apology or acknowledgement

I composed a complaint letter and asked why I hadn't been informed of these risks, and why other options for delivery had not been discussed. I was fobbed off with a standard generic reply that they were sorry for the unfortunate outcome, but my level of care had been adequate. I was livid. This wasn't 'unfortunate'. This was a known high-risk patient who had been seen fortnightly for 40 weeks with a known macrosomic baby.

There was absolutely no acknowledgement that I had a right to self-determine. No one cared or recognized that there was a deficiency in my care. I was concerned that if people didn't recognize the problem, no positive changes would be made. And if no positive changes were going to be made, then this would happen again. So, my goal became to ensure that others didn't endure what I did, and that the right discussions should occur regarding options and risks between doctors and patients, making decisions together.

Lawsuit and Supreme Court judgment

My journey through the Scottish courts was long and arduous. We failed on every count, largely because my obstetrician's omissions were consistent with a 'responsible body of medical opinion' (Montgomery v. Lanarkshire Health Board, 2010). So, I appealed to the Supreme Court in London, where they assembled a full bench of seven judges. They were taking this matter seriously and I was finally heard. The General Medical Council intervened at the appeal, highlighting the good medical practice guidelines from the era of Sam's birth, and emphasizing the need for doctors and patients to make their decisions together.

In 2015, the Supreme Court handed down its judgment. All seven judges unanimously agreed with me (Montgomery v. Lanarkshire Health Board, 2015). The ethical guidance regarding valid consent was now passed into law.

Lord Reed held:

> The doctor is therefore under a duty to take reasonable care to ensure that the patient is aware of any material risks involved in any recommended treatment, and of any reasonable alternative. The test for materiality is whether, in the circumstances of the particular case, a reasonable person in the patient's position would be likely to attach significance to the risk, or the doctor is or should reasonably be aware that the particular patient would be likely to attach significance to it.

Finally, my voice was heard and understood. This was a real victory, not only for Sam but for every patient in the UK. Although it took nearly 16 years, I am pleased that it concluded in the Supreme Court so every UK patient can benefit.

Recent evolution from informed consent to SDM

While most laws governing healthcare communication and decision making still require only traditional informed consent, there is an ongoing evolution towards SDM. Because clinicians' use of PtDAs is more specific, measurable, and achievable than the use of SDM, many laws focus specifically on PtDAs. Lawmakers have deployed three types of legislative and regulatory initiatives to encourage SDM. First, they categorically mandate clinicians to use SDM and PtDAs in certain situations. Second, they offer payment incentives for practising SDM. Third, they offer liability protection for using certified PtDAs as part of SDM.

Mandates to use SDM and PtDAs

Medicare is a federal government health insurance programme that covers 64 million Americans. It is administered by the Centers for Medicare and Medicaid Services (CMS). Since 2015, CMS has increasingly required SDM with evidence-based PtDAs as an essential Medicare condition for payment. CMS is doing this because it recognizes that most healthcare is preference-sensitive and value-laden. That means whether treatment is 'right' or 'beneficial' for a patient is not only a matter of clinical expertise. It equally depends on the patient's values, preferences, and goals. So, CMS wants to ensure that patients understand the risks, benefits, and alternatives to the healthcare that they receive and for which CMS pays.

Since 2015, CMS has issued four national coverage determinations (NCDs) that require SDM. Under these mandates, coverage eligibility is determined not only by laboratories and examinations but also by better-informed patient choice. CMS first included this new payment rule in its 2015 NCD on low-dose computed tomography scanning, a preventative diagnostic screening for long-time smokers (CMS, 2015). It even created a billing code and payment for the SDM visit separate from the billing code and payment for the computed tomography scan itself.

After the mandate for low-dose computed tomography, CMS issued three more NCDs mandating SDM as an essential condition of coverage. In 2016, CMS included even stronger SDM requirements for left-atrial appendage closure therapy (CMS, 2016). In 2018, CMS included SDM requirements for implanted cardioverter–defibrillators (CMS, 2018). In 2023, CMS included SDM requirements for percutaneous transluminal angioplasty of the carotid artery concurrent with stenting (CMS, 2023).

In addition to these four NCD mandates, CMS has seriously considered extending SDM requirements to other interventions and procedures like transcatheter aortic valve replacement (CMS, 2019). It has also announced plans to continue expanding SDM requirements to include more Medicare-covered services and procedures (Pope, 2025). Furthermore, this mandate model is being replicated at the state level. The Washington State Health Care Authority purchases healthcare for over 2 million Medicaid beneficiaries and almost 1 million state government employees. Analogous to Medicare NCDs, the Health Care Authority requires using 'certified' PtDAs in its provider contracts. Unique in the USA, the Health Care Authority has a PtDA certification process (Washington State, 2013). And it has certified nearly 50 PtDAs (Washington State Health Care Authority, 2024).

Unfortunately, despite the nearly 10-year track record of Medicare promulgating mandates to use SDM, we have little data on their success. More than a dozen studies show that clinician compliance is abysmally poor (Pope, 2025). And while non-compliance with NCD eligibility requirements violates serious healthcare fraud laws, Medicare has not enforced its mandates. Indeed, there has been significant pressure from the professional societies on CMS to relax or repeal the mandates. Further, just as with government mandates for informed consent, legally requiring SDM by predicating Medicare reimbursement on compliance, mandating SDM could result in clinicians following the 'letter of the law' at the expense of a robust SDM process that truly reflects patients' values and preferences.

Payment incentives for SDM

In addition to imposing mandates to use SDM, Medicare has also incorporated SDM as a quality measure benchmark within two other programmes: (1) the Merit-based Incentive Payment System (MIPS) and (2) the Medicare Shared Savings Program (MSSP). In contrast to the NCD mandates, these programmes do not categorically require SDM. But providers who use SDM can increase their payments.

MIPS is a programme that determines Medicare payment adjustments. Clinicians can get a payment bonus, a payment penalty, or no payment adjustment. There are four performance categories that affect a provider's future Medicare payments: (1) quality, (2) improvement activities, (3) promoting interoperability, and (4) cost. Using SDM can increase a provider's score in the improvement activities category and potentially total payments (CMS, 2024a, CMS, 2024b). But because this category counts the least and carries a high data collection burden, it may not effectively incentivize any real focus on SDM (Elwyn et al., 2023).

MSSP is an alternative payment programme in which providers, hospitals, and suppliers form an accountable care organization to share financial and medical responsibility for a defined patient population. CMS gives accountable care organizations a share in any savings generated by more efficient healthcare delivery. To determine an accountable care organization's eligibility for shared payments, CMS established dozens of quality performance standards. One is SDM. Accountable care organizations must 'define, establish, implement, evaluate, and periodically update processes to ... promote patient engagement'. Those processes must address 'beneficiary engagement and shared decision-making that takes into account the beneficiaries' unique needs, preferences, values, and priorities' (CMS, 2024c).

Liability incentives to use SDM and PtDAs

Finally, in addition to mandates and payment incentives, some jurisdictions have used liability incentives. To incentivize the use of SDM, Washington State enacted legislation that encourages SDM as an alternative means of informed consent (Washington State, 2007). It promotes this policy by offering a higher degree of protection against a failure to inform lawsuit if SDM with a 'certified patient decision aid' is used as part of an alternate informed consent process.

The statute specifies that a patient's signed 'acknowledgement of SDM' constitutes prima facie evidence that the patient gave his or her informed consent to the treatment administered. The patient has 'the burden of rebutting this by clear and convincing evidence'. Thus, if a 'certified' PtDA is used and the patient alleges that the physician failed to obtain their informed consent, she must confidently establish (greater than 80%) that her consent was not informed. This stands in contrast to the usual preponderance of the evidence standard, under which a patient would have to show that her consent was probably (greater than 50%) not informed.

Only Washington State provides formal legal safe harbour liability protection. However, clinicians in other states may be able to earn similar liability protection by using a PtDA because using a PtDA effectively serves as evidence that the clinician made all the necessary and appropriate disclosures. At least five instructive studies found that using a PtDA provides greater protection against a determination of malpractice than either the clinician's word or a medical record note about the provision of information (Barry et al., 2008; Brodney et al., 2018; Schoenfeld et al., 2019; Pope, 2022; Srinivas et al., 2023). In short, using a PtDA is powerful evidence that the clinician has fulfilled their legal duties of informed consent.

Furthermore, while PtDAs can most obviously mitigate liability from negligent non-disclosure, they can also mitigate liability from most other types of medical malpractice claims—from misdiagnosis to administration of incorrect medications (Pope, 2022). This provides a strong legal incentive to use PtDAs.

Ongoing legal reform efforts

Apart from the mandates, payment incentives, and liability incentives described above, few laws require or incentivize SDM, although it might appear otherwise. First, over the past decade, various governmental and private organizations have issued dozens of endorsements and position statements regarding SDM. But these are non-binding guidelines and recommendations. Second, the term 'SDM' has increasingly appeared in statutes and regulations. However, because it is typically undefined, 'SDM' is often interpreted to mean nothing more than traditional informed consent. In short, SDM implementation remains seldom, incomplete, infrequent, stagnant, elusive, and rare. There is a 'significant and sustained adoption problem' (Bravo et al., 2022). Yet two emerging and expanding initiatives may better drive change.

Certification of PtDAs

It is difficult for regulators to legally require PtDAs without first assuring they are evidence-based, accurate, up to date, understandable, and free from bias and conflicts of interest. Certification incentivizes PtDA use by assuring clinicians, patients, and payers that the PtDA meets these quality criteria.

The Washington State legal liability legislation described above had anticipated the emergence of a 'national certifying organization' for PtDAs because that was explicitly called for in the 2010 Affordable Care Act (Affordable Care Act, 2010). However, when the federal government failed to implement that part of the Affordable Care Act, Washington State moved forward on its own. It developed certification criteria, built a certification process, and started certifying PtDAs in 2016. Today, it has certified nearly 50 (Washington State Health Care Authority, 2024). Yet, as with the Medicare programmes at the federal level, there is still little evidence of the impact certification is having.

Growing focus on SDM in healthcare regulation

Medicare has not been the only federal agency promoting SDM. In 2021, the Food and Drug Administration prohibited breast implant manufacturers from selling to providers unless the provider uses a 'patient decision checklist' (Food and Drug Administration, 2021). The provider must review this checklist with the prospective patient to help ensure the patient understands the risks, benefits, and other information about the breast implant device. The patient must be given the opportunity to initial and sign the patient decision checklist and it must be signed by the physician implanting the device. While not exactly a PtDA, this tool entails more structured communication than traditional informed consent.

While research with human subjects lies outside the clinical treatment setting, it is instructive to note that in 2024, the Food and Drug Administration joined with the US Department of Health and Human Services Office of Human Research Protections to issue new regulations titled 'Enhancing Understanding in Informed Consent' (Food and Drug Administration, 2024). They address not only 'what' information to present to but also 'how' to present that information. They recommend visual aids and other strategies to enhance understanding.

Developments also continue at the state level. Massachusetts requires its Center for Health Information and Analysis to maintain a 'consumer health information website' that is 'designed to assist consumers in making informed decisions regarding their medical care' and that includes 'patient decision aids' (Massachusetts, 2012). The Minnesota Department of Health incorporates SDM principles into its certification requirements for Health Care Homes (Minnesota, 2010). Legislation in New Jersey calls for creation and distribution of a 'SDM tool' for maternity care hospitals and licensed birthing centres (New Jersey, 2024), and legislation in Washington calls for the creation and distribution of an 'SDM tool' to 'assist behavioural health providers when discussing medication treatment options for patients with alcohol use disorder' (Washington State, 2024).

Conclusion

The law is an important lever that can help reduce and eliminate barriers to the wider adoption of SDM in clinical practice. Current and emerging legal incentives and penalties are helping to drive the evolution from a one-way, disclosure-oriented informed consent to a two-way, participation-oriented SDM process. Still, the law may be better equipped to regulate the process of informed consent, with its emphasis on unidirectional physician disclosures. It may be more difficult to craft legal rules that ensure genuine SDM.

REFERENCES

Affordable Care Act. 2010. Pub. L. No. 111-148 §§ 3021 & 3056, codified at 42 U.S.C. §§ 1395jjj(b)(2)(G) & 299b-36.

American Law Institute. 2023. Restatement of the law third, torts: medical malpractice, tentative draft no. 1. Available at: https://www.ali.org/publications/restatement-law-third/torts-medical-malpractice

Australian Commission on Safety and Quality in Health Care. 2021. National safety and quality health service standards. Available at: https://www.safetyandquality.gov.au/

Barry, M.J., Wescott, P.H., Reifler E.J., Chang, Y., Moulton, B.W. 2008. Reactions of potential jurors to a hypothetical malpractice suit alleging failure to perform a prostate specific antigen test. *J Law Med Ethics*, **36**, 396–402.

Beauchamp, T. L. 2011. Informed consent: its history, meaning, and present challenges. *Cam Q Healthc Ethics*, **20**, 515–523.

Bravo, P., Härter, M., McCaffery, K., Giguère, A., Hahlweg, P., Elwyn, G. 2022. Editorial: 20 years after the start of international shared decision-making activities: is it time to celebrate? *Z Evid Fortbild Qual Gesundhwes*, **171**, 1–4.

Brodney, S., Wescott, P.H., Moulton, B.W, Hartmann, K., Chang, Y., Barry, M.J. 2018. *J Law Med Ethics*, **46**, 967–974.

Canterbury v. Spence. 1972. 464 F.2d 772 (D.C. Cir.).

Centers for Medicare and Medicaid Services. 2015. Decision memo for screening for lung cancer with low dose computed tomography (LCDT) (CAG-00439N). Available at: https://www.cms.gov/medicare-coverage-database/view/ncacal-decision-memo.aspx?proposed=N&NCAId=274

Centers for Medicare and Medicaid Services. 2016. Decision memo for implantable cardioverter defibrillators (CAG-00157R4). Available at: https://www.cms.gov/medicare-coverage-database/details/nca-decision-memo.aspx?NCAId=288

Center for Medicare and Medicaid Services. 2018. Decision memo for percutaneous left atrial appendage (LAA) closure therapy (CAG-00445N). Available at: https://www.cms.gov/medicare-coverage-database/details/nca-decisionmemo.aspx?NCAId=281

Center for Medicare and Medicaid Services. 2019. Transcatheter aortic valve replacement (TAVR) (CAG-00430R). Available at: https://www.cms.gov/medicare-coverage-database/view/ncacal-decision-memo.aspx?proposed=N&NCAId=293

Center for Medicare and Medicaid Services. 2023. Percutaneous transluminal angioplasty (PTA) of the carotid artery concurrent with stenting (CAG-00085R8). Available at: https://www.cms.gov/medicare-coverage-database/view/ncacal-decision-memo.aspx?proposed=N&ncaid=311

Centers for Medicare and Medicaid Services. 2024a. Merit-Based Incentive Payment System and alternative payment model incentive. 42 C.F.R. §§ 414.1300–414.1465. Available at: https://www.ecfr.gov/current/title-42/chapter-IV/subchapter-B/part-414/subpart-O

Centers for Medicare and Medicaid Services. 2024b. Quality payment program: improvement activities: traditional MIPS requirements. Available at: https://qpp.cms.gov/mips/improvement-activities

Centers for Medicare and Medicaid Services. 2024c. Shared Savings Program eligibility requirements: required processes and patient-centeredness criteria. 42 C.F.R. § 425.112(b). Available at: https://www.ecfr.gov/current/title-42/chapter-IV/subchapter-B/part-425/subpart-B/section-425.112

Coulter, A. 2018. *National Strategies for Implementing Shared Decision Making*. Bertelsmann Stiftung.

Cruzan v. Director, Missouri Department of Health. 1990. 497 U.S. 261.

Elwyn, G., Burstin, H., Barry, M. J., et al. 2018. A proposal for the development of national certification standards for patient decision aids in the US. *Health Policy*, **122**, 703–706.

Elwyn, G., Sierpe, A., Forcino R. 2023. Do payment programs incentivize shared decision making in US healthcare? *Patient Educ Couns*, **113**, 107798.

Food and Drug Administration. 2021. FDA strengthens safety requirements and updates study results for breast implants. Available at: https://www.fda.gov/news-events/press-announcements/fda-strengthens-safety-requirements-and-updates-study-results-breast-implants

Food and Drug Administration. 2023. Mammography Quality Standards Act: final rule. *Federal Register*, **89**, 15126–15167.

Food and Drug Administration. 2024. Key information and facilitating understanding in informed consent; draft guidance for sponsors, investigators, and institutional review boards. *Federal Register*, **88**, 15094–15096.

General Medical Council. 2020. Decision making and consent. Available at: https://www.gmc-uk.org/professional-standards

Gusfield, J. R. 1967. Moral passage: the symbolic process in public designations of deviance. *Soc Prob*, **15**, 175–188.

Himmelfarb, C. R. D., Beckie, T. M., Allen, L. A. 2023. Shared decision-making and cardiovascular health: a scientific statement from the American Heart Association. *Circulation*, **148**, 912–931.

Koch, V. G. 2024a. Reforming informed consent to include comprehension: a proposal to promote equity in medical decision-making. *Cardozo L Rev De Novo*, **24**, 8–15.

Koch, V. G. 2024b. Reimagining informed consent: from disclosure to comprehension. *UC Irvine Law Rev*, **14**, 894–935.

Lamb, M. 2017. Montgomery: a symbolic or substantive change to the law. *NELR*, **5**, 25–29.

Le Gallez, I., Skopek, J., Liddell, K. 2022. Montgomery's legal and practical impact: a systematic review at 6 years. *J Eval Clin Pract*, **28**, 690–702.

Légaré, F., Harter, M., Stiggelbout, A. M., et al. 2020. Choosing treatments and the role of shared decision-making. In: *Achieving Person-Centered Health Systems: Evidence, Strategies, and Challenges*, pp. 283–316. Cambridge University Press.

Lu, Y., Elwyn, G., Moulton, B. W., et al. 2022. Shared decision-making in the U.S.: evidence exists, but implementation science must now inform policy for real change to occur. *Z Evid Fortbild Qual Gesundhwes*, **171**, 144–149.

Massachusetts. 2012. General Laws Annotated 12C § 20.

McCulloch v. Forth Valley Health Board. 2023. UKSC 26.

Minnesota. 2010. Administrative Rule 4764.0040.

Montgomery v. Lanarkshire Health Board. 2010. CSOH 104.

Montgomery v. Lanarkshire Health Board. 2015. UKSC 11, AC 1430.

Natanson v. Kline. 1960. 354 P.2d 670 (Kansas).

New Jersey. 2024. A.B. 1799.

Pope, T. M. 2017. Certified patient decision aids: solving persistent problems with informed consent law. *J Law Med Ethics*, **45**, 12–40.

Pope, T. M. 2019. Informed consent requires understanding: complete disclosure is not enough. *Am J Bioeth*, **19**, 27–28.

Pope, T. M. 2022. Patient decision aids improve patient safety and reduce medical liability risk. *Maine Law Rev*, **74**, 73–100.

Pope, T. M. 2025. Medicare mandates for shared decision making: linking payment to patient preferences. *Ann Health Law Life Sci*, **34**, 143–188.

Pope, T. M., Hexum, M. 2014. Legal briefing: informed consent in the clinical context. *J Clin Ethics*, **25**, 152–175.

Rozovsky, F. A. 2024. *Consent to Treatment: A Practical Guide*, 5th edition. Wolters Kluwer.

Ryan, R. E., Hill, S. 2024. Decision aids: challenges for practice when we have confidence in effectiveness. *Cochrane Database Syst Rev*, **1**, ED000164.

Sawicki, N. N. 2023. The politics of informed consent and the limits of the first amendment. *JAMA*, **329**, 1635–1636.

Schoenfeld, E. M., Mader, S., Houghton, C. 2019. The effect of shared decisionmaking on patients' likelihood of filing a complaint or lawsuit: a simulation study. *Ann Emerg Med*, **74**, 126–136.

Sidaway v. Board of Governors of the Bethlem Royal Hospital and the Maudsley Hospital. 1985. AC 871.

Srinivas, S., Newton, I. G., Waradzyn, M., Kothary, N., Keller, E. J. 2023. Patient decision aids before informed consent conversations for image-guided procedures: controlled trials at two institutions. *Am J Roentgenol*, **220**, 272–281.

Stacey, D., Lewis, K. B., Smith, M., et al. 2024. Decision aids for people facing health treatment or screening decisions. *Cochrane Database Syst Rev*, **1**, CD001431.

Vermont. 2013. Statutes Annotated 18 § 5283.

Washington State. 2007. Revised Code of Washington § 7.70.060.

Washington State. 2013. Washington Administrative Code §§ 182.60.005 to 182.60.030.

Washington State. 2024. HB 2319.

Washington State Health Care Authority. 2024. Patient decision aids (PDAs). Available at: https://www.hca.wa.gov/about-hca/programs-and-initiatives/making-informed-health-care-decisions/patient-decision-aids-pdas#what-pdas-has-hca-certified

66

Where do we go from here?

International priorities for shared decision making practice and research

Natalie Joseph-Williams, Glyn Elwyn, Libby Humphris, and Adrian Edwards

Background

Across the previous 65 chapters, we have learned much about *things that work* to support shared decision making (SDM) in different contexts, *challenges* that endure to limit its true potential, and *key priorities* for more successful, widespread, and equitable implementation. These have been presented by patients, clinicians, allied health professionals, health and care managers, policymakers, legal experts, and academic researchers.

In this final chapter, we assemble this compendium of learning to reflect briefly on the remaining challenges and present a clear direction for SDM research and implementation over the next decade—with the ultimate ambition of ensuring every patient can 'walk together' with their professionals on their healthcare journey.

Remaining challenges

The fact that we have 65 chapters written by health professionals working across multiple specialties and disciplines across so many countries shows that SDM is happening more now than a decade ago. The learning described in this book reinforces and builds on what we know works to support SDM implementation:

- Legal mandates.
- Policy support.
- Professional bodies supporting SDM through accreditation and standards.
- Guidelines.
- Patient organizations promoting SDM.
- Access to high-quality patient decision support tools (e.g. patient decision aids, checklists, counselling, and question prompts).
- Patient preparation for SDM.
- Accessible learning and training packages for healthcare professionals.
- Undergraduate/postgraduate teaching and continued professional training.

The consistent message throughout this book is that aligned *multi-level implementation strategies* are essential—they must target the micro (patients and healthcare professionals), meso (teams and systems), and macro (policy, standards, legislation) levels to be successful.

Despite this wealth of knowledge, widespread implementation continues to be problematic; *key challenges* remain, such as how can we better:

- Support a more diverse range of patients to feel able to take part in SDM and to achieve equity of experience for all patients
- Understand the limits of SDM
- Support local initiatives while coordinating implementation efforts to encourage spread and sustainability
- Integrate SDM into existing technology systems and harness new technology
- Create sustainable patient decision aids that remain up to date as evidence changes
- Routinely measure and capture SDM that occurs within and between visits and between various care pathways
- Support patients with increasingly complex health issues and multimorbidity to be involved in SDM
- Understand the impact of SDM on outcomes such as duration of healthcare encounter, health status, health resource utilization, and economic outcomes.

International priorities for SDM research and implementation

In the third edition, Elwyn and Edwards described a '*path* towards customized care'. We may have passed significant milestones already, but we are still on this journey, and with the goal of continuous

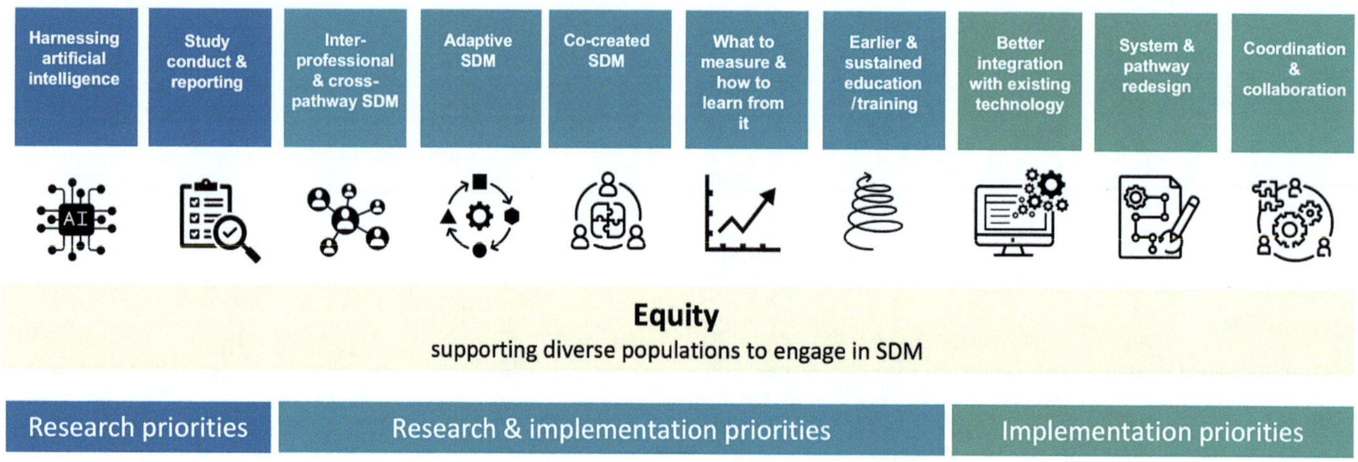

Figure 66.1 Ten priority areas for SDM research and implementation.

improvement, we will remain on this journey for some time. Where do we go from here? What new roadblocks do we need to be aware of? Is there an alternative route we could take to make the journey easier?

What are the top ten international priorities for SDM?

Over 150 specific priorities have been identified throughout this book relating to research, implementation, or both. We grouped the pertinent priorities from each chapter into descriptive themes. This allowed us to see what these priorities were and how often they are mentioned. It was also important to consider the priorities within the likely landscape of healthcare over the next few decades[1] (World Health Organization, 2020; The Health Foundation, 2023; IESE Business School, 2024):

- Ageing population with increased multimorbidities.
- Health inequalities widening.
- Growth of digital technology.
- Changing patient expectations.
- Lack of resource and capacity in healthcare systems.
- Workforce recruitment and retention issues.
- Economic climates leading to increased push for efficiencies and cost-cutting.
- Volume and profit-driven systems remain, yet we see the increasing importance of value-based initiatives.

The top ten priorities for SDM research and implementation are presented below (see Figure 66.1 for specific questions and topics).

1. Harnessing artificial intelligence

Artificial intelligence (AI) has dramatically developed over the past decade. Public awareness is no longer confined to personal assistant home devices, targeted advertisements, or film recommendations—people are becoming aware that healthcare systems also harness AI, particularly in diagnostics and remote monitoring. AI could also support personalized medicine and SDM (Abbasgholizadeh Rahimi et al., 2022). It could support evidence summarization automation—is this the answer to sustainable patient decision aids perhaps? It could be used for training and evaluation, automating real-time feedback. But for AI to be successfully used in SDM, we must ensure patients know how this technology will be used, why it will improve their experience, and proactively address concerns around privacy and inclusivity.

2. Study conduct and reporting—improved consistency and transparency

The number of SDM studies has increased significantly in the last decade. The 2024 update of the Cochrane review of patient decision aids identified a further 104 studies since 2017 and implementation studies have demonstrated the spread of SDM into routine settings (Stacey et al., 2024). Yet variations in outcome reporting remain, and the inadequate detail provided about implementation strategies often limits transferability of learning. Further, limited evidence remains for key outcomes that are increasingly important to resource-stretched healthcare services, including clinic time, cost–benefit analysis, resource utilization and economic benefits, and health outcomes; these could be critical for adoption of SDM.

Key priorities for SDM study conduct and reporting include increased use of the SUNDAE reporting guidelines (Sepucha et al., 2018), SDM core outcomes set (using COMET methodology (COMET Initiative, n.d.)), standardized and comprehensive reporting of implementation studies (e.g. StaRI (Equator Network, n.d.)), and the inclusion of currently under-researched outcomes that could support adoption into routine settings.

3. Whole-team and cross-pathway SDM—acknowledging and redefining the SDM 'team'

A recurring word used across the clinical specialties and allied disciplines chapters is 'team'. SDM is based on the principles of partnership. We know that it involves professionals, patients, and sometimes their family members, and key models have recognized this 'team' approach to SDM discussions.

However, the accounts from routine practice highlight the importance of training entire teams. In systems that lack continuity in care, patients could interact with different team members over time for

1 We acknowledge this context will differ and additional factors will be present locally and depend on the funding structure for a country's health system. This summarizes key universal issues.

the same issue. It is, at best, frustrating, at worst, disempowering, for patients to encounter team members with varying degrees of SDM receptiveness or skills within a care pathway. Further, the breadth of the 'team' has not been fully appreciated. The reality is that many patients are under the care of multiple teams at one time for a specific issue—how do we bring these together as one 'team' supporting the patient through their journey rather than operating as distinct teams with varying approaches to SDM or duplication in efforts?

We need to understand more about the benefits of training whole teams, how SDM tasks can be shared within and across care pathways, what training, tools, and systems are required for cross-pathway SDM, and if and how we can measure such distributed decisions and processes.

4. Adaptive SDM—making SDM available to everyone

'One size does not fit all' in SDM. The process should be tailored to fit the patient, context, and the decision. However, reading these chapters has made it evident just how important this mantra is. It raises questions about whether we have truly grasped the level of adaptation that is needed for SDM to be truly inclusive.

One thing is clear from the work across multiple disciplines and specialties—we know how to use SDM to support discrete choices, and we know how to modify the process slightly so that it fits the context. However, we need much more than minor modifications to existing approaches. If we want to support a broader range of decisions for diverse populations, we need *adaptive* theories, models, training, tools, measurements, and implementation strategies.

The chapters have identified key areas where *adaptive SDM* is needed, and work has already begun to understand what is required for these different contexts and populations beyond slight modifications that tailor existing approaches. Work is now required to further develop, evaluate, and implement these adaptive approaches. Still, a critical first step is to raise awareness of key areas that require adaptation—these are summarized in Figure 66.2.

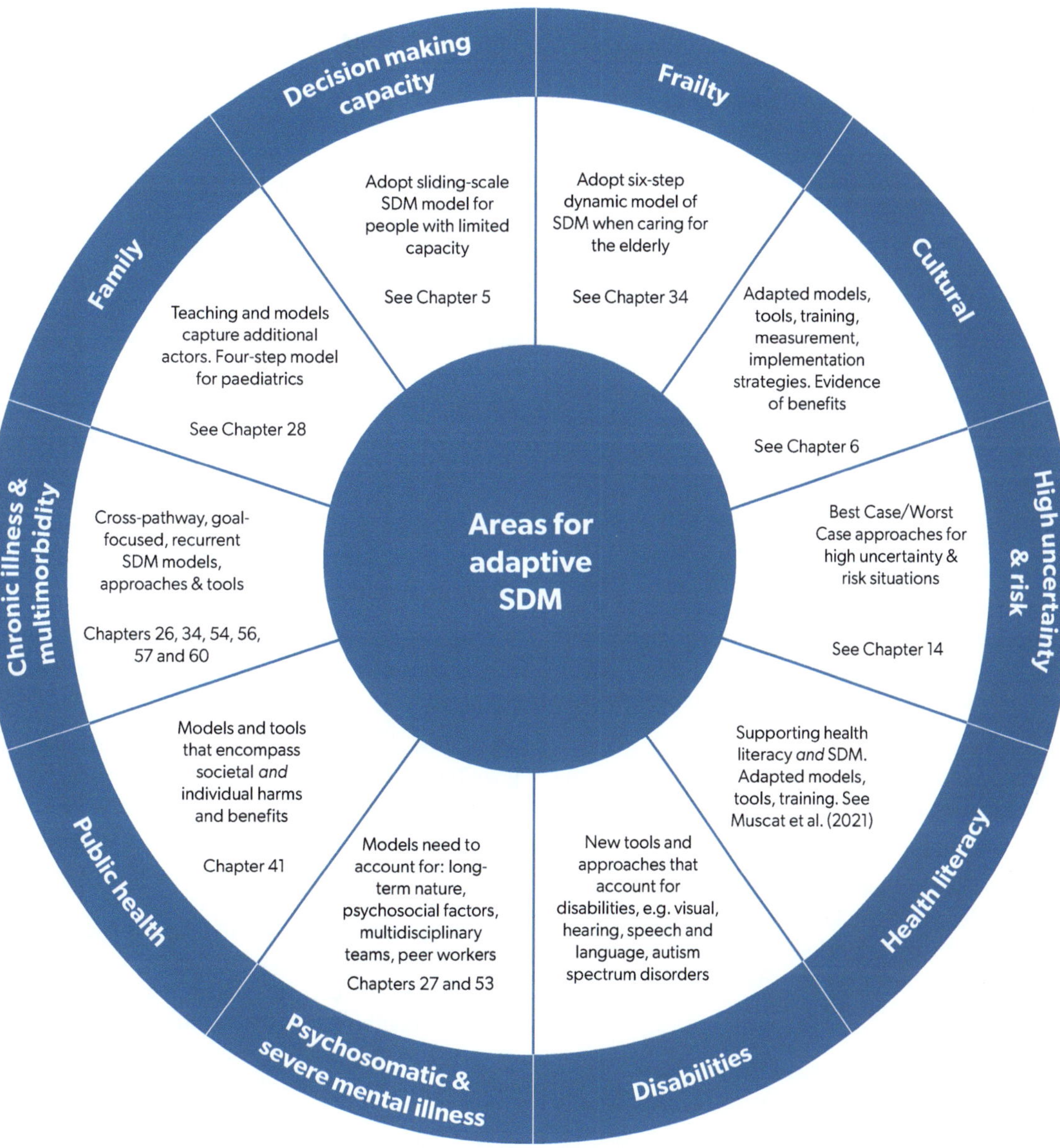

Figure 66.2 Key areas for adaptive SDM.

5. Co-created models, interventions, measures, research, and implementation—partnership beyond intervention design

In a book about SDM, we expect to see 'better co-production' as a key priority for improvement. Yet this reflects the evolving and expanding role of patient partners, underpinned by increased recognition of public involvement and engagement. Even at the time of publishing the third edition of this book, patient involvement tended to focus on issues of intervention content and design. While patients have typically contributed to SDM intervention development, fewer SDM models and measurement tools have been truly co-produced with patients, and even fewer effectiveness or implementation studies. The involvement of diverse populations is even more limited.

Diverse patients should play a critical role in co-production across the research-to-impact pathway—overseeing project governance, prioritizing research questions, identifying outcome measures that matter to them, reviewing existing evidence, supporting new data collection and analysis, identifying key recommendations, and informing implementation strategies. Supporting a diverse range of patients to be equal partners in co-producing SDM models, interventions, measures, research, and implementation is a key priority.

6. What gets measured gets 'improved'—using measurement to support sustainable SDM

'What gets measured gets done.' It is no secret in change management that when things are measured, people are more likely to take action to achieve something, and SDM implementation is no different. Various implementation studies have shown that measurement can be key in whether SDM is adopted and embedded into care systems. Thinking of the broader context, we will increasingly work in resource-poor systems where any new investment for SDM (whether that be staffing, budget allocation, technical support to embed tools in digital systems, commitment to rearrange care pathways, etc.) will need to demonstrate the potential for benefits and sustainable impact.

Taking this common saying further: 'What gets measured gets improved.' When people can see how they are doing, they not only strive to make improvements, but they can also track progress. However, the remaining question from many disciplines is 'What should we measure?' Accepting that 'not everything important is measurable, and not everything measurable is important', we can do more to support SDM. As such, key future priorities should include:

- Greater consensus on what to measure
- Working out how the measurement can be integrated into routine learning systems that are not research study dependent with finite timeframes.

It is nice to know how many people felt involved in decisions at one time point. Still, what is even better is knowing that progress is being made, more and more patients feel included over time, that we are not missing key populations, and if we are, that improvements and support can be targeted to the right areas.

7. SDM training and education across the learning continuum—earlier, regular, and sustained exposure

The benefits of teaching and training are clear. Beyond knowledge and skills, they are critical for changing attitudes, increasing buy-in, and supporting routine implementation. However, what is evident from the chapters in this book is that earlier, regular, and continued exposure is needed.

One seminar will not enable students to deal with the complexities of doing SDM in practice. One workshop for professionals will not support continued improvement or sustained SDM. Earlier exposure for students cements the idea that care should be centred around individuals and provides a frame for all other learning. Across a spiral curriculum, they will deepen their understanding of the skills and the complexities of SDM (including adaptive contexts). Continued professional development opportunities will then refresh and reinforce learning and support professionals to adapt the approach as they specialize and continually improve.

We now need to understand and demonstrate how we can include SDM at the earliest point in healthcare curricula, embed a spiral curriculum with regular exposure, support continued professional development during increasing specialization, and to examine benefits of this approach.

8. Better integration and use of existing technology

Existing digital systems have been effectively used to support SDM, including integrating patient decision aids into online patient portals and sharing electronic health records with patients, allowing them the option to provide real-time feedback. However, despite the potential, we see reports of under-utilization due to critical barriers.

At the most rudimentary level, these systems do not 'speak to each other'. Even in small geographical areas, different providers under the same national healthcare system are using different digital systems—incompatible systems jeopardize the ambitions of cross-pathway SDM, and the work required to embed SDM tools and routine measurement across all these systems would be exponential. There are also areas of potential that are yet to be explored. For example, how can registries populated from routine data be used to help populate SDM tools and inform conversations with patients about outcomes, risks, and benefits?

Key priorities include understanding the opportunities and challenges of existing digital systems, exploring how they can be used to support SDM, and understanding what we need to do to make sure they help patients and the teams.

9. Commitment to system and pathway redesign—not expecting patients to engage in systems not designed for SDM

Most SDM implementation strategies aim to make it easy to integrate the approaches and tools into existing care pathways. Ideally, this is achieved with changes that are minimally disruptive. This sounds ideal from a change management perspective and motivates people to get on board, but have we been avoiding the elephant in the room?

Most care pathways have not been designed with person-centred care in mind. Their focus is on diagnosis and patient through-flow. Take elective surgery. The patient is referred, and then they wait; maybe 2 months, perhaps 6 months, increasingly over 12 months in some systems. Some patients call this the void, where they wait in solitude. Even if the patient found the initial motivation to seek care, this often wanes over time and leaves the patient feeling disengaged. They eventually see the surgeon they were referred to, an event that many patients call the 'point of no return'. They are on the surgery conveyor belt, and they will not get off it until it ends, even if another less invasive option might have been possible for them.

Another issue is time and space to think about options. While some evidence shows that SDM does not significantly increase length of encounters, we should recognize this will depend on the starting point of the teams. If the pathway includes a 30-minute appointment, the consultation could be restructured to enable the SDM process to take place, while still covering the critical clinical aspects of history taking and diagnosis. If a team is only working with 10 minutes and has high patient demand, this does not provide much margin to include the additional SDM tasks, particularly within the context of patients with increasingly complex health issues or in adaptive SDM situations where patients might require additional support to engage (e.g. lower level of health literacy).

Critically, we often ask patients to fully engage in systems that, due to their design, can unintentionally disengage or disempower patients. Principles of good communication underpin SDM, and this should be just as evident in communication about referrals as it is when patients are making specific treatment choices. We cannot expect patients to fully engage at certain points of the care pathway when the rest of the care pathway does not foster the same engagement, or in situations that do not allow time and space to think about options.

W. Edwards Deming said: 'Every system is perfectly designed to get the results it gets.' A key priority will be for organizations to understand when pathway redesign is required and commit to designing workflows that genuinely foster the principles of person-centred care from start to finish, provide adequate time for SDM, and adequately utilize staff across the care pathway.

10. What will it take for SDM to become the new normal? Coordination and collaboration to deliver what we know works

The chapters report various approaches that work to embed SDM, yet most areas struggle to achieve routine, widespread, and sustainable implementation. What will it take for SDM to become the new normal?

Most implementation case studies (international and speciality/discipline specific) acknowledge the vital roles of legislation, policy, professional standards, and guidelines. However, *limited coordination* of SDM roll-out plans, education, training, decision support tool development, and measurement are consistently reported as challenges to progressing and sustaining SDM in routine practice. *Limited collaboration* is also reported as a key challenge. The chapters highlight the problems associated with siloed implementation efforts, particularly when increasing numbers of patients are being supported by multidisciplinary teams across different care pathways (see priority '5. Co-created models, interventions, measures, research, and implementation').

They report the duplicated or, at worst, wasted efforts that occur with lack of coordination and when people do not collaborate within or between organizations. Instead of reinventing the wheel and starting from scratch, the chapters highlight the role better coordination and collaboration could play in speeding up SDM adoption, and in supporting continued improvement and sustainable SDM that adapts to the changing context.

Key implementation priorities include understanding the role centralized coordination can play in sustainable SDM, including which implementation strategies would benefit from this, and fostering collaboration and shared learning by establishing SDM networks and community of practice. Crucially, we need to understand how we can achieve better coordination and collaboration, while still allowing for regional, local, and patient-level adaptations, which we also know are important for implementation.

A note on equity

Equity underpins all ten priorities. Whether the priority is earlier SDM education for healthcare students, pathway redesign, or harnessing AI, we must focus on supporting patients who are yet to be heard, on those most at risk of being unequal partners in decision making, populations most at risk for unequal health outcomes, and those who need additional support to work together with their healthcare professionals. If we do not ask these questions, we risk promoting disparities in healthcare experiences and not reaching those who need our support the most.

See Box 66.1 for our patient perspective.

Box 66.1 Patient perspective

As SDM becomes more integral to healthcare, conducting diverse and in-depth research to understand the needs and expectations of patients will be crucial for enhancing engagement, trust, and outcomes.

A key research priority is exploring how SDM is perceived and experienced by patients with varying levels of health literacy and digital literacy. Health literacy is a significant factor in how patients understand and participate in medical decision making, and low health literacy can be a significant barrier. Studies should investigate the specific needs of patients with low health literacy, identifying effective strategies to make medical information more accessible and comprehensible.

Cultural differences also play an essential role in how patients perceive and engage with SDM, and research could provide a richer understanding of these variations. In some cultures, family members play a significant role in healthcare decisions, while in others, patients may defer heavily to clinicians. Research into culturally tailored approaches to SDM could help healthcare providers create inclusive practices that respect diverse cultural perspectives and values, thus strengthening the SDM experience for all patients.

The whole-team approach to SDM is critical to ensuring everyone is on the same page. This requires us to go back to the start of a clinician's career. SDM should be embedded within the curriculum from day one for all students and continued throughout their career to update them on emerging SDM themes and new evidence. This should not be aimed solely at medical students; the use of SDM by allied healthcare professionals is just as important in improving 'whole-team' approaches.

AI and predictive analytics is another promising area. AI could provide patients with personalized outcomes of different treatment options based on their medical history, preferences, and specific conditions. By integrating predictive analytics into SDM tools, researchers could explore whether providing patients with more tailored, data-driven insights enhances their understanding and satisfaction with the decision making process. However, research will need to explore patients' trust and comfort with AI-generated information, ensuring that these technologies support—not hinder—meaningful communication with healthcare providers.

Understanding how SDM can be optimized for patients with chronic conditions, often with multiple comorbidities, or those undergoing long-term treatment is also important. Chronic illness often requires continuous management and complex decisions, making SDM particularly valuable. However, long-term treatment can be overwhelming for patients, and research could focus on identifying the best ways to maintain patient engagement and satisfaction over time. This may include exploring the use of decision aids, or digital platforms that reinforce the patient's role in their care decisions while adjusting to evolving health needs.

Finally, co-production across the whole research cycle is vital to ensure that all the above priorities are patient-centred. Public involvement can enrich SDM research, helping break down barriers to include diverse populations and ensuring that the research addresses the real-world needs and preferences of patients. By involving patients and the public from the outset, researchers can co-create more relevant, equitable, and impactful studies that reflect the complexities of patient experiences. This collaborative approach not only enhances the quality and applicability of research but also fosters trust and ownership among participants, empowering them to actively contribute to the development of healthcare solutions that truly benefit them.

Ultimately, by prioritizing patient-centred research and incorporating diverse perspectives, we can ensure that SDM evolves to meet the needs of all patients, fostering better healthcare experiences and outcomes for everyone.

A way forward

In 10 years, we may be able to check off some of these priorities. Yet, we will continue to explore others alongside evolving healthcare systems, population needs, and geopolitical and economic climates.

For now, we should focus on coordinated, co-created, cross-pathway SDM that is adaptive, equitable, capitalizes on new and existing technology, and demonstrates benefits that matter to patients, professionals, and systems.

REFERENCES

Abbasgholizadeh Rahimi, S., Cwintal, M., Huang, Y., et al. 2022. Application of artificial intelligence in shared decision making: scoping review. *JMIR Med Inform*, **10**, e36199.

COMET Initiative. n.d. Core Outcome Measures in Effectiveness Trials. Available at: https://www.comet-initiative.org/

Equator Network. n.d. Standards for Reporting Implementation Studies (StaRI) statement. Available at: https://www.equator-network.org/reporting-guidelines/stari-statement/

IESE Business School, University of Navarra. 2024. The future of healthcare: 5 challenges for 2030. Available at: https://www.iese.edu/insight/articles/healthcare-challenges-future/

Muscat, D. M., Shepherd, H. L., Nutbeam, D., Trevena, L., McCaffery, K. J. 2021. Health literacy and shared decision-making: exploring the relationship to enable meaningful patient engagement in healthcare. *J Gen Intern Med*, **36**, 521–524.

Sepucha, K. R., Abhyankar, P., Hoffman, A. S., et al. 2018. Standards for UNiversal reporting of patient Decision Aid Evaluation studies: the development of SUNDAE Checklist. *BMJ Qual Saf*, **27**, 380–388.

Stacey, D., Lewis, K. B., Smith, M., et al. 2024. Decision aids for people facing health treatment or screening decisions. *Cochrane Database Syst Rev*, **1**, CD001431.

The Health Foundation. 2023. Nine major challenges facing health and care in England. https://www.health.org.uk/publications/long-reads/nine-major-challenges-facing-health-and-care-in-england

World Health Organization. 2020. Urgent health challenges for the next decade. Available at: https://www.who.int/news-room/photo-story/photo-story-detail/urgent-health-challenges-for-the-next-decade

Index

For the benefit of digital users, indexed terms that span two pages (e.g., 52–53) may, on occasion, appear on only one of those pages.

Tables, figures, and boxes are indicated by an italic *t*, *f*, and *b* following the page number.